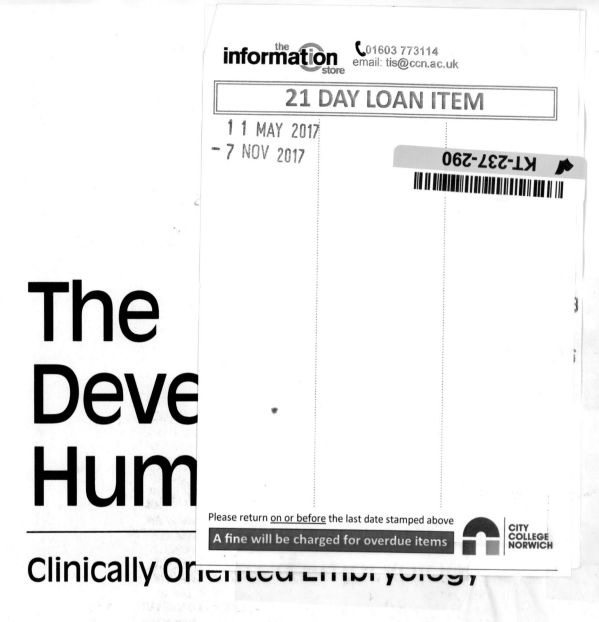

the information ⓘ store

☏ 01603 773114
email: tis@ccn.ac.uk

21 DAY LOAN ITEM

1 1 MAY 2017
− 7 NOV 2017

KT-237-290

Please return <u>on or before</u> the last date stamped above

A fine will be charged for overdue items

CITY
COLLEGE
NORWICH

The Deve Hum

Clinically Oriented Embryology

176 816

The Developing Human

Clinically Oriented Embryology

KEITH L. MOORE, B.A., M.Sc., Ph.D., F.I.A.C., F.R.S.M.

Professor of Anatomy and Cell Biology
Faculty of Medicine, University of Toronto
Toronto, Ontario, Canada

Visiting Professor of Clinical Anatomy
Department of Anatomy, Faculty of Medicine
University of Manitoba
Winnipeg, Manitoba, Canada

NORWICH CITY COLLEGE LIBRARY		
Stock No	176816	
Class	612.64 MOO	
Cat.	Proc.	3WL 05

T.V.N. PERSAUD, M.D., Ph.D., D.Sc., F.R.C.Path. (Lond.).

Professor and Head, Department of Anatomy
Professor of Pediatrics and Child Health
Associate Professor of Obstetrics, Gynecology and
    Reproductive Sciences
University of Manitoba, Faculties of Medicine and Dentistry

Consultant in Pathology and Clinical Genetics
Health Sciences Centre
Winnipeg, Manitoba, Canada

W. B. SAUNDERS COMPANY *Philadelphia/London/Toronto/Montreal/Sydney/Tokyo*
Harcourt Brace Jovanovich, Inc.

W.B. SAUNDERS COMPANY
Harcourt Brace Jovanovich, Inc.

The Curtis Center
Independence Square West
Philadelphia, PA 19106

Library of Congress Cataloging-in-Publication Data

Moore, Keith L.
    The developing human: clinically oriented embryology / Keith L. Moore, T.V.N. Persaud. — 5th ed.
        p.   cm.
    Includes bibliographical references and index.
    ISBN 0-7216-4662-X
    1. Embryology, Human.   2. Anomalies, Human.   I. Persaud, T.V.N.   II. Title.
    [DNLM: 1. Embryology.   QS 604 M822d]
    QM601.76   1993
    612.6′4 — dc20
    DNLM/DLC
                                                                                            92-49327

Front cover: Photograph of a 13-week-old human fetus. Courtesy of Professor Jean Hay, Department of Anatomy, Faculty of Medicine, University of Manitoba, Winnipeg, Canada.

International Edition ISBN 0-7216-4803-7

THE DEVELOPING HUMAN — Clinically Oriented Embryology   ISBN   0-7216-4662-X

Copyright © 1993, 1988, 1982, 1977, 1973 by W.B. Saunders Company.

All rights reserved. No part of this publication may be reproduced or transmitted in any form or by any means, electronic, mechanical, including photocopy, recording, or any information storage and retrieval system, without permission in writing from the publisher.

Printed in the United States of America.

Last digit is the print number: 9   8   7   6   5   4   3   2   1

To our wives, children and grandchildren

Preface

Two decades have passed since this book was first published. The fifth edition welcomes *Dr. T.V.N. (Vid) Persaud,* Professor and Head of the Department of Anatomy at the University of Manitoba with whom I have worked for many years. He is also a Professor of Pediatrics and Child Health and an Associate Professor of Obstetrics, Gynecology and Reproductive Sciences. An award-winning teacher of embryology and gross anatomy, Dr. Persaud is conducting modern research in embryology using molecular biological techniques. The contents of this edition will reflect his basic and clinical knowledge, and his vigour.

The book has been thoroughly updated to reflect the expanded significance of embryology and teratology in the education of medical and other students in the health professions. We have attempted to make the book an easy-to-read account of human development before birth. Every chapter has been thoroughly revised to reflect new findings in research and their clinical implications. Recent advances in developmental biology affecting knowledge about the causes of birth defects and prenatal management of fetuses have been carefully woven into the comprehensive clinically oriented text. In accordance with current trends in medical education, more clinical comments and problem solving questions have been added to prepare students for problem-based learning sessions.

Many new illustrations, including high resolution ultrasound images of embryos and fetuses, and scanning electron micrographs of human embryos, have been added to make it easier for students to understand the dynamics of developmental processes.

The chapters are organized so that they present a systematic and logical approach to explain how the embryo develops. The first chapter introduces the reader to the scope and importance of embryology, the historical background of the discipline, and the nomenclature for describing embryos. The next four chapters cover the pre-embryonic and embryonic periods, beginning with the formation of gametes and ending with the formation of basic organs and systems. The development of specific organs and systems is then described in a systematic manner, following chapters dealing with the highlights of the fetal period, the placenta and fetal membranes, and the causes of human congenital anomalies. At the end of each chapter are lists of references which contain classic works and the most recent research publications. This updating of references will be appreciated by serious students and those who wish to use the book as a reference text.

Many of our colleagues have helped with the preparation of this edition; it is a pleasure to record our indebtedness to them. Dr. Michael Wiley and Dr. David Cormack, Department of Anatomy and Cell Biology, Faculty of Medicine, University of Toronto, Toronto, Ontario; Dr. Margaret W. Thompson, Professor Emeritus, Department of Molecular and Medical Genetics, University of Toronto, Toronto, Ontario; Dr. Eugene Daniels, Department of Anatomy, McGill University, Montreal, Quebec; Dr. Raymond Gasser, Louisiana State University School of Medicine, New Orleans, Louisiana; Dr. A.E. Chudley, Professor of Pediatrics and Child Health, Director of Clinical Genetics, Health Sciences Centre, University of Manitoba, Winnipeg, Manitoba; Dr. E.A. Lyons, Professor of Radiology and Obstetrics and Gynecology and Chairman and Head of the Department of Radiology, Health Sciences Centre, University of Manitoba, Winnipeg, Manitoba, Canada; and Prof. Dr. K. Hinrichsen, Rühr-Universität Bochum, Institut für Anatomie, Medizinische Fakultät, Germany. Those who have contributed photographs are individually acknowledged in the figure legends. Sari O'Sullivan of Toronto modified old illustrations and prepared some new ones. Barbara Clune in Winnipeg, and Marion Moore in Toronto, did all the word processing and helped with the review of the manuscript. Lawrence McGrew, Medical Editor and Lorraine Kilmer, Manager of the Editorial, Design, and Production Team, W.B. Saunders Company and their colleagues have been most helpful with our work. To all these people, we extend our sincere thanks. Last, but not least, we thank our wives, Marion and Gisela, for their tolerance and support.

KEITH L. MOORE
T.V.N. PERSAUD

Contents

4

Formation of the Human Embryo
THE THIRD WEEK

5

Development of Tissues, Organs, and Body Form
THE FOURTH TO EIGHTH WEEKS

6

The Fetal Period
THE NINTH WEEK TO BIRTH

7

The Placenta and Fetal Membranes

8

Human Birth Defects

9

Body Cavities, Primitive Mesenteries, and the Diaphragm

10

The Branchial or Pharyngeal Apparatus

11

The Respiratory System

12
The Digestive System

13
The Urogenital System

14
The Cardiovascular System

15
The Skeletal System

16
The Muscular System

Introduction

Interest in developing humans before they are born is widespread, largely because of curiosity about our beginnings and the desire to improve the quality of human life. The intricate processes by which a baby develops from a single cell are miraculous, and few events are more exciting than a mother viewing her fetus during an ultrasound examination. The adaptation of a newborn infant to its new environment is also exhilarating to witness.

Human development is a continuous process that begins when an **oocyte** (ovum) from a female is fertilized by a **sperm** (spermatozoon) from a male. Cell division, cell migration, programmed cell death, differentiation, growth, and cell rearrangement transform the *fertilized oocyte*, a highly specialized cell called a **zygote**, into a multicellular adult human being. Although most developmental changes occur during the embryonic and early fetal periods, some important changes occur during the later periods of development: infancy, childhood, adolescence, and adulthood.

DEVELOPMENTAL PERIODS

Although it is customary to divide human development into *prenatal* (before birth) and *postnatal* (after birth) periods, it is important to realize that birth is merely a dramatic event during development resulting in a change in environment. **Development does not stop at birth.** Important developmental changes, in addition to growth, occur after birth, e.g., the development of teeth and female breasts. The brain triples in weight between birth and 16 years. Most developmental changes are completed by the age of 25.

The Prenatal Period

The obvious developmental changes occurring before birth are illustrated in the *Timetables of Human Prenatal Development* (Figs. 1–1 and 1–2). This developmental calendar is based on the examination of many embryos and fetuses by the authors and on studies by Streeter (1942), Gasser (1975), Persaud and colleagues (1985), O'Rahilly and Müller (1987),

Butler and Juurlink (1987), and Shiota (1991). Study of these timetables reveals that the most striking advances in development occur during the third to eighth weeks, which is known as the *embryonic period*. The following terms are commonly used in discussions of developing humans during the prenatal period.

Abortion (L. *abortio*, to miscarry). This term refers to the birth of an embryo or a fetus before it is *viable* (capable of living outside the uterus). *Threatened abortion* is a common complication in about 25 per cent of clinically apparent pregnancies. Despite every effort to prevent abortion, about one-half of these pregnancies ultimately abort (Callen, 1988). All terminations of pregnancy that occur naturally or are induced before 20 weeks are abortions. A *complete abortion* is one in which all the products of conception (p. 6) have been expelled from the uterus.

About 15 per cent of all recognized pregnancies end in *spontaneous abortions* (i.e., they occur naturally), usually during the first 12 weeks. Legally induced abortions, often called *elective abortions*, are usually produced by suction curettage (evacuation of the embryo and its membranes by suction from the uterus). Some abortions are induced because of the mother's poor health or to prevent the birth of a severely malformed child (e.g., one without most of its brain). A *missed abortion* is the retention of a conceptus in the uterus after death of the embryo or fetus.

Abortus. This term refers to the products of an abortion (i.e., the embryo/fetus and its associated membranes, such as the amnion and chorionic sac). An embryo or nonviable fetus and its membranes weighing less than 500 gm is called an abortus, but often one refers to them as aborted embryos or fetuses.

Oocyte (ovum). This term refers to the female germ or sex cell. When mature, the oocyte is often called an ovum (L. egg). A "blighted ovum" refers to an embryo that is dead; other products of conception (e.g., the chorionic [gestational] sac) may remain alive for several weeks.

Zygote (Gr. *zygōtos*, yoked together). This cell results from fertilization of an oocyte by a sperm.
Text continued on page 6

TIMETABLE OF HUMAN PRENATAL DEVELOPMENT
1 to 6 weeks

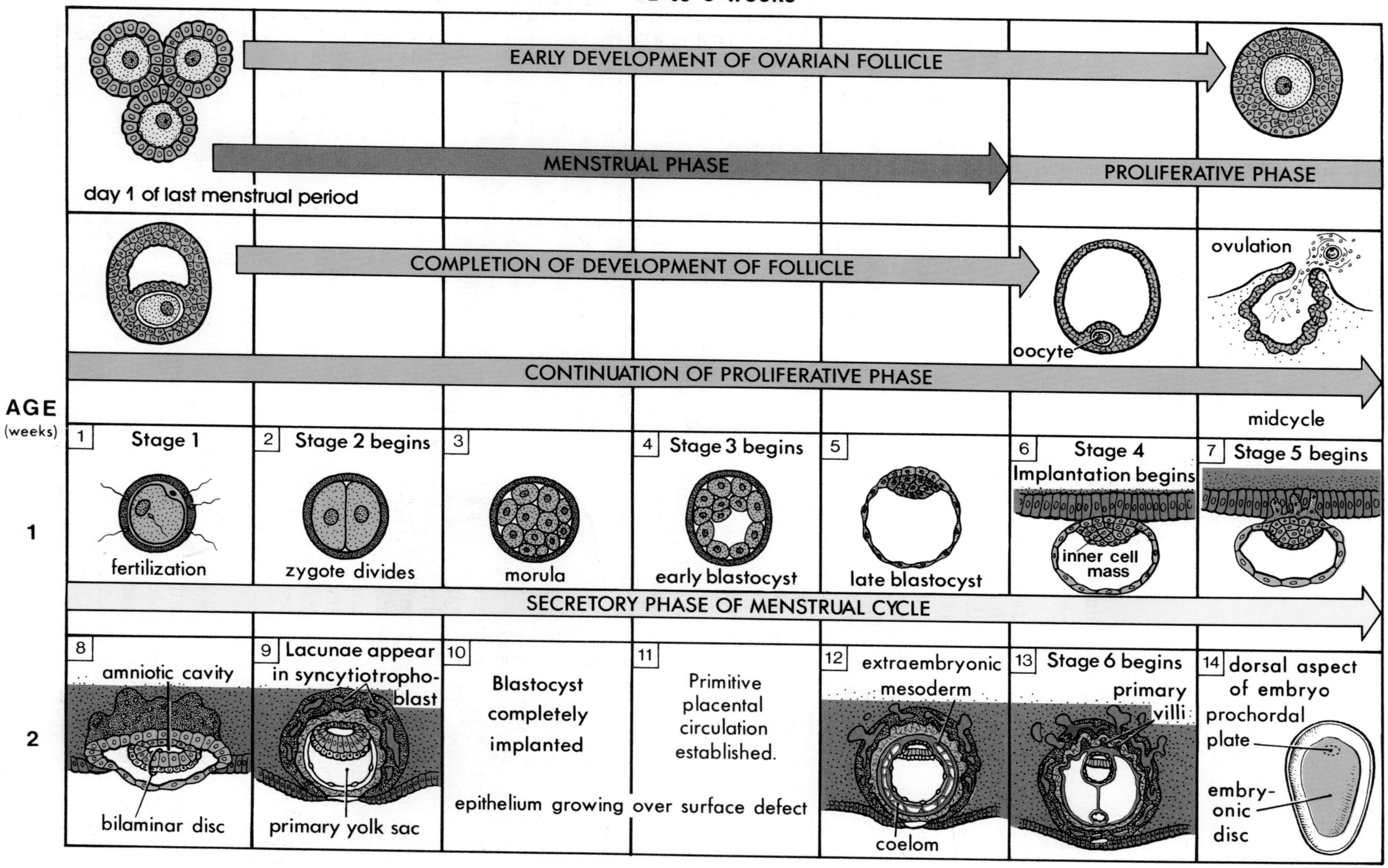

EARLY DEVELOPMENT OF OVARIAN FOLLICLE

MENSTRUAL PHASE

COMPLETION OF DEVELOPMENT OF FOLLICLE

PROLIFERATIVE PHASE

CONTINUATION OF PROLIFERATIVE PHASE

SECRETORY PHASE OF MENSTRUAL CYCLE

ovulation

midcycle

day 1 of last menstrual period

oocyte

AGE (weeks)

1

2

1	Stage 1	2	Stage 2 begins	3		4	Stage 3 begins	5		6	Stage 4 Implantation begins	7	Stage 5 begins
	fertilization		zygote divides		morula		early blastocyst		late blastocyst		inner cell mass		

| 8 | amniotic cavity / bilaminar disc | 9 | Lacunae appear in syncytiotrophoblast / primary yolk sac | 10 | Blastocyst completely implanted | 11 | Primitive placental circulation established. | 12 | extraembryonic mesoderm / coelom | 13 | Stage 6 begins / primary villi | 14 | dorsal aspect of embryo / prochordal plate / embryonic disc |

epithelium growing over surface defect

2

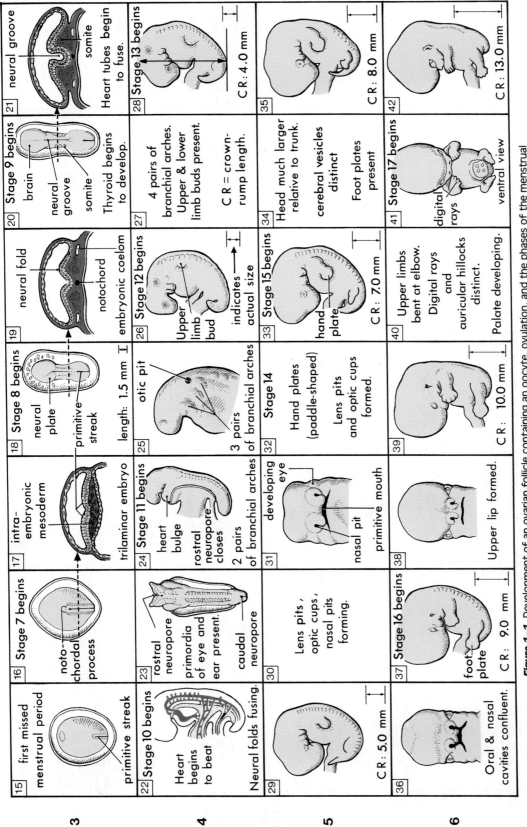

Figure 1–1. Development of an ovarian follicle containing an oocyte, ovulation, and the phases of the menstrual cycle are illustrated first. *Human development begins at fertilization,* about 14 days after the onset of the last menstruation. Cleavage of the zygote in the uterine tube, implantation of the blastocyst, and early development of the embryo are also shown. The main features of developmental stages in human embryos are illustrated. For a full discussion of embryonic development, see Chapter 5. Beginning students should make no attempt to memorize these tables or the stages (e.g., that Stage 3 begins on day 4 and Stage 5 on day 7).

15 first missed menstrual period

primitive streak

16 Stage 7 begins

noto-chordal process

17 intra-embryonic mesoderm

trilaminar embryo

18 Stage 8 begins

neural plate

primitive streak

length: 1.5 mm

19 neural fold

notochord

embryonic coelom

20 Stage 9 begins

brain

neural groove

somite

Thyroid begins to develop.

21 neural groove

somite

Heart tubes begin to fuse.

22 Stage 10 begins

Heart begins to beat

Neural folds fusing.

23 rostral neuropore

primordia of eye and ear present.

caudal neuropore

24 Stage 11 begins

heart bulge

rostral neuropore closes

2 pairs of branchial arches

25 3 pairs of branchial arches

otic pit

26 Stage 12 begins

Upper limb bud

indicates actual size

27 4 pairs of branchial arches.

Upper & lower limb buds present.

C R = crown-rump length.

28 Stage 13 begins

C R : 4.0 mm

29 C R : 5.0 mm

30 Lens pits, optic cups, nasal pits forming.

31 developing eye

nasal pit

primitive mouth

32 Stage 14

Hand plates (paddle-shaped)

Lens pits and optic cups formed.

33 Stage 15 begins

hand plate

C R : 7.0 mm

34 Head much larger relative to trunk.

cerebral vesicles distinct

Foot plates present

35 C R : 8.0 mm

36 Oral & nasal cavities confluent.

37 Stage 16 begins

foot plate

C R : 9.0 mm

38 Upper lip formed.

39 C R : 10.0 mm

40 Upper limbs bent at elbow.

Digital rays and auricular hillocks distinct.

Palate developing.

41 Stage 17 begins

digital rays

ventral view

42 C R : 13.0 mm

3

4

5

6

TIMETABLE OF HUMAN PRENATAL DEVELOPMENT
7 to 38 weeks

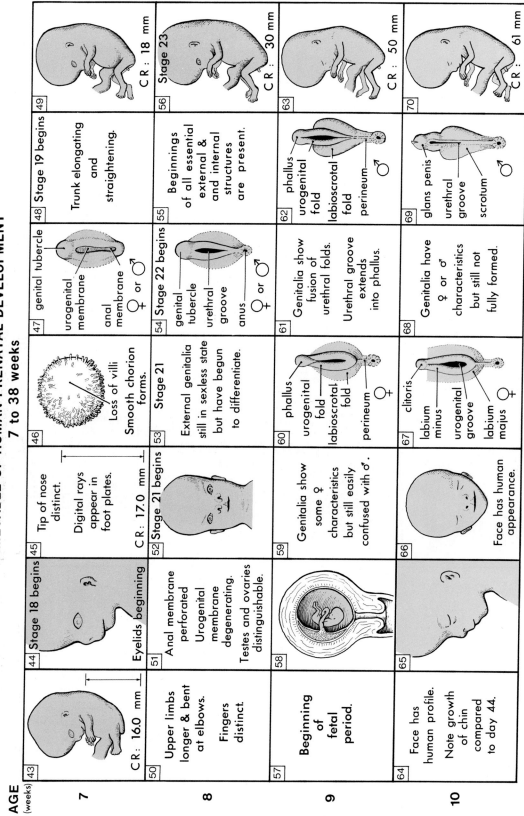

AGE (weeks)

7

43 — Stage 18 begins. CR: 16.0 mm

44 — Stage 18 begins

45 — Tip of nose distinct. Digital rays appear in foot plates. CR: 17.0 mm

46 — Loss of villi. Smooth chorion forms.

47 — genital tubercle, urogenital membrane, anal membrane ♀ or ♂

48 — Stage 19 begins. Trunk elongating and straightening.

49 — CR: 18 mm

8

50 — Upper limbs longer & bent at elbows. Fingers distinct.

51 — Eyelids beginning. Anal membrane perforated. Urogenital membrane degenerating. Testes and ovaries distinguishable.

52 — Stage 21 begins

53 — Stage 21. External genitalia still in sexless state but have begun to differentiate.

54 — Stage 22 begins. genital tubercle, urethral groove, anus ♀ or ♂

55 — Beginnings of all essential external and internal structures are present.

56 — Stage 23. CR: 30 mm

9

57 — Beginning of fetal period.

58

59 — Genitalia show some ♀ characteristics but still easily confused with ♂.

60 — phallus, urogenital fold, labioscrotal fold, perineum ♀

61 — Genitalia show fusion of urethral folds. Urethral groove extends into phallus.

62 — phallus, urogenital fold, labioscrotal fold, perineum ♂

63 — CR: 50 mm

10

64 — Face has human profile. Note growth of chin compared to day 44.

65

66 — Face has human appearance.

67 — clitoris, labium minus, urogenital groove, labium majus ♀

68 — Genitalia have ♀ or ♂ characteristics but still not fully formed.

69 — glans penis, urethral groove, scrotum ♂

70 — CR: 61 mm

4

The Fetal Period

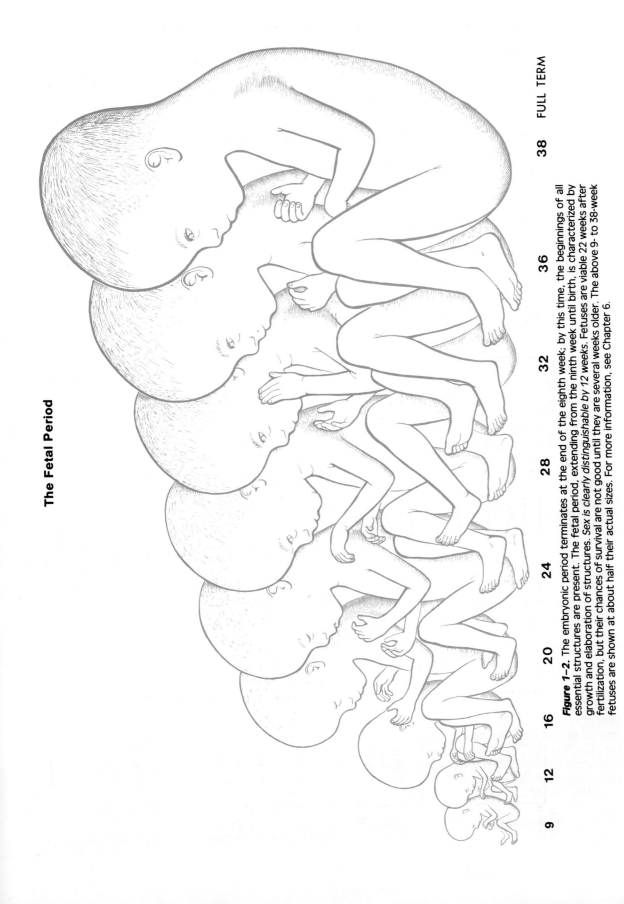

Figure 1–2. The embryonic period terminates at the end of the eighth week; by this time, the beginnings of all essential structures are present. The fetal period, extending from the ninth week until birth, is characterized by growth and elaboration of structures. *Sex is clearly distinguishable by 12 weeks.* Fetuses are viable 22 weeks after fertilization, but their chances of survival are not good until they are several weeks older. The above 9- to 38-week fetuses are shown at about half their actual sizes. For more information, see Chapter 6.

9 12 16 20 24 28 32 36 38 FULL TERM

A zygote is the beginning of a new human being. The expression "fertilized ovum" refers to the zygote, but it is not appropriate for scientific presentations.

Cleavage. This term refers to the series of mitotic divisions of the zygote that result in the formation of cells called *blastomeres.* At each succeeding cleavage division, the blastomeres become smaller.

Morula (L. *morus*, mulberry). The blastomeres change their shape and tightly align themselves against each other to form a compact ball of cells. This phenomenon, known as *compaction*, is probably mediated by cell surface adhesion glycoproteins (Gilbert, 1991). When 12 or more blastomeres have formed, the spherical group of cells is called a morula. It was given this name because of its resemblance to the fruit of the mulberry tree. This stage occurs three to four days after fertilization, just as the developing human is about to enter the uterus (see Fig. 1–1).

Blastocyst (Gr. *blastos*, germ + *kystis*, bladder). After the morula enters the uterus from the uterine tube, a fluid-filled cavity develops inside it; this converts the morula into a blastocyst. Its centrally located cells, called the **embryoblast** or *inner cell mass*, will form the embryo.

Gastrula. During gastrulation (transformation of the blastocyst into a gastrula), a three-layered or trilaminar embryonic disc forms (third week). The three germ layers of the gastrula (ectoderm, mesoderm, and endoderm) subsequently differentiate into all the embryo's tissues and organs.

Neurula. During neurulation, the period during which the neural plate forms and closes to form the *neural tube* (fourth week), the embryo is sometimes called a neurula. The neural tube gives rise to the central nervous system (brain and spinal cord).

Embryo. This term refers to the developing human during its early stages of development. The term is not usually used until the middle of the second week. The *embryonic period* extends to the end of the eighth week, at which time the beginnings of all major structures are present.

Conceptus. This term refers to the embryo and its membranes, i.e., *the products of conception* or fertilization. It includes all structures that develop from the zygote, both embryonic and extraembryonic. Hence, it includes the embryo as well as the fetal part of the placenta and its associated membranes, e.g., the amnion and chorionic sac (see Chapter 7).

Fetus (L. offspring). After the embryonic period, the developing human is called a fetus. During the *fetal period* (ninth week to birth), differentiation and growth of the tissues and organs formed during the embryonic period occur. Although developmental changes are not so dramatic as those occurring during the embryonic period, they are very important because they enable the tissues and organs to function. The rate of body growth is remarkable, especially during the third and fourth months, and weight gain is phenomenal during the terminal months.

Primordium (L. *primus*, first + *ordior*, to begin). This term refers to the first indication of an organ or structure, i.e., its earliest stage of development. The term *anlage* has a similar meaning, e.g., the primordium or anlage of the upper limb appears as a bud on about day 26 (see Chapter 5).

Miscarriage. This is a lay term that refers to an interruption of pregnancy during the later stages of pregnancy (i.e., spontaneous expulsion of the products of conception after the twentieth week). In medical descriptions, it is common to use the term *premature birth* for the expulsion of a mature fetus.

Trimester. This is a period of *three calendar months.* Obstetricians commonly divide the nine-month period of gestation (stages of intrauterine development) into three trimesters. The most critical stages of development occur during the first trimester.

The Postnatal Period

The changes occurring after birth are more or less familiar to most people. Explanations of frequently used developmental periods and terms follow.

Infancy (babyhood). This period refers to the earliest period of extrauterine life, *roughly the first year* after birth. The first four weeks are designated as the newborn or *neonatal period.* Transition from intrauterine to extrauterine existence requires many changes, especially in the cardiovascular and respiratory systems. If a newborn infant, or *neonate*, survives the first crucial moments after birth, his or her chances of living are usually good. The body as a whole grows particularly rapidly during infancy; total length increases by about one-half and weight is usually trebled. By the age of one year most children have six to eight teeth. For details of development during infancy, see Behrman (1992).

Childhood. This is the period from about 13 months until 12 to 13 years. The primary (deciduous) teeth continue to appear and are later replaced by the secondary (permanent) teeth. During early childhood there is active ossification (formation of bone), but as the child becomes older, the rate of growth slows down. Just before puberty, however, growth accelerates; this is known as the *prepubertal growth spurt.*

Puberty. This is the period, usually between the ages of 12 and 15 years in girls and 13 and 16 years in boys, during which the *secondary sexual characteristics develop.* The stages of pubertal development follow a consistent pattern for individuals and are defined by the development of primary and secondary sexual characteristics (pubic hair and breasts in females; pubic hair and growth of the external genitalia in males). The legal ages of *presumptive puberty* are 12 years in girls and 14 years in boys.

Adolescence. This is the period from about 12 to 17 years that is characterized by rapid physical and sexual maturation. It extends from the earliest signs of sexual maturity, or *pubertal development*, until the attainment of physical, mental, and emotional maturity. During adolescence, the ability to reproduce is achieved. The general growth rate decelerates as this period terminates, but growth of some structures accelerates (e.g., the female breasts and male genitalia).

Adulthood. This period is generally reached between the ages of 18 and 21 years. Ossification and growth are virtually completed during early adulthood, 21 to 25 years; thereafter, developmental changes occur very slowly.

SCOPE OF EMBRYOLOGY

Embryology literally means the study of embryos (third to eighth week, inclusive); however, the term generally refers to prenatal development, i.e., the study of both embryos and fetuses. The term *developmental anatomy* refers to the prenatal and postnatal periods of development. There are no essential differences between these two stages of development. Prenatal development is more rapid and results in more striking changes, but the developmental mechanisms of the two periods are similar. The study of abnormal development (anomalies or birth defects) is called *teratology*. This branch of embryology is concerned with the various genetic and environmental factors that disturb normal development (see Chapter 8).

SIGNIFICANCE OF EMBRYOLOGY

The study of embryology advances knowledge concerning the beginnings of human life and the changes occurring during development before birth. Knowledge of the developing human is of practical value in helping to understand the normal relationships of body structures and the causes of congenital anomalies. In other words, *embryology illuminates anatomy* and explains how normal relations and abnormalities develop. Knowledge physicians have of normal development and of the causes of congenital anomalies is necessary for giving the embryo and fetus the greatest possible chance of developing normally.

Much of the modern practice of *obstetrics* involves what could be called **applied embryology**. Embryological topics of special interest to obstetricians are ovulation, oocyte and sperm transport, fertilization, implantation, fetal-maternal relations, fetal circulation, critical periods of development, and causes of birth defects. In addition to caring for the mother, obstetricians must guard the health of the embryo and fetus. The significance of embryology is readily apparent to pediatricians because many of their patients have congenital anomalies resulting from maldevelopment, e.g., diaphragmatic hernia, spina bifida, and congenital heart disease. *Developmental defects cause most deaths during infancy.* Knowledge of the development of structure and function is essential to understanding the physiological changes that occur during the newborn period and for helping babies in distress.

Progress in surgery, especially in the prenatal and pediatric age groups, has made knowledge of human development more clinically significant. *Surgical treatment of the fetus is now possible* (Harrison et al., 1990). The understanding and correction of most congenital anomalies (e.g., cleft palate and cardiac defects) depend upon knowledge of normal development and of the deviations that have occurred. An understanding of common congenital anomalies and their causes also enables physicians, dentists, and others to explain the developmental basis of abnormalities, often dispelling parental guilt feelings.

Physicians and other health care professionals who are aware of common abnormalities and their embryological basis approach unusual situations with confidence rather than surprise. For example, when it is realized that the renal artery represents only one of several vessels originally supplying the kidney during development, the frequent variations in number and arrangement of renal vessels are understandable and not unexpected.

HISTORICAL GLEANINGS

If I have seen further, it is by standing on the shoulders of giants.
—*Sir Isaac Newton,*
English mathematician, 1643–1727

This statement, made over 300 years ago, emphasizes that each new study of a problem rests on a base of knowledge established by earlier investigators. The theories of every age offer explanations based on the knowledge and experience of the investigators of the period. Although we should not consider them final, we should appreciate, rather than scorn, these ideas. People have always been interested in knowing how they originated, how they were born, and why some people develop abnormally. Ancient people, filled with curiosity, developed many answers to these questions.

Ancient Views About Embryology

A brief Sanskrit treatise on ancient Indian embryology is thought to have been written in 1416 B.C. This scripture of the Hindus, called *Garbha Upanishad*, describes ancient ideas concerning the embryo. It states, "From the conjugation of blood and semen the embryo comes into existence. During the period favorable for conception, after the sexual intercourse, (it) becomes a *Kalada* (one-day-old embryo). After remaining seven nights, it becomes a vesicle. After a fortnight, it becomes a spherical mass. After a month, it becomes a firm mass. After two months, the head is formed. After three months, the limb regions appear." Although the dates of appearance of the structures are inaccurate, the sequence is correct. The scripture further states that, "During the seventh month, (it) becomes endowed with life."

The **Greeks** made many important contributions to the science of embryology (Persaud, 1984, Horder et al., 1986, Dunstan, 1990). The first recorded embryological studies are in the books of **Hippocrates** (Fig. 1–3), the famous Greek physician of the fifth century B.C. who is regarded by many as the *Father of Medicine*. In order to understand how the human embryo develops, he recommended, "Take twenty or more eggs and let them be incubated by two or more hens. Then each day from the second to that of hatching, remove an egg, break it, and examine it. You will find exactly as I say, for the nature of the bird can be likened to that of man."

In the fourth century B.C., **Aristotle** wrote a treatise on embryology in which he described development of the chick and other embryos. Embryologists regard Aristotle as *The Founder of Embryology* despite the fact that he promoted the idea that the embryo developed from a formless mass, which he described as a "less fully concocted seed with a nutritive soul and all bodily parts." This arose from menstrual blood after activation by the male semen. The same erroneous idea appeared in the Sanskrit treatise on ancient Indian embryology described earlier. **Galen** (second century A.D.) wrote a book entitled *On the Formation of the Foetus*, in which he described the development and nutri-

tion of fetuses and the structures that we now call the allantois, amnion, and placenta.

Embryology In The Middle Ages

Growth of science was slow during the medieval period, and few high points of embryological investigation undertaken during this time are known to us. It is, however, cited in the *Koran* or *Qur'an* (seventh century A.D.), The Holy Book of the Muslims, that human beings are produced from a mixture of secretions from the male and female. Several references are made to the creation of a human being from a *nutfa* (small drop). It is also stated that the resulting organism settles in the womb like a seed, six days after its beginning. (The human blastocyst begins to implant in the uterus about six days after fertilization.) Reference is also made to the leech-like appearance of the early embryo. (The four-week embryo shown looks like a leech or bloodsucker.) The embryo is also said to resemble a "chewed substance." (The somites of older embryos somewhat resemble teethmarks in a chewed substance.) For more information about embryological references in the Koran, see Moore (1986) and Musallam (1990).

A concise treatise entitled *De humana natura* is attributed to **Constantinus Africanus** (Circa 1020–1087 A.D.) of Salerno. He gave the West a great number of classical learnings in readable Latin through his many translations of the Greek, Roman, and Arabic scholars. Constantinus Africanus described the composition and sequential development of the embryo in relation to the planets and each month of pregnancy, a concept unknown in antiquity (Burnett, 1990).

The Renaissance

During the fifteenth century, **Leonardo da Vinci** made accurate drawings of dissections of the pregnant uterus containing a fetus (Fig. 1–4). He introduced the quantitative approach by making measurements of prenatal growth. According to Brockliss (1990), the embryological revolution began with the publication of Harvey's book *De generatione animalium* in 1651. He believed that the male seed, after entering the womb, became metamorphosed into an egg-like substance from which the embryo developed. **Harvey** was greatly influenced by one of his professors at the University of Padua, *Fabricius of Aquapendente*, who was the first to study embryos from different species of animals. Harvey examined chick embryos with simple lenses and made many observations, especially on the circulation of blood. He also studied development of the fallow deer but, when unable to observe early stages, concluded that embryos were secreted by the uterus.

Early microscopes were simple (Fig. 1–5), but they opened an exciting new field of observation. In 1672 **de Graaf** observed little chambers in the rabbit's uterus and concluded that they could not have been secreted by the uterus but must have come from the organs that he called ovaries. Undoubtedly, the little chambers de Graaf described were blastocysts. He also described vesicular ovar-

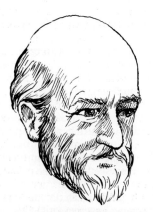

Figure 1–3. Copy of a drawing by Hippocrates, "the Father of Medicine" (460–377 B.C.). He placed medicine on a scientific foundation. In addition to the Hippocratic oath attributed to him, he wrote several books in anatomy, including one in embryology.

ian follicles, which are still sometimes called *graafian follicles* in his honor.

Malpighi, in 1675, studying what he believed were unfertilized hen's eggs, observed early embryos. As a result, he thought the egg contained a miniature chick. In 1677 **Hamm** and **Leeuwenhoek**, using an improved microscope, first observed human sperms (spermatozoa), but they misunderstood the sperm's role in fertilization. They thought the sperm contained a miniature, preformed human being (Fig. 1–6) that enlarged when it was deposited in the female genital tract.

Wolff, in 1759, refuted both versions of the *preformation theory* after observing parts of the embryo develop from "globules" (developing embryonic tissues). He examined unincubated eggs and could not see the embryos described by Malpighi. He proposed the *layer concept*, whereby division of the zygote produces layers of cells (now called the embryonic disc) from which the embryo develops. His ideas formed the basis of the theory of *epigenesis*, which states that development results from growth and differentiation of specialized cells. The preformation controversy finally ended around 1775 when **Spallanzani** showed that both the ovum and sperm were necessary for initiating the development of a new individual. From his experiments, including artificial insemination in dogs, Spallanzani concluded that the sperm was the fertilizing agent that initiated the developmental processes.

In 1818, **Saint Hilaire** and his son made the first significant studies of congenital anomalies. They performed experiments in animals that were designed to produce developmental defects, initiating what is now known as *the science of teratology*.

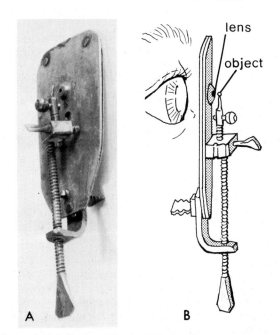

Figure 1–5. *A*, Photograph of a 1673 Leeuwenhoek microscope. *B*, Drawing of a lateral view illustrating its use. The object was held in front of the lens on the point of the short rod, and the screw arrangement was used to adjust the object under the lens. After the development of this crude instrument, embryologists were able to observe the early stages of development.

In 1827, about 150 years after the discovery of the sperm, **von Baer** described the oocyte in the ovarian follicle of a dog. He also observed dividing zygotes in the uterine tube and blastocysts in the uterus. He contributed much knowledge about the origin of tissues and organs from the layers described by Malpighi. His significant and far-reaching contributions resulted in his later being regarded as *The Father of Modern Embryology*. Great advances were made in embryology when the **cell theory**, stating that the body was composed of cells and cell products, was established in 1839 by **Schleiden** and **Schwann**. This concept soon led to the realization that the embryo developed from a single cell, the *zygote*, which underwent many cell divisions as the tissues and organs of the embryo formed.

O'Rahilly (1988) noted the significant impact of His' contributions to the study of human embryology. **Wilhelm His** (1831–1904) developed improved techniques for fixation of tissues, sectioning them with a microtome, staining of tissues, and reconstruction of embryos. His method of graphic reconstruction paved the way for producing three-dimensional, stereoscopic, and computer-generated images of embryos. In 1887, inspired by His' work, **Franklin P. Mall** (1862–1917) began his collection of human embryos, which forms the basis of the *Carnegie Collection* that is known throughout the world. It is now in the National Museum of Health and Medicine of the Armed Forces Institute of Pathology in Washington, D.C.

Wilhelm Roux (1850–1924) pioneered analytical experimental studies on the physiology of development in amphibia, which was pursued further by **Hans Spemann**

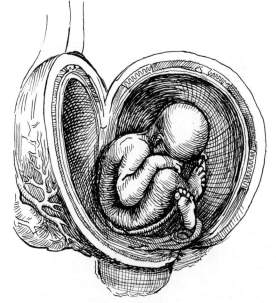

Figure 1–4. Reproduction of Leonardo da Vinci's drawing made in the fifteenth century A.D., showing a fetus in a uterus that has been incised and opened.

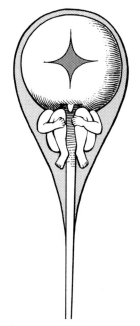

Figure 1–6. Copy of a seventeenth century drawing of a sperm by Hartsoeker. The miniature human being within it was thought to enlarge after the sperm entered an ovum. Other embryologists at this time thought the oocyte contained a miniature human being that enlarged when it was stimulated by a sperm.

(1869–1941). For his discovery of the phenomenon of primary induction, i.e., how one tissue determines the fate of another, *Spemann received the Nobel Prize in 1935.* Over the decades, scientists have been attempting to isolate the substances that are transmitted from one tissue to another, causing induction. Recent studies suggest that endogenous *retinoic acid,* a hydrophobic molecule that specifically binds to nuclear receptors, is a likely *morphogen* that induces the normal pattern of embryonic structures (Eichele, 1989; Slack, 1991).

One of the most revolutionary developments in the history of human reproduction is the technique of *in vitro fertilization* (p. 33), pioneered by **Edwards** and **Steptoe**, which in 1978 led to the birth of Louise Brown, the first "test tube baby." Since then, thousands of infertile couples throughout the world have experienced the miracle of birth because of this new technology.

Chromosomes, Genetics, and Human Development

In 1859, **Darwin** published a book, *On the Origin of Species,* in which he emphasized the hereditary nature of variability among members of a species as an important factor in evolution. The principles of heredity were developed in 1865 by an Austrian monk named **Gregor Mendel**, but medical scientists and biologists did not understand the significance of these principles in the study of mammalian development for many years.

Flemming observed chromosomes in 1878 and suggested their probable role in fertilization. In 1883, **von Beneden** observed that mature germ cells have a reduced number of chromosomes. He also described some features of meiosis, the process whereby the chromosome number is reduced. In 1902, **Sutton** and **Boveri** declared independently that the behavior of the chromosomes during germ cell formation and fertilization agreed with Mendel's principles of inheritance. In the same year, **Garrod** reported *alcaptonuria* as the first example of mendelian inheritance in human beings. Many consider Garrod to be the *Father of Medical Genetics.*

It was soon realized that the zygote contains all the genetic information necessary for directing the development of a new human being. The first significant observations on human chromosomes were made in 1912, when **von Winiwarter** reported that there were 47 chromosomes in the cells of the body. In 1923, **Painter** concluded that 48 was the correct number; this conclusion was widely accepted until 1956 when **Tjio** and **Levan** reported finding only 46 chromosomes in embryonic cells. Their descriptions and photomicrographs were so superior to those of previous workers that few cytologists doubted the accuracy of their chromosome counts. *Chromosome studies were soon used in medicine* in a number of important ways (e.g., chromosome mapping, clinical diagnosis, and prenatal diagnosis; Thompson et al., 1991).

Once the normal chromosomal pattern was firmly established, it soon became evident that some persons with congenital abnormalities had an abnormal number of chromosomes. A new era in medical genetics resulted from the demonstration by **Lejeune** and associates in 1959 that infants with mongolism (now called the *Down syndrome*) have 47 chromosomes instead of the usual 46 in their body cells. It is now known that chromosomal aberrations are a significant cause of congenital anomalies and embryonic death (see Chapter 8).

Recent advances in **molecular biology** have led to the development of sophisticated techniques for studying embryonic development. The application of *recombinant DNA technology,* chimeric models, and transgenic mice are now widely used in research laboratories to address such diverse problems as the genetic regulation of morphogenesis, the temporal and regional expression of specific genes, and how cells are committed to form the various parts of the embryo. For the first time we are beginning to understand how, when, and where selected genes are activated and expressed in the embryo during normal and abnormal development (Goodwin, 1988; Rossant and Joyner, 1989; Cherfas, 1990; and Rusconi, 1991). *Endogenous retinoic acid* has been identified as an important regulatory substance in embryonic development. Apparently it acts as a transcriptional activator for specific genes and is involved in embryonic patterning (Eichele, 1989).

DESCRIPTIVE TERMS

The terminology in this book is based on the third edition of *Nomina Embryologica* which was

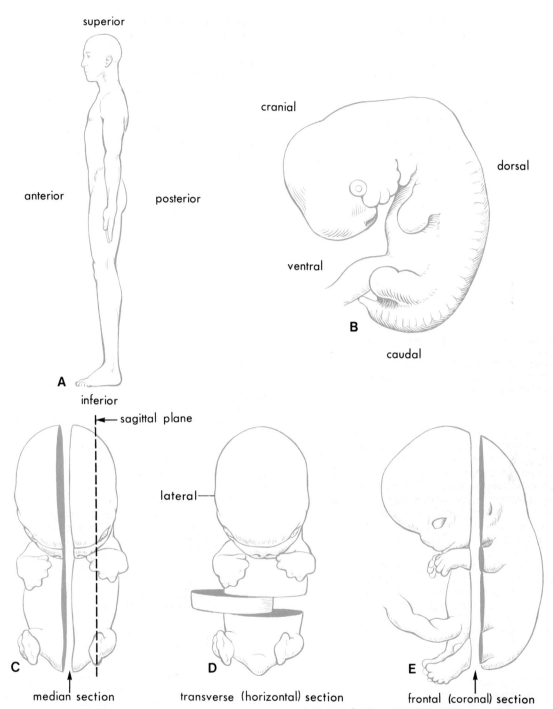

Figure 1-7. Drawings illustrating descriptive terms of position, direction, and planes of the body. *A*, Lateral view of an adult in the anatomical position. *B*, Lateral view of a five-week embryo. *C* and *D*, Ventral views of six-week embryos. *E*, Lateral view of a seven-week embryo. In describing development, it is necessary to use words denoting the position of one part to another or to the body as a whole. For example, the vertebral column (backbone) develops in the dorsal part of the embryo, and the sternum (breast bone) develops ventral to it in the ventral part of the embryo.

published as part of the sixth edition of Nomina Anatomica (Warwick, 1989). Officially recognized terms are used in the present work, but for clarity, other commonly used ones appear in parentheses, e.g., uterine tube (fallopian tube). In anatomy several terms relating to position and direction are used, and reference is made to various planes of the body. All descriptions of the adult are based on the assumption that the body is erect, with the upper limbs by the sides and the palms directed anteriorly (Fig. 1–7*A*). This is called the **anatomical position**. The terms anterior or ventral and posterior or dorsal are used to describe the front or back of the body or limbs and the relations of structures within the body to one another. When describing embryos, the terms dorsal and ventral are used (Fig. 1–7*B*).

Superior and inferior are used to indicate the relative levels of different structures (Fig. 1–7*A*). For embryos, the terms cranial (cephalic) and caudal are used to denote relationships to the head and tail, respectively (Fig. 1–7*B*). Distances from the source of attachment of a structure are designated as proximal or distal, e.g., in the lower limb the knee is proximal to the ankle and the ankle is distal to the knee.

The Planes of the Body

The *median plane* is the vertical plane passing through the midline of the body. Median sections divide the body into right and left halves (Fig. 1–7*C*). The terms *lateral* and *medial* refer to structures that are respectively farther from or nearer to the median plane of the body. A *sagittal plane* is any vertical plane passing through the body parallel to the median plane (Fig. 1–7*C*). A transverse or *horizontal plane* refers to any plane that is at right angles to both the median and frontal planes (Fig. 1–7*D*). A frontal or *coronal plane* is any vertical plane that intersects the median plane at a right angle (Fig. 1–7*E*); it divides the body into anterior (ventral) and posterior (dorsal) parts.

CLINICALLY ORIENTED QUESTIONS FOR PROBLEM-BASED LEARNING SESSIONS

1. At what stage does a new human being start to develop? When do developmental stages end?
2. What is the human organism called at the beginning of its development? Why is this an appropriate term? Could it be referred to as a conceptus?
3. How does a conceptus differ from an abortus?
4. What sequence of events occurs during puberty? Are they the same in males and females? What are the respective ages of presumptive puberty in males and females?
5. How do the terms embryology and teratology differ"? Are these studies applicable to clinical investigations?

The answers to these questions are given on page 458.

References and Suggested Reading[1]

Behrman RE: *Nelson Textbook of Pediatrics*, 14th ed. Philadelphia, WB Saunders, 1992, pp 14–39.

Biggers JD: Arbitrary partitions of prenatal life. *Human Reprod* 5:1, 1990.

Brockliss LWB: The embryological revolution in the France of Louis XIV: the dominance of ideology. *In* Dunstan GR (ed): *The Human Embryo: Aristotle and the Arabic and European Traditions.* Exeter, University of Exeter Press, 1990.

Burnett CSF: The planets and the development of the embryo. *In* Dunstan GR (ed): *The Human Embryo: Aristotle and the Arabic and European Traditions.* Exeter, University of Exeter Press, 1990.

Butler H, Juurlink BHJ: *An Atlas for Staging Mammalian and Chick Embryos.* Boca Raton, CRC Press, 1987.

Callen PW: *Ultrasonography in Obstetrics and Gynecology*, 2nd ed, Philadelphia, WB Saunders, 1988.

Cherfas J: Embryology gets down to the molecular level. *Science* 250:33, 1990.

De Pomerai D: *From Gene to Animal*, 2nd ed. New York, Cambridge University Press, 1991.

Dunstan GR (ed): *The Human Embryo: Aristotle and the Arabic and European Traditions.* Exeter, University of Exeter Press, 1990.

Eichele G: Retinoids and vertebrate limb pattern formation. *Trends in Genet* 5:246, 1989.

Gasser R: *Atlas of Human Embryos.* Hagerstown, Harper & Row, 1975.

Gilbert SF: *Developmental Biology*, 3rd ed. Sunderland, Sinauer Associates, 1991.

Goodwin BC: Problems and prospects in morphogenesis. *Experientia* 44:633, 1988.

Harrison MR, Golbus MS, Filly RA: *The Unborn Patient: Prenatal Diagnosis and Treatment.* Philadelphia, WB Saunders, 1990.

---

[1] In this and other chapters, the references include not only those cited in the text, but ones that are classic (e.g., Streeter, 1942) and others that will be helpful to those who wish more details about embryology and related subjects.

Hawkins J: *Gene Structure and Expression*, 2nd ed. New York, Cambridge University Press, 1991.

Horder TJ, Witkowski JA, Wylie CC (eds): *A History of Embryology*. Cambridge, Cambridge University Press, 1986.

Meyer AW: *The Rise of Embryology*. Stanford, Stanford University Press, 1939.

Moore KL: A scientist's interpretation of references to embryology in the Qur'an. *JIMA 18*:15, 1986.

Moore KL: *The Sex Chromatin*. Philadelphia, WB Saunders, 1966.

Musallam B: The human embryo in arabic scientific and religious thought. *In* Dunstan GR (ed): *The Human Embryo: Aristotle and the Arabic and European Traditions*. Exeter, University of Exeter Press, 1990.

Needham J: *A History of Embryology*, 2nd ed. Cambridge, Cambridge University Press, 1959.

Oppenheimer JM: Problems, concepts and their history. *In* BH Willier, PA Weiss, and V Hamburger (eds): *Analysis of Development*. New York, Hafner Publishing, 1971.

O'Rahilly R: One hundred years of human embryology. *In* Kalter H (ed): *Issues and Reviews in Teratology*, vol. 4, New York, Plenum Press, 1988, pp 81–128.

O'Rahilly R, Müller F: *Developmental Stages in Human Embryos*. Washington, D.C., Carnegie Institution of Washington, 1987.

Persaud TVN: *Early History of Human Anatomy*. Springfield, Charles C Thomas, 1984.

Persaud TVN: *Problems of Birth Defects: From Hippocrates to Thalidomide and After*. Baltimore, University Park Press, 1977.

Persaud TVN, Chudley AE, Skalko RG: *Basic Concepts in Teratology*. New York, Alan R. Liss, 1985.

Rossant J, Joyner AL: Towards a molecular-genetic analysis of mammalian development. *Trends in Genet 5*:277, 1989.

Rusconi S: Transgenic regulation in laboratory animals. *Experientia 47*:866, 1991.

Shiota K: Development and intrauterine fate of normal and abnormal human conceptuses. *Cong Anomalies 31*:67, 1991.

Slack JMW: *From Egg to Embryo*, 2nd ed. New York, Cambridge University Press, 1991.

Streeter GL: Developmental horizons in human embryos. Description of age group XI, 13 to 20 somites, and age group XII, 21 to 29 somites. *Contrib Embryol Carnegie Inst 30*:211, 1942.

Thompson MW, McInnes RR, Willard HF: *Thompson & Thompson's Genetics In Medicine*, 5th ed. Philadelphia, WB Saunders, 1991.

Warwick R: *Nomina Anatomica*, 6th ed. Edinburgh, Churchill Livingstone, 1989.

Willis RA: *The Borderland of Embryology and Pathology*, 2nd ed. London, Butterworth, 1962.

2

The Beginning of Human Development

THE FIRST WEEK

He who sees things grow from the beginning will have the finest view of them.
— Aristotle, Greek philosopher and scientist 384–322 B.C.

Human development begins at conception or fertilization,[1] the process during which a male gamete or sperm (spermatozoon) unites with a female gamete or oocyte (ovum) to form a single cell called a **zygote** (Gr. *zygōtos*, yoked together). This highly specialized, totipotent cell marked the beginning of each of us as a unique individual. Although large, the zygote is just visible to the unaided eye as a tiny speck. It contains chromosomes and genes (units of genetic information) that are derived from the mother and father. The unicellular organism, known as a zygote, divides many times and becomes progressively transformed into a multicellular human being through cell division, migration, growth, and differentiation (Gilbert, 1991). Before describing the beginning of development, it is helpful to give brief outlines of gametogenesis and the male and female reproductive systems.

GAMETOGENESIS

Gametogenesis (*gamete or germ cell formation*) is the process of formation and development of specialized generative cells called **gametes** or germ cells. This process, involving the chromosomes and cytoplasm of the gametes, *prepares the sex cells for fertilization* (union of male and female gametes). During gametogenesis, the chromosome number is reduced by half and the shape of the cells is altered. The sperm (spermatozoon) and oocyte (ovum), the male and female gametes, are highly *specialized sex cells* (Fig. 2–1). They contain half the number of chromosomes (haploid number) present in somatic (body) cells. The number of chromosomes is reduced during **meiosis**, a special type of cell division that occurs during gametogenesis. This maturation process is called *spermatogenesis* in males and *oogenesis* in females (Fig. 2–2). The history of male and female gamete formation is different, but the sequence is the same. It is the timing of events during meiosis that differs in the two sexes.

Meiosis

This is a special type of cell division that takes place in germ cells only (Fig. 2–2). During gametogenesis, two meiotic divisions occur. The **first meiotic division** is often called the reduction division because the chromosome number is reduced from diploid (Gr. double) to haploid (Gr. single). *Homologous chromosomes*[2] (one from each parent) pair during prophase and then separate during anaphase, with one representative of each pair going to each pole. The X and Y chromosomes are not homologs but have homologous segments at the tips of their short arms. They pair in these regions only. By the end of the first meiotic division, each new cell formed (secondary spermatocyte or secondary oocyte) has the *haploid chromosome number*, i.e., half the number of chromosomes of the preceding cell (primary spermatocyte or primary oocyte). This separation or disjunction of

---

[1] Although development begins at conception (formation of the zygote), the stages and duration of pregnancy in clinical medicine are often calculated from the commencement of the mother's last normal menstrual period, which is about 14 days before conception.

[2] Homologous chromosomes (homologs) are pairs of chromosomes of one type, one inherited from each parent.

14

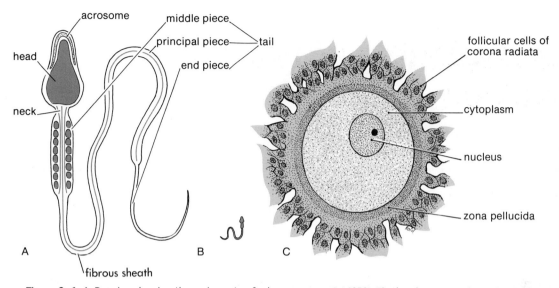

Figure 2–1. *A*, Drawing showing the main parts of a human sperm (× 1250). The head, composed mostly of the nucleus, is partly covered by the acrosome, an organelle containing enzymes that have an important role during fertilization (see Fig. 2–14). The sperm tail consists of three regions: the middle piece, principal piece, and end piece. The mitochondria in the middle piece are believed to generate the energy for sperm motility. *B*, A sperm drawn to about the same scale as the oocyte. Because sperms were regarded as parasites at one time, they were given the name spermatozoa ("semen animals"). *C*, Drawing of a human secondary oocyte (× 200) surrounded by the zona pellucida and the corona radiata. The corona radiata is composed of follicular cells that accompany the oocyte during ovulation.

paired homologous chromosomes is the *physical basis of segregation*, the separation of allelic genes during meiosis.

The **second meiotic division** follows the first division without a normal interphase; i.e., without an intervening step of DNA replication. Each chromosome (consisting of two parallel strands called chromatids) divides and each half, or *chromatid*, is drawn to a different pole; thus, the haploid number of chromosomes (23) is retained, and each daughter cell formed by meiosis has the reduced haploid number of chromosomes, with one representative of each chromosome pair. The second meiotic division is similar to an ordinary mitosis except that the chromosome number of the cell entering the second meiotic division is haploid. For more information about meiosis, see Thompson et al. (1991).

The Importance of Meiosis. The significance of meiosis is that it provides for *constancy of the chromosome number* from generation to generation by reducing the number from diploid to haploid, thereby producing haploid gametes (germ cells). Meiosis also allows random *assortment of maternal and paternal chromosomes* among the gametes. By relocating segments of the maternal and paternal chromosomes, *crossing over of chromosome segments* "shuffles"

the genes and thereby produces a recombination of genetic material. Disturbances of meiosis during gametogenesis, e.g., *nondisjunction* (Fig. 2–3), result in the formation of chromosomally abnormal gametes. If involved in fertilization, these cells with numerical chromosome abnormalities cause abnormal development such as occurs in the Down syndrome (see Chapter 8, Table 8–2).

Spermatogenesis

The term spermatogenesis refers to the entire sequence of events by which primitive germ cells called *spermatogonia* are transformed into spermatozoa, which are usually called sperms for brevity. This maturation process begins at puberty (13 to 16 years) and continues into old age. The **spermatogonia**, which have been dormant in the seminiferous tubules of the testes since the fetal period, begin to increase in number at puberty. After several mitotic divisions, the spermatogonia grow and undergo gradual changes that transform them into **primary spermatocytes** (Fig. 2–2), the largest germ cells in the seminiferous tubules of the testis (Moore, 1992).

Each primary spermatocyte subsequently undergoes a reduction division (called the first meiotic

NORMAL GAMETOGENESIS

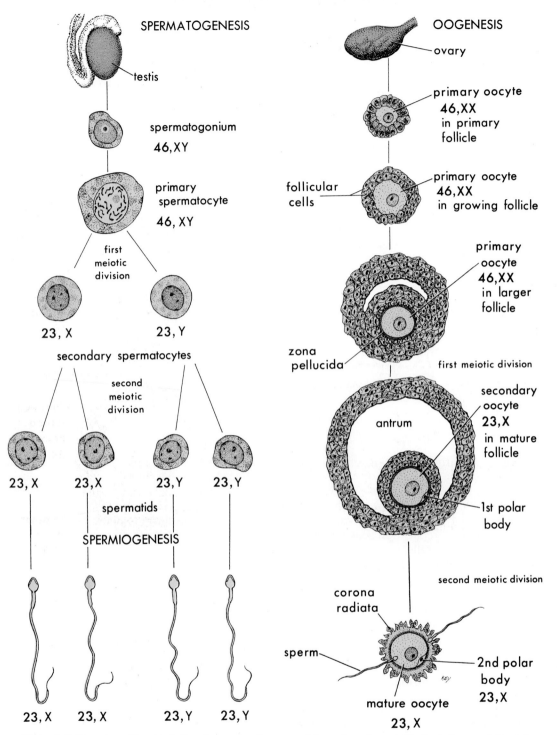

Figure 2-2. Normal gametogenesis. Drawings comparing spermatogenesis and oogenesis. Oogonia are not shown in this figure because all oogonia differentiate into primary oocytes before birth. The chromosome complement of the germ cells is shown at each stage. The number designates the total number of chromosomes including the sex chromosome(s) shown after the comma. Note that: (1) following the two meiotic divisions, the diploid number of chromosomes, 46, is reduced to the haploid number, 23; (2) four sperms form from one primary spermatocyte whereas only one mature oocyte results from maturation of a primary oocyte; and (3) the cytoplasm is conserved during oogenesis to form one large cell, the mature oocyte or ovum. The polar bodies are small, nonfunctional cells that eventually degenerate.

ABNORMAL GAMETOGENESIS

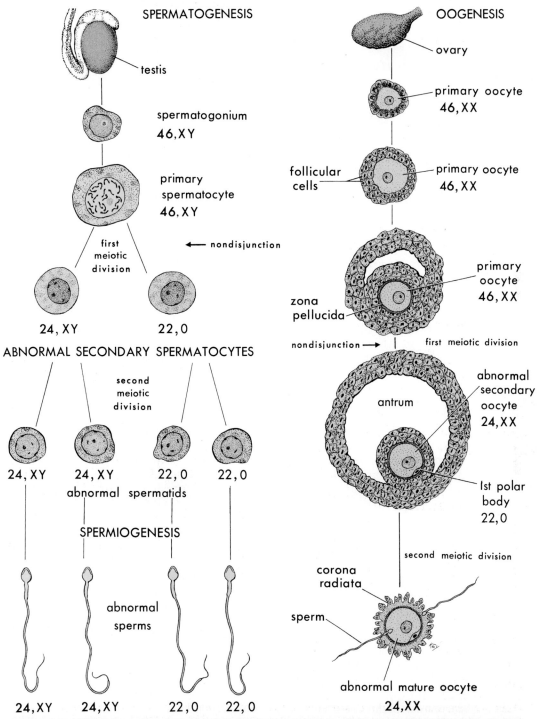

SPERMATOGENESIS

OOGENESIS

testis

ovary

spermatogonium
46,XY

primary oocyte
46,XX

primary spermatocyte
46,XY

follicular cells

primary oocyte
46,XX

first meiotic division

← nondisjunction

zona pellucida

primary oocyte
46,XX

24,XY

22,0

nondisjunction →

first meiotic division

ABNORMAL SECONDARY SPERMATOCYTES

second meiotic division

antrum

abnormal secondary oocyte
24,XX

24,XY

24,XY

22,0

22,0

abnormal spermatids

1st polar body
22,0

SPERMIOGENESIS

second meiotic division

corona radiata

abnormal sperms

sperm

24,XY

24,XY

22,0

22,0

abnormal mature oocyte
24,XX

Figure 2–3. Abnormal gametogenesis. Drawings showing how nondisjunction, an error in cell division, results in an abnormal chromosome distribution in germ cells. (Although nondisjunction of sex chromosomes is illustrated, a similar defect may occur during division of autosomes.) When nondisjunction occurs during the first meiotic division of spermatogenesis, one secondary spermatocyte contains 22 autosomes plus an X and a Y chromosome, and the other one contains 22 autosomes and no sex chromosome. Similarly, nondisjunction during oogenesis may give rise to an oocyte with 22 autosomes and two X chromosomes (as shown) or in one with 22 autosomes and no sex chromosomes.

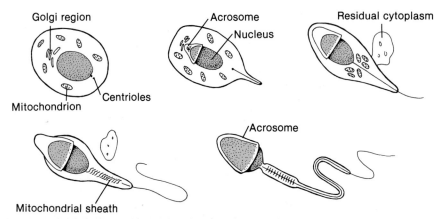

Figure 2–4. Drawings illustrating the last phase of spermatogenesis, known as *spermiogenesis*. During this process the rounded spermatids are transformed into elongated sperms (spermatozoa). Note the loss of cytoplasm, the development of the tail, and the formation of the acrosome. The acrosome, derived from the Golgi region of the spermatid, contains enzymes that are released at the beginning of the fertilization process and assist the sperm in penetrating the corona radiata and zona pellucida surrounding the secondary oocyte (see Fig. 2–14). The mitochondria arrange themselves end to end in the form of a tight helix, forming a collarlike mitochondrial sheath. Note that the excess cytoplasm is shed during spermiogenesis.

division) to form two haploid **secondary spermato-cytes** that are about half the size of primary spermato-cytes. Subsequently, these secondary spermatocytes undergo a *second meiotic division* to form four haploid **spermatids** that are about half the size of secondary spermatocytes. The spermatids are gradually transformed into four mature sperms by a differentiation process known as **spermiogenesis** (Fig. 2–4). The entire process of spermatogenesis, which includes spermiogenesis, takes about two months (60 to 64 days). The sperms are stored and become functionally mature in the *epididymis*, the first part of the duct of the testis.

The Mature Sperm (Figs. 2–1*A*, 2–4, and 2–13). This is a free-swimming, actively motile germ cell consisting of a *head* and a *tail*. The junction between the head and tail is called the *neck*. The head forms most of the bulk of the sperm and contains the *haploid nucleus*. The anterior two thirds of the nucleus is covered by the **acrosome** (acrosomal cap), a caplike organelle or saccule containing more than ten different enzymes, including hyaluronidase and acrosin. When released, these enzymes facilitate sperm penetration of the corona radiata and zona pellucida during fertilization (Fig. 2–14).

The *tail of the sperm* consists of three segments: the middle piece (midpiece), the principal piece, and the end piece. The tail provides the motility of the sperm, which assists in its transport to the site of fertilization. The middle piece contains mitochondria which provide the adenosine triphosphate (ATP) necessary for activity. The fibrous sheath is believed to promote the lashing movements of the tail (Cormack, 1987; Oura and Toshimori, 1990).

Oogenesis

The term oogenesis (ovogenesis) refers to the entire sequence of events by which primitive germ cells called **oogonia** are transformed into mature oocytes (ova). This maturation process begins before birth and is completed after sexual maturity has been reached during puberty (p. 6).

Prenatal Maturation of Oocytes. During early fetal life, oogonia proliferate by mitotic division. *All oogonia enlarge to form primary oocytes before birth*; for this reason, no oogonia are shown in Figures 2–2 and 2–3. As a **primary oocyte** forms, connective tissue cells (ovarian stromal cells) surround it and form a single layer of flattened, follicular, epithelial cells. The primary oocyte enclosed by this layer of cells constitutes a *primordial follicle* (Fig. 2–7*A*).

As the primary oocyte enlarges during puberty, the flattened, follicular, epithelial cells become cuboidal in shape and then columnar, forming a *primary follicle* (Fig. 2–2). The primary oocyte soon becomes surrounded by a covering of amorphous, acel-lular, glycoprotein material called the **zona pellucida** (Fig. 2–7*B*). Scanning electron microscopy of the surface of the zona pellucida reveals a regular meshlike appearance with intricate fenestrations, not unlike Swiss cheese. When the primary follicle has more than one layer of cuboidal follicular cells, it is called a growing or *secondary follicle*.

Primary oocytes begin the first meiotic division before birth, but completion of prophase does not occur until adolescence. The primary oocytes remain in suspended prophase (dictyotene) for several years until sexual maturity and the reproductive cycles begin during puberty. The follicular cells surrounding the primary oocyte are believed to secrete a substance called the *oocyte maturation inhibitor* (OMI) which keeps the meiotic process of the oocyte arrested (Scott and Hodgen, 1990).

Postnatal Maturation of Oocytes. Beginning during puberty, usually one follicle matures each month and ovulation occurs, except when oral contraceptives (birth control pills) are used. The long duration of the first meiotic division (up to 45 years) may account in part for the relatively high frequency of meiotic errors, such as *nondisjunction* (failure of paired chromatids to dissociate), that occur with increasing maternal age. The primary oocytes in suspended prophase I (dictyotene) are vulnerable to environmental agents (e.g., radiation). *No primary oocytes form after birth in females*, in contrast to the continuous production of primary spermatocytes in males after puberty.

As mentioned, the primary oocytes remain dormant in the ovarian follicles until puberty. As a follicle matures, the primary oocyte increases in size. Shortly before ovulation, the primary oocyte completes the first meiotic division. Unlike the corresponding stage of spermatogenesis, however, the division of cytoplasm is unequal. The **secondary oocyte** receives almost all the cytoplasm (Fig. 2–2), and the *first polar body* receives hardly any. The first polar body is a small, nonfunctional cell that soon degenerates. At ovulation, the nucleus of the secondary oocyte begins the second meiotic division but progresses only to metaphase, when division is arrested. If a sperm penetrates the secondary oocyte (Fig. 2–14), the second meiotic division is completed, and most cytoplasm is again retained by one cell, the oocyte (Fig. 2–2). The other cell, the *second polar body*, is a small, nonfunctional cell that soon degenerates. As soon as the second polar body is extruded, maturation of the oocyte is complete. The mature oocyte is commonly referred to as an **ovum**.

There are about two million primary oocytes in the ovaries of a newborn female infant but many regress during childhood, so that by adolescence, no more than 40 thousand remain. Of these, only about 400 become secondary oocytes and are expelled at ovulation (p. 23) during the reproductive period. Few, if any, of these oocytes become mature (Scott and Hodgen, 1990). The number of oocytes that ovulate is greatly reduced in women who take contraceptive pills because the hormones in them prevent ovulation from occurring.

Comparison of Male and Female Gametes

The sperm and secondary oocyte are dissimilar in several ways because of their adaptation for specialized roles in reproduction. The oocyte is a massive cell as compared with the sperm and is immotile (Fig. 2–1), whereas the microscopic sperm is highly motile. The oocyte is surrounded by the zona pellucida and a layer of follicular cells called the *corona radiata* (Fig. 2–1C). The oocyte also has an abundance of cytoplasm containing yolk granules, which provide nutrition (e.g., protein) to the dividing zygote during the first week of development.

The sperm bears little resemblance to an oocyte or any other cell because of its sparse cytoplasm and specialization for motility. With respect to sex chromosome constitution, there are *two kinds of normal sperm* (Fig. 2–2), 23, X and 23, Y, whereas there is only *one kind of normal ovum*, 23, X. In the foregoing descriptions, and in Figures 2–2 and 2–3, the numbers 23 and 46 indicate the total number of chromosomes in the complement, including the sex chromosomes. For example, the number 23 is followed by a comma and an X or Y to indicate the sex chromosome constitution; e.g., 23, X indicates that there are 23 chromosomes in the complement, made up of 22 autosomes and 1 sex chromosome (an X in this case). The difference in the sex chromosome complement of sperms forms *the basis of primary sex determination*.

Abnormal Gametes

The ideal maternal age for reproduction is generally considered to be from 18 to 35 years of age. The likelihood of chromosomal abnormalities in the embryo increases significantly after the mother is 35 years of age. In older mothers, there is an appreciable risk of Down syndrome or some other form of trisomy in the infant (see Chapter 8). The likelihood of a fresh *gene mutation* (change in DNA) also increases with age. The older the parents are at the time of conception, the more likely they are to have accumulated mutations that the embryo might inherit. For fathers of children with fresh mutations, such as the one causing *achondroplasia* (see Fig. 8–10), this age relationship has continually been demonstrated (Stoll et al., 1982). This relationship does not hold for all dominant mutations and is not an important consideration in older mothers. For a full discussion of gene mutations, see Thompson et al. (1991).

Numerical Chromosomal Abnormalities in Gametes. During meiosis, homologous chromosomes sometimes fail to separate and go to opposite poles of the germ cell. As a result of this error of cell division, known as *nondisjunction*, some gametes have 24 chromosomes and others have only 22 (Fig. 2–3). If a gamete with 24 chromosomes fuses with a normal one with 23 chromosomes during fertilization, a zygote with 47 chromosomes forms (see Fig. 8–1). This condition is called **trisomy** because of the presence of three representatives of a particular chromosome, instead of the usual two. If a gamete with only 22 chromosomes fuses with a normal one, a zygote with 45 chromosomes forms. This condition is known as *monosomy* because only one representative of the particular chromosome pair is present. For a description of the clinical conditions associated with numerical disorders of chromosomes, see Chapter 8 and Thompson et al. (1991).

Morphological Abnormalities of Gametes. Up to 10 per cent of the sperms in an ejaculate may be grossly abnormal (e.g., with two heads or tails), but it is generally believed that they do not fertilize oocytes due to lack of normal motility. Most, if not all, morphologically abnormal sperms are unable to pass through the mucus in the cervical canal. X-rays, severe allergic reactions, and certain antispermatogenic agents have been reported to increase the percentage of abnormally shaped sperms in man. Such sperms are not believed to affect fertility unless their number exceeds 20 per cent (Cormack, 1987).

Although some oocytes have two or three nuclei, these germ cells die before maturity. Similarly, some ovarian follicles contain two or more oocytes, but this phenomenon is infrequent. Although such compound follicles could result in multiple births, it is believed most of them never mature and expel the oocytes at ovulation.

STRUCTURE OF THE UTERUS

A brief description of the structure of the uterus is presented as a basis for understanding reproductive cycles and implantation of the blastocyst. The **uterus** (L., womb) is a thick-walled, pear-shaped organ that varies considerably in size (Fig. 2–5A). It averages 7 to 8 cm in length, 5 to 7 cm in width at its superior part, and 2 to 3 cm in thickness. The uterus consists of two main parts, the *body* and the *cervix*. The rounded superior part of the body is called the *fundus*. (For details about the clinical anatomy of the uterus, including illustrations, see Moore, 1992.)

The walls of the body of the uterus consist of three layers (Fig. 2–5A): (1) a very thin outer serosa or *perimetrium*; (2) a thick, smooth muscle layer or myometrium; and (3) a thin, inner layer or *endometrium*. The perimetrium is a peritoneal layer that is firmly attached to the myometrium. At the peak of its development, the **endometrium** is 4 to 5 mm thick. During the secretory phase of the menstrual cycle (Fig. 2–6), *three layers of the endometrium* can be distinguished (Fig. 2–5B): (1) a thin, superficial, *compact layer* consisting of densely packed, stromal cells

around the straight necks of the glands; (2) a thick *spongy layer* composed of edematous stroma containing the dilated, tortuous bodies of the glands; and (3) a thin *basal layer* containing the blind ends of the glands. The latter deep layer has its own blood supply and is not sloughed off during menstruation. The compact and spongy layers, known collectively as the *functional layer*, disintegrate and are shed at menstruation and after parturition (delivery of a baby).

The Uterine Tubes (Fig. 2–5A). The uterine tubes (fallopian tubes), 10 to 12 cm long and 1 cm in diameter, extend laterally from the *cornua* or horns of the uterus. The uterine tubes carry oocytes from the ovaries and sperms from the uterus to the fertilization site in the *ampulla of the uterine tube*. The uterine tube also conveys the dividing zygote to the uterine cavity. Each tube opens at its proximal end into the cornu or horn of the uterus and, at its distal end, into the peritoneal cavity near the ovary. For descriptive purposes, *the uterine tube is divided into four parts*: infundibulum, ampulla, isthmus, and uterine part (Moore, 1992).

FEMALE REPRODUCTIVE CYCLES

Commencing at puberty and normally continuing throughout the reproductive years, human females undergo monthly reproductive cycles (sexual cycles), involving activities of the hypothalamus of the brain, cerebral hypophysis (pituitary gland), ovaries, uterus, uterine tubes, vagina, and mammary glands. These cycles prepare the reproductive system for pregnancy. A *gonadotropin-releasing hormone* (GnRH) that is synthesized by neurosecretory cells in the hypothalamus is carried by the *hypophyseal portal system* to the anterior lobe of the cerebral hypophysis. **GnRH** controls the secretion of the two hormones produced by this gland which act on the ovaries. As will be described, *follicle stimulating hormone* (**FSH**) stimulates the development of ovarian follicles and *luteinizing hormone* (**LH**) serves as the "trigger" for ovulation (release of the secondary oocyte). These hormones also stimulate growth of the endometrium.

The Ovarian Cycle

The gonadotropins (FSH and LH) produce cyclic changes in the ovaries (development of follicles, ovulation, and formation of a corpus luteum) known as the ovarian cycle. During each cycle, FSH promotes growth of several primary follicles; however, usually only one of these develops into a mature follicle and

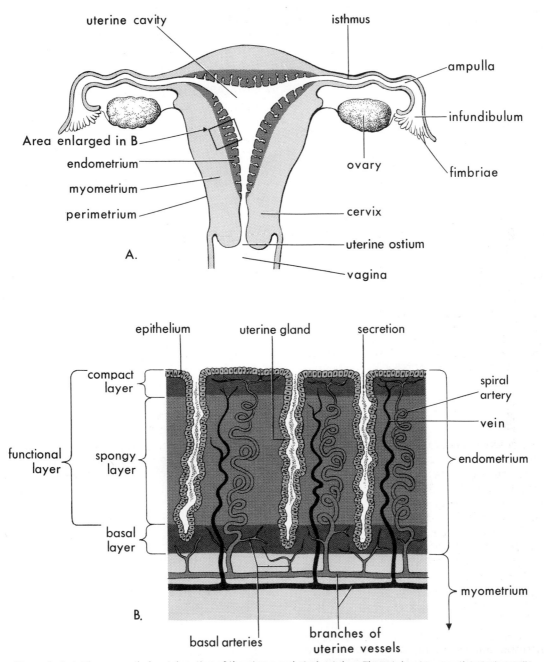

Figure 2–5. *A*, Diagrammatic frontal section of the uterus and uterine tubes. These tubes traverse the uterine wall and open onto its internal surface. The ovaries and vagina are also illustrated.*B*, Enlargement of the area outlined in *A*. The functional layer of the endometrium is sloughed off during menstruation (Fig. 2–6), the monthly endometrial shedding and discharge of bloody fluid (menses) from the uterus.

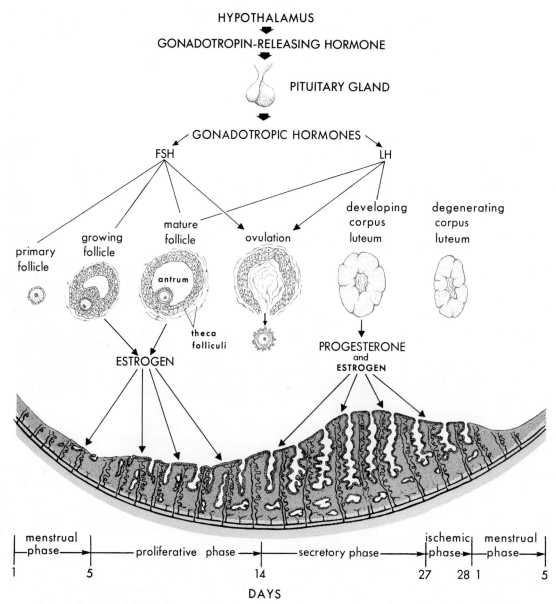

HYPOTHALAMUS

GONADOTROPIN-RELEASING HORMONE

PITUITARY GLAND

GONADOTROPIC HORMONES

FSH   LH

primary
follicle

growing
follicle

mature
follicle

antrum

theca
folliculi

ovulation

developing
corpus
luteum

degenerating
corpus
luteum

ESTROGEN

PROGESTERONE
and
ESTROGEN

menstrual
phase

proliferative   phase

secretory phase

ischemic
phase

menstrual
phase

1   5   14   27   28 1   5

DAYS

Figure 2–6. Schematic drawing illustrating the interrelations of the hypothalamus of the brain, cerebral hypophysis or pituitary gland, ovaries, and endometrium. One complete menstrual cycle and the beginning of another are shown. Changes in the ovaries, called the ovarian cycle, are promoted by the gonadotropic hormones (FSH and LH). Hormones from the ovaries (estrogens and progesterone) then promote changes in the structure and function of the endometrium, called the menstrual cycle. Thus, the cyclical activity of the ovary is intimately linked with changes in the uterus. The ovarian cycles are under the rhythmic endocrine control of the adenohypophysis of the pituitary gland, which in turn is controlled by gonadotropin-releasing hormone (GnRH) produced by neurosecretory cells in the hypothalamus of the brain.

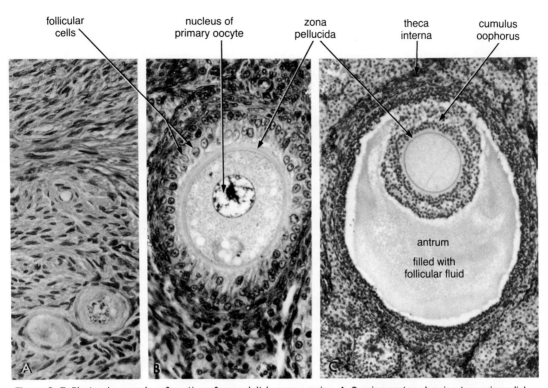

Figure 2–7. Photomicrographs of sections from adult human ovaries. *A,* Ovarian cortex showing two primordial follicles containing primary oocytes that have completed the prophase of the first meiotic division and have entered the dictyotene stage, a "resting" stage between prophase and metaphase (× 250). *B,* Growing follicle containing a primary oocyte, surrounded by the zona pellucida and a stratified layer of follicular cells (× 250). *C,* An almost mature follicle with a large antrum. The oocyte, embedded in the cumulus oophorus, does not show a nucleus because it has been sectioned tangentially (× 100). (From Lesson CR, Leeson TS, Paparo AA: *Text/Atlas of Histology.* Philadelphia, WB Saunders, 1988.)

ruptures through the surface of the ovary, expelling its oocyte (Figs. 2–9 to 2–11). Hence, several follicles degenerate each month.

Follicular Development. Development of an ovarian follicle is characterized by: (1) growth and differentiation of the primary oocyte, (2) proliferation of follicular cells, (3) formation of the zona pellucida, and (4) development of a connective tissue capsule, the *theca folliculi* (Gr. *theke,* box), from the ovarian stroma (Fig. 2–6). The follicular cells divide actively, producing a stratified layer around the oocyte (Fig. 2–7*B*). The ovarian follicle soon becomes oval and the oocyte eccentric in position because proliferation of the follicular cells occurs more rapidly on one side. Subsequently, fluid-filled spaces appear around the cells; these spaces soon coalesce to form a single large cavity, the *antrum,* containing follicular fluid (Fig. 2–7*C*). When the antrum forms, the ovarian follicle is called a vesicular or *secondary follicle.* The primary oocyte is pushed to one side of the follicle where it is surrounded by a mound of follicular cells, the *cumulus oophorus,* that projects into the antrum (Figs. 2–7 and 2–8). The follicle continues to enlarge until it reaches maturity and forms a bulge on the surface of the ovary. It is now called a *mature follicle* (graafian follicle).

The early development of ovarian follicles is induced by FSH but the final stages of maturation require LH as well. Growing follicles produce **estrogen,** a hormone that regulates development and function of the reproductive organs. The vascular *theca interna* produces the follicular fluid and some estrogen. Its cells also secrete *androgens* that pass to the follicular (granulosa) cells which convert them into estrogen (Cormack, 1987). Some estrogen is also produced by widely scattered groups of stromal secretory cells, known collectively as the *interstitial gland of the ovary.*

Ovulation (Figs. 2–6 and 2–9 to 2–11). Around midcycle (14 days in an "average" 28-day cycle),

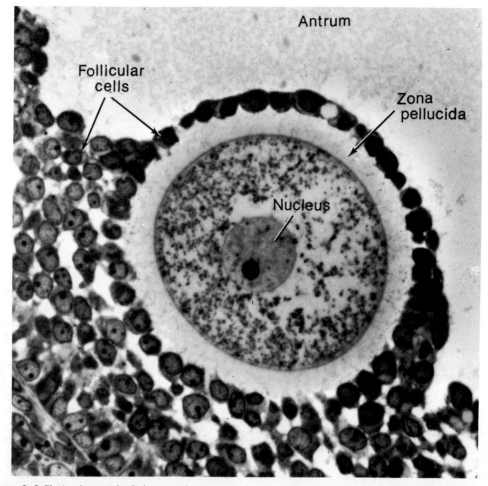

Figure 2–8. Photomicrograph of a human primary oocyte in a secondary follicle surrounded by follicular cells of the cumulus oophorus. The zona pellucida is a refractile, deeply staining layer of uniform thickness. It is a gellike, neutral glycoprotein that protects the oocyte. The follicular cells around the antrum form the membrana granulosa. (From Bloom W, Fawcett DW: *A Textbook of Histology*, 10th ed. Philadelphia, WB Saunders, 1975. Courtesy of L Zamboni.)

under the influence of FSH and LH, the ovarian follicle undergoes a sudden growth spurt, producing a cystic swelling or bulge on the surface of the ovary. A small, oval, avascular spot, the *stigma*, soon appears on this swelling (Fig. 2–9A). Prior to ovulation, the secondary oocyte and some cells of the cumulus oophorus detach from the interior of the distended follicle (Fig. 2–9B). The influence of LH during ovulation is much more important than FSH.

Ovulation is triggered by a surge of LH production (Fig. 2–12). Ovulation usually follows the LH peak by 12 to 24 hours. The **LH surge**, elicited by the high estrogen level in the blood, appears to cause the stigma to balloon out, forming a vesicle. The stigma then ruptures, expelling the secondary oocyte with the follicular fluid (Figs. 2–9D and 2–10). Expulsion of the oocyte is the result of intrafollicular pressure and

possibly by the contraction of smooth muscle in the theca externa due to stimulation by prostaglandins (Beck et al., 1985). The expelled secondary oocyte is surrounded by the zona pellucida and one or more layers of follicular cells, which quickly become radially arranged as the *corona radiata* and a cumulus layer (Figs. 2–1C and 2–9C), forming the oocyte-cumulus complex (Talbot, 1985). The LH surge also seems to induce resumption of the first meiotic division of the primary oocyte; hence, mature ovarian follicles contain secondary oocytes (Fig. 2–9A and B).

A variable amount of abdominal pain called *mittelschmerz* (Ger. *mittel*, mid + *schmerz*, pain), accompanies ovulation in some women. In these cases ovulation results in some bleeding into the peritoneal cavity, which results in sudden constant pain in the inferolateral part of the abdo-

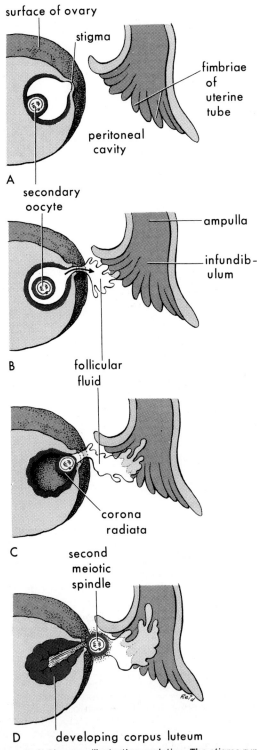

A

surface of ovary

stigma

fimbriae of uterine tube

peritoneal cavity

secondary oocyte

B

ampulla

infundib-ulum

follicular fluid

C

corona radiata

second meiotic spindle

D   developing corpus luteum

Figure 2–9. Diagrams illustrating ovulation. The stigma ruptures and the secondary oocyte is expelled with the follicular fluid.

men. Mittelschmerz may be used as a sign of ovulation, but there are better ones; e.g., the basal body temperature usually shows a slight drop followed by a sustained rise. Some women do not ovulate due to an inadequate release of gonadotropins; as a result, they are unable to become pregnant in the usual way. In some of these patients *ovulation can be induced* by the administration of gonadotropins or an ovulatory agent (clomiphene citrate). This drug stimulates the release of pituitary gonadotropins (FSH and LH) which usually results in maturation of several ovarian follicles and multiple ovulations. The incidence of multiple pregnancy increases up to tenfold when ovulation is induced. Apparently, the fine control of FSH output is not present in these cases and multiple ovulations occur, leading to multiple pregnancies and, often, spontaneous abortions.

The Corpus Luteum (Figs. 2–6, 2–9*D*, and 2–10). Shortly after ovulation, the walls of the follicle and the theca folliculi collapse and are thrown into folds. Under LH influence, they develop into a glandular structure known as the corpus luteum, which secretes mainly *progesterone*, but also produces some estrogen. These hormones, particularly progesterone, cause the endometrial glands to secrete and generally prepare the endometrium for blastocyst implantation (see Fig. 3–1). If the ovum is fertilized, the corpus luteum enlarges to form a *corpus luteum of pregnancy* and increases its hormone production. When pregnancy occurs, degeneration of the corpus luteum is prevented by *human chorionic gonadotropin* (hCG), a hormone secreted by the syncytiotrophoblast of the chorion, which is rich in LH (see Fig. 3–6).

The corpus luteum of pregnancy remains functionally active throughout the first 20 weeks of pregnancy. By this time the placenta has assumed the production of the estrogen and progesterone necessary for the maintenance of pregnancy (see Chapter 7). If the ovum is not fertilized, the corpus luteum begins to involute and degenerate about 10 to 12 days after ovulation. It is then called a *corpus luteum of menstruation*. The corpus luteum is subsequently transformed into white scar tissue called a *corpus albicans*.

The Menstrual Cycle

The hormones produced by the ovarian follicles and the corpus luteum (estrogen and progesterone) produce changes in the endometrium of the uterus (Fig. 2–6). These cyclic changes constitute the *endometrial cycle*, commonly referred to as the menstrual cycle or period because **menstruation** (a flow of blood from the uterus) is an obvious event. The normal endometrium is a mirror of the ovarian cycle because it responds in a consistent manner to the fluctuating concentrations of ovarian hormones. It is common to

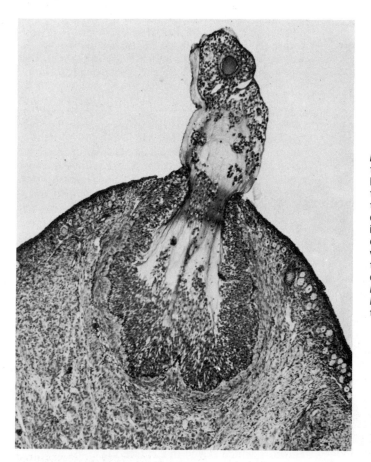

Figure 2-10. Photomicrograph of a section of an ovary taken just after rupture of an ovarian follicle during ovulation. The secondary oocyte, previously torn away from the cumulus oophorus (Fig. 2–9D), has been carried with the gelatinous follicular fluid out of the follicle and the ovary into the peritoneal cavity. The follicular cells adhering to the secondary oocyte constitute the corona radiata. Ovulation occurs through a small opening that develops when the stigma ruptures (Fig. 2–9B). Expulsion takes 1 to 2 seconds and is not an explosive process as once thought. (From Page EW, Villee CA, Villee DB: *Human Reproduction. Essentials of Reproductive and Perinatal Medicine*, 3rd ed. Philadelphia, WB Saunders, 1981. Courtesy of Dr Richard J Blandau.)

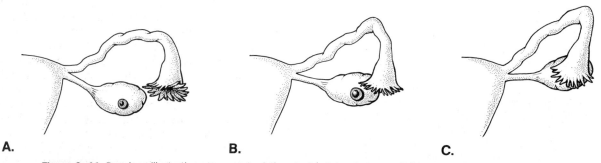

A.   B.   C.

Figure 2-11. Drawings illustrating movement of the uterine tube during ovulation. Note that the fimbriated infundibulum of the tube becomes closely applied to the ovary. Its fingerlike fimbriae move back and forth over the ovary and "sweep" the secondary oocyte into the infundibulum as soon as it is expelled from the ovarian follicle and ovary during ovulation (see Figs. 2–9 and 2–10).

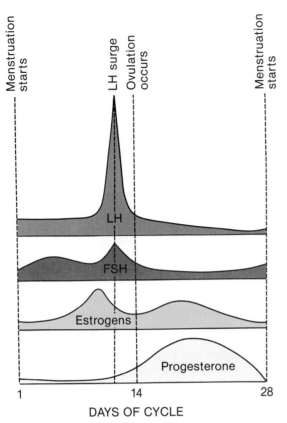

Figure 2–12. A diagram illustrating the blood levels of various hormones during the menstrual cycle (see Fig. 2–6). FSH stimulates the ovarian follicles to develop and produce estrogens. The level of estrogens rises to a peak just before the LH surge induces ovulation. Ovulation normally occurs 24 to 36 hours after the LH surge. If fertilization does not occur, the blood levels of circulating estrogens and progesterone fall. This hormone withdrawal causes the endometrium to regress and menstruation to start again.

describe "average" 28-day menstrual cycles, but they can vary in length by several days in normal women. In 90 per cent of healthy women, the length of the cycles ranges between 23 and 35 days. Almost all these variations result from alterations in the duration of the proliferative phase of the cycle.

The typical reproductive cycles illustrated in Figure 2–6 are not always realized because the ovary may not produce a mature follicle and ovulation does not occur. In *anovulatory cycles* the endometrial changes are minimal; the proliferative endometrium develops as usual, but because there is no ovulation and no corpus luteum formation, the endometrium does not progress to the secretory phase. It remains in the proliferative phase until menstruation begins. Anovulatory cycles may result from ovarian hypofunction but they are commonly produced by administering sex hormones. The estrogen, with or without progesterone, in *birth control pills* acts on the hypothalamus and cerebral hy-

pophysis, resulting in an inhibition of secretion of GnRH and gonadotropic hormones (FSH and LH) that are essential for ovulation to occur. Suppression of ovulation is the basis for the success of birth control pills. In most cases, when no other method of contraception is used, the interval between cessation of *oral contraception* and the occurrence of pregnancy is 12 months.

Phases of the Menstrual Cycle. The ovarian hormones cause cyclic changes in the structure of the reproductive tract, notably the endometrium. Although the menstrual cycle is divided into three phases for descriptive purposes (Fig. 2–6), it must be stressed that *the menstrual cycle is a continuous process*; each phase gradually passes into the next one.

The Menstrual Phase. The first day of menstruation is the beginning of the menstrual cycle. The functional layer of the uterine wall is sloughed off and discarded with the menstrual flow, which usually lasts four to five days. Menstrual flow consists of small amounts of blood combined with small pieces of endometrial tissue.

The Proliferative Phase. The proliferative (estrogenic, follicular) phase, lasting about nine days, coincides with the growth of ovarian follicles and is controlled by estrogen secreted by these follicles. There is a two- to threefold increase in the thickness of the endometrium during this phase of repair and proliferation. Early during this phase, the surface epithelium reforms and covers the endometrium. The glands increase in number and length and the spiral arteries elongate.

The Secretory Phase. The secretory (progestational or progravid) phase, lasting about 13 days, coincides with the formation, functioning, and growth of the corpus luteum. The progesterone produced by the corpus luteum stimulates the glandular epithelium to secrete a material rich in glycogen (hence the name, secretory phase). The glands become wide, tortuous, and saccular, and the endometrium thickens due to the influence of progesterone and estrogen from the corpus luteum and partly as a result of the increased fluid in the stroma. As the spiral arteries grow into the spongy and compact layers, they become increasingly coiled (Figs. 2–5*B* and 2–6). If the oocyte released at ovulation is fertilized, the blastocyst normally begins to implant in the endometrium on about the sixth day of the secretory phase (Fig. 2–18); i.e., on the twentieth day of a 28-day menstrual cycle (Fig. 2–6).

If fertilization does not occur, the secretory endometrium enters an *ischemic phase* during the last day of the secretory phase (Fig. 2–6). The ischemia (reduction in blood supply) gives the endometrium a pale appearance and occurs as the spiral arteries constrict intermittently. This arterial constriction results from the decreasing secretion of hormones, primarily progesterone, by the degenerating corpus luteum. In addition to vascular changes, the hormone withdrawal results in a stoppage of glandular secretion, a loss of interstitial fluid, and a marked shrinking of the endometrium. Toward the end of the ischemic phase, the spiral arteries become constricted for longer periods. Eventually, blood begins to seep through their ruptured walls into the surrounding connective tissue (stroma). Small pools of blood soon form and break through the endometrial surface, resulting in bleeding into the uterine lumen and the beginning of another menstrual phase and cycle.

As small pieces of the endometrium become detached and pass into the uterine cavity, the torn ends of the arteries bleed into the uterine cavity, resulting in a loss of 20 to 80 ml of blood. Eventually, over three to five days, the entire compact layer and most of the spongy layer of the endometrium are discarded in the *menses* (menstrual flow). The remnants of the spongy layer and the basal layer remain to undergo regeneration during the subsequent proliferative phase of the endometrium. Consequently, the cyclic hormonal activity of the ovary is intimately linked with cyclic histological changes in the endometrium (Fig. 2–6).

If pregnancy occurs, the menstrual cycles stop and the endometrium passes into a *pregnancy phase*. With the termination of pregnancy, the ovarian and menstrual cycles resume after a variable period (usually six to ten weeks if the woman is not breast-feeding her baby). If pregnancy does not occur, the reproductive cycles normally continue until the end of a woman's reproductive life, usually between the ages of 47 and 52.

TRANSPORTATION OF GAMETES

Oocyte Transport (Figs. 2–5*A*, 2–9, 2–10, and 2–11). At ovulation, the secondary oocyte is expelled from the ovarian follicle and the ovary with the escaping follicular fluid. During ovulation the fimbriated end of the uterine tube becomes closely applied to the ovary. The fingerlike *fimbriae* move back and forth over the ovary and "sweep" the secondary oocyte into the infundibulum of the uterine tube. The oocyte then passes into the ampulla of the tube mainly by gentle waves of peristalsis that pass down the tube toward the uterus. The nature of oocyte transport through the uterine tube is extremely complex and involves many factors that are poorly understood (Egarter, 1990; Beer, 1991).

Sperm Transport. From their storage site in the epididymis, and possibly in the ampulla of the ductus (vas) deferens, the sperms are transported to the urethra by peristaltic contractions of the thick muscular coat of the ductus deferens (Moore, 1992). From 200 to 600 million sperms are deposited on the cervix and in the fornix of the vagina during sexual intercourse (Figs. 2–5*A* and 2–13). The sperms pass by movements of their tails through the cervical canal. The enzyme *vesiculase*, produced by the seminal vesicles, coagulates some of the *semen* (fluid containing sperms) and forms a vaginal plug that may prevent the backflow of semen into the vagina. At the time of ovulation the cervical mucus increases in amount and becomes less viscid, making it more favorable for sperm transport.

Passage of sperms through the uterus and uterine tubes results mainly from muscular contractions of the walls of these organs. *Prostaglandins* in the semen are thought to stimulate uterine motility at the time of intercourse and assist in the movement of sperms through the uterus and uterine tubes to the site of fertilization in the ampulla of the tube. *Fructose* in the semen, secreted by the seminal vesicles, is an energy source for the sperms (see Barratt and Cooke, 1991 for details).

It is not known how long it takes sperms to reach the fertilization site, but the time of transport is probably short. Settlage and colleagues (1973) found a few motile sperms in the ampulla of the uterine tube five minutes after their deposition near the uterine ostium (external os), but some sperms took up to 45 minutes to complete the journey. Only about 200 sperms reach the fertilization site. Most sperms degenerate and are resorbed by the female genital tract.

Sperm Counts. During evaluation of male fertility, an analysis of the semen is made (Comhaire et al., 1992). The average volume of the ejaculate is about 3.5 ml, and the sperms account for less than 10 per cent of the semen or seminal fluid. The remainder of the ejaculate consists of the secretions of the accessory glands of the male reproductive tract, i.e., seminal vesicles (60 per cent), bulbourethral glands (10 per cent), and prostate (30 per cent). In normal males there are usually more than 100 million sperms per ml of semen. Although there is much variation in individual cases, men whose semen contains 20 million sperms per ml, or 50 million in the total specimen, are probably fertile. A man with less than 10 million sperms per ml of semen is likely to be sterile, especially when the specimen contains immotile and abnormal sperms. Thus, in assessing fertility potential, the total number and the motility of the sperms in the ejaculate are taken into consideration. Following deferentectomy or *vasectomy* (sterilization consisting of cutting and ligating each ductus deferens), there are no sperms in the ejaculate, but the amount of seminal fluid is the same.

Fertilization Site. The usual site of fertilization is the *ampulla of the uterine tube*, its longest and widest part (Figs. 2–5*A* and 2–9). If the oocyte is not fertilized here, it slowly passes along the tube to the uterus

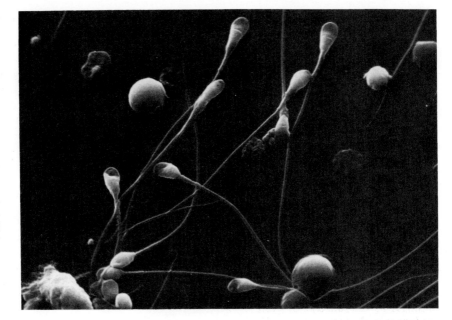

Figure 2–13. Scanning electron micrograph of several human sperms. Each of these male gametes consists of a head and a long tail. The head is formed principally by the nucleus, which contains the genetic traits transmitted by the male to the zygote during fertilization. The tail provides the motility that assists in the transport of the sperm to the fertilization site. (From Page EW, Villee CA, Villee DB: *Human Reproduction. Essentials of Reproductive and Perinatal Medicine,* 3rd ed. Philadelphia, WB Saunders, 1981. Courtesy of JE Flechon and ESE Hafez.)

where it degenerates and is resorbed. Although fertilization may occur in other parts of the uterine tube, it does not occur in the uterus.

VIABILITY OF GAMETES

Oocytes. Studies on early stages of development indicate that oocytes are usually fertilized within 12 hours after expulsion from the follicles at ovulation. In vitro observations have shown that the human secondary oocyte cannot be fertilized after 24 hours and that it degenerates shortly thereafter.

Sperms. Most sperms probably do not survive for more than 48 hours in the female genital tract. Some sperms are stored in folds of the mucosa of the cervix and are gradually released into the cervical canal and pass through the uterus into the uterine tubes. The short-term storage of sperms in the cervix provides a gradual release of sperms and thereby increases the chances of fertilization (Hafez, 1978). After being frozen to low temperatures, semen may be kept for many years (Sathananthan et al., 1987, 1988). Children have been born to women who have been artificially inseminated with semen that had been stored for several years.

MATURATION OF SPERMS

The Capacitation of Sperms. Freshly ejaculated sperms are unable to fertilize oocytes. They must undergo a *period of conditioning* lasting about seven hours during a process called capacitation. During this period a glycoprotein coat and seminal proteins are removed from the surface of the sperm's acrosome (Fig. 2–1A). Capacitated sperms show no morphological changes but they are more active (Wassarman, 1987). Sperms are usually capacitated in the uterus or uterine tubes by substances secreted by these parts of the female genital tract. During *in vitro fertilization* (p. 33), capacitation is induced by incubating the sperms in a defined media for several hours (Yanagimachi, 1981). Completion of capacitation permits the acrosome reaction to occur.

The Acrosome Reaction of Sperms. This reaction must be completed before the sperm can fuse with the ovum. When capacitated sperms come into contact with the corona radiata surrounding a secondary oocyte (Fig. 2–14A), they undergo changes that result in the development of perforations in the acrosome (Figs. 2–1A and 2–14B). Multiple point fusions of the plasma membrane of the sperm and the external acrosomal membrane occur. Breakdown of the membranes at these sites produces apertures. These changes, known as the acrosome reaction, are associated with the release of enzymes, including *hyaluronidase* and *acrosin,* from the acrosome that facilitate fertilization.

FERTILIZATION

The *pre-embryonic period* begins when an oocyte is fertilized. Fertilization is a sequence of events that

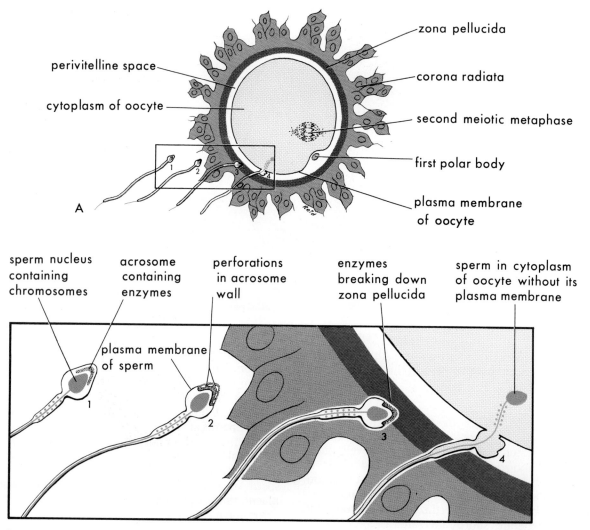

zona pellucida

perivitelline space

corona radiata

cytoplasm of oocyte

second meiotic metaphase

first polar body

plasma membrane
of oocyte

A

sperm nucleus
containing
chromosomes

acrosome
containing
enzymes

perforations
in acrosome
wall

enzymes
breaking down
zona pellucida

sperm in cytoplasm
of oocyte without its
plasma membrane

plasma membrane
of sperm

B

Figure 2–14. Diagrams illustrating the acrosome reaction and a sperm penetrating an oocyte during fertilization. The detail of the area outlined in *A* is given in *B*. 1, Sperm during capacitation, a period of conditioning that occurs in the female reproductive tract. 2, Sperm undergoing the acrosome reaction during which perforations form in the acrosome. 3, Sperm digesting a path through the zona pellucida by the action of enzymes released from the acrosome. 4, Sperm after entering the cytoplasm of the oocyte. Note that : (1) the plasma membranes of the sperm and oocyte have fused, and (2) the head and tail of the sperm have entered the oocyte, leaving the sperm's plasma membrane attached to the oocyte's plasma membrane.

begins with contact between a sperm and a secondary oocyte (Fig. 2–14*A*) and ends with the fusion of the nuclei of the sperm and ovum and the intermingling of maternal and paternal chromosomes (Fig. 2–15). Carbohydrate binding molecules on the surface of the gametes are possibly involved in the process of fertilization through gamete recognition and fusion of the cells (Boldt et al., 1989). The fertilization process lasts about 24 hours and occurs as follows (Figs. 2–14 and 2–15).

Phases of Fertilization

1. *Passage of the sperm through the corona radiata* (Figs. 2–14 and 2–15). The dispersal of the follicular cells of the corona radiata appears to result mainly from the action of the enzyme *hyaluronidase* released from the acrosome. Tubal mucosal enzymes also appear to assist this sperm enzyme. Movements of the tail of the sperm also help it to penetrate the corona radiata.

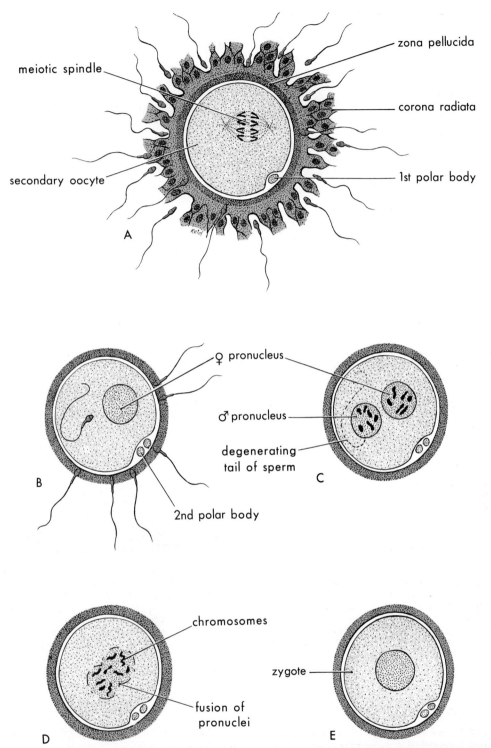

meiotic spindle

zona pellucida

corona radiata

secondary oocyte

1st polar body

A

♀ pronucleus

♂ pronucleus

degenerating
tail of sperm

B

C

2nd polar body

chromosomes

zygote

fusion of
pronuclei

D

E

Figure 2-15. Diagrams illustrating fertilization, the procession of events beginning when the sperm contacts the secondary oocyte's plasma membrane and ending with the intermingling of maternal and paternal chromosomes at metaphase of the first mitotic division of the zygote. *A*, Secondary oocyte surrounded by several sperms. (Only four of the 23 chromosome pairs are shown.) *B*, The corona radiata has disappeared; a sperm has entered the oocyte and the second meiotic division has occurred, forming a mature ovum. The nucleus of the ovum is now called the female pronucleus. *C*, The sperm head has enlarged to form the male pronucleus. *D*, The pronuclei are fusing. *E*, The zygote has formed. It contains 46 chromosomes, the diploid number of human chromosomes.

2. *Penetration of the zona pellucida by the sperm* (Figs. 2–14 and 2–15). The formation of a pathway through the zona pellucida also results from the action of enzymes released from the acrosome. The enzymes *acrosin* and *neuraminidase* appear to cause lysis of the zona pellucida, thereby forming a path for the sperm to follow to the oocyte. Once the first sperm passes through the zona pellucida, a *zona reaction* occurs in this amorphous layer that makes it impermeable to other sperms. This reaction is believed to result from the action of lysosomal enzymes released by cortical granules near the plasma membrane of the secondary oocyte. The contents of these granules, which are released into the perivitelline space (Fig. 2–14*A*), also cause changes in the plasma membrane of the oocyte that make it impermeable to sperms (Yanagimachi, 1981; Chen and Sathananthan, 1986; Wassarman, 1987).

Although several sperms may begin to penetrate the zona pellucida, usually only one sperm enters the ovum and fertilizes it. Two sperms may participate in fertilization during an abnormal process known as *dispermy*. The resulting triploid embryos (69 chromosomes) may appear quite normal, but they nearly always abort. A few triploid infants have been born but all died shortly after birth (Carr, 1971).

3. *Fusion of the oocyte and sperm cell membranes.* The plasma membranes of the oocyte and sperm fuse and soon break down at the area of fusion. The head and tail of the sperm enter the cytoplasm of the oocyte, but the sperm's plasma membrane remains behind (Fig. 2–14*B*).

4. *Completion of the second meiotic division of the secondary oocyte.* After entry of the sperm, the secondary oocyte completes its second meiotic division, forming a mature oocyte (ovum) and a second polar body (Fig. 2–15*B*). The nucleus of the mature oocyte is known as the **female pronucleus**.

5. *Formation of the male pronucleus.* Within the cytoplasm of the oocyte the nucleus in the head of the sperm enlarges to form the **male pronucleus**. During this process the tail of the sperm degenerates (Fig. 2–15*C*). Morphologically, the male and female pronuclei are indistinguishable. During growth of the pronuclei, they replicate their DNA.

6. *The male and female pronuclei contact each other,* lose their nuclear membranes, and fuse to form a new cell called the **zygote** (Fig. 2–15*D* and *E*). Fertilization is completed within 24 hours of ovulation. Within 24–48 hours after fertilization an immunosuppressant protein, known as the *early pregnancy factor* (EPF), appears in the maternal serum. EPF forms the basis of pregnancy tests during the first week of development (Nahhas and Barnea, 1990).

The Results of Fertilization

Restoration of the Diploid Chromosome Number. Fusion of the two haploid gametes produces a zygote, a diploid cell with 46 chromosomes, the usual number in human somatic cells. The zygote is the beginning or primordium of a new human being.

Species Variation. Because half the chromosomes in the zygote come from the mother and half from the father, the zygote contains a new combination of chromosomes different from that in the cells of either parent. This mechanism forms the basis of *biparental inheritance* and variation of the human species. Meiosis allows independent assortment of maternal and paternal chromosomes among the germ cells. *Crossing over of chromosomes*, by relocating segments of the maternal and paternal chromosomes, "shuffles" the genes, thereby producing a recombination of genetic material.

Primary Sex Determination. The embryo's chromosomal sex is determined at fertilization by the kind of sperm (X or Y) that fertilizes the ovum; hence, it is the father rather than the mother whose gamete determines the sex of the embryo. Fertilization by an X-bearing sperm produces an XX zygote which normally develops into a female, whereas fertilization by a Y-sperm produces an XY zygote which normally develops into a male.

Preselection of the Sex of the Embryo. Because the sex of the embryo is determined by whether the sperm contributes an X or a Y chromosome to the zygote and because X and Y sperms are formed in equal numbers, the expectation is that the sex ratio at fertilization (*primary sex ratio*) would be 1.00 (100 boys per 100 girls). It is well known, however, that there are more male babies than female babies born in all countries. In North America, for example, the sex ratio at birth (*secondary sex ratio*) is about 1.05 (105 boys per 100 girls).

Various in vitro techniques have been developed in an attempt to separate X and Y sperms using: (1) the differential swimming abilities of the two types of sperm, (2) different speeds of migration in an electric field, and (3) microscopic differences in the X and Y sperms. The use of a selected sperm sample in artificial insemination may produce the desired sex. Others claim that the timing and management of sexual intercourse can enable a couple to choose the sex of their child. A study of 3,668 births, for example, found that the proportion of male births was higher when sexual intercourse occurred two or more days after ovulation than when it occurred at or near ovulation (Harlap, 1979); however, no method of controlling the human embryo's sex has been shown to change the sex ratio consistently.

Initiation of Cleavage of the Zygote. Fertilization activates the zygote and initiates development by stimulating the zygote to undergo a series of rapid mitotic divisions called cleavage. An unfertilized oocyte degenerates about 24 hours after fertilization. Cleavage of an unfertilized ovum may occur through a process known as *parthenogenesis*; this may occur naturally or be artificially induced. Parthenogenesis is a normal event in some species; for example, some eggs laid by a queen bee are not fertilized but develop parthenogenetically. In a few other species (e.g., rabbits), an unfertilized ovum can be induced experimentally to undergo parthenogenetic development. *No verified case of parthenogenesis has occurred in humans*, but an embryo could develop by fusion of a secondary oocyte with the second polar body. These embryos, however, would not likely survive because they would probably contain lethal genes that would result in their death and early abortion.

In Vitro Fertilization (IVF) and "Embryo" Transfer

Fertilization of secondary oocytes in vitro (L., in glass) and transfer of the dividing zygotes ("cleaved embryos") into the uterus have provided an opportunity for many sterile women (e.g., due to tubal occlusion) to bear children (Steinkampf et al., 1992). The first of these IVF babies was born in 1978. Since then, many thousand pregnancies have occurred using this technique and its modifications, especially *gamete intrafallopian transfer* (Steptoe and Edwards, 1978; Edwards, 1990). The steps involved during in vitro fertilization and "embryo" transfer are as follows:

1. Ovarian follicles are stimulated to grow and mature by the administration of gonadotropins to the patient.

2. Several secondary oocytes are aspirated from mature ovarian follicles (Fig. 2-11*B*). This process is performed during *laparoscopy* (viewing the contents of the abdominal cavity with a laparoscope) just prior to ovulation.

3. The oocytes are placed in a test tube or Petri dish containing a special culture medium.

4. Sperms are added almost immediately (Chen and Sathananthan, 1986).

5. Fertilization of the oocytes and cleavage of the zygotes are monitored microscopically (Fig. 2-17).

6. Dividing zygotes ("cleaved embryos") during the four- to eight-cell stage (Figs. 2-16*B* and *C* and 2-17) are transferred to the uterus via the cervical canal. The probability of a successful pregnancy is enhanced by implanting two or three dividing zygotes. Obviously, the chances of multiple pregnancies are higher than when pregnancy results from normal ovulation and passage of the morula into the uterus via the uterine tube. The incidence of spontaneous abortion of transferred embryos is also higher than normal (Ben-Rafael et al., 1988). Preimplantation zygotes and blastocysts resulting from in vitro fertilization can be preserved for long periods by freezing them with a cryoprotectant solution such as glycerol or 1,2-propanediol (*cryopreservation*). Successful transfer of dividing zygotes ("cleaved embryos") and blastocysts to the uterus after thawing is now a common practice (Fugger et al., 1991; Hartshorne et al., 1991).

Assisted In Vivo Fertilization

A technique enabling fertilization to occur in the uterine (fallopian) tube is called *gamete intrafallopian transfer* (GIFT). It involves superovulation (similar to that used for IVF), oocyte retrieval, sperm collection, and laparoscopic placement of several oocytes and many sperms into the uterine tubes. Using this technique, fertilization occurs in the ampulla, its usual location. For a description of GIFT and other assisted in vivo techniques, see Dooley et al. (1988) and Edwards (1990).

CLEAVAGE OF THE ZYGOTE

Cleavage consists of repeated mitotic divisions of the zygote, resulting in a rapid increase in the number of cells (Fig. 2-16). First, the zygote divides into two cells known as **blastomeres**; these cells then divide into four blastomeres, eight blastomeres, and so on. Cleavage normally occurs as the zygote passes along the uterine tube toward the uterus (see Fig. 2-20). The zygote is still contained within the jellylike, rather thick zona pellucida; hence, an increase in cells occurs without an increase in the cytoplasmic mass. Division of the zygote into blastomeres begins about 30 hours after fertilization. Subsequent divisions follow one another, forming progressively smaller blastomeres (Fig. 2-16*D*). The blastomeres change their shape and tightly align themselves against each other to form a compact ball of cells known as the morula. This phenomenon, known as **compaction**, is probably mediated by cell surface adhesion glycoproteins (Gilbert, 1991). Compaction permits greater cell-to-cell interaction and is a prerequisite for segregation of the internal cells that form the embryoblast or inner cell mass of the blastocyst (Fig. 2-16). The spherical **morula** (L. *morus*, mulberry), a solid ball of 12 or more blastomeres, forms about three days after fertilization and enters the uterus. It was given its name because of its resemblance to the fruit of the mulberry tree.

If *nondisjunction* (failure of two members of a chromosome pair to dissociate during cell division) occurs during early cleavage division of a zygote, an embryo with two or more cell lines with different chromosome complements is produced. Such individuals in whom numerical mosaicism is present are termed *mosaics*; for example, a zygote with an additional chromosome 21 might lose the extra chromosome during an early division of the zygote into blastomeres. Consequently, some cells of the embryo would have a normal chromosome complement and others would have an additional chromosome 21. In general, individuals who are mosaic for a given trisomy, such as *mosaic Down syndrome*, are less severely affected than those with the usual nonmosaic condition (Thompson et al, 1991).

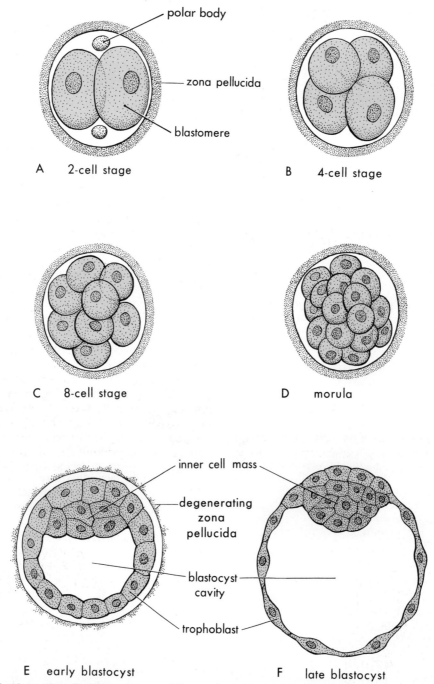

Figure 2-16. Drawings illustrating cleavage of the zygote and formation of the blastocyst. *A to D* show various stages of cleavage. Compaction of the blastomeres results in the formation of a morula. The period of the morula begins at the 12- to 16-cell stage and ends when the blastocyst forms, which occurs when there are 50 to 60 blastomeres present. *E and F* are sections of blastocysts. The zona pellucida has disappeared by the late blastocyst stage (five days). The polar bodies shown in *A* are small, nonfunctional cells that soon degenerate. Cleavage of the zygote and formation of the morula occur as the dividing zygote passes along the uterine tube (Fig. 2-20). Blastocyst formation normally occurs in the uterus. Although cleavage increases the number of cells, called blastomeres, the daughter cells become smaller than the parent cells. As a result, there is no increase in the size of the blastocyst until the zona pellucida degenerates. The blastocyst then enlarges considerably. The inner cell mass, or embryoblast, gives rise to the tissues and organs of the embryo.

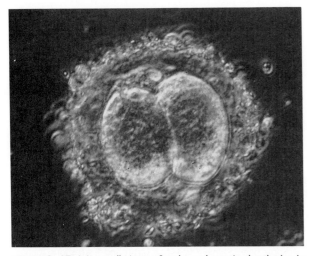

Figure 2-17. A two-cell stage of a cleaved zygote developing in vitro. Observe that it is surrounded by many sperms. The dividing zygote is observed until the eight-cell stage and it is then placed in the uterus. To increase the chances of pregnancy, three or four cleaved zygotes are inserted. (Courtesy of Dr. Maria T. Zenzes and Dr. Peng Wang, In Vitro Fertilization Program, Toronto Hospital, Toronto, Ontario, Canada.)

FORMATION OF THE BLASTOCYST

Shortly after the morula enters the uterus (about four days after fertilization), spaces appear between the central blastomeres of the morula. Fluid soon passes through the zona pellucida into these spaces from the uterine cavity. As the fluid increases, it separates the blastomeres into two parts: (1) a thin outer cell layer (or "mass") called the **trophoblast** (Gr. *trophe*, nutrition) which gives rise to part of the placenta, and (2) a group of centrally located blastomeres, known as the inner cell mass (or **embryoblast**), which gives rise to the embryo.

The fluid-filled spaces within the blastocyst soon fuse to form a single, large *blastocyst cavity* (Figs. 2-16 and 2-18). At this stage of development, the conceptus is called a **blastocyst** (blastula). The inner cell mass (or embryoblast) now projects into the blastocyst cavity and the trophoblast forms the wall of the blastocyst. After the blastocyst has floated in the uterine secretions for about two days, the zona pellucida gradually degenerates and disappears (Figs. 2-16E and 2-18A). This permits the blastocyst to increase rapidly in size. While floating freely in the uterus, it derives its nourishment from the secretions of the uterine glands.

About six days after fertilization (about day 20 of a 28-day menstrual cycle), the blastocyst attaches to the endometrial epithelium, usually adjacent to the inner cell mass that represents the *embryonic pole* (Fig. 2-19A). As soon as it attaches to this epithelium, the trophoblast starts proliferating rapidly. It gradually differentiates into two layers: (1) an inner *cytotrophoblast* (cellular trophoblast), and (2) an outer *syncytiotrophoblast* (syncytial trophoblast) consisting of a multinucleated protoplasmic mass in which no cell boundaries can be observed (Fig. 2-19B). Both in

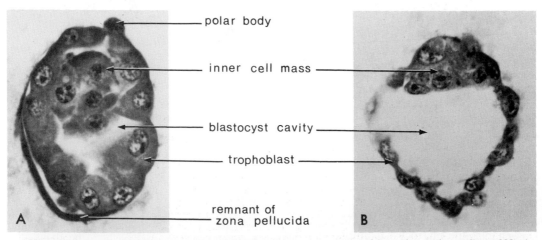

polar body

inner cell mass

blastocyst cavity

trophoblast

remnant of zona pellucida

A   B

Figure 2-18. Photomicrographs of sections of human blastocysts recovered from the uterine cavity (× 600). *A,* Four days: the blastocyst cavity is just beginning to form and the zona pellucida is deficient over part of the blastocyst. *B,* Four and a half days: the blastocyst cavity has enlarged and the inner cell mass and trophoblast are clearly defined. The zona pellucida has disappeared. (From Hertig AT, Rock, J, Adams EC: *Am J Anat 98*:435, copyright © 1956. Reprinted by permission of Wiley-Liss, a division of John Wiley & Sons, Inc. Courtesy of Carnegie Institution of Washington.)

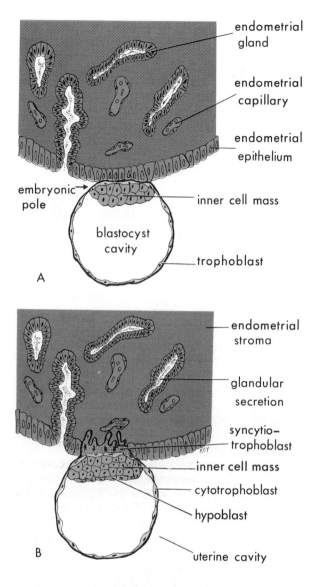

endometrial gland

endometrial capillary

endometrial epithelium

embryonic pole

inner cell mass

blastocyst cavity

trophoblast

A

endometrial stroma

glandular secretion

syncytio-trophoblast

inner cell mass

cytotrophoblast

hypoblast

B

uterine cavity

Figure 2–19. Drawings of sections illustrating the attachment of the blastocyst to the endometrial epithelium and the early stages of its implantation. *A*, Six days: the trophoblast is attached to the endometrial epithelium at the embryonic pole of the blastocyst. *B*, Seven days: the syncytiotrophoblast has penetrated the epithelium and has started to invade the endometrial stroma (connective tissue). Some people have difficulty interpreting illustrations such as these because, in histological studies, it is conventional to draw the endometrial epithelium upward; whereas, in embryological studies, the embryo is usually shown with its dorsal surface upward. Because the embryo implants on its future dorsal surface, it would appear upside-down if the histological convention were followed. In this book, the histological convention is followed when the endometrium is the dominant consideration (e.g., Fig. 2–5*B*), and the embryological convention is used when the developing embryo is the center of interest, as in these illustrations.

intrinsic and extracellular matrix factors modulate, in carefully timed sequences, the differentiation of the trophoblast (Aplin, 1991).

The fingerlike processes of the syncytiotrophoblast extend through the endometrial epithelium and invade the endometrial connective tissue (stroma). By the end of the first week, the blastocyst is superficially implanted in the compact layer of the endometrium and is deriving its nourishment from the eroded maternal tissues (Fig. 2–19*B*). The syncytiotrophoblast produces the substances that erode the maternal tissues. This enables the blastocyst to implant in the endometrium. *At about seven days*, a flattened layer of cells called the *hypoblast* (primitive endoderm) appears on the surface of the inner cell mass facing the blastocyst cavity (Fig. 2–19*B*).

Abnormal Zygotes, Blastocysts, and Spontaneous Abortion

At least 15 per cent of zygotes die and blastocysts abort. Early implantation of the blastocyst is a critical period of development that may fail to occur due to inadequate production of progesterone and estrogen by the corpus luteum (Fig. 2–6). Another 30 per cent of women abort very early, unaware that they were pregnant. Clinicians occasionally see a patient who states that her last menstrual period was delayed by several days and her last menstrual flow was unusually profuse. Very likely such patients have had an early spontaneous abortion; thus, the overall *early spontaneous abortion rate* is thought to be about 45 per cent (Rubin and Farber, 1988).

Preimplantation Diagnosis of Genetic Disorders. Using currently available techniques of micromanipulation and DNA amplification, a dividing zygote known to be at risk

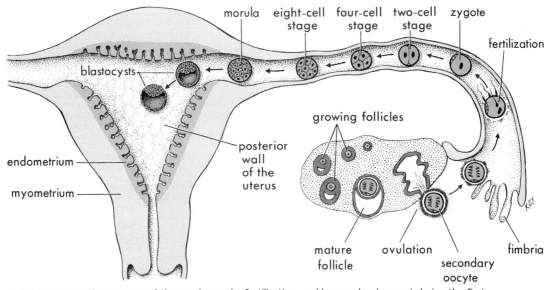

Figure 2–20. Diagrammatic summary of the ovarian cycle, fertilization, and human development during the first week. Stage 1 of development begins with fertilization and ends when the zygote forms. Stage 2 (days two to three) comprises the early stages of cleavage (from 2 to about 16 cells or the morula). Stage 3 (days four to five) consists of the free, unattached blastocyst. Stage 4 (days five to six) is represented by the blastocyst attaching to the posterior wall of the uterus, a common site of implantation. The blastocysts have been sectioned to show their structure.

for a specific genetic disorder could theoretically be diagnosed before implantation (Thompson et al., 1991). An application of this technology has already been made. Sex can be determined from one blastomere taken from a six- to eight-cell dividing zygote and analyzed by DNA amplification of sequences from the Y chromosome. This procedure has been used to detect female embryos during IVF in cases in which a male embryo would be at risk for a serious X-linked disorder (Handyside et al., 1990).

Early spontaneous abortions occur for a variety of reasons, one being the presence of chromosomal abnormalities in the zygote. Carr and Gedeon (1977) estimated that about half of all known spontaneous abortions occur because of chromosomal abnormalities. Hertig and associates (1959), while examining blastocysts recovered from early pregnancies, found several clearly defective dividing zygotes ("cleaved embryos") and blastocysts. Some were so abnormal survival would not have been likely. The early loss of embryos, once called *pregnancy wastage*, appears to represent a disposal of abnormal conceptuses that could not have developed normally, i.e., a natural screening of embryos. Without this "screening," about 12 per cent instead of 2 to 3 per cent of newborn infants would likely be congenitally malformed (Warkany, 1981).

SUMMARY OF THE FIRST WEEK OF HUMAN DEVELOPMENT

The pre-embryonic period of human development begins at fertilization, but several important events

have to happen before this process can take place (e.g., gametogenesis). Oocytes are produced by the ovary (*oogenesis*) and are expelled from it during *ovulation*. The fimbriae of the uterine tube sweep the oocyte into the ampulla where it may be fertilized.

Sperms are produced in the seminiferous tubules of the testes (*spermatogenesis*) and are stored in the epididymis. Ejaculation of semen during sexual intercourse results in the deposit of millions of sperms in the vagina around the uterine ostium. Several hundred sperms pass through the uterus and enter the uterine tubes. Many of them surround a secondary oocyte if it is present. When a secondary oocyte is contacted by a sperm, it completes the second meiotic division. As a result, a mature oocyte or ovum and a second polar body are formed. The nucleus of the mature ovum constitutes the *female pronucleus*.

After the sperm enters the ovum's cytoplasm, the head of the sperm separates from the tail and enlarges to become the *male pronucleus*. Fertilization is complete when the pronuclei fuse and the maternal and paternal chromosomes intermingle during metaphase of the first mitotic division of the **zygote**, the cell that gives rise to a human being. As it passes along the uterine tube, the zygote undergoes **cleavage** (a series of mitotic divisions) into a number of smaller cells called *blastomeres* (Fig. 2–20). About three days after fertilization, a ball of 12 or more blastomeres, called a *morula*, enters the uterus.

A cavity soon forms in the morula, converting it into a **blastocyst** consisting of: (1) an *inner cell mass or embryoblast*, which gives rise to the embryo, (2) a *blastocyst cavity*, and (3) a thin outer layer of cells, the **trophoblast**. The trophoblast encloses the inner cell mass and blastocyst cavity and later forms the embryonic part of the placenta. Four to five days after fertilization, the zona pellucida disappears and the blastocyst attaches to the endometrial epithelium. The syncytiotrophoblastic cells then invade the endometrial epithelium and underlying endometrial stroma. Concurrently, the *hypoblast* begins to form on the deep surface of the inner cell mass. By the end of the first week, the blastocyst is superficially implanted in the endometrium.

CLINICALLY ORIENTED QUESTIONS FOR PROBLEM-BASED LEARNING SESSIONS

1. What is the main cause of numerical aberrations of chromosomes? Define this process. What is the usual result of this abnormal chromosomal mechanism?
2. During in vitro cleavage of a zygote, all blastomeres of a morula were found to have an extra set of chromosomes. Explain how this could happen. Can such a morula develop into a viable fetus?
3. In infertile couples, the inability to conceive is attributable to some factor in the woman or the man. What is a major cause of (a) female infertility and (b) male infertility?
4. Some people have a mixture of cells with 46 and 47 chromosomes (e.g., some Down syndrome patients are *mosaics*). How do mosaics form? Would children with mosaic Down syndrome have the same stigmata as other infants with this condition? At what stage of development does mosaicism develop? Can this chromosomal abnormality be diagnosed before birth?
5. A young woman who feared that she might be pregnant asked about the so-called "morning after pills" (*postcoital birth control pills*). What would you tell her? Would termination of such an early pregnancy be considered an abortion?

The answers to these questions are given on page 458.

References and Suggested Reading

Aplin JD: Implantation, trophoblast differentiation and hemochorial placentation: mechanistic evidence *in vivo* and *in vitro*. *J Cell Sci* 99:681, 1991.

Austin CR: Membrane fusion events in fertilization. *J Reprod Fertil* 44:155, 1975.

Barratt CLR, Cooke ID: Sperm transport in the human female reproductive tract–a dynamic interaction. *Int J Androl* 14:394, 1991.

Beatty RA: *Parthenogenesis and Polyploidy in Mammalian Development*. Cambridge, Cambridge University Press, 1957.

Beck F, Moffat DB, Davies DP: *Human Embryology*, 2nd ed. Oxford, Blackwell Scientific Publications, 1985.

Beer E: Egg transport through the oviduct. *Am J Obstet Gynecol* 165:483, 1991.

Ben-Rafael Z, Fateh M, Flickinger GL, Tureck R, Blasco L, Mastroianni Jr, L: Incidence of abortion in pregnancies after *in vitro* fertilization and embryo transfer. *Obstet Gynecol* 71:297, 1988.

Biggers JD: New observations on the nutrition of the mammalian oocyte and the preimplantation embryo. *In* Blandau RJ (ed): *The Biology of the Blastocyst*. Chicago, University of Chicago Press, 1971.

Boldt J, Howe AM, Parkerson JB, Gunter LE, Kuehn E: Carbohydrate involvement in sperm-egg fusion in mice. *Biol Reprod* 40:887, 1989.

Brackett BG, Seitz HM, Rocha G, Mastroianni L: The mammalian fertilization process. *In* Moghissi KS and Hafez ESE (eds): *Biology of Mammalian Fertilization and Implantation*. Springfield, Charles C Thomas, 1972, pp 165–184.

Carr DH: Chromosome studies on selected spontaneous abortions: Polyploidy in man. *J Med Genet* 8:164, 1971.

Carr DH, Gedeon M: Population cytogenetics of human abortuses. *In* Hook EB, Porter IH (eds): *Population Cytogenetics: Studies in Humans*. New York, Academic Press, 1977.

Chandley AC: Meiosis in man. *Trends Genet* 4:79–83, 1988.

Chapman MG, Grudzinskas JG, Chard T (eds): *Implantation. Biological and Clinical Aspects*. Berlin, Springer Verlag, 1988.

Chen CM, Sathananthan AH: Early penetration of human sperm through the vestments of human egg *in vitro*. *Arch Androl* 16:183, 1986.

Clermont Y, Trott M: Kinetics of spermatogenesis in mammals: Seminiferous epithelium cycle and spermatogonial renewal. *Physiol Rev* 52:198, 1972.

Comhaire FH, Huysse S, Hinting A, Vermeulen L, Schoonjans F: Objective semen analysis: has the target been reached? *Human Reprod* 7:237, 1992.

Cormack DH: *Ham's Histology*, 9th ed. Philadelphia, JB Lippincott, 1987.

Cumming DC, Cumming CE, Kieren DK: Menstrual mythology and sources of information about menstruation. *Am J Obstet Gynecol* 164:472, 1991.

Dooley M, Lim-Howe D, Savros M, Studd JWW: Early experience with gamete intrafallopian transfer (GIFT) and direct intraperitoneal insemination (DIPT). *J Royal Soc Med 81*:637, 1988.

Edwards RG: Fertilization of human eggs in vitro: Morals, ethics, and the law. *Q Rev Biol 49*:3, 1974.

Edwards RG: A decade of *in vitro* fertilization. *Research in Reprod 22*:1, 1990.

Edwards RG, Steptoe PC: Current status of *in vitro* fertilization and implantation of human embryos. *Lancet 2*:1265, 1983.

Egarter C: The complex nature of egg transport through the oviduct. *Am J Obstet Gynecol 163*:687, 1990.

Elstein M: Cervix and cervical barrier. *In* Ludwig H, Tauber PF (eds): *Human Fertilization.* Stuttgart, Georg Thieme, 1978.

Fugger EP, Bustillo M, Dorfmann AD, Schulman JD: Human preimplantation embryo cryopreservation: selected aspects. *Human Reprod 6*:131, 1991.

Gilbert SF: *Developmental Biology.* Sunderland, Sinauer Associates, 1991.

Hafez ESE: *Human Reproductive Physiology.* Ann Arbor, Michigan, Ann Arbor Science Publishers, 1978.

Hafez ESE: *Human Ovulation. Mechanisms, Prediction, Detection and Induction.* Amsterdam, North Holland Publishing Co, 1979.

Handyside AH, Kontogianni EH, Hardy K, Winston RML: Pregnancies from biopsied human preimplantation embryos sexed by Y-specific DNA amplification. *Nature 344*:768, 1990.

Harlap S: Gender of infants conceived on different days of the menstrual cycle. *New Eng J Med 300*:1445, 1979.

Hartshorne GM, Elder K, Crow J, Dyson H, Edwards RG: The influence of in vitro development upon post-thaw survival and implantation of cryopreserved human blastocysts. *Human Reprod 6*:136, 1991.

Hertig AT, Adams EC, Mulligan WJ: On the preimplantation stages of the human ovum: A description of four normal and four abnormal specimens ranging from the second to the fifth day of development. *Contrib Embryol Carnegie Inst 35*:199, 1954.

Hertig AT, Rock J: Two human ova of the previllous stage, having a developmental age of about seven and nine days respectively. *Contrib Embryol Carnegie Inst 31*:65, 1945.

Hertig AT, Rock J, Adams EC: A description of 34 human ova within the first seventeen days of development. *Am J Anat 98*:435, 1956.

Hertig AT, Rock J, Adams EC, Menkin MC: Thirty-four fertilized human ova, good, bad, and indifferent, recovered from 210 women of known fertility. *Pediatrics 23*:202, 1959.

Leeson CR, Leeson TS, Paparo A: *Text/Atlas of Histology.* Philadelphia, WB Saunders, 1988.

Ludwig H, Tauber PF: *Human Fertilization.* Stuttgart, Georg Thieme Publishers, 1978.

Moore KL: *Clinically Oriented Anatomy,* 3rd ed. Baltimore, Williams & Wilkins, 1992.

Nahhas F, Barnea E: Human embryonic origin of early pregnancy factor before and after implantation. *Am J Reprod Immunol 22*:105, 1990.

O'Rahilly R: *Developmental Stages in Human Embryos. Part A. Embryos of the First Three Weeks (Stages 1 to 9).* Washington, DC, Carnegie Institution of Washington, 1973.

Oura C, and Toshimori K: Ultrastructural studies on the fertilization of mammalian gametes. *In Rev Cytol 122*:105, 1990.

Page EW, Villee CA, Villee DB: *Human Reproduction: Essentials of Reproductive and Perinatal Medicine,* 3rd ed. Philadelphia, WB Saunders, 1981.

Rock J, Hertig AT: The human conceptus during the first two weeks of gestation. *Am J Obstet Gynecol 55*:6, 1948.

Rubin E, Farber JL: *Pathology.* Philadelphia, JB Lippincott, 1988.

Sathananthan AH, Trounson A, Freeman L: Morphology and fertilizability of frozen human oocytes. *Gamete Res 16*:343, 1987.

Sathananthan AH, Trounson A, Freeman L: The effects of cooling human oocytes. *Human Reprod 3*:968, 1988.

Scott Jr, RT, Hodgen GD: The ovarian follicle: life cycle of a pelvic clock. *Clin Obstet Gynecol 33*:551, 1990.

Settlage DSF, Motoshima M, Tredway DR: Sperm transport from the external cervical os to the fallopian tubes in women. *Fertil Steril 24*:655, 1973.

Sidhu KS, Guraya SS: Current concepts in gamete receptors for fertilization in mammals. *In Rev Cytol 127*:253, 1991.

Steinkampf MP, Kretzer PA, McElroy E, Conway-Myers BA: A simplified approach to in vitro fertilization. *J Reprod Med 37*:199, 1992.

Steptoe PC, Edwards RG: Birth after implantation of a human embryo. *Lancet ii*:36, 1978.

Stoll C, Roth MP, Bigel P: A re-examination of paternal age effect on the occurrence of new mutants for achondroplasia. *Prog Clin Biol Res 104*:419, 1982.

Talbot P: Sperm penetration through oocyte investments in mammals. *Am J Anat 174*:331, 1985.

Thompson MW, McInnes RR, Willard HF: *Thompson & Thompson Genetics in Medicine,* 5th ed. Philadelphia, WB Saunders, 1991.

Warkany J: Prevention of congenital malformations. *Teratology 23*:175, 1981.

Wassarman PM: The biology and chemistry of fertilization. *Science 235*:553, 1987.

Wood C, Trounson A (eds): *Clinical In Vitro Fertilization,* 2nd ed. New York, Springer Verlag, 1989.

Yanagimachi R: Specificity of sperm-egg interaction. *In* Edidin M, Johnson MM (eds): *The Immunobiology of the Gametes.* Cambridge, Cambridge University Press, 1977.

Yanagimachi R: Mechanisms of fertilization in mammals. *In* Mastroianni Jr, L, Biggers JD (eds): *Fertilization and Embryonic Development In Vitro.* New York, Plenum Press, 1981, pp 81–82.

Zaneveld LJD: Capacitation of spermatozoa. *In* Ludwig H, Tauber PF (eds): *Human Fertilization.* Stuttgart, Georg Thieme Publishers, 1978.

3

Formation of the Bilaminar Embryonic Disc

THE SECOND WEEK

Implantation of the blastocyst is completed during the second week of the pre-embryonic period. As this crucial process takes place, morphological changes occur in the inner cell mass (or embryoblast) that produce a bilaminar embryonic disc composed of two layers, embryonic epiblast and hypoblast (Fig. 3–1A). As described in Chapter 4, the **embryonic disc** gives rise to the germ layers of the embryo (ectoderm, mesoderm, and endoderm). Other structures that form during the second week are the amniotic cavity, amnion, yolk sac, connecting stalk, and chorionic sac.

COMPLETION OF IMPLANTATION AND EARLY EMBRYONIC DEVELOPMENT

Implantation of the blastocyst commences at the end of the first week (see Fig. 2–19) and is completed by the end of the second week. The actively erosive **syncytiotrophoblast** invades the endometrial stroma (connective tissue framework), which supports the capillaries and glands. As this occurs, the blastocyst slowly embeds itself in the endometrium. Using in vitro culture techniques, the attachment of human blastocysts to monolayer cultures of uterine epithelium has been studied. The blastocysts attach to the endometrial layer at their embryonic pole; and, from this region, trophoblast cells displace endometrial cells in the central part of the implantation site (Lindenberg et al., 1989). The stromal cells around the implantation site become laden with glycogen and lipids and assume a polyhedral appearance. Some of these *decidual cells* degenerate adjacent to the penetrating syncytiotrophoblast and provide a rich source of embryonic nutrition.

As the blastocyst implants, more **trophoblast** contacts the endometrium and differentiates into two layers (Fig. 3–1A): (1) the *cytotrophoblast*, a layer of mononucleated cells which is mitotically active and forms new cells that migrate into the increasing mass of syncytiotrophoblast, and (2) the *syncytiotrophoblast*, which rapidly becomes a large, thick, multinucleated mass in which no cell boundaries are discernible (Fig. 3–1B). As cells of the cytotrophoblast proliferate, they migrate into the mass of syncytiotrophoblast and fuse, lose their cell membranes, and become part of this multinucleated zone. The syncytiotrophoblast begins to produce human chorionic gonadotrophin (hCG) which enters the maternal blood and forms the basis for *pregnancy testing* (Filly, 1988). Highly sensitive radioimmune assays are available to detect hCG. The antibodies used in these tests are specific for the beta subunit of the hormone (Filly, 1988). Enough hCG is produced by the syncytiotrophoblast at the end of the second week to give a positive pregnancy test even though the woman is probably unaware she is pregnant. See also the discussion of the early pregnancy factor (EPF) on p. 32.

Formation of the Amniotic Cavity, Amnion, Bilaminar Embryonic Disc, and Yolk Sac

As implantation of the blastocyst progresses, a small cavity appears at the embryonic pole between the embryoblast and trophoblast. This space is the primordium of the **amniotic cavity** (Fig. 3–1A). Soon, amniogenic cells called *amnioblasts* delaminate from the cytotrophoblast and organize to form a membrane, known as the **amnion**, that encloses the amniotic cavity (Fig. 3–1B and C).

Concurrently, morphological changes occur in the embryoblast that result in the formation of a flattened, essentially circular, bilaminar plate of cells called the **embryonic disc**. The thick disc consists of

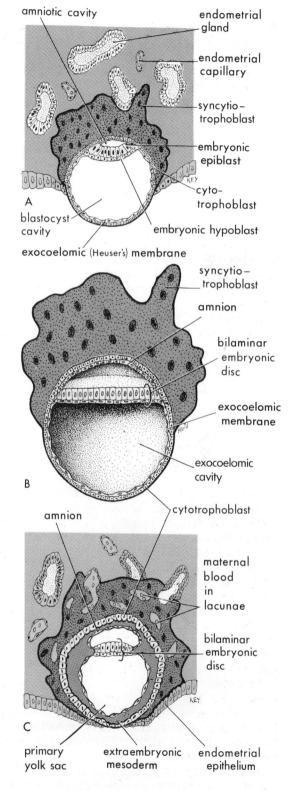

Figure 3–1. Drawings illustrating implantation of a blastocyst in the endometrium. The actual size of the conceptus is about 0.1 mm. *A,* Drawing of a section through a blastocyst partially implanted in the endometrium (about eight days). Note the slitlike amniotic cavity. *B,* An enlarged, three-dimensional sketch of a slightly older blastocyst after removal from the endometrium. Note the extensive syncytiotrophoblast at the embryonic pole and the much larger amniotic cavity. *C,* Drawing of a section through a blastocyst of about nine days implanted in the endometrium. (Based on Hertig and Rock, 1945.) Note the lacunae (spaces) appearing in the syncytiotrophoblast; these soon communicate with the endometrial vessels. The type of implantation illustrated here, in which the blastocyst becomes completely embedded in the endometrium, is called *interstitial implantation.*

two layers: (1) the *epiblast*, consisting of high columnar cells related to the amniotic cavity, and (2) the *hypoblast*, consisting of cuboidal cells adjacent to the blastocyst cavity. The epiblast forms the floor of the amniotic cavity and is continuous peripherally with the amnion (Fig. 3–1B). Cells migrate from the hypoblast and form a thin, *exocoelomic membrane*

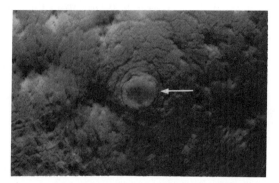

Figure 3–3. Photograph of the endometrial surface of the uterus, showing the implantation site of the human embryo of about 12 days shown in Figure 3–4. The implanted conceptus produces a small elevation (*arrow*) (× 8). (From Hertig AT, Rock J: *Contr Embryol Carneg Instn* 29:127, 1941. Courtesy of the Carnegie Institution of Washington.)

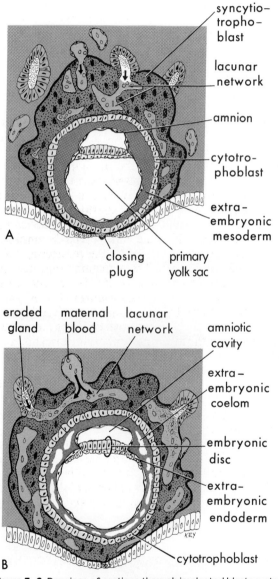

Figure 3–2. Drawings of sections through implanted blastocysts. *A*, 10 days; *B*, 12 days. (Based on Hertig and Rock, 1941.) This stage of development is characterized by the communication of lacunae that are filled with maternal blood. In *B*, note that large cavities have appeared in the extraembryonic mesoderm, forming the primordium of the extraembryonic coelom.

(Fig. 3–1B) that is continuous with the hypoblast.[1] It surrounds the blastocyst cavity which is now called the *exocoelomic cavity*. The exocoelomic membrane and cavity soon become modified to form the *primary yolk sac* (primitive yolk sac). The embryonic disc now lies between the amniotic cavity and the primary yolk sac. Cells, probably from the hypoblast, give rise to a layer of loosely arranged tissue, called the **extraembryonic mesoderm,**[2] around the amnion and primary yolk sac (Fig. 3–1C).

The Lacunar Stage of Trophoblast Development (Fig. 3–1C). As the amnion, bilaminar embryonic disc, and primary yolk sac form, isolated spaces called *lacunae* appear in the syncytiotrophoblast. These soon become filled with a mixture of maternal blood from ruptured endometrial capillaries and secretions from eroded endometrial glands. This nutritive fluid, sometimes called *embryotroph*, passes to the embryonic disc by diffusion. The openings of the eroded uterine vessels into the lacunae represent the beginning of the uteroplacental circulation. When maternal blood flows into the syncytiotrophoblastic lacunae, its nutritive substances become available to the extraembryonic tissues over the large surface of the syncytiotrophoblast. As both arterial and venous branches of the maternal blood vessels communicate with the syncytiotrophoblastic lacunae, blood circulation is established. Oxygenated blood passes into the lacunae from the *spiral arteries* in the endometrium,

---

[1] The origin of the exocoelomic membrane in the human embryo is thought to be derived from the hypoblast (Luckett, 1978).

[2] From studies in the rhesus monkey, there is evidence for the formation of extraembryonic mesoderm from the hypoblast (Enders and King, 1988).

and deoxygenated blood is removed from them via the endometrial veins (see Fig. 2–5B).

The ten-day conceptus is completely embedded in the endometrium (Fig. 3–2A). For about two days, a defect exists in the endometrial epithelium that is indicated by a *closing plug* composed of a fibrinous coagulum of blood. By day 12 an almost completely regenerated epithelium covers the endometrial defect (Fig. 3–2B). The implanted blastocyst now produces a minute elevation on the endometrial surface that protrudes into the uterine cavity (Figs. 3–2 to 3–4).

By the twelfth day adjacent syncytiotrophoblastic lacunae have fused to form *lacunar networks* (Fig. 3–2B), which give the syncytiotrophoblast a sponge like appearance (Figs. 3–4 and 3–5). The lacunar networks, particularly obvious around the embryonic pole, are the primordium of the *intervillous space* of the placenta (see Fig. 4–11C). The endometrial capillaries around the implanted embryo first become congested and dilated to form *sinusoids*, and then the syncytiotrophoblast erodes them. Maternal blood seeps in and out of the lacunar networks, establishing a *primitive uteroplacental circulation*. The degenerated endometrial stromal cells and glands, together with the maternal blood, provide a rich source of material for embryonic nutrition. Examination of Figures 3–1 and 3–2 shows that growth of the bilaminar embryonic disc is slow compared with growth of the trophoblast.

Because the placenta contains about 50 per cent paternal genes, it is, strictly speaking, a homograft in the uterus. The failure of maternal tissue to reject the conceptus has puzzled embryologists and immunologists for some time. It has been suggested that the syncytiotrophoblast lacks *transplantation antigens* and the conceptus is not rejected for this reason (Lala et al., 1984; Rodger and Drake, 1987; Saji et al., 1989). Another view is that the trophoblast cells, which protect the fetus from the immunological properties of the mother, may be resistant to natural killer cells and lymphokine-activated killer cells, thereby providing a protective barrier for the fetus. Recent experiments have suggested that the chorion may also help to protect the fetus from the immune reaction of the mother (Chaouat, 1990).

As changes occur in the trophoblast and endometrium, the extraembryonic mesoderm increases (Fig. 3–2A), and isolated coelomic spaces appear within it (Figs. 3–2B and 3–4B). These spaces rapidly fuse to form a large, isolated cavity called the **extraembryonic coelom** (Fig. 3–5A). This fluid-filled cavity surrounds the amnion and yolk sac except where they are attached to the chorion by the connecting stalk (Fig. 3–5). As the extraembryonic coelom forms, the primary yolk sac decreases in size and a smaller, *secondary yolk sac* forms. It is often referred to simply as the **yolk sac**. This smaller sac is formed by cells that mi-

grate from the hypoblast of the embryonic disc inside the primary yolk sac (Figs. 3–2B and 3–5A). The yolk sac contains fluid but no yolk. It appears to have a role in the selective transfer of the nutritive fluid to the embryonic disc. The trophoblast absorbs the fluid from the lacunar networks in the endometrium (Fig. 3–2B).

DEVELOPMENT OF THE CHORIONIC SAC

The end of the second week is characterized by the appearance of *primitive chorionic villi* (Figs. 3–5 and 3–6). Proliferation of cytotrophoblast cells produces local masses that extend into the syncytiotrophoblast. These cellular projections form *primary chorionic villi* which represent the first stage in the development of the chorionic villi of the placenta (Figs. 3–5 and 3–6).

The extraembryonic coelom splits the extraembryonic mesoderm into two layers (Fig. 3–5): (1) *extraembryonic somatic mesoderm*, lining the trophoblast and covering the amnion, and (2) *extraembryonic splanchnic mesoderm*, surrounding the yolk sac. The extraembryonic somatic mesoderm and the two layers of trophoblast constitute the **chorion** (Fig. 3–5A). *The chorion forms the wall of the chorionic sac*, within which the embryo and its amniotic and yolk sacs are suspended by the connecting stalk (Figs. 3–5B and 3–6B). The extraembryonic coelom is now called the *chorionic cavity*. The amniotic sac (with the embryonic epiblast forming its "floor") and the yolk sac (with the embryonic hypoblast forming its "roof") are analogous to two balloons pressed together (site of the bilaminar embryonic disc) and suspended by a cord (the connecting stalk) from the inside of a larger balloon (the chorionic sac).

The 14-day embryo still has the form of a flat, bilaminar embryonic disc, but the hypoblastic cells in a localized area are now columnar and form a thickened, circular area called the **prochordal plate** (Fig. 3–5B and C). This plate indicates the future site of the mouth and is an important *organizer of the head region*. It indicates the cranial region of the embryo and will later form the endodermal layer of the bilaminar *oropharyngeal (buccopharyngeal) membrane* (see Fig. 4–6C).

IMPLANTATION SITES OF THE BLASTOCYST

Implantation of the blastocyst usually occurs in the endometrium of the uterus. If implantation occurs elsewhere, a misplaced or *ectopic pregnancy* results (Figs. 3–7 and 3–8). Serious complications usually

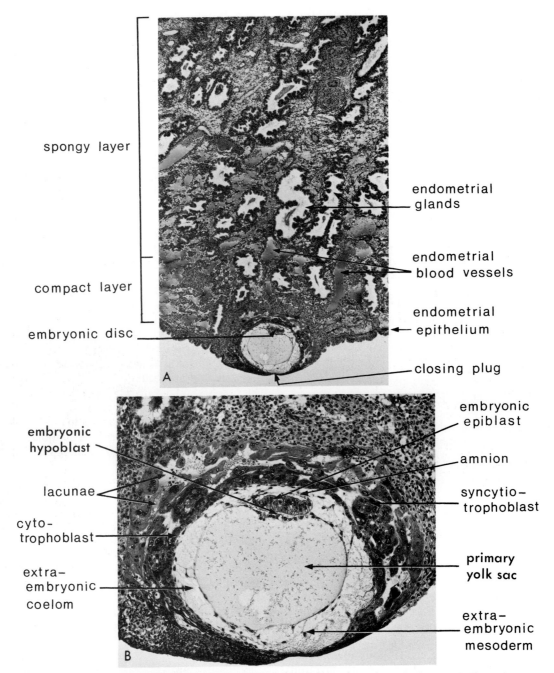

spongy layer

endometrial
glands

endometrial
blood vessels

compact layer

endometrial
epithelium

embryonic disc

closing plug

A

embryonic
epiblast

embryonic
hypoblast

amnion

lacunae

syncytio-
trophoblast

cyto-
trophoblast

primary
yolk sac

extra-
embryonic
coelom

extra-
embryonic
mesoderm

B

Figure 3–4. *A*, Section through the implantation site of the 12-day embryo shown in Figure 3–3. The embryo is embedded in the compact layer of the endometrium (✕ 30). *B*, Higher magnification of the conceptus and surrounding endometrium (✕ 100). Lacunae containing maternal blood are visible in the syncytiotrophoblast. (From Hertig AT, Rock J: *Contr Embryol Carneg Instn 29*:127, 1941. Courtesy of the Carnegie Institution of Washington.)

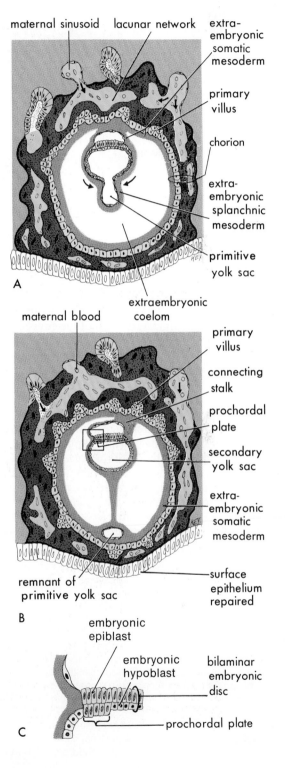

Figure 3–5. Drawings of sections through implanted human embryos, based mainly on Hertig et al, 1956. *Note:* (1) the defect in the surface epithelium of the endometrium has disappeared; (2) a small secondary yolk sac has formed inside the primary yolk sac; (3) a large cavity, the extraembryonic coelom, now surrounds the yolk sac and amnion except where the amnion is attached to the chorion by the connecting stalk; and (4) the extraembryonic coelom splits the extraembryonic mesoderm into two layers: extraembryonic somatic mesoderm lining the trophoblast and covering the amnion, and the extraembryonic splanchnic mesoderm around the yolk sac. The trophoblast and extraembryonic somatic mesoderm together form the chorion, which eventually gives rise to the fetal part of the placenta. *A*, 13 days, illustrating the decrease in relative size of the primary yolk sac and the early appearance of primary chorionic villi. *B*, 14 days, showing the newly formed, secondary yolk sac and the location of the prochordal plate in its roof. *C*, Detail of the prochordal plate area outlined in *B*.

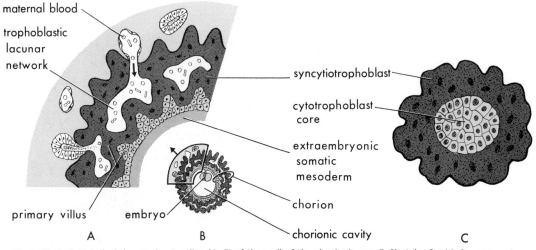

Figure 3–6. *A,* Detail of the section (outlined in *B*) of the wall of the chorionic sac. *B,* Sketch of a 14-day conceptus illustrating the chorionic sac and the shaggy appearance created by the primary chorionic villi (× 6). *C,* Drawing of a transverse section through a primary chorionic villus (× 300). Development at the end of the second week is characterized by the appearance of primary chorionic villi (see also Fig. 3–5).

develop in a few weeks and a spontaneous abortion may occur or surgical removal of the conceptus may be necessary (Fig. 3–7).

Intrauterine Implantation Sites. The blastocyst usually implants superiorly in the endometrium of the body of the uterus, slightly more often on the posterior than on the anterior wall (Fig. 3–8). Implantation of a blastocyst in the inferior segment of the uterus near the internal ostium results in *placenta previa,* a placenta that partially or completely covers the internal opening of the uterus. Placenta previa may cause bleeding due to premature separation of the placenta during pregnancy or at delivery of the fetus. Intrauterine pregnancy can be detected by highly sensitive radioimmune assays of hCG (p. 40) as early as the end of the second week.

Extrauterine Implantation Sites (Figs. 3–7 to 3–9). The blastocyst may implant outside the uterus. These implantations are referred to as **ectopic pregnancies** (Filly, 1988); 95 to 97 per cent of ectopic implantations occur in the uterine tube. *Most tubal pregnancies are in the ampulla or isthmus* (Figs. 2–5*A* and 3–8*A* and *B*). The incidence of tubal pregnancy varies from 1 in 80 to 1 in 250 pregnancies depending on the socioeconomic level of the population (Page et al., 1981). The highest rates of ectopic pregnancy are in women 35 years of age or older and in women who are nonwhite (Rubin, 1983); however, "all women of childbearing age are at risk of harboring an ectopic gestation" (Filly, 1988). A woman with a tubal pregnancy has signs and symptoms of pregnancy (e.g., misses her menstrual period). She may also experience abdominal pain and tenderness due to distention of the uterine tube and irritation of the pelvic perito-

neum and abnormal bleeding. The pain may be confused with *appendicitis* if the pregnancy is in the right uterine tube. Ectopic pregnancies produce hCG at a slower rate than normally implanted pregnancies (Cartwright and DiPietro, 1984); consequently, assays may give false-negative tests if performed too early. *Endovaginal (intravaginal) sonography* is very helpful in detecting ectopic pregnancies (Filly, 1988; Ash et al., 1991).

There are several causes of tubal pregnancy, but they are often related to factors that delay or prevent transport of the dividing zygote to the uterus; e.g., blockage caused by scarring resulting from infection in the abdominopelvic cavity (e.g., *pelvic inflammatory disease*). Ectopic tubal pregnancies usually result in rupture of the uterine tube and hemorrhage into the peritoneal cavity during the first eight weeks, followed by death of the embryo. Tubal rupture and hemorrhage constitute a threat to the mother's life and are therefore of major clinical importance. The affected tube and conceptus are surgically removed (Figs. 3–7 and 3–9).

When blastocysts implant in the isthmus of the uterine tube (Figs. 2–5*A* and 3–8*D*), the tube tends to rupture early because this part is narrow and relatively unexpandable. Abortion of the embryo from this site often results in extensive bleeding, probably because of the rich anastomoses between ovarian and uterine vessels in this area (Moore, 1992). When blastocysts implant in the intramural or uterine part of the tube (Fig. 3–8*E*; see also Fig. 2–5*A*), they may develop into fetuses (12 to 16 weeks) before expulsion occurs. When an *intramural tubal pregnancy* ruptures, it usually bleeds profusely. Blastocysts that implant in the ampulla (Fig. 3–7) or in the fimbriae of the uterine tube are often expelled into the peritoneal cavity where they commonly implant in the rectouterine pouch (Fig. 3–10).

Simultaneous intrauterine and extrauterine pregnancies are unusual (no greater than 1 in 7000; Filly, 1988). The

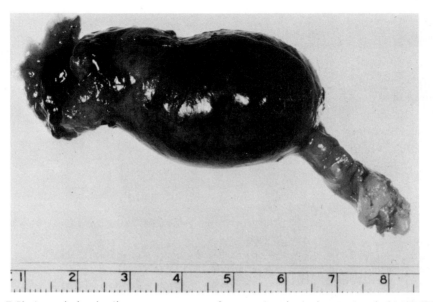

Figure 3–7. Photograph showing the gross appearance of an unruptured ectopic pregnancy located in the ampulla of the uterine tube. When the chorionic sac distends the tube, partial separation of the placenta and rupture of the tube often occur. Spurts of blood escape from the ruptured tube and its infundibulum (shown at the left). Tubal rupture and the associated hemorrhage constitute a threat to the mother's life. (From Page EW, Villee CA, Villee DB: *Human Reproduction. Essentials of Reproductive and Perinatal Medicine*, 3rd ed. Philadelphia, WB Saunders, 1981.)

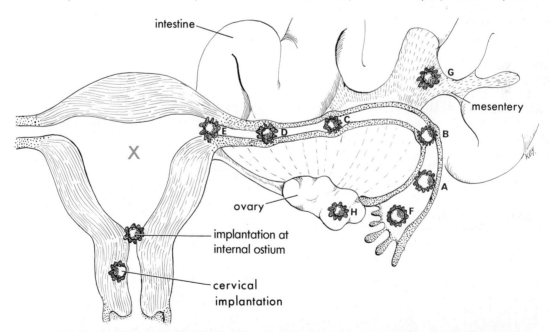

Figure 3–8. Drawing illustrating various implantation sites of the blastocyst; the usual site in the posterior wall of the uterus is indicated by an X. The approximate order of frequency of ectopic implantations is indicated alphabetically (A, most common to H, least common). A to F, Tubal pregnancies. G, Abdominal pregnancy. H, Ovarian pregnancy. Tubal pregnancies are the most common type of ectopic pregnancy.

uterine tube chorionic sac

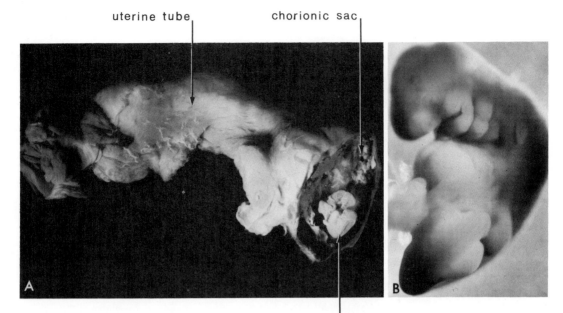

embryo

Figure 3–9. Photographs of a tubal pregnancy. *A*, The uterine tube has been surgically removed and sectioned to show the conceptus implanted in the mucous membrane (× 3). *B*, Enlarged photograph of the normal-appearing, four-week embryo (× 13). Ectopic pregnancies occur most often in the ampulla of the uterine tube (Fig. 3–8*A*). This serious condition may be caused by a delay in the passage of the dividing zygote along the tube. Ectopic tubal pregnancy results in death of the embryo and usually sudden, massive bleeding from the ruptured tube. (Photographed by Professor Jean Hay, Department of Anatomy, University of Manitoba, Winnipeg, Canada.)

ectopic pregnancy is masked initially by the presence of the uterine pregnancy. Usually, the ectopic pregnancy can be terminated, e.g., by surgical removal of the involved uterine tube without interfering with the intrauterine pregnancy (Fig. 3–7). *Cervical implantations* are unusual (Fig. 3–8). Some of these pregnancies in the cervix are not recognized

embryo

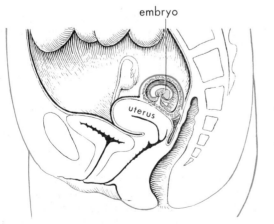

Figure 3–10. Drawing illustrating an abdominal pregnancy. Although a blastocyst expelled from the uterine tube may attach to any organ or to the mesentery of the intestines, it commonly attaches to the peritoneum of the rectouterine pouch.

because the conceptus is aborted during early gestation. In other cases, the placenta becomes firmly attached to the fibrous and muscular parts of the cervix, often resulting in bleeding and subsequent surgical intervention, e.g., *hysterectomy* (excision of the uterus).

Spontaneous early abortion of an embryo and its membranes implanted in the uterine tube may result in implantation of the conceptus in the ovary or in other organs or mesenteries (Figs. 3–8 and 3–10), but ovarian and abdominal pregnancies are very uncommon. Bleeding from these ectopic sites usually results in *intra-abdominal hemorrhage* and severe abdominal pain. Most of these cases are discovered during abdominal exploration of a presumed tubal pregnancy. In exceptional cases, an *abdominal pregnancy* may progress to full term, and the fetus may be delivered alive. Usually, however, an abdominal pregnancy creates a serious condition because the placenta attaches to abdominal organs and causes considerable bleeding. In very unusual cases, an abdominal fetus dies and is not detected; the fetus becomes calcified, forming a so-called stone fetus or lithopedion (Gr. *lithos*, stone, + *paidion*, child).

SPONTANEOUS ABORTION OF EARLY EMBRYOS

Abortion is commonly defined as the termination of pregnancy before 20 weeks' gestation; i.e., before the period of viability of the embryo or fetus. Most abortions of em-

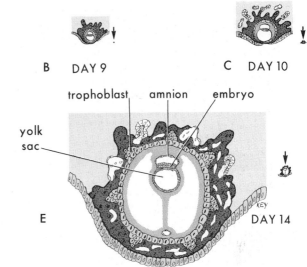

A   DAY 8

B   DAY 9

C   DAY 10

trophoblast   amnion   embryo

yolk
sac

Figure 3–11. Drawings of sections of human blastocysts during the second week illustrating the rapid expansion of the trophoblast and the relatively minute size of the conceptuses (× 25); the sketches indicated by the arrows show the actual size of the blastocysts. Obviously, an aborted conceptus would be difficult to detect in the menstrual fluid.

D   DAY 12

E   DAY 14

bryos during the first three weeks occur spontaneously; i.e., they are not induced. *Sporadic and recurrent spontaneous abortions* are two of the most common gynecological problems (Coulam et al., 1990; Thom et al., 1992). The frequency of early abortions is difficult to establish because they often occur before women are aware that they are pregnant. An abortion just after the first missed period is very likely to be mistaken for a delayed menstruation. Detection of the conceptus in the menses (menstrual blood) is very difficult because of its small size (Fig. 3–11).

Study of most early spontaneous abortions resulting from medical problems reveal abnormal conceptuses. Hertig et al. (1959) studied 34 early embryos recovered from women of known fertility and found ten of them so abnormal that they probably would have aborted spontaneously by the end of the second week of development. Hertig (1967) estimated that of the 70 to 75 per cent of blastocysts that implant, only 58 per cent survive to the end of the second week. He further estimated that 16 per cent of this latter group would be abnormal and would abort in a week or so.

The incidence of chromosomal abnormalities in early spontaneous abortions in one study was about 61 per cent (Boué et al., 1975). Summarizing the data of several studies, Carr and Gedeon (1977) estimated that 50 per cent of all known spontaneous abortions result from chromosomal abnormalities. The higher incidence of early abortions in older women probably results from the increasing frequency of *nondisjunction of chromosomes* during oogenesis (see Fig. 2–3 and Table 8–3). It has been estimated that from one third to one half of all zygotes never become blastocysts and implant. Failure of blastocysts to implant may result from a poorly developed endometrium; but, in many cases, there are probably lethal chromosomal abnormalities in the zygote that cause the abortion. Shepard et al.

(1988) found a higher incidence of spontaneous abortuses with *neural tube defects* (p. 63), cleft lip, and cleft palate, as well as other malformations, than in newborns and induced abortuses.

SUMMARY OF IMPLANTATION

Implantation of the blastocyst begins at the end of the first week and is completed by the end of the second week. The process may be summarized as follows:

1. The zona pellucida degenerates (day 5). Its disappearance results from enlargement of the blastocyst and degeneration caused by enzymatic lysis. The lytic enzymes are released from the acrosomes of the many sperms that surround and partially penetrate the zona pellucida.

2. The blastocyst attaches to endometrial epithelium (day 6).

3. The trophoblast begins to differentiate into two layers, syncytiotrophoblast and cytotrophoblast (day 7).

4. The syncytiotrophoblast erodes endometrial tissues (capillaries, glands, stroma) and the blastocyst starts to embed in the endometrium (day 8).

5. Blood-filled lacunae appear in the syncytiotrophoblast (day 9).

6. The blastocyst sinks beneath the endometrial epithelium (day 10).

6. The blastocyst sinks beneath the endometrial epithelium (day 10).

7. Lacunar networks form by fusion of adjacent lacunae (days 10 and 11).

8. The syncytiotrophoblast continues to erode endometrial blood vessels, allowing maternal blood to seep into and out of the lacunar networks, thereby establishing a *primitive uteroplacental circulation* (days 11 and 12).

9. The defect in the endometrial epithelium gradually disappears as the surface epithelium is repaired (days 12 and 13).

10. Primary chorionic villi develop (days 13 and 14).

Inhibition of Implantation. The administration of relatively large doses of estrogens ("morning-after pills") for five days, beginning 72 hours after sexual intercourse, will usually prevent pregnancy by inhibiting implantation of the blastocyst. *Diethylstilbestrol*, given daily in high dosage (25 mg) for five to six days, may also accelerate passage of the dividing zygote along the uterine tube (Kalant et al., 1990). Normally, the endometrium progresses to the secretory phase of the menstrual cycle as the zygote forms, undergoes cleavage, and enters the uterus. The large amount of estrogen disturbs the normal balance between estrogen and progesterone that is necessary for preparation of the endometrium for implantation of the blastocyst (see Fig. 2–6). Postconception administration of hormones to prevent implantation of the blastocyst is often used in cases of sexual assault or leakage of a condom but is contraindicated for routine contraceptive use. The controversial "abortion pill" *RU486* used in France also destroys the conceptus by interrupting implantation due to interference with the hormonal environment of the developing embryo.

An *intrauterine device* (IUD) inserted into the uterus through the vagina and cervix usually interferes with implantation by causing a local inflammatory reaction. Some IUDs contain progesterone that is slowly released and interferes with the development of the endometrium so that implantation is unlikely to occur.

SUMMARY OF THE SECOND WEEK OF HUMAN DEVELOPMENT

Rapid proliferation and differentiation of the trophoblast are important features of the second week of development (Fig. 3–11). These processes occur as the blastocyst implants in the endometrium. The various endometrial changes resulting from the adaptation of these tissues to implantation of the blastocyst are known collectively as the **decidual reaction** (see Chapter 7). Concurrently, the primary yolk sac forms and extraembryonic mesoderm arises from the internal surface of the cytotrophoblast. The extraembryonic coelom forms from spaces that develop in the extraembryonic mesoderm (Fig. 3–4). This coelom later becomes the chorionic cavity (Fig. 3–6B). The primary yolk sac becomes smaller and gradually disappears as the secondary yolk sac develops.

As these changes occur, the following developments are recognizable: (1) the amniotic cavity appears as a space between the cytotrophoblast and the embryoblast; (2) the inner cell or embryoblast differentiates into a **bilaminar embryonic disc** consisting of *epiblast*, related to the amniotic cavity, and *hypoblast*, adjacent to the blastocyst cavity; and (3) the **prochordal plate** develops as a localized thickening of the hypoblast, indicating the future cranial region of the embryo and the site of the future mouth. It is also an important organizer of the head region.

CLINICALLY ORIENTED QUESTIONS FOR PROBLEM-BASED LEARNING SESSIONS

1. Is it advisable to do a radiological examination of a healthy, 22-year-old female's chest during the last week of her menstrual cycle? Are birth defects likely to develop in her conceptus if she happens to be pregnant?

2. A woman who was sexually assaulted during her fertile period was given large doses of estrogen twice daily for five days to interrupt a possible pregnancy. If fertilization had occurred, what do you think would be the mechanism of action of this hormone? What do laypeople call this type of medical treatment? Is this what the media refer to as the "abortion pill"? If not, explain the method of action of this pill. How early can a pregnancy be detected?

3. A 23-year-old woman reported severe lower abdominal pain to her physician. She said that she had missed two menstrual periods. A diagnosis of ectopic pregnancy was made. What techniques might be used to enable this diagnosis to be made with certainty? What is the most likely site of the extrauterine gestation? How do you think the physician would likely treat the condition?

4. A 30-year-old woman had an appendectomy toward the end of her menstrual cycle; 8½ months later she had a child with a congenital anomaly of the brain. Could the surgery have produced the congenital anomaly? Explain the basis for your views. You may wish to refer to Chapter 8.
5. A 42-year-old woman finally became pregnant after many years of trying to conceive. She was concerned about the development of her baby. What would the physician likely tell her? Can women over 40 have normal babies? What tests and diagnostic techniques would likely be performed?

The answers to these questions are given on page 459.

References and Suggested Reading

Ash KM, Lyons ES, Levi CS, Lindsay DJ: Endovaginal sonographic diagnosis of ectopic twin gestation. *J Ultrasound Med 10*:497, 1991.

Billington WD: Trophoblast. *In* Philipp EE, Barnes J, Newton M (eds): *Scientific Foundations of Obstetrics and Gynecology.* London, William Heinemann, 1970.

Blandau RJ (ed): *The Biology of the Blastocyst.* Chicago, University of Chicago Press, 1971.

Boronow RC, McElin TW, West RH, Buckingham JC: Ovarian pregnancy. *Am J Obstet Gynecol 91*:1095, 1965.

Boué J, Boué A, Lazar P: Retrospective and prospective epidemiological studies of 1500 karyotyped spontaneous abortions. *Teratology 12*:11, 1975.

Böving BG: Implantation mechanisms. *In* Hartmann CG (ed): *Mechanisms Concerned with Conception.* New York, Pergamon Press, 1963.

Carr DH: Chromosome studies in selected spontaneous abortions. III. Early pregnancy loss. *Obstet Gynecol. 37*:750, 1971.

Carr DH, Gedeon M: Population cytogenetics of human abortuses. *In* Hook EB, Porter IH (eds): *Population Cytogenetics: Studies in Humans.* New York, Academic Press, 1977.

Cartwright PS, DiPietro DL: Ectopic pregnancy: Changes in serum human chorionic gonadotropin concentration. *Obstet Gynec 63*:76, 1984.

Chaouat G: *The Immunology of the Fetus.* Boca Raton, CRC Press, 1990.

Chapman MG, Grudzinskas JG, Chard T (eds): *Implantation: Biological and Clinical Aspects.* Berlin, Springer Verlag, 1988.

Coulam CB, Faulk WP, McIntyre JA: Spontaneous and recurrent abortions. *In* Quilligan EJ, Zuspan FP (eds): *Current Therapy in Obstetrics and Gynecology,* vol. 3. Philadelphia, WB Saunders, 1990.

Coulam CG: Epidemiology of recurrent spontaneous abortion. *Am J Reprod Immunol 26*:23, 1991.

Cowchock S: Autoantibodies and fetal wastage. *Am J Reprod Immunol 26*:38, 1991.

Enders AC, King BF: Formation and differentiation of extraembryonic mesoderm in the rhesus monkey. *Am J Anat 181*:327, 1988.

Filly RA: The first trimester. *In* Callen PW (ed): *Ultrasonography In Obstetrics and Gynecology,* 2nd ed. Philadelphia, WB Saunders, 1988, p 21.

Filly RA: Ectopic pregnancy. *In* Callen PW (ed): *Ultrasonography in Obstetrics and Gynecology,* 2nd ed. Philadelphia, WB Saunders, 1988, p 447.

Gilbert SF: *Developmental Biology,* 3rd ed. Sunderland, Sinauer Associates, 1991.

Hertig AT: The overall problem in man. *In* Benirschke K (ed): *Comparative Aspects of Reproductive Failure.* New York, Springer Verlag, 1967.

Hertig AT: *Human Trophoblast.* Springfield, Ill., Charles C Thomas, 1968.

Hertig AT, Rock J: Two human ova of the previllous stage, having a developmental age of about eleven and twelve days respectively. *Contrib Embryol Carnegie Inst 29*:127, 1941.

Hertig AT, Rock J: Two human ova of the pre-villous stage, having a developmental age of about seven and nine days respectively. *Contrib Embryol Carnegie Inst 31*:65, 1945.

Hertig AT, Rock J: Two human ova of the pre-villous stage, having a developmental age of about eight and nine days, respectively. *Contrib Embryol Carnegie Inst 33*:169, 1949.

Hertig AT, Rock, J, Adams EC: A description of 34 human ova within the first seventeen days of development. *Am J Anat 98*:435, 1956.

Hertig AT, Rock J, Adams EC, Menkin MC: Thirty-four fertilized human ova, good, bad and indifferent, recovered from 210 women of known fertility. *Pediatrics 23*:202, 1959.

Kalant H, Roschlau WHE, Hickie RA: *Essentials of Medical Pharmacology.* Toronto, BC Decker, 1990.

Lala PK, Kearns M, Colavincenzo V: Cells of the fetomaternal interface: their role in the maintenance of viviparous pregnancy. *Am J Anat 170*:501, 1984.

Li TC, Tristram A, Hill AS, Cooke ID: A review of 254 ectopic pregnancies in a teaching hospital in the Trent region, 1977–1990. *Human Reprod 6*:1002, 1991.

Lindenberg G, Hyttel P, Sjogren A, Greve T: A Comparative study of attachment of human, bovine and mouse blastocysts to uterine epithelial monolayer. *Human Reprod 4*:446, 1989.

Lindsay DJ, Lovett IS, Lyons EA, Levi CS, Zheng X-H, Holt SC, Daschefsky SM: Endovaginal sonography: yolk sac diameter and shape as a predictor of pregnancy outcome in the first trimester. *Radiology 183*:115, 1992.

Luckett WP: The origin of extraembryonic mesoderm in the early human and rhesus monkey embryos. *Anat Rec 169*:369, 1971.

Luckett WP: Amniogenesis in the early human and rhesus monkey embryos. *Anat Rec 175*:375, 1973.

Luckett WP: Origin and differentiation of the yolk sac and extraembryonic mesoderm in presomite human and rhesus monkey embryos. *Am J Anat 152*:59, 1978.

Moore KL: *Clinically Oriented Anatomy,* 3rd ed. Baltimore, Williams & Wilkins, 1992.

Page EW, Villee CA, Villee DB: *Human Reproduction. Essentials of Reproductive and Perinatal Medicine,* 3rd ed. Philadelphia, WB Saunders, 1981.

Reid DE: Obstetric hemorrhage in late pregnancy and post partum. *In* Reid DE, Ryan KJ, Benirschke K: *Principles and Management of Human Reproduction.* Philadelphia, WB Saunders, 1972.

Reid DE, Benirschke K: Ectopic pregnancy. *In* Reid DE, Ryan KJ,

Benirschke K: *Principles and Management of Human Reproduction.* Philadelphia, WB Saunders, 1972.

Rodger JC, Drake BL: The enigma of the fetal graft. *American Scientist 75*:51, 1987.

Rubin GL: Ectopic pregnancy in the United States: 1970 through 1978. *J Amer Med Assoc 249*:1725, 1983.

Saji F, Kameda T, Koyama M, Matsuzaki N, Negoro T, Tanizawa O: Impaired susceptibility of human trophoblast to MHC nonrestricted killer cells: Implication in the maternal-fetal relationship. *Am J Reprod Immunol 19*:108, 1989.

Shepard TH, Fantel AG, Mirkes PE: Collection and scientific use of human embryonic and fetal material. *In* Kalter H (ed): *Issues and Reviews in Teratology*, vol. 4, 1988.

Stander RW: Abdominal pregnancy. *Clin Obstet Gynecol 5*:1065, 1962.

Streeter GL: Developmental horizons in human embryos. Description of age group XI, 13 to 20 somites, and age group XII, 21 to 29 somites. *Contrib Embryol Carnegie Inst 30*:211, 1942.

Thom DH, Nelson LM, Vaughan TL: Spontaneous abortion and subsequent adverse birth outcomes. *Am J Obstet and Gynecol 166*:111, 1992

Formation of the Human Embryo

THE THIRD WEEK

This is the *beginning of the embryonic period* that terminates at the end of the eighth week. Rapid development of the embryo from the embryonic disc, as the result of numerous morphogenetic events, is characterized by the formation of the primitive streak, notochord, and three **germ layers** from which all embryonic tissues and organs develop (Figs. 4–1 and 4–2). The third week of development occurs during the week following the first missed menstrual period; i.e., five weeks after the onset of the last normal menstrual period (LNMP) (see Figure 1–1).

Cessation of menstruation is often the first indication that a woman may be pregnant, but missing a period is not a certain sign of pregnancy; for example, delay of menstruation may result from severe emotional shock or illness. Relatively simple and rapid tests are now available for detecting pregnancy. Most tests depend on the presence of an *early pregnancy factor* (EPF) in the maternal serum (Nahhas and Barnea, 1990) and *human chorionic gonadotropin* (hCG), a hormone produced by the syncytiotrophoblast and excreted in the mother's urine. EPF can be detected 24 to 48 hours after fertilization, and the production of hCG is sufficient to give a positive indication of pregnancy early in the second week of development (Filly, 1988). Early confirmation of pregnancy is also possible with ultrasound techniques (Kurtz and Needleman, 1988). About three weeks after conception and approximately five weeks after the LNMP, a normal pregnancy can be detected with ultrasonography (Filly, 1988). A frequent symptom of pregnancy is nausea and vomiting, which may occur by the end of the third week though the time of onset is variable. Slight bleeding at the expected time of menstruation does not rule out pregnancy because there may be a slight loss of blood, in some cases, from the implantation site of the blastocyst. This *implantation bleeding* results from leakage of blood into the uterine cavity from disrupted endometrial blood vessels around the implanted blastocyst. When such bleeding is interpreted as menstruation, an error occurs in determining the expected delivery date of the baby.

GASTRULATION: FORMATION OF GERM LAYERS

The process by which the bilaminar embryonic disc is converted into a trilaminar embryonic disc is called gastrulation. It is the *beginning of morphogenesis* (development of body form) and the most significant event occurring during the third week. Gastrulation, which establishes the three **germ layers** of the embryo, begins with formation of the primitive streak (Figs. 4–1 and 4–2). Each of the germ layers (ectoderm, mesoderm, and endoderm) gives rise to specific tissues and organs. *Ectoderm* gives rise to the epidermis, nervous system, and various other structures (see Fig. 5–5). *Endoderm* is the source of the epithelial linings of the respiratory passages and the digestive tract, including the glandular cells of associated organs, such as the liver and pancreas. *Mesoderm* gives rise to smooth muscular coats, connective tissues, and the vessels supplying tissues and organs. Mesoderm is also the source of blood cells and bone marrow, the skeleton, striated muscles, and the reproductive and excretory organs.

Formation of the primitive streak, notochord, and germ layers are the important processes occurring during **gastrulation**. During this stage of development, the embryo may be referred to as a *gastrula*.

The Primitive Streak

At the beginning of the third week, an opacity, formed by a thickened linear band of epiblast known as the primitive streak, appears caudally in the median plane of the dorsal aspect of the embryonic disc (Figs. 4–1 and 4–2). The primitive streak results from the proliferation and migration of cells of the epiblast to the median plane of the embryonic disc.

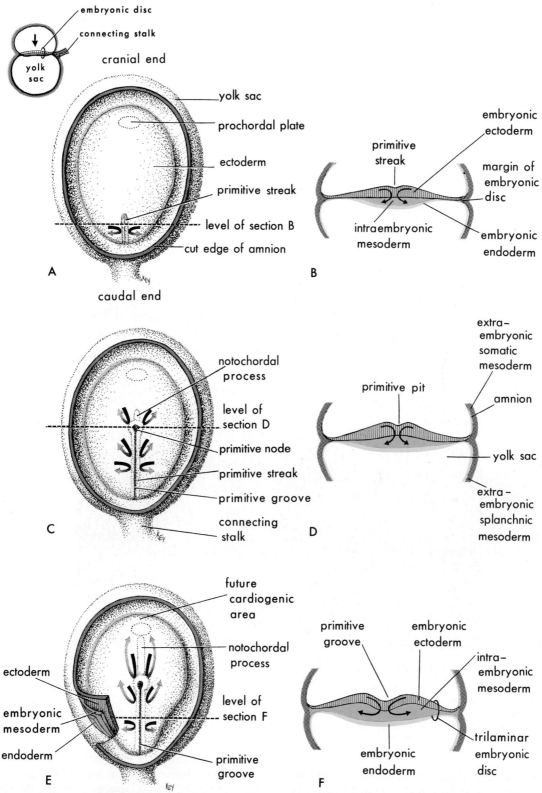

Figure 4–1. Drawings illustrating formation of the trilaminar embryonic disc (days 15 to 16). The small sketch at the upper left is for orientation; the arrow indicates the dorsal aspect of the embryonic disc as shown in *A*. The arrows in all other drawings indicate invagination and migration of mesenchymal cells between the ectoderm and endoderm. *A, C,* and *E,* Dorsal views of the embryonic disc early in the third week, exposed by removal of the amnion. *B, D,* and *F,* Transverse sections through the embryonic disc at the levels indicated. The prochordal plate, indicating the head region, is indicated by a broken outline because it is a thickening of endoderm that cannot be seen from the dorsal surface.

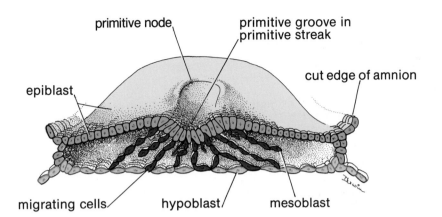

A.

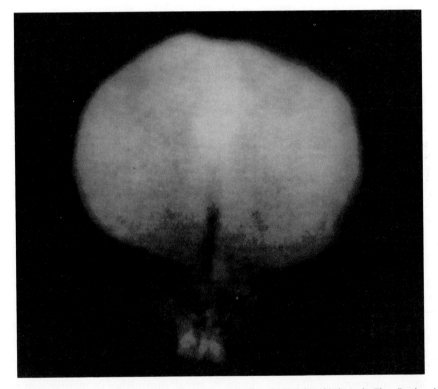

B.

Figure 4–2. *A,* Drawing of the cranial half of the embryonic disc during the third week. The disc has been cut transversely to show the migration of mesenchymal cells from the primitive streak to form mesoblast that soon organizes to form the intraembryonic mesoderm. This illustration also shows that most of the embryonic endoderm also arises from the epiblast. Most of the hypoblastic cells are displaced to extraembryonic regions, such as the wall of the yolk sac. *B,* Photograph of a human embryo of about 16 days. The primitive streak is clearly visible (Courtesy of Dr. Kohei Shiota, Professor of Anatomy and Chairman, Faculty of Medicine, Kyoto University, Kyoto, Japan).

The cells from both sides of the disc meet to form the primitive streak. As the primitive streak elongates by addition of cells to its caudal end, its cranial end proliferates to form a *primitive node* or knot (Figs. 4–1*C* and 4–3*B*). Concurrently, a *narrow primitive groove* develops in the primitive streak that is continuous with a depression in the primitive node known as the *primitive pit* (Figs. 4–1*C* and 4–2). When the primitive streak appears, it is possible to identify the embryo's craniocaudal axis, its cranial and caudal ends, its dorsal and ventral surfaces, and its right and left sides. The primitive groove and pit result from the

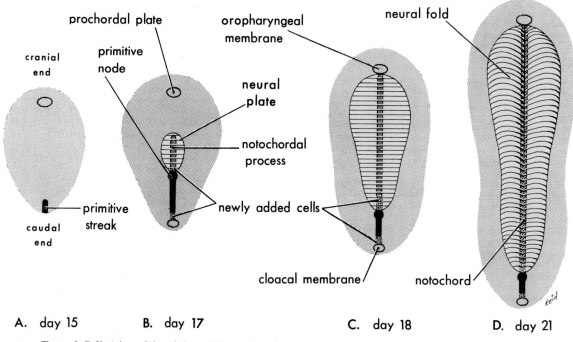

Figure 4–3. Sketches of dorsal views of the embryonic disc showing how it lengthens and changes shape during the third week. The primitive streak lengthens by addition of cells at its caudal end; the notochordal process lengthens by migration of cells from the primitive node. The notochordal process and adjacent mesoderm induce the overlying embryonic ectoderm to form the neural plate, the primordium of the central nervous system. Observe that, as the notochordal process elongates, the primitive streak shortens. At the end of the third week the notochordal process is transformed into the notochord (see Figs. 4–5 and 4–6). Note that the embryonic disc is originally egg-shaped but soon becomes pear-shaped and then slipperlike as the notochord develops.

invagination (a turning inward) of epiblastic cells (see arrows in Fig. 4–1).

Shortly after the primitive streak appears, cells leave its deep surface and form a loose network of embryonic connective tissue called *mesenchyme* or mesoblast (Fig. 4–2*A*). It forms the supporting tissues of the embryo; e.g., most connective tissues of the body and the stromal components of all glands. Some mesenchymal tissue forms a layer known as the **intraembryonic mesoderm** (Fig. 4–1*B*). Some cells from the primitive streak also displace the hypoblast and form the **intraembryonic endoderm**. As soon as the primitive streak begins to produce intraembryonic mesoderm, the epiblast is referred to as the **intraembryonic ectoderm.** Under the influence of various embryonic growth factors (Slack, 1987; Tabin, 1991), the mesenchymal cells leaving the primitive streak migrate widely and have the potential to proliferate and differentiate into diverse types of cells; e.g., fibroblasts, chondroblasts, and osteoblasts. In summary, cells of the epiblast, through the process of gas-

trulation, give rise to all three germ layers in the embryo, which are the primordia of all tissues and organs.

Fate of the Primitive Streak. The primitive streak actively forms intraembryonic mesoderm until the end of the fourth week; thereafter, production of mesoderm and mesenchyme slows down. The primitive streak diminishes in relative size and becomes an insignificant structure in the sacrococcygeal region of the embryo (Fig. 4–3*D*). Normally the primitive streak undergoes degenerative changes and disappears.

Remnants of the primitive node may persist and give rise to a tumor known as a *sacrococcygeal teratoma* (Fig. 4–4). As they are derived from pleuripotent primitive streak cells, these tumors contain various types of tissue containing elements of the three germ layers in incomplete stages of differentiation. Sacrococcygeal teratoma is the most common tumor in the newborn period and has an incidence of about 1 in 35,000 to 40,000 newborns (Holzgreve et al., 1991).

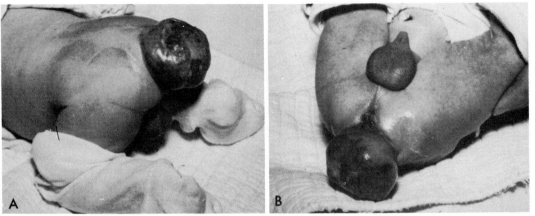

Figure 4–4. Photographs of an infant with a large sacrococcygeal teratoma, probably of primitive streak origin. These tumors are more common in females than in males, and they often become malignant during infancy. (Courtesy of Dr. Jan Hoogstraten, Children's Centre, Winnipeg, Canada.)

The Notochordal Process and Notochord

Some mesenchymal cells migrate cranially from the primitive node and form a median cellular cord known as the **notochordal process** (Fig. 4–1*C* and *E*). It soon acquires a lumen known as the *notochordal canal*. This process grows cranially between the ectoderm and endoderm until it reaches the *prochordal (prechordal) plate*, a small, circular area of columnar endodermal cells (see Figs. 3–5*C*, 4–3*B*, and 4–5). The hollow, rodlike, notochordal process can extend no farther because the prochordal plate is firmly attached to the overlying ectoderm. These fused germ layers form the *oropharyngeal membrane* located at the future site of the mouth (Fig. 4–6*C*).

Some mesenchymal cells from the primitive streak and notochordal process migrate laterally and cranially between the ectoderm and mesoderm until they reach the margins of the embryonic disc. There, these cells are continuous with the extraembryonic mesoderm covering the amnion and yolk sac (Fig. 4–1*D*). Most extraembryonic mesoderm is derived from the cytotrophoblast (see Chapter 3), but, as in other mammals, some arises from the primitive streak (Luckett, 1978). Some cells from the primitive streak migrate cranially on each side of the notochordal process and around the prochordal plate. Here, they meet cranially to form *cardiogenic mesoderm* in the **cardiogenic area** (Fig. 4–1*E*) where the heart (Gr. *kardia*) begins to develop at the end of the third week (p. 65).

Caudal to the primitive streak there is a circular area known as the *cloacal membrane*, which indicates the future site of the anus (Figs. 4–3 and 4–5*E*). The embryonic disc remains bilaminar here and at the *oropharyngeal membrane* because the embryonic ec-toderm and endoderm are fused at these sites, thereby preventing migration of mesenchymal cells between them. By the middle of the third week, intraembryonic mesoderm separates the ectoderm and endoderm everywhere except: (1) at the oropharyngeal membrane cranially, (2) in the median plane cranial to the primitive node where the notochordal process extends, and (3) at the cloacal membrane caudally.

Formation of the Notochord. (Figs. 4–3 and 4–6). The notochord is a cellular rod that develops by transformation of the notochordal process. *The notochord defines the primitive axis of the embryo* and gives it some rigidity. It also indicates the future site of the vertebral column. The notochord develops as follows:

1. As the notochordal process elongates, the primitive pit extends into it, forming a *notochordal canal* (Fig. 4–5*B* to *E*). The notochordal process is now a tubular column of cells that extends cranially from the primitive node to the prochordal plate.

2. The floor of the notochordal process fuses with the underlying embryonic endoderm.

3. The fused regions gradually undergo degeneration, resulting in the formation of openings in the floor of the notochordal process. They bring the notochordal canal into communication with the yolk sac (Fig. 4–6*B*).

4. The openings rapidly become confluent and the notochordal canal disappears (Fig. 4–6*C*). The primitive pit persists for a while as the *neurenteric canal*. The remains of the notochordal process form a flattened, grooved plate known as the *notochordal plate* (Fig. 4–6*D*).

5. Beginning at the cranial end, the notochordal cells proliferate and the notochordal plate infolds to form the *notochord* (Fig. 4–6*F* and *G*).

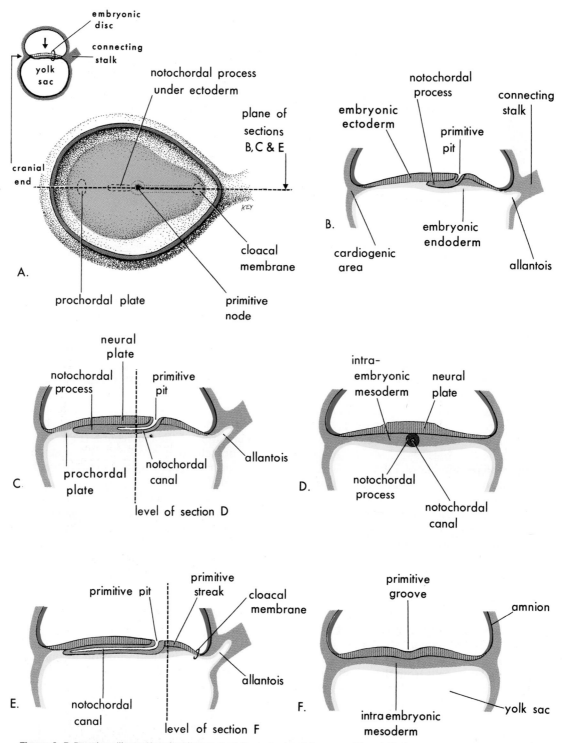

Figure 4–5. Drawings illustrating development of the notochordal process. The small sketch at the upper left is for orientation; the short arrow indicates the dorsal aspect of the embryonic disc. *A*, Dorsal view of the embryonic disc (about 16 days) exposed by removal of the amnion. The notochordal process is shown as if it were visible through the embryonic ectoderm. *B, C,* and *E*, Median sections, at the plane shown in *A*, illustrating successive stages in the development of the notochordal process and canal. Stages shown in *C* and *E* occur at about 18 days. *D* and *F*, Transverse sections through the embryonic disc at the levels shown.

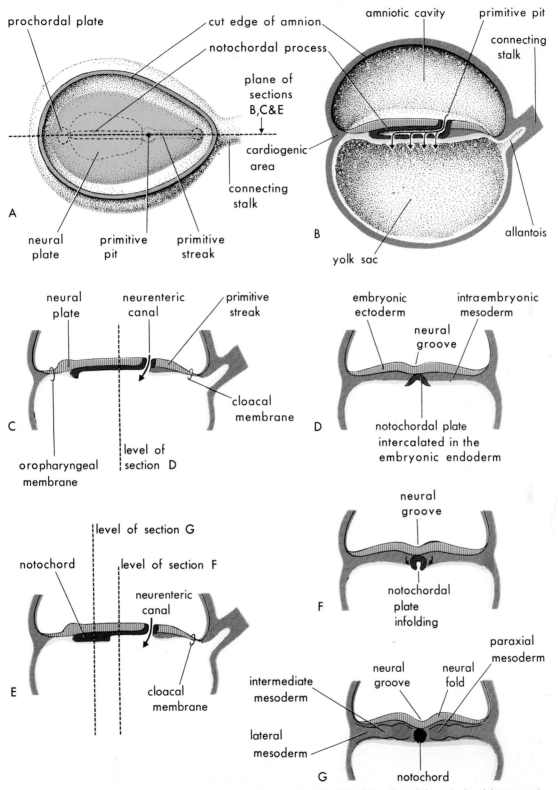

Figure 4–6. Drawings illustrating development of the notochord by transformation of the notochordal process. *A*, Dorsal view of the embryonic disc (about 18 days) exposed by removing the amnion. *B*, Three-dimensional median section of the embryo. *C* and *E*, Similar sections of slightly older embryos. *D*, *F*, and *G*, Transverse sections of the trilaminar embryonic disc.

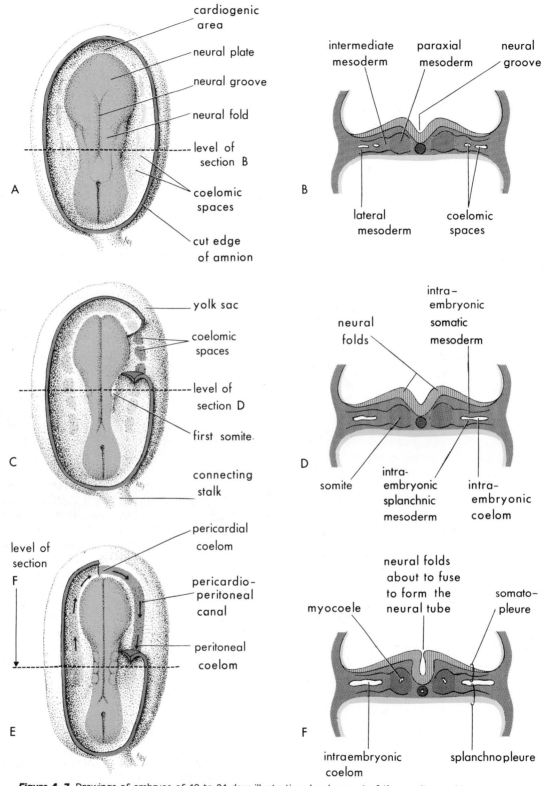

Figure 4–7. Drawings of embryos of 19 to 21 days illustrating development of the somites and intraembryonic coelom. A, C, and E, Dorsal view of the embryo exposed by removal of the amnion. B, D, and F, Transverse sections through the embryonic disc at the levels shown. A, Presomite embryo of about 18 days. C, An embryo of about 20 days showing the first pair of somites. A portion of the somatopleure on the right has been removed to show the isolated coelomic spaces in the lateral mesoderm. E, A three-somite embryo (about 21 days) showing the horseshoe-shaped intraembryonic coelom exposed on the right by removal of a portion of the somatopleure.

6. The notochord becomes detached from the embryonic endoderm, which again becomes a continuous layer that forms the roof of the yolk sac (Figs. 4–6*G* and 4–7*B*, *D*, and *F*).

Fate of the Notochord. The notochord is the structure around which the vertebral column forms (see Chapter 15). It extends from the oropharyngeal membrane to the primitive node. The notochord degenerates and disappears as the vertebral bodies form, but it persists as the *nucleus pulposus* of each intervertebral disc (see Fig. 15–5). The developing notochord induces the overlying ectoderm to form the neural plate (Figs. 4–3, 4–5, and 4–8), the primordium of the central nervous system. A small passage, the *neurenteric canal*, temporarily connects the amniotic cavity and the yolk sac (Fig. 4–6*C* and *E*). When development of the notochord is complete, the neurenteric canal normally obliterates.

In very uncommon cases the neurenteric canal persists, giving rise to a congenital anomaly in which the central canal of the spinal cord is connected to the lumen of the intestine, a derivative of the cavity of the yolk sac (see Fig. 5–1). In addition, both benign and malignant tumors arising from human notochordal tissue have been reported (Horowitz, 1977).

THE ALLANTOIS

The allantois (Gr. *allas*, sausage) appears on about day 16 as a small, sausagelike diverticulum (outpouching) from the caudal wall of the yolk sac and extends into the connecting stalk (Fig. 4–5*B*, *C*, and *E*). The allantois in embryos of reptiles, birds, and some mammals has a respiratory function and/or acts as a reservoir for urine during embryonic life. The allantois remains very small in human embryos but is involved with early blood formation and associated with development of the urinary bladder (see Fig. 13–9). As the bladder enlarges, the allantois becomes the urachus and is represented in adults as the *median umbilical ligament* (see Fig. 13–16 for urachal malformations). The blood vessels of the allantois become the umbilical arteries and veins.

Allantoic cysts, remnants of the extraembryonic portion of the allantois, are usually found between the fetal umbilical vessels and can be detected by sonography. They are most commonly detected in the proximal part of the umbilical cord, near its insertion in the ventral abdominal wall.

NEURULATION

The processes involved in the formation of the neural plate and neural folds and the closure of these folds to form the neural tube is called neurulation. These processes are completed by the end of the fourth week when closure of the caudal neuropore occurs (see Fig. 5–8). During neurulation, the embryo may be referred to as a *neurula*.

The Neural Plate and Neural Tube

As the notochord develops, the embryonic ectoderm over it thickens to form the *neural plate* (Figs. 4–3 and 4–5 to 4–8). Neural plate formation is induced by the developing notochord. The ectoderm of the neural plate, called neuroectoderm, gives rise to the **central nervous system (CNS)**, which consists of the brain and spinal cord. Neuroectoderm also gives rise to various other structures (see Fig. 5–5).

The elongated neural plate at first corresponds precisely in length to the underlying notochord; thus, it appears cranial to the primitive node and dorsal to the notochord and the mesoderm adjacent to it (Fig. 4–3*B*). As the notochord elongates, the neural plate broadens and eventually extends cranially as far as the oropharyngeal membrane (Figs. 4–3*C* and 4–6*C*). Eventually, it extends beyond the notochord. On about the eighteenth day, the neural plate invaginates along its central axis to form a longitudinal median *neural groove* that has neural folds on each side of it (Figs. 4–3*D* and 4–6 to 4–8). The *neural folds* become particularly prominent at the cranial end of the embryo. These enlarged neural folds are the *first signs of brain development* (Fig. 4–7*A*).

The Neural Tube. By the end of the third week, the *neural folds* have begun to move together and fuse, converting the neural plate into a neural tube (Figs. 4–7*F* and 4–8*D*). Neural tube formation is a complex, multifactorial process involving extrinsic forces (Smith and Schoenwolf, 1991). The neural tube has openings at its cranial and caudal ends called the rostral and caudal *neuropores*, respectively (see Fig. 5–8*A*). The neural tube soon separates from the surface ectoderm. The free edges of the surface ectoderm fuse so that this layer becomes continuous over the neural tube and back of the embryo (Fig. 4–8*D*). Subsequently, the surface ectoderm differentiates into the epidermis of the skin. Neurulation is completed during the fourth week when the cranial and caudal neuropores close (see Fig. 5–8).

The Neural Crest

As the neural folds fuse to form the neural tube, some neuroectodermal cells lying along the crest of each neural fold lose their epithelial affinities and attachments to neighboring cells (Fig. 4–8). As the neural tube separates from the surface ectoderm,

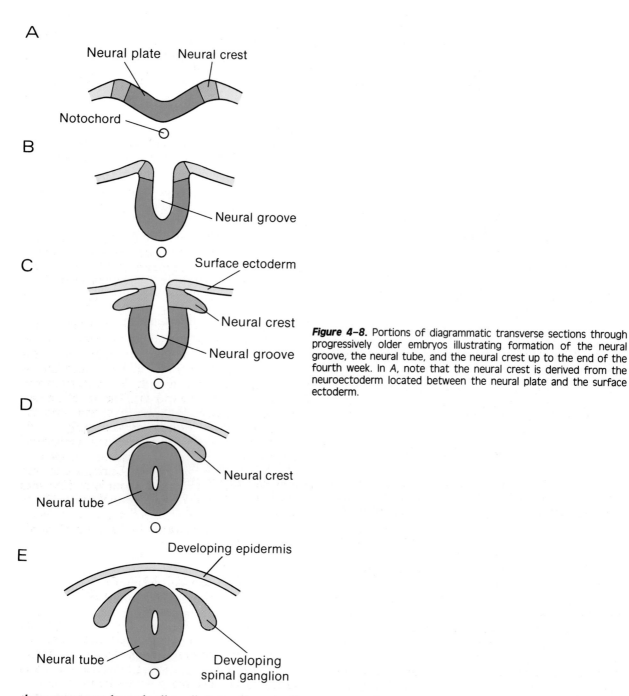

Figure 4-8. Portions of diagrammatic transverse sections through progressively older embryos illustrating formation of the neural groove, the neural tube, and the neural crest up to the end of the fourth week. In *A*, note that the neural crest is derived from the neuroectoderm located between the neural plate and the surface ectoderm.

these neuroectodermal cells, called **neural crest cells**, migrate ventrolaterally on each side of the neural tube. They soon form an irregular flattened mass, called the **neural crest**, between the neural tube and the overlying surface ectoderm. The neural crest soon separates into right and left parts that migrate to the dorsolateral aspects of the neural tube where they give rise to the sensory ganglia of the spinal and cranial nerves. Many neural crest cells migrate in lateral and ventral directions and disperse within the mesenchyme. Although these cells are difficult to identify, special tracer techniques have revealed that they disseminate widely and have important derivatives.

Derivatives of the Neural Crest (see Figs. 5–5 and 18–8). Neural crest cells give rise to the spinal ganglia (dorsal root ganglia) and the ganglia of the autonomic nervous system. The ganglia of cranial nerves V, VII, IX, and X are also partly derived from neural crest cells. In addition to forming ganglion cells, neural crest cells form the sheaths of nerves (Schwann cells) and the meningeal covering of the brain and spinal cord (at least the pia mater and arachnoid). They also contribute to the formation of pigment cells, the suprarenal (adrenal) medulla, and several skeletal and muscular components in the head (see Chapter 10).

Congenital Anomalies Resulting From Abnormal Neurulation

Because the neural plate, primordium of the CNS, appears during the third week and gives rise to neural folds and the beginning of the neural tube, disturbance of neurulation may result in severe abnormalities of the brain and spinal cord (see Figs. 18–12D and 18–15 to 18–18). *Neural tube defects* (NTDs) are among the most common congenital anomalies (Filly, 1991). The incidence of these anomalies has been estimated to be as high as 16 per 10,000 births in the eastern United States (Greenberg et al., 1983). *Meroanencephaly* (*anencephaly*), or partial absence of the brain, is the most severe defect and is also the most common anomaly affecting the CNS. Available evidence suggests that the primary disturbance (e.g., a teratogenic drug; see Chapter 8) affects the neuroectoderm, resulting in failure of the neural folds to fuse and form the neural tube in the brain and/or spinal cord regions. This results in meroanencephaly (p. 412) and *spina bifida cystica* (p. 395).

DEVELOPMENT OF SOMITES

As the notochord and neural tube form, the intraembryonic mesoderm on each side of them proliferates to form a thick, longitudinal column of *paraxial mesoderm* (Fig. 4–6G). Each column is continuous laterally with the *intermediate mesoderm*, which gradually thins laterally into a layer of *lateral mesoderm*. The lateral mesoderm is continuous with the extraembryonic mesoderm covering the yolk sac and amnion. Toward the end of the third week, the paraxial mesoderm differentiates and begins to divide into paired cuboidal bodies called **somites** (Gr. *soma*, body). These blocks of mesoderm are located on each side of the developing neural tube and notochord (Fig. 4–7C to E). About 38 pairs of somites form during the *somite period of development* (days 20 to 30).

By the end of the fifth week, 42 to 44 pairs are present. The somites form distinct surface elevations on the embryo (see Figs. 4–7E and 5–9) and are somewhat triangular in transverse section. A slitlike cavity, the myocoele, appears within each somite (Fig. 4–7F), but it is unimportant and soon disappears. Because the somites are so prominent during the fourth and fifth weeks, they are used as one of the

criteria for determining an embryo's age (see Table 5–1).

The somites first appear in the future occipital region of the embryo. They soon appear craniocaudally and give rise to most of the *axial skeleton* (the bones of the head, neck, and trunk) and associated musculature, as well as to the adjacent dermis of the skin (see Chapters 15 and 20). The first pair of somites appears at the end of the third week (Fig. 4–7C) a short distance caudal to the cranial end of the notochord. Subsequent pairs form in a craniocaudal sequence.

DEVELOPMENT OF THE INTRAEMBRYONIC COELOM

The intraembryonic coelom (cavity) first appears as small, isolated, *coelomic spaces* in the lateral mesoderm and the cardiogenic (heart-forming) mesoderm (Fig. 4–7A and B). These spaces soon coalesce to form a single horseshoe-shaped cavity in the mesoderm called the *intraembryonic coelom* (Fig. 4–7E). The intraembryonic coelom divides the lateral mesoderm into two layers (Fig. 4–7D): a somatic or *parietal layer* continuous with the extraembryonic mesoderm covering the amnion and a splanchnic or *visceral layer* continuous with the extraembryonic mesoderm covering the yolk sac. The somatic mesoderm and overlying embryonic ectoderm form the embryonic body wall or *somatopleure* (Fig. 4–7F) whereas the splanchnic mesoderm and embryonic endoderm form the embryonic gut wall or *splanchnopleure* (wall of primitive gut). During the second month, the intraembryonic coelom is divided into three body cavities: (1) the *pericardial cavity*, (2) the *pleural cavities*, and (3) the *peritoneal cavity*. For a description of these divisions of the intraembryonic coelom, see Chapter 9.

EARLY DEVELOPMENT OF THE CARDIOVASCULAR SYSTEM

At the beginning of the third week, angiogenesis (Gr. *angeion*, vessel, + *genesis*, production), or blood vessel formation, begins in the extraembryonic mesoderm covering the yolk sac, connecting stalk, and chorion. Embryonic blood vessels begin to develop about two days later. The early formation of the cardiovascular system is correlated with the absence of a significant amount of yolk in the ovum and yolk sac and the consequent urgent need for blood vessels to bring nourishment and oxygen to the embryo from the maternal circulation via the placenta (Fig. 4–10). At the end of the second week embryonic nutrition is obtained from the maternal blood by diffusion

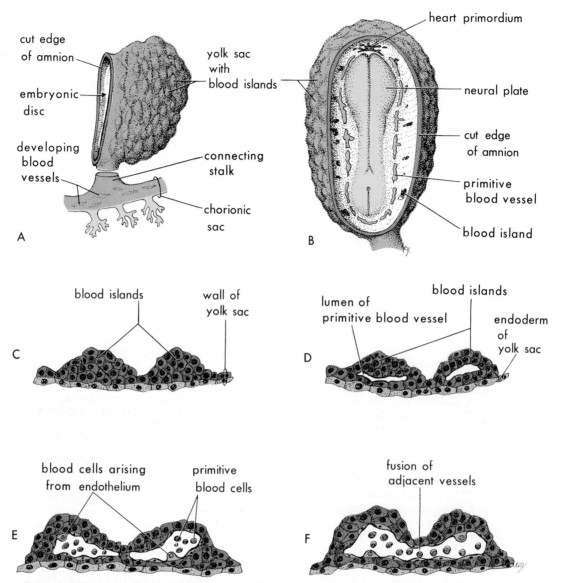

Figure 4–9. Successive stages in the development of blood and blood vessels. *A,* The yolk sac and a portion of the chorionic sac (about 18 days). *B,* Dorsal view of the embryo exposed by removing the amnion. *C to F,* Sections of blood islands showing progressive stages in the development of blood and blood vessels.

through the extraembryonic coelom and yolk sac. During the third week a primitive placental circulation develops (Figs. 4–10 and 4–11).

Angiogenesis and Hematogenesis

Blood vessel and blood formation in the embryo and extraembryonic membranes during the third week may be summarized as follows (Fig. 4–9):

1. Mesenchymal cells known as *angioblasts* aggregate to form isolated angiogenic cell clusters known as **blood islands**. Small cavities appear within the blood islands by confluence of intercellular clefts.

2. Angioblasts flatten to form *endothelial cells* that arrange themselves around these cavities and form the primitive endothelium.

3. These endothelial-lined cavities soon fuse to form networks of endothelial channels.

4. Vessels extend into adjacent areas by endothelial budding and fusion with other vessels.

Primitive Blood Cells and Plasma. Blood develops from endothelial cells as the vessels develop on the

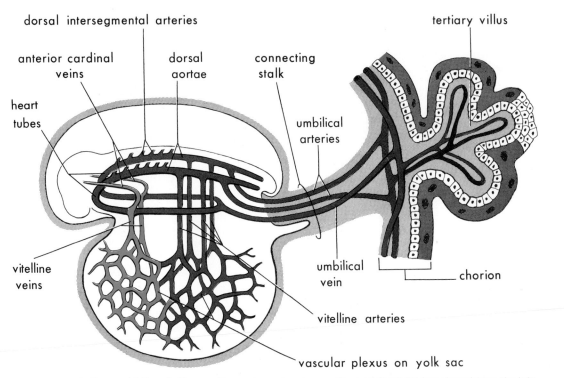

Figure 4–10. Diagram of the primitive cardiovascular system in an embryo of about 20 days viewed from the left side. Observe the transitory stage of paired symmetrical vessels. Each heart tube continues dorsally into a dorsal aorta that passes caudally. Branches of the aortae are: (1) umbilical arteries establishing connections with vessels in the chorion, (2) vitelline arteries to the yolk sac, and (3) dorsal intersegmental arteries to the body of the embryo. An umbilical vein returns blood from the chorion and divides into right and left umbilical veins within the embryo. Vessels on the yolk sac form a vascular plexus that is connected to the heart tubes by vitelline veins. The anterior cardinal veins return blood from the head region. The umbilical vein is shown in red to indicate that it carries oxygenated blood and nutrients from the chorion (embryonic part of the placenta to the embryo). The arteries are colored medium red to indicate that they are carrying partially deoxygenated blood and waste products to the chorionic villi.

yolk sac and allantois at the end of the third week (Fig. 4–9E). Blood formation does not begin in the embryo until the fifth week. It occurs first in various parts of the embryonic mesenchyme, chiefly the liver, and later in the spleen, bone marrow, and lymph nodes. The mesenchymal cells surrounding the primitive endothelial blood vessels differentiate into the muscular and connective tissue elements of the vessels. (For more details, see Schwartz et al., 1990 and Navaratnam, 1991).

The Primitive Cardiovascular System. The heart and great vessels form from mesenchymal cells in the cardiogenic area (Figs. 4–6B and 4–9B). Paired, longitudinal, endothelial-lined channels called *endothelial heart tubes* develop before the end of the third week and begin to fuse into a primitive **heart tube** (see Fig. 14–6). By the end of the third week, the endothelial heart tubes have fused to form a single, tubular heart, which is joined to blood vessels in the embryo, connecting stalk, chorion, and yolk sac to form a primitive cardiovascular system (Fig. 4–10). By the end of the third week, the blood is circulating, and the heart begins to beat on the twenty-first or twenty-second day (about five weeks after LNMP). The cardiovascular system is thus the first organ system to reach a functional state. The embryonic heartbeat can be detected ultrasonographically with a Doppler during the fifth week (seven weeks after LNMP).

DEVELOPMENT OF CHORIONIC VILLI

Shortly after the *primary chorionic villi* appear at the end of the second week (see Fig. 3–6), they begin to branch. Early in the third week, mesenchyme grows into the primary villi, forming a core of loose connective tissue. The villi at this stage (called *secondary chorionic villi*) cover the entire surface of the chorionic sac (Fig. 4–11A and B). Soon, some mesenchymal cells in the villi differentiate into blood capillaries, which fuse to form arteriocapillary venous networks (embryos 15 to 20 days old).

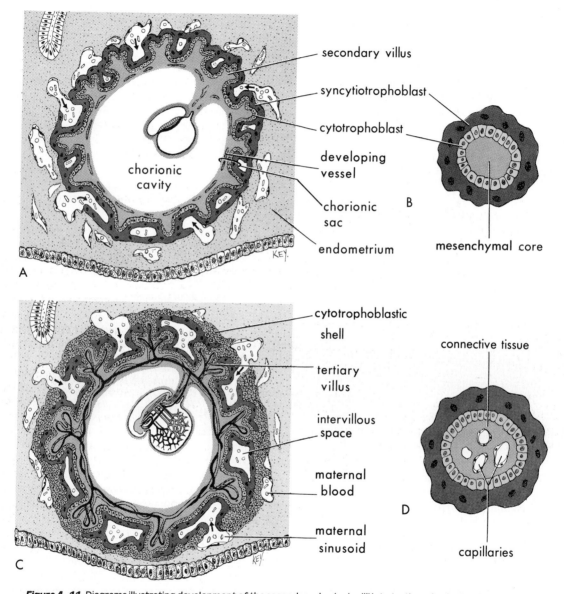

secondary villus

syncytiotrophoblast

cytotrophoblast

developing vessel

chorionic sac

endometrium

chorionic cavity

mesenchymal core

B

cytotrophoblastic shell

tertiary villus

intervillous space

maternal blood

maternal sinusoid

connective tissue

capillaries

D

Figure 4–11. Diagrams illustrating development of the secondary chorionic villi into tertiary chorionic villi. Formation of the placenta is also shown. *A*, Sagittal section of an embryo (about 16 days). *B*, Section of a secondary chorionic villus. *C*, Section of an implanted embryo (about 21 days). *D*, Section of a tertiary chorionic villus. The fetal blood in the capillaries is separated from the maternal blood surrounding the villus by the placental membrane composed of the endothelium of the capillary, mesenchyme, cytotrophoblast, and syncytiotrophoblast.

After blood vessels have developed in the villi, they are called *tertiary chorionic villi* or stem villi (Figs. 4–10 and 4–11*D*). The vessels in these **stem villi** soon become connected with the embryonic heart via vessels that differentiate in the mesenchyme of the chorion and connecting stalk (Fig. 4–10). By the end of the third week, embryonic blood begins to flow slowly through the capillaries in the chorionic villi. Oxygen and nutrients in the maternal blood in the intervillous space diffuse through the walls of the villi (*placental membranes*) and enter the embryo's blood. Carbon dioxide and waste products diffuse from blood in the fetal capillaries through the walls of the villi into the maternal blood.

Concurrently, cytotrophoblast cells of the chorionic villi proliferate and extend through the syncytiotrophoblastic layer to form a **cytotrophoblastic shell** (Fig. 4–11*C*), which attaches the chorionic sac to the endometrium. Villi that are attached to the maternal tissues via the cytotrophoblastic shell are called *stem villi* (anchoring villi). The villi that grow from the sides of the stem villi are called *branch villi*, and it is through them that the main exchange of material between the blood of the mother and the embryo takes place (see Chapter 7).

Abnormal Growth of the Trophoblast. Sometimes the embryo dies and the chorionic villi do not complete their development; i.e., they do not become vascularized to form tertiary villi. Instead they form cystic swellings which resemble a bunch of grapes. They exhibit variable degrees of trophoblastic proliferation and are known as a *hydatiform mole*. Excessive amounts of hCG are produced. About two per cent of these moles develop into malignant, trophoblastic lesions called **choriocarcinomas**. Some of them follow spontaneous abortions and others occur after normal deliveries. Choriocarcinomas invariably metastasize (spread) by way of the bloodstream to various sites; e.g., the lungs and brain (Rubin and Farber, 1988).

SUMMARY OF THE THIRD WEEK OF HUMAN DEVELOPMENT

Major changes occur in the embryo as the bilaminar embryonic disc is converted into a trilaminar embryonic disc during a process known as **gastrulation**. These changes begin with the appearance of the primitive streak.

Primitive Streak Formation (Figs. 4–1 and 4–2) The primitive streak appears at the beginning of the third week as a thickening of the embryonic epiblast at the caudal end of the embryonic disc. It results from the migration of epiblastic cells to the median plane of the embryonic disc. Invagination of epiblastic cells from the primitive streak gives rise to mesenchymal cells that migrate ventrally, laterally, and cranially between the epiblast and hypoblast. As soon as the primitive streak begins to produce mesenchymal cells, the epiblast layer becomes known as the embryonic ectoderm and the hypoblast as the embryonic endoderm. The mesenchymal cells produced by the primitive streak soon organize into a third germ layer, the *intraembryonic mesoderm*. Cells from the primitive streak migrate to the edges of the embryonic disc where they join the *extraembryonic mesoderm* covering the amnion and yolk sac. By the end of the third week, mesoderm exists between the ectoderm and endoderm everywhere, except at the oropharyngeal membrane, in the median plane occupied by the notochord (a derivative of the notochordal process), and at the cloacal membrane.

Notochord Formation (Figs. 4–1, 4–3, 4–5, and 4–6). Early in the third week, mesenchymal cells arising from the primitive node of the primitive streak form the *notochordal process* which extends cranially from the primitive node as a rod of cells between the ectoderm and endoderm. The primitive pit extends into the notochordal process to form a *notochordal canal*. When fully developed, the notochordal process extends from the primitive node to the prochordal plate. Openings develop in the floor of the notochordal canal that soon coalesce, leaving a *notochordal plate*. The notochordal plate soon infolds to form the notochord. The notochord forms the primitive axis of the embryo around which the axial skeleton forms.

Neural Tube Formation (Figs. 4–3 and 4–5 to 4–8). The neural plate appears as a thickening of the embryonic ectoderm cranial to the primitive node. The *neural plate* is induced to form by the developing notochord and the mesenchyme adjacent to it. A longitudinal *neural groove* develops in the neural plate, which is flanked by *neural folds*. Fusion of the folds forms the neural tube. The process of neural plate formation and its infolding to form the *neural tube* is called neurulation.

Neural Crest Formation (Fig. 4–8). As the neural folds form and fuse to form the neural tube, neuroectodermal cells migrate ventrolaterally to form the neural crest between the surface ectoderm and the neural tube. The neural crest soon divides into two cell masses that give rise to the sensory ganglia of the cranial and spinal nerves. Other neural crest cells migrate from the neural tube and give rise to various other structures (see Figs. 5–5 and 18–8).

Somite Formation (Fig. 4–7). The mesoderm on each side of the notochord thickens to form longitudinal columns of paraxial mesoderm. Division of these paraxial mesodermal columns into pairs of somites begins cranially by the end of the third week. The somites are compact aggregates of mesenchymal cells from which cells migrate to give rise to the vertebrae, ribs, and axial musculature. During the third week, the number of somites present is a reliable indicator of the age of the embryo.

Intraembryonic Coelom Formation (Fig. 4–7). The coelom (cavity) within the embryo arises as isolated spaces in the lateral mesoderm and in the cardiogenic mesoderm. These coelomic spaces subsequently coalesce to form a single, horseshoe-shaped cavity that eventually gives rise to the body cavities (e.g., the peritoneal cavity).

Blood and Blood Vessel Formation (Figs. 4–9 and 4–10). Blood vessels first appear on the yolk sac, around the allantois, and in the chorion. They develop within the embryo shortly thereafter. Spaces, known as *blood islands*, appear within aggregations of mesenchyme, which soon become lined with endothelium derived from the mesenchymal cells. These primitive vessels unite with other vessels to form a *primitive cardiovascular system*. At the end of the third week, the heart is represented by paired endothelial heart tubes that are joined to blood vessels in the embryo and in the extraembryonic membranes (yolk sac, umbilical cord, and chorionic sac). The primitive blood cells are derived mainly from the endothelial cells of blood vessels in the walls of the yolk sac and allantois.

Chorionic Villi Formation (see Figs. 3–5 and 4–11). Primary chorionic villi become secondary chorionic villi as they acquire mesenchymal cores. Before the end of the third week, capillaries develop in the villi, transforming them into tertiary chorionic villi. Cytotrophoblastic extensions from these stem villi join to form a cytotrophoblastic shell that anchors the chorionic sac to the endometrium. The rapid development of chorionic villi during the third week greatly increases the surface area of the chorion for the exchange of nutrients and other substances between the maternal and embryonic circulations.

CLINICALLY ORIENTED QUESTIONS FOR PROBLEM-BASED LEARNING SESSIONS

1. A 30-year-old woman became pregnant two months after discontinuing use of birth control pills. About three weeks later she had an early spontaneous abortion. How do the hormones in these pills affect the ovarian and menstrual cycles? What might have caused the abortion? What would the physician likely have told this patient?

2. A 25-year-old woman with a history of regular menstrual cycles was five days overdue on menses. Due to mental distress related to the abnormal bleeding and the undesirability of a possible pregnancy, the doctor decided to do a menstrual extraction or uterine evacuation. The tissue removed was examined for evidence of a pregnancy. Would a highly sensitive radioimmune assay have detected pregnancy at this early stage? What findings would indicate an early pregnancy? How old would the products of conception be?

3. What major organ systems undergo early development during the third week? What severe congenital anomaly might result from teratological factors (Chapter 8) acting during this period of development?

4. A female infant was born with a large tumor situated between her rectum and sacrum. A diagnosis of *sacrococcygeal teratoma* was made and the mass was surgically removed. What is the probable embryological origin of this tumor? Explain why these tumors often contain various types of tissue derived from all three germ layers. Does an infant's sex make him or her more susceptible to the development of one of these tumors?

5. Is ultrasonography any value in assessing pregnancy during the third week? What structures might be recognizable? If a pregnancy test is negative, is it safe to assume that the woman is not pregnant? Could an extrauterine gestation be present?

The answers to these questions are given on page 459.

References and Suggested Reading

Amaya E, Musci TJ, Kirschner AW: Expression of a dominant negative mutant of the FGF receptor disrupts mesoderm formation in Xenopus embryos. *Cell 66*:257, 1991.

Beddington RSP: The origin of the foetal tissues during gastrulation in the rodent. *In* Johnson MH (ed): *Development In Mammals.* New York, Elsevier, 1983.

Bessis M: The blood cells and their formation. *In* Brachet J, Mirsky AE (eds): *The Cell,* vol. 5. New York, Academic Press, 1961.

Boué J, Boué A, Lazar P: Retrospective and prospective epidemiological studies of 1500 karyotyped spontaneous abortions. *Teratology 12*:11, 1975.

Carr DH: Chromosomes and abortion. *Adv Hum Genet 2*:201, 1971.

Cooke J: The early embryo and the formation of body pattern. *American Scientist 76*:35, 1988.

Filly RA: Ectopic pregnancy. *In* Callen PW (ed): *Ultrasonography in Obstetrics and Gynecology,* 2nd ed. Philadelphia, WB Saunders, 1988.

Filly RA: The fetus with a CNS Malformation: Ultrasound Evaluation. *In* Harrison MR, Golbus MS, Filly RA (eds): *The Unborn Patient. Prenatal Diagnosis and Treatment,* 2nd ed. Philadelphia, WB Saunders, 1991.

Gilbert SF: *Developmental Biology,* 3rd ed. Sunderland, Sinauer Associates, 1991.

Goldstein RB, Callen PW: Ultrasound evaluation of the fetal thorax and abdomen. *In* Callen PW (ed): *Ultrasonography in Obstetrics and Gynecology,* 2nd ed. Philadelphia, WB Saunders, 1988.

Greenberg F, James LM, Oakley GP: Estimates of birth prevalence rates of spina bifida in the United States from computer generated maps. *Am J Obstet Gynecol 145*:570, 1983.

Guthrie S: Horizontal and vertical pathways in neural induction. *Trends in Neurosciences 14*:123, 1991.

Hamilton WJ, Boyd JD: Development of the human placenta. *In* Philipp EE, Barnes J, Newton M (eds): *Scientific Foundations of Obstetrics and Gynecology.* London, William Heinemann, 1970.

Hertig AT: Angiogenesis in the early human chorion and in the primary placenta of the macaque monkey. *Contrib Embryol Carnegie Inst 25*:37, 1935.

Holzgreve W, Flake AW, Langer JC: The fetus with sacrococcygeal teratoma. *In* Harrison MR, Golbus MS, Filly RA (eds): *The Unborn Patient. Prenatal Diagnosis and Treatment,* 2nd ed. Philadelphia, WB Saunders, 1991.

Horowitz T: *The Human Notochord. A Study of Its Development and Regression, Variations and Pathogenic Derivative, Chordoma.* Indianapolis, Limited Private Printing, 1977.

Jacobson AG, Sater AK: Features of embryonic induction. *Development 104*:341, 1988.

Jacobson M: *Developmental Neurobiology,* 2nd ed. New York, Plenum Press, 1989.

Keller R, Danilchick M: Regional expression, pattern and timing of convergence and extension during gastrulation of *Xenopus laevis. Development 103*: 193, 1988.

Kratochwil K: Embryonic Induction. *In* Yamada KM (ed): *Cell Interactions and Development.* New York, John Wiley & Sons, 1982.

Kurtz AB, Needleman L: Ultrasound assessment of fetal age. *In:* Callen PW (ed): *Ultrasonography in Obstetrics and Gynecology,* 2nd ed. Philadelphia, WB Saunders, 1988, pp 47–64.

Luckett WP: Origin and differentiation of the yolk sac and extraembryonic mesoderm in presomite human and rhesus monkey embryos. *Am J Anat 152*:59, 1978.

Marx J: How embryos tell heads from tails. *Science 254*:1586, 1991.

Nahhas F, Barnea E: Human embryonic origin of early pregnancy factor before and after implantation. *Am J Reprod Immunol 22*:105, 1990.

Navaratnam V: Organization and reorganization of blood vessels in embryonic development. *Eye 5:(Pt.2)*:147, 1991.

Nieuwkoop PD, Albers B: The role of competence in the craniocaudal segregation of the central nervous system. *Develop Growth & Differ 32*:23, 1990.

O'Rahilly R: The manifestation of the axes of the human embryo. *Z Anat Entwicklungsgesch 132*:50, 1970.

O'Rahilly R, Müller F: *Developmental Stages in Human Embryos.* Washington, Carnegie Institute of Washington, 1987.

Placzek M, Tessier-Lavigne M, Yamada T, Jessell T, Dodd J: Mesodermal control of neural cell identity: floor plate induction by the notochord. *Science 250*:985, 1990.

Rohrer H: The role of growth factors in the control of neurogenesis. *Eur J Neurosci 2*:1005, 1990.

Rubin R, Farber JL: *Pathology.* Philadelphia, JB Lippincott Company, 1988.

Schoenwolf GC, Smith JL: Mechanisms of neurulation: traditional viewpoint and recent advances. *Development 109*:243, 1990.

Schwartz SM, Heimark RL, Majesky MW: Developmental mechanisms underlying pathology of arteries. *Physiol Rev 70*:117, 1990.

Slack JMW: We have a morphogen! *Nature 327*:553, 1987.

Smith JL, Schoenwolf GC: Further evidence of extrinsic forces in bending of the neural plate. *J Comp Neurol 307*:225, 1991.

Springer M: Die Canalis neurentericus beim Menschen. *Z Kinderchir 11*:183, 1972.

Tabin CJ: Retinoids, homeoboxes, and growth factors: Toward molecular models for limb development. *Cell 66*:199, 1991.

Taeusch HW, Ballard RB, Avery ME (eds): *Schaffer and Avery's Diseases of the Newborn,* 6th ed. Philadelphia, WB Saunders, 1991.

Weston JA: Regulation of neural crest cell migration and differentiation. *In* Yamada KM, (ed): *Cell Interactions and Development.* New York, John Wiley & Sons, 1982.

Wilson KM: A normal human ovum of 16 days development, the Rochester ovum. *Contrib Embryol Carnegie Inst 31*:103, 1945.

5

Development of Tissues, Organs, and Body Form

THE FOURTH TO EIGHTH WEEKS

These five weeks constitute most of the **embryonic period** (third to eighth weeks). The beginnings of all major external and internal structures are established during this time. By the end of this period, all the main organ systems have begun to develop but the function of most of them is minimal. As the organs form, the shape of the embryo changes; and, by the eighth week, the embryo has a distinctly human appearance.

PHASES OF DEVELOPMENT

Human development may be divided into three essential phases, which, to some extent, are interrelated. The first of these is *growth* (increase in size), which involves cell division and the elaboration of cell products. The second process is *morphogenesis* (development of form), which includes mass cell movements. Morphogenesis is an elaborate process during which many complex interactions occur in an orderly sequence (Cooke, 1988). The movement of cells allows them to interact with each other during the formation of tissues and organs. *Differentiation* is the third phase of development (maturation of physiological processes). Completion of this process results in the formation of tissues and organs that are able to perform specialized functions. Because the organ systems develop during the fourth to eighth weeks, exposure of embryos to **teratogens** during this period may cause major congenital defects. A teratogen is an agent (e.g., drugs and viruses) that produces or raises the incidence of congenital anomalies. They act during the stage of active differentiation of an organ or tissue (see Chapter 8).

FOLDING OF THE EMBRYO

A significant event in the establishment of body form is folding of the flat trilaminar embryonic disc into a somewhat cylindrical embryo. This folding occurs in both the median and horizontal planes and results from rapid growth of the embryo, particularly of its central nervous system (Fig. 5–1). The growth rate at the sides of the embryonic disc fails to keep pace with the rate of growth in the long axis as the embryo increases rapidly in length. As a result, folding of the embryo occurs. Folding at the cranial and caudal ends and at the sides occurs simultaneously. Concurrently, there is relative constriction at the junction of the embryo and the yolk sac (Fig. 5–1).

Folding of the Embryo in the Median Plane

Folding of the ends of the embryo ventrally produces head and tail folds that result in the cranial and caudal regions moving ventrally as if on hinges (Fig. 5–1A_2 to D_2).

The Head Fold (Figs. 5–1 and 5–2). By the end of the third week, the neural folds in the cranial region have thickened to form the primordium of the brain. Initially, the primitive brain projects dorsally into the amniotic cavity. Later, the developing forebrain grows cranially beyond the oropharyngeal membrane

---

Figure 5–1. Drawings of embryos during the fourth week illustrating folding in the median and horizontal planes. A_1, Dorsal view of an embryo at the beginning of the fourth week. The continuity of the intraembryonic coelom and extraembryonic coelom is illustrated on the right side by removal of a portion of the embryonic ectoderm and mesoderm (also see Fig. 5–3). B_1, C_1, and D_1, Lateral views of embryos at about 24, 26, and 28 days, respectively. A_2 to D_2, Longitudinal sections at the plane shown in A_1. A_3 to D_3, Transverse sections at the levels indicated in A_1 to D_1.

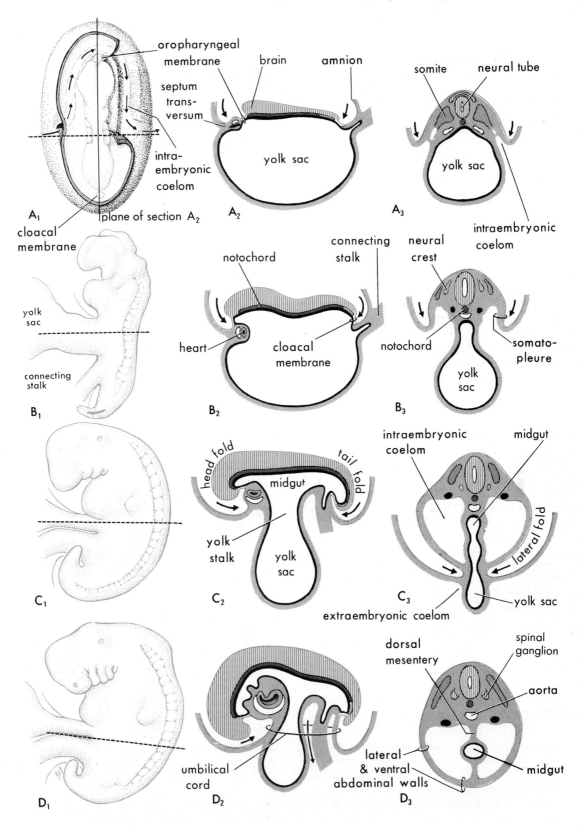

oropharyngeal membrane

brain

amnion

septum transversum

intraembryonic coelom

A_1

plane of section A_2

cloacal membrane

yolk sac

A_2

somite

neural tube

yolk sac

A_3

intraembryonic coelom

yolk sac

connecting stalk

B_1

notochord

connecting stalk

neural crest

heart

cloacal membrane

B_2

notochord

somatopleure

yolk sac

B_3

head fold

tail fold

midgut

intraembryonic coelom

midgut

C_1

yolk stalk

yolk sac

C_2

lateral fold

extraembryonic coelom

yolk sac

C_3

dorsal mesentery

spinal ganglion

aorta

umbilical cord

lateral & ventral abdominal walls

midgut

D_1

D_2

D_3

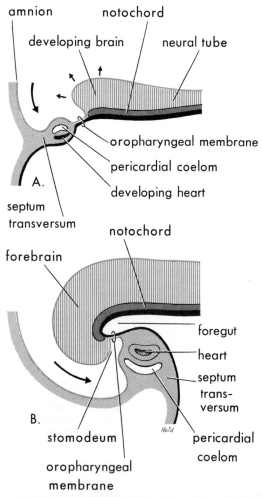

Figure 5–2. Drawings of longitudinal sections of the cranial region of embryos early and late during the fourth week showing the effect of the head fold on the position of the heart and other structures. *A*, Early in the fourth week (about 22 days). *B*, Later in the fourth week (about 26 days). Note that the septum transversum, heart, pericardial coelom, and oropharyngeal membrane turn under onto the ventral surface. Observe also that part of the yolk sac is incorporated into the embryo as the foregut.

and overhangs the developing heart. Concomitantly, the *septum transversum* (a transverse septum of mesoderm), primitive heart, pericardial coelom (cavity), and oropharyngeal membrane move onto the ventral surface of the embryo. During longitudinal folding, part of the yolk sac is incorporated into the embryo as the *foregut* (primordium of the pharynx, etc.; see Chapter 12). It lies between the caudal part of the brain and the heart (Fig. 5–2*B*). The oropharyngeal membrane separates the foregut from the *stomodeum* (primitive mouth or oral cavity). After folding, the septum transversum lies caudal to the heart where it subsequently develops into the *central tendon of the diaphragm* (see Fig. 9–7).

The head fold also affects the arrangement of the intraembryonic coelom (primordium of the body cavities). Before folding, the coelom consists of a flattened, horseshoe-shaped cavity (Fig. 5–1A_1). After folding, the pericardial coelom lies ventrally, and pericardioperitoneal canals run dorsally over the septum transversum and join the peritoneal coelom, a derivative of the intraembryonic coelom (Fig. 5–3*B*). At this stage, the peritoneal coelom communicates widely on each side with the extraembryonic coelom. The peritoneal coelom is the primordium of the peritoneal cavity (see Figs. 9–3 and 12–4*A*).

The Tail Fold (Figs. 5–1 and 5–4). Folding of the caudal end of the embryo results primarily from growth of the distal part of the neural tube (developing spinal cord). As the embryo grows, the tail region projects over the *cloacal membrane* (future site of the anus). During folding, part of the yolk sac is incorporated into the embryo as the *hindgut* (primordium of descending colon, etc.; see Chapter 12). The terminal part of the hindgut soon dilates slightly to form the *cloaca* (primordium of the urinary bladder and rectum; see Chapters 12 and 13). Before folding, the primitive streak lies cranial to the cloacal membrane (Fig. 5–4*A*); after folding, it lies caudal to this structure (Fig. 5–4*B*). After folding, the connecting stalk (primordium of the umbilical cord) is attached to the ventral surface of the embryo, and the *allantois* (p. 61) is partially incorporated into the embryo (Fig. 5–4*B*).

Folding of the Embryo in the Horizontal Plane

Folding of the sides of the embryo produces right and left *lateral folds* (Fig. 5–1A_3 to D_3). The primordium of each lateral body wall folds toward the median plane, rolling the edges of the embryonic disc ventrally and forming a roughly cylindrical embryo. As the abdominal walls form, part of the yolk sac is incorporated into the embryo as the *midgut* (primordium of the small intestine, etc.; see Chapter 12). Concurrently, the connection of the midgut with the yolk sac is reduced to a narrow *yolk stalk*. After folding, the region of attachment of the amnion to the ventral surface of the embryo is reduced to a relatively narrow umbilical region (Figs. 5–1C_2 and D_2 and 5–8*C*). As the *umbilical cord* forms from the connecting stalk, ventral fusion of the lateral folds reduces the region of communication between the intraembryonic and extraembryonic coeloms to a narrow communication (see long arrow in Fig. 5–1D_2). As the amniotic cavity expands and obliterates most of the extraembryonic coelom or chorionic cavity, the amnion forms the epithelial covering of the umbilical cord (Fig. 5–1D_2 and see Fig. 7–17).

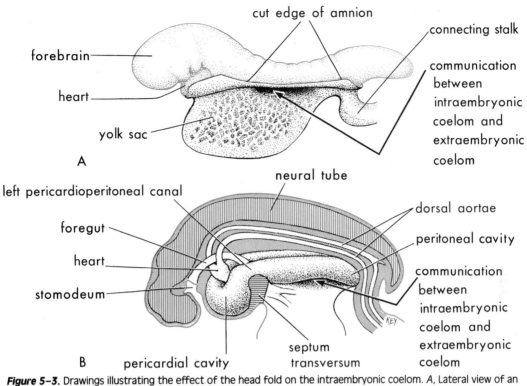

Figure 5-3. Drawings illustrating the effect of the head fold on the intraembryonic coelom. *A,* Lateral view of an embryo (24 to 25 days) during folding, showing: (1) the large forebrain, (2) the ventral position of the heart, and (3) the communication between the intraembryonic and extraembryonic parts of the coelom. *B,* Schematic drawing of an embryo (26 to 27 days) after folding, showing: (1) the pericardial cavity ventrally, (2) the pericardioperitoneal canals running dorsally on each side of the foregut, and (3) the peritoneal cavity (coelom) in communication with the extraembryonic coelom.

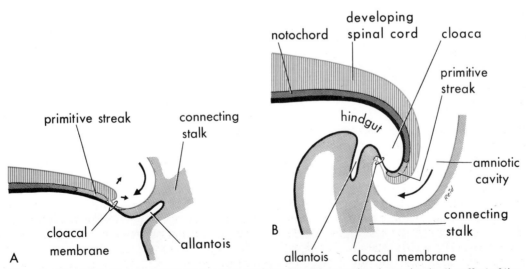

Figure 5-4. Drawings of longitudinal sections of the caudal region of four-week embryos showing the effect of the tail fold on the position of the cloacal membrane and other structures. *A,* Beginning of the fourth week. *B,* End of the fourth week. Note that part of the yolk sac is incorporated into the embryo as the hindgut and that the terminal part of the hindgut soon dilates to form the cloaca. Observe the change in position of the primitive streak, allantois, cloacal membrane, and connecting stalk.

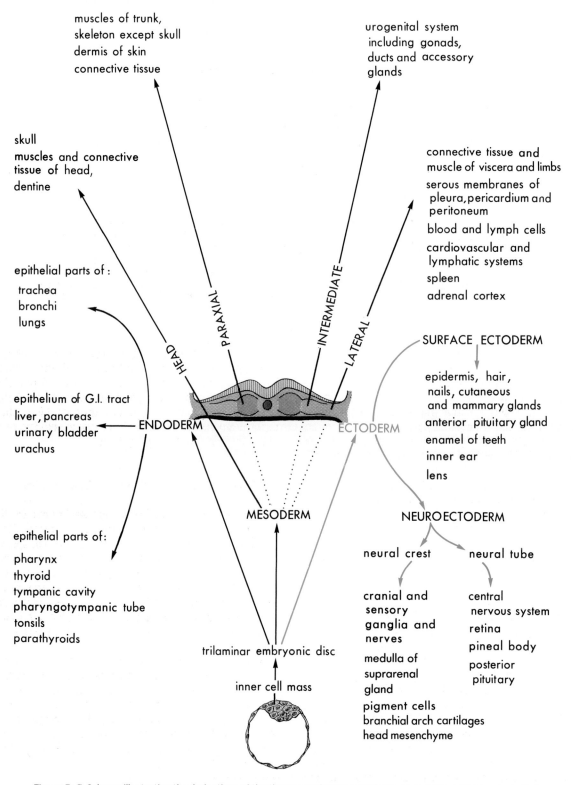

muscles of trunk,
skeleton except skull
dermis of skin
connective tissue

urogenital system
including gonads,
ducts and accessory
glands

skull
muscles and connective
tissue of head,
dentine

connective tissue and
muscle of viscera and limbs
serous membranes of
  pleura, pericardium and
  peritoneum
blood and lymph cells
cardiovascular and
  lymphatic systems
spleen
adrenal cortex

epithelial parts of :
  trachea
  bronchi
  lungs

PARAXIAL

INTERMEDIATE

LATERAL

HEAD

SURFACE ECTODERM

epidermis, hair,
nails, cutaneous
and mammary glands
anterior pituitary gland
enamel of teeth
inner ear
lens

epithelium of G.I. tract
liver, pancreas
urinary bladder
urachus

ENDODERM

ECTODERM

MESODERM

NEUROECTODERM

epithelial parts of:

pharynx
thyroid
tympanic cavity
pharyngotympanic tube
tonsils
parathyroids

neural crest

neural tube

cranial and
sensory
ganglia and
nerves

medulla of
suprarenal
gland

pigment cells
branchial arch cartilages
head mesenchyme

central
  nervous system
retina
pineal body
posterior
  pituitary

trilaminar embryonic disc

inner cell mass

Figure 5–5. Scheme illustrating the derivatives of the three germ layers: ectoderm, endoderm, and mesoderm. Cells from these layers make contributions to the formation of the different tissues and organs; e.g., the endoderm forms the epithelial lining of the gastrointestinal tract, and the mesoderm gives rise to its connective tissues and muscles.

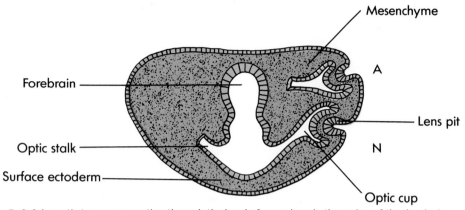

Figure 5-6. Schematic transverse section through the head of an embryo in the region of the developing eyes to illustrate inductive tissue interaction. At the normal site *N*, the optic cup and its precursor, the optic vesicle, have acted on the surface ectoderm of the head to induce formation of a lens pit, the primordium of the lens. On the opposite side, the optic stalk was cut and the optic vesicle removed. As a result, no lens placode (first indication of the lens) developed. At the abnormal site *A*, the optic vesicle removed from the right side was inserted deep to the skin. Here, along with the optic cup, it acted on the surface ectoderm to induce the formation of a lens pit.

GERM LAYER DERIVATIVES

The three germ layers (ectoderm, mesoderm, and endoderm) formed during gastrulation in the third week give rise to the primordia of all the tissues and organs during the fourth to eighth weeks (Fig. 5–5). The specificity of the germ layers, however, is not rigidly fixed. The cells of each germ layer divide, migrate, aggregate, and differentiate in rather precise patterns as they form the various organ systems (*organogenesis*). The main germ layer derivatives are as follows (Fig. 5–5).

Ectoderm. This layer gives rise to the central nervous system (brain and spinal cord), the peripheral nervous system, the sensory epithelia of the eye, ear, and nose, the epidermis and its appendages (hair and nails), the mammary glands, the cerebral hypophysis (pituitary gland), the subcutaneous glands, and the enamel of teeth. *Neural crest cells*, derived from neuroectoderm, give rise to the cells of the spinal, cranial (CNs V, VII, IX, and X), and autonomic ganglia; ensheathing cells of the peripheral nervous system; pigment cells of the dermis; muscle, connective tissues, and bone of branchial arch origin (see Chapter 10); the suprarenal (adrenal) medulla; and the meninges (coverings) of the brain and spinal cord.

Mesoderm. This layer gives rise to connective tissue, cartilage, bone, striated and smooth muscles, the heart, blood and lymph vessels and cells, the kidneys, ovaries and testes, the genital ducts, serous membranes lining the body cavities (pericardial, pleural, and peritoneal), the spleen, and the cortex of the suprarenal gland.

Endoderm. This layer gives rise to the epithelial lining of the gastrointestinal and respiratory tracts, the parenchyma of the tonsils, thyroid and parathyroid glands, thymus, liver, and pancreas, the epithelial lining of the urinary bladder and most of the urethra, and the epithelial lining of the tympanic cavity, tympanic antrum, and auditory tube.

CONTROL OF EMBRYONIC DEVELOPMENT[1]

Development results from genetic plans in the chromosomes. Knowledge of the genes or hereditary units that control human development is still sparse. Most information about developmental processes has come from studies in other organisms, especially *Drosophila* and mice, because of ethical problems associated with the use of human embryos for laboratory studies. For a discussion of the molecular genetics of mammalian development, see Thompson et al. (1991).

Most developmental processes depend upon a precisely coordinated interaction of genetic and environmental factors. Several control mechanisms guide differentiation and ensure synchronized development; e.g., tissue interactions, regulated migration of cells and cell colonies, controlled proliferation, and programmed cell death (England, 1990). Each system

[1] We are grateful to Dr. Michael Wiley, Associate Professor of Anatomy and Cell Biology, Faculty of Medicine, University of Toronto, for his assistance in preparing this section.

of the body has its own developmental pattern, but most processes of morphogenesis are similar and relatively simple. Underlying all these changes are basic regulating mechanisms (Cooke, 1988). *Embryonic development is essentially a process of growth and increasing complexity of structure and function.* Growth is achieved by mitosis together with the production of extracellular matrices; whereas, complexity is achieved through morphogenesis and differentiation.

The cells that make up the tissues of very early embryos are pleuripotential, which under different circumstances are able to follow more than one pathway of development. This broad developmental potential becomes progressively restricted as tissues acquire the specialized features necessary for increasing their sophistication of structure and function. Such restriction presumes that choices must be made in order to achieve tissue diversification. At present, most evidence indicates that these choices are determined not as a consequence of cell lineage but, rather, in response to cues from the immediate surroundings, including the adjacent tissues. As a result, the architectural precision and coordination that are often required for the normal function of an organ appear to be achieved by the interaction of its constituent parts during development.

The interaction of tissues during development is a recurring theme in embryology (Guthrie, 1991). The interactions that lead to a change in the course of development of at least one of the interactants are termed *inductions*. Numerous examples of such inductive interactions can be found in the literature; for example, during development of the eye, the optic vesicle is believed to induce the development of the lens from the surface ectoderm of the head. When the optic vesicle is absent, the eye fails to develop (Fig. 5–6). Moreover, if the optic vesicle is removed and placed in association with surface ectoderm that is not usually involved in eye development, lens formation can be induced. Clearly then, development of a lens is dependent on the ectoderm acquiring an association with a second tissue. In the presence of the neuroectoderm of the optic vesicle, the surface ectoderm of the head adopts a pathway of development that it would not otherwise have taken. In a similar fashion, many of the morphogenetic tissue movements that play such important roles in shaping the embryo also provide for the changing tissue associations fundamental to inductive tissue interactions.

The fact that one tissue can influence the developmental pathway adopted by another tissue presumes that a signal passes between the two interactants. The precise nature of the signal is not known; however,

the mechanism of signal transfer appears to vary with the specific tissues involved. In some cases, the signal appears to take the form of a diffusible molecule, such as retinoic acid (Eichele, 1990; Ruberte et al., 1990), that passes from the inductor to the reacting tissue (Fig. 5–7A). In others, the message appears to be mediated through a nondiffusible, extracellular matrix secreted by the inductor and with which the reacting tissue comes into contact (Fig. 5–7B). In still other cases, the signal appears to require that physical contacts occur between the inducing and responding tissues (Fig. 5–7C). Regardless of the mechanism of intercellular transfer involved, the signal is translated into an intracellular message that influences the genetic activity of the responding cells.

Laboratory studies have established that the signal can be relatively nonspecific in some interactions. Under experimental conditions, the role of the natural inductor in a variety of interactions has been shown to be mimicked by a number of heterologous tissue sources and, in some instances, even by a variety of cell-free preparations. These studies suggest that the specificity of a given induction is a property of the reacting tissue rather than of the inductor. Inductions should not be thought of as isolated phenomena. Often they occur in a sequential fashion that results in the orderly development of a complex structure; for example, following induction of the lens by the optic vesicle, the lens induces the development of the cornea from the surface ectoderm and adjacent mesenchyme. This ensures the formation of component parts appropriate in size and relationship for the function of the organ. In other systems, there is evidence that the interactions between tissues are reciprocal. During development of the kidney, for instance, the ureteric bud induces the formation of tubules in the metanephric mesoderm (see Chapter 13). This mesoderm, in turn, induces branching of the ureteric bud that results in the development of the collecting tubules and calices of the kidney.

The ability of the reacting system to respond to an inducing stimulus is not unlimited. Most inducible tissues appear to pass through a transient, but more or less sharply delimited, physiological state in which they are competent to respond to an inductive signal from the neighboring tissue. Because this state of receptiveness is limited in time, a delay in the development of one or more components in an interacting system may lead to failure of an inductive interaction. Regardless of the signal mechanism employed, inductive systems seem to have the common feature of close proximity between the interacting tissues. Experimental evidence has demonstrated that interactions may fail if the interactants are too widely sepa-

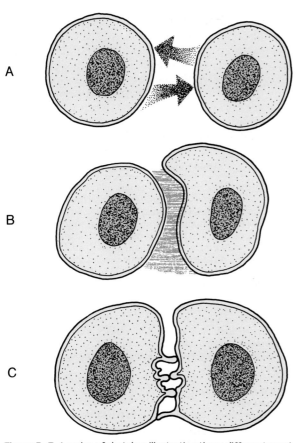

Figure 5–7. A series of sketches illustrating three different possible methods of transmission of signal substances in inductive cell interactions. *A*, Diffusion of signal substances. The signal appears to take the form of a diffusible molecule that passes from the inductor to the reacting tissue. *B*, Matrix-mediated interaction. The signal is mediated through a nondiffusible, extracellular matrix secreted by the inductor with which the reacting tissue comes in contact. *C*, Cell contact-mediated interaction. The signal requires physical contact between the inducing and responding tissues. (Modified from Grobstein C: *Adv Cancer Res 4*:187, 1956, and Saxen L: *In* Tarin D (ed): *Tissue Interactions in Carcinogenesis.* London, Academic Press, 1972.)

rated. Consequently, inductive processes appear to be limited in space as well as by time. Because tissue induction plays such a fundamental role in ensuring the orderly formation of precise structure, failed interactions can be expected to have drastic developmental consequences (e.g., congenital defects, such as absence of the lens of the eye).

HIGHLIGHTS OF THE FOURTH TO EIGHTH WEEKS

The following descriptions summarize the main developmental events and changes in external form (O'Rahilly and Müller, 1987). The details of organ formation are given with descriptions of the various systems in Chapters 11 to 20. Criteria for estimating developmental stages in human embryos are listed in Table 5–1.

The Fourth Week

At the beginning of the fourth week, the embryo is almost straight, and the somites produce conspicuous surface elevations (Fig. 5–8). By the middle of the fourth week, the neural tube is formed opposite the somites, but it is widely open at the rostral and caudal neuropores (Fig. 5–9*A*). By 24 days, the first, or mandibular, arch and the second, or hyoid, arch are distinct (Fig. 5–8*C* and *D*). The major portion of the first arch will give rise to the mandible (lower jaw); and a rostral extension of it, the maxillary prominence, will contribute to the maxilla (upper jaw). The embryo is now slightly curved due to the head and tail folds, and the heart produces a large ventral prominence (Figs. 5–8*C* and 5–10).

Three pairs of pharyngeal or *branchial arches* are visible by 26 days (Figs. 5–8*D* and 5–11), and the rostral neuropore is closed. The *forebrain* produces a prominent elevation of the head, and folding of the embryo in the median plane has given the embryo a characteristic C-shaped curvature. *Upper limb buds* become recognizable by day 26 or 27 as small swellings on the ventrolateral body walls (Fig. 5–8*D* and *E*). The *otic pits*, the primordia of the internal ears, are also clearly visible. The fourth pair of branchial arches and the *lower limb buds* are visible by the end of the fourth week (Figs. 5–8*E* and 5–12). Ectodermal thickenings indicating the future lenses of the eyes, called *lens placodes*, are visible on the sides of the head. By the end of the fourth week, the *attenuated tail* is a characteristic feature (Figs. 5–11 and 5–12).

The Fifth Week

During this week, changes in body form are minor compared with those that occurred during the fourth week, but growth of the head exceeds that of other regions (Figs. 5–13 and 5–14*A*). Head growth is mainly caused by the rapid development of the brain. The face soon contacts the heart prominence. The second, or hyoid, arch overgrows the third and fourth arches, forming the *cervical sinus*.

Text continued on page 84

Table 5-1. CRITERIA FOR ESTIMATING DEVELOPMENTAL STAGES IN HUMAN EMBRYOS

Age (Days)	Figure Reference	Carnegie Stage	No. of Somites	Length (mm)*	Main External Characteristics†
20–21	5–1A_1	9	1–3	1.5–3.0	*Flat embryonic disc. Deep neural groove and prominent neural folds. One to three pairs of somites present.* Head fold evident.
22–23	5–8*A* 5–8*B* 5–9	10	4–12	2.0–3.5	*Embryo straight or slightly curved.* Neural tube forming or formed opposite somites, but widely open at rostral and caudal neuropores. First and second pairs of branchial arches visible.
24–25	5–8*C* 5–10	11	13–20	2.5–4.5	*Embryo curved owing to head and tail folds.* Rostral neuropore closing. Otic placodes present. Optic vesicles formed.
26–27	5–8*D* 5–11	12	21–29	3.0–5.0	*Upper limb buds appear.* Rostral neuropore closed. Caudal neuropore closing. Three pairs of branchial arches visible. Heart prominence distinct. Otic pits present.
28–30	5–12	13	30–35	4.0–6.0	*Embryo has C-shaped curve.* Caudal neuropore closed. Upper limb buds are flipper-like. Four pairs of branchial arches visible. Lower limb buds appear. *Otic vesicles* present. Lens placodes distinct. Attenuated *tail* present.
31–32	5–13 5–14*A*	14	‡	5.0–7.0	*Upper limbs are paddle-shaped.* Lens pits and nasal pits visible. Optic cups present.
33–36	5–14*B*	15		7.0–9.0	*Hand plates formed; digital rays present.* Lens vesicles present. Nasal pits prominent. *Lower limbs are paddle-shaped.* Cervical sinuses visible.
37–40		16		8.0–11.0	*Foot plates formed.* Pigment visible in retina. Auricular hillocks developing.
41–43	5–14*C* 5–15	17		11.0–14.0	*Digital rays clearly visible in hand plates.* Auricular hillocks outline future auricle of external ear. Trunk beginning to straighten. Cerebral vesicles prominent.
44–46		18		13.0–17.0	*Digital rays clearly visible in foot plates.* Elbow region visible. Eyelids forming. Notches between the digital rays in the hands. Nipples visible.
47–48	5–16 5–17*A*	19		16.0–18.0	*Limbs extend ventrally.* Trunk elongating and straightening. Midgut herniation prominent.
49–51	5–17*B* 5–18	20		18.0–22.0	*Upper limbs longer and bent at elbows. Fingers distinct but webbed.* Notches between the digital rays in the feet. Scalp vascular plexus appears.
52–53	5–19*A* 5–20	21		22.0–24.0	*Hands and feet approach each other. Fingers are free and longer.* Toes distinct but webbed. Stubby tail present.
54–55		22		23.0–28.0	*Toes free and longer.* Eyelids and auricles of external ears more developed.
56	5–19*B* 5–21	23		27.0–31.0	*Head more rounded and shows human characteristics.* External genitalia still have sexless appearance. Distinct bulge still present in umbilical cord, caused by herniation of intestines. *Tail has disappeared.*

* The embryonic lengths indicate the usual range, but they do not indicate the full range within a given stage, especially when specimens of poor quality are included. In stages 10 and 11, the measurement is greatest length (*GL*); in subsequent stages crown-rump (*CR*) measurements are given (Fig. 5–23).

† Based on Streeter (1942, 1945, 1948, and 1951), Nishimura et al. (1974), O'Rahilly and Müller (1987), and Shiota (1991).

‡ At this and subsequent stages, the number of somites is difficult to determine and so is not a useful criterion.

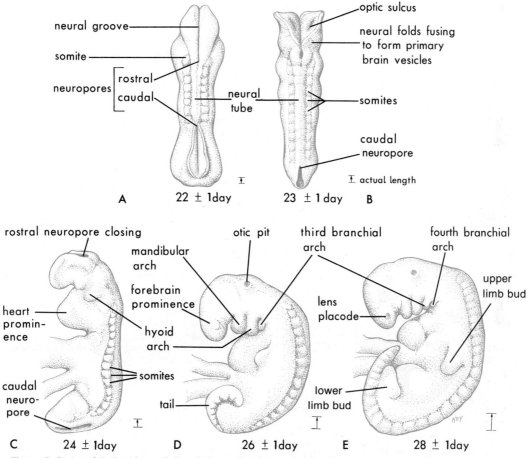

Figure 5-8. *A* and *B*, Drawings of dorsal views of embryos early in the fourth week showing 8 to 12 somites, respectively. *C, D,* and *E,* Lateral views of older embryos showing 16, 27, and 33 somites, respectively. The rostral neuropore is normally closed by 25 to 26 days, and the caudal neuropore is usually closed by the end of the fourth week.

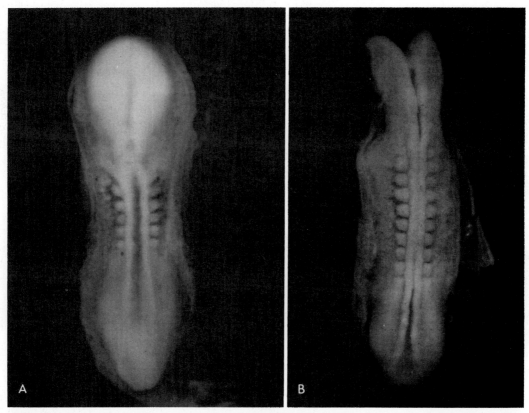

Figure 5–9. Photographs of embryos early in the fourth week. In *A*, the embryo is essentially straight; whereas in *B*, the embryo is slightly curved. In *A*, the neural groove is deep and is open throughout its entire extent. In *B*, the neural tube has formed opposite the somites but is widely open at the rostral and caudal neuropores. (Courtesy of Professor Hideo Nishimura, Kyoto University, Kyoto, Japan.)

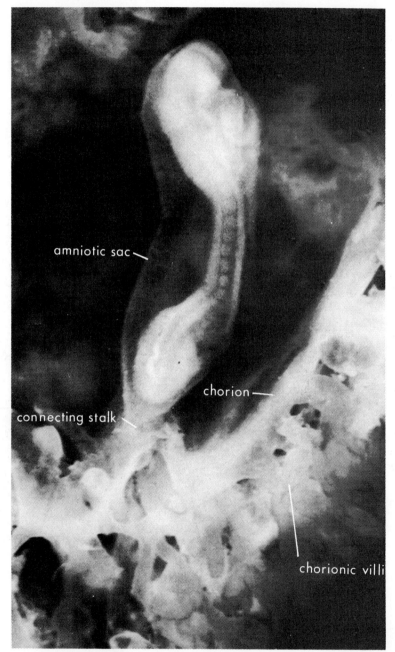

Figure 5–10. Photograph of a human embryo with 13 somites (24 to 25 days). Observe the ventral prominence produced by the primitive heart (see also Fig. 5–8C). The embryo lies within its amniotic sac and is attached to the chorion by the connecting stalk. Note the well-developed chorionic villi. (Courtesy of Professor E. Blechschmidt, University of Göttingen, Göttingen, Germany.)

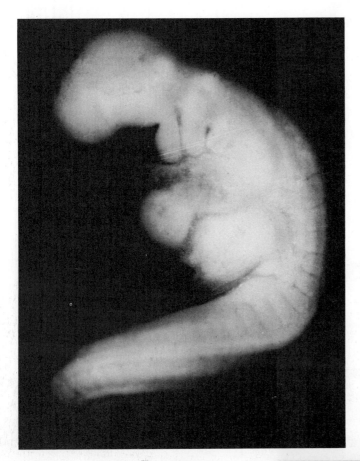

Figure 5-11. Photograph of a human embryo of about 26 days. Three pairs of branchial or pharyngeal arches are visible. The upper limb bud has begun to develop but is not visible in this photograph. Observe the forebrain prominence, mandibular arch, primitive heart, and the long curved tail (see also Fig. 5-8D). Actual size: 3 to 5 mm. (Courtesy of Dr. Kazumasa Hoshino, former Professor of Anatomy and Director of the Congenital Anomaly Center, Faculty of Medicine, Kyoto University, Kyoto, Japan.)

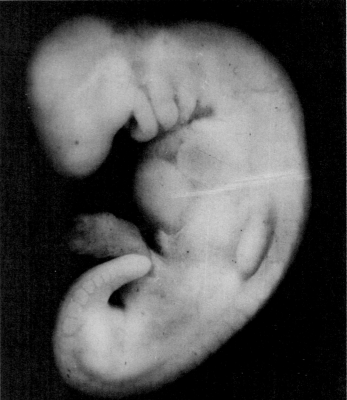

Figure 5-12. Photograph of a 28-day-old human embryo. The embryo has a characteristic C-shaped curvature, four branchial or pharyngeal arches, and upper and lower limb buds. The lower limb is not recognizable in this photograph. The heart prominence is easily recognized. The curled, attenuated tail with its somites is a characteristic feature of this stage. Actual size: 4.0 mm. (Courtesy of Professor Hideo Nishimura, Kyoto University, Kyoto, Japan.)

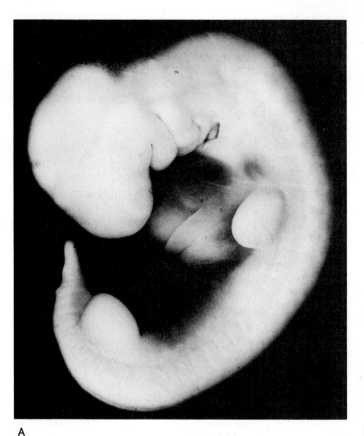

A

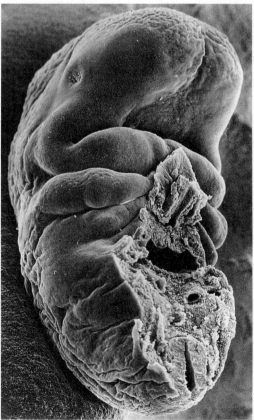

B

Figure 5–13. *A*, Photograph of an embryo of about 32 days. The upper limb buds are paddle-shaped, and the lower limb buds appear as flipperlike outgrowths (see also Fig. 5–14*A*). Four pairs of branchial or pharyngeal arches are visible. The fourth arch is small. Actual size: 7.0 mm. (Courtesy of Dr. Kazumasa Hoshino, former Professor of Anatomy and Director of the Congenital Anomaly Center, Faculty of Medicine, Kyoto University, Kyoto, Japan.) *B*, Scanning electron micrograph of the craniofacial region of a human embryo of about 32 days (Stage 14, 6.8 mm). The rostral neuropore is closed and three pairs of branchial or pharyngeal arches are present. The maxillary and mandibular prominences of the first arch are clearly delineated. Observe the stomodeum located between the prominent forebrain and the fused mandibular prominences. (Courtesy of Professor K. Hinrichsen, Ruhr-Universität Bochum, Federal Republic of Germany).

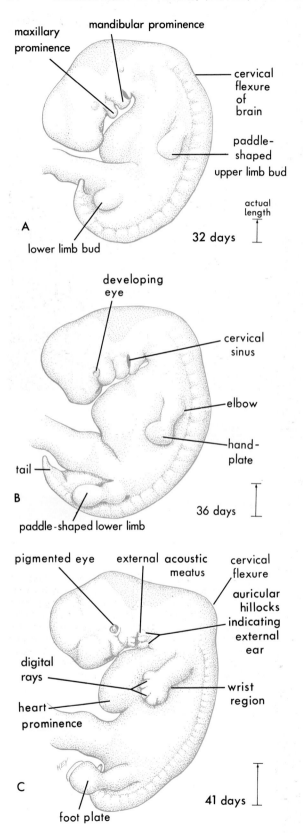

A 32 days

maxillary prominence
mandibular prominence
cervical flexure of brain
paddle-shaped upper limb bud
actual length
lower limb bud

B 36 days

developing eye
cervical sinus
elbow
hand-plate
tail
paddle-shaped lower limb

C 41 days

pigmented eye
external acoustic meatus
cervical flexure
auricular hillocks indicating external ear
digital rays
heart prominence
wrist region
foot plate

The upper limbs begin to show some regional differentiation as the elbows and *hand plates* develop (Fig. 5–13*B*). The primordia of the digits, called *digital rays*, begin to develop at 33 days (see Fig. 15–13*C*). It has been reported that embryos in the fifth week show spontaneous movements, such as twitching of the trunk and limbs.

The Sixth Week

The upper limbs show rapid regional differentiation during the sixth week (Figs. 5–14*B* and *C* and 5–15). The elbow and wrist regions are clearly identifiable, and the *digital rays* indicating the future digits (fingers) are visible externally. Note that development of the lower limbs occurs somewhat later than that of the upper limbs. Several small swellings develop around the branchial groove between the first two branchial arches (Fig. 5–14*C*). This groove becomes the *external acoustic meatus* (L. a passage), and the swellings around it fuse to form the auricle of the external ear. Largely because retinal pigment has formed, the eye is now obvious (Figs. 5–14*C* and 5–15). The head is now much larger relative to the trunk and is more bent over the *heart prominence*. This head position results from bending of the brain in the cervical region. The trunk and neck have begun to straighten. It has been reported that embryos during the sixth week show reflex responses to touch.

The Seventh Week

The communication between the primitive gut and yolk sac is now reduced to a relatively small duct, the *yolk stalk*. The intestines enter the extraembryonic coelom in the proximal portion of the umbilical cord. This process, called *umbilical herniation*, is a normal event in the embryo (Fig. 5–17). The limbs undergo considerable change during the seventh week. Notches appear between the digital rays in the hand plates, clearly indicating the future digits (Figs. 5–16 and 5–17*A*).

The Eighth Week

At the beginning of the final week of the embryonic period, the digits of the hand are short and noticeably webbed (Fig. 5–17*B* and 5–18). Notches are now clearly visible between the digital rays of the feet and

Figure 5–14. Drawings of lateral views of embryos during the fifth and sixth weeks. Note that development of the upper limb precedes development of the lower limb buds by several days. Observe the digital rays in the hand plate at 41 days. They indicate where the digits will develop.

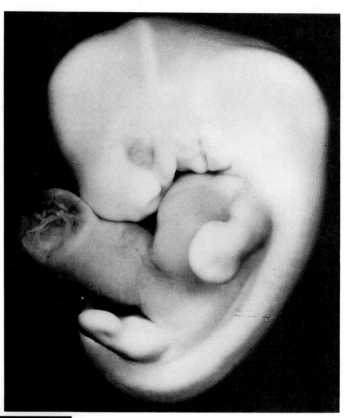

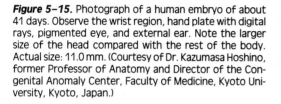

Figure 5–15. Photograph of a human embryo of about 41 days. Observe the wrist region, hand plate with digital rays, pigmented eye, and external ear. Note the larger size of the head compared with the rest of the body. Actual size: 11.0 mm. (Courtesy of Dr. Kazumasa Hoshino, former Professor of Anatomy and Director of the Congenital Anomaly Center, Faculty of Medicine, Kyoto University, Kyoto, Japan.)

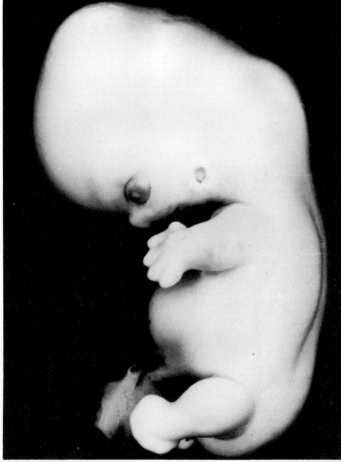

Figure 5–16. Photograph of a human embryo of about 48 days. Actual size: 18.0 mm. Observe the well-developed eye and the notches between the digital rays in the developing hand. Note that the developing external ear is set low on the head. The ventral abdominal prominence is produced mainly by the liver. (Courtesy of Dr. Kazumasa Hoshino, former Professor of Anatomy and Director of the Congenital Anomaly Center, Faculty of Medicine, Kyoto University, Kyoto, Japan.)

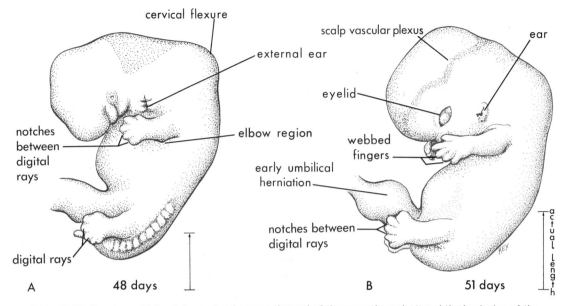

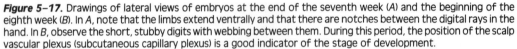

Figure 5–17. Drawings of lateral views of embryos at the end of the seventh week (*A*) and the beginning of the eighth week (*B*). In *A*, note that the limbs extend ventrally and that there are notches between the digital rays in the hand. In *B*, observe the short, stubby digits with webbing between them. During this period, the position of the scalp vascular plexus (subcutaneous capillary plexus) is a good indicator of the stage of development.

Figure 5–18. Photograph of a human embryo of about 51 days. Actual size: 22.0 mm. Observe the webbed digits and the notches between the digital rays of the foot. Note the pigmented eye, the developing eyelids, and the remnant of the tail. (Courtesy of Dr. Kazumasa Hoshino, former Professor of Anatomy and Director of the Congenital Anomaly Center, Faculty of Medicine, Kyoto University, Kyoto, Japan.)

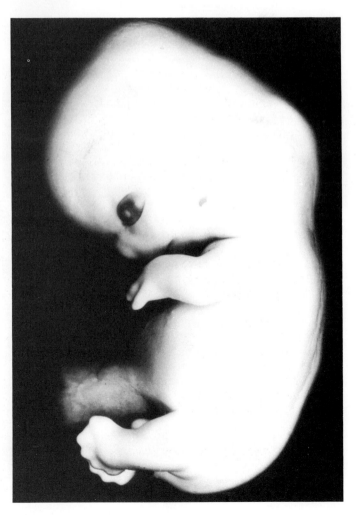

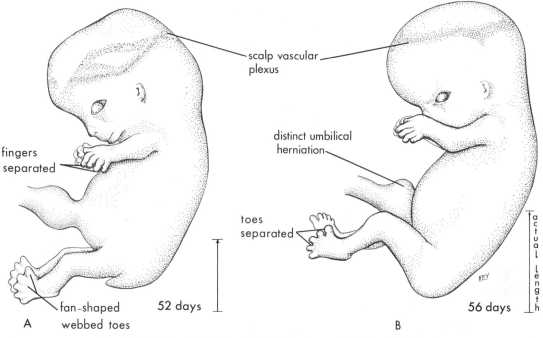

Figure 5–19. Drawings of lateral views of embryos during the eighth week.

the tail is still present but stubby (Fig. 5–19A). The *scalp vascular plexus* has appeared and forms a characteristic band around the head. By the end of the eighth week, all the regions of the limbs are apparent, and the digits have lengthened and are separated. Purposeful limb movements first occur during this week. All evidence of the tail disappears by the end of the eighth week (Figs. 5–19B and 5–21). The scalp vascular plexus now forms a band near the vertex (crown) of the head.

By the end of the eighth week, the embryo has distinct human characteristics; however, the head is still disproportionately large, constituting almost half of the embryo. The neck region has become established and the eyelids are more obvious. The intestines are still within the proximal portion of the umbilical cord (Figs. 5–19 to 5–21). Early in the eighth week the eyes are open; but, toward the end of the week, the eyelids often begin to unite by epithelial fusion. The auricles of the external ears begin to assume their final shape but are still low-set on the head. Although sex differences exist in the appearance of the external genitalia, they are not distinct enough to permit accurate sexual identification by laypersons.

ESTIMATION OF EMBRYONIC AGE

Determination of the starting date of a pregnancy may be difficult, partly because it depends on the mother's memory of an event that occurred several weeks before she realized she was pregnant. Two reference points are commonly used for estimating gestational or embryonic age: (1) the onset of the last normal menstrual period (LNMP), and (2) the probable time of fertilization (conception). In about 20 per cent of women, the estimation of gestational age from the menstrual history alone is unreliable. The probability of error in establishing LNMP is highest in women who become pregnant after cessation of oral contraception because the interval between discontinuance of the hormones and the onset of ovulation is highly variable. In addition, slight uterine bleeding (or "spotting"), which sometimes occurs after implantation of the blastocyst, may be incorrectly regarded as menstruation. Other contributing factors may include *oligomenorrhea* (scanty menstruation), pregnancy in the postpartum period (i.e., after childbirth), and use of intrauterine devices (IUDs). Despite these possible sources of error, LNMP is commonly used by clinicians to estimate the age of embryos and is a reliable criterion in most cases. Ultrasound assessment of the size of the chorionic (gestational) sac and its contents (Fig. 5–22) enables clinicians to obtain an accurate estimate of the date of conception (Kurtz and Needleman, 1988; Lyons and Levi, 1991).

It must be emphasized that the zygote does not form until about two weeks after LNMP. Consequently, 14 ± two days must be deducted from the so-called gestational or "menstrual" age to obtain the actual or fertilization age of an embryo. The day fertilization occurs is the most accurate reference point for estimating age; this is commonly calculated from the estimated time of ovulation because the ovum is usually fertilized within 12 hours after ovulation. Because it may be important to know the fertilization age of

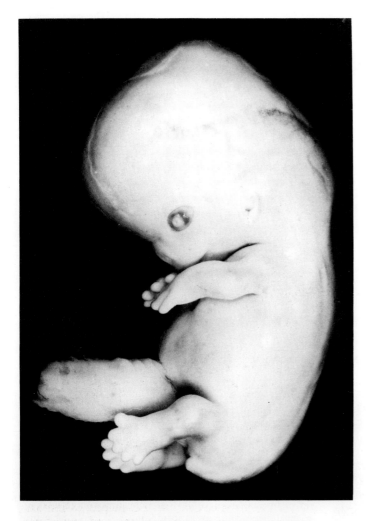

Figure 5–20. Photograph of a human embryo of about 52 days. Actual size: 23.0 mm. Observe that the digits are separated. Note that the feet are fan-shaped and that the digits are webbed. Observe that a stubby tail is still present (Courtesy of Dr. Kazumasa Hoshino, former Professor of Anatomy and Director of the Congenital Anomaly Center, Faculty of Medicine, Kyoto University, Kyoto, Japan.)

an embryo (e.g., for determining its sensitivity to teratogenic agents [see Chapter 8]), all statements about age should indicate the reference point used, i.e., days after LNMP or after the estimated time of fertilization.

Estimates of the age of recovered embryos (e.g., after spontaneous abortion) are determined from their external characteristics and measurements of their length (Table 5–1 and Fig. 5–23). Size alone may be an unreliable criterion because some embryos undergo a progressively slower rate of growth prior to death. The appearance of the developing limbs is a very helpful criterion for estimating embryonic age.

Methods of Measuring Embryos

Because embryos of the third and early fourth weeks are straight (Figs. 5–9, 5–22*A*, and 5–23*A*), measurements of them indicate the greatest length (GL). The sitting height, or crown-rump length (CRL), is most frequently used for older embryos (Figs. 5–22 and 5–23 *B* and *C*). In those with greatly flexed heads, the CRL is actually a neck-rump measurement (Fig. 5–23*C*). Standing height, or crown-heel length (CHL), is sometimes measured for eight-week-old embryos. As CHL of formalin-fixed embryos may be difficult to determine because their limbs are not easy to straighten, they should be measured as shown in Figure 5–23*D*. Because the length of an embryo is only one criterion for establishing age (Table 5–1), one should not refer to a 5-mm stage embryo (O'Rahilly and Müller, 1987). The *Carnegie Embryonic Staging System* is used internationally (Table 5–1); its usage enables comparisons to be made between the findings of one person and those of another.

The size of an embryo in a pregnant woman can be estimated using ultrasound measurements. *Transvaginal sonography* permits an earlier and more accurate measure-

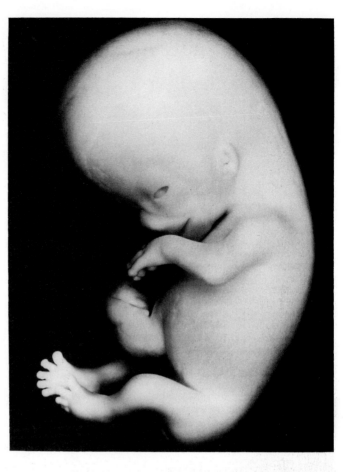

Figure 5–21. Photograph of a human embryo of about 56 days. Actual size: 30.0 mm. Observe that the upper and lower limbs are well formed and that the digits of the hands and feet are separated. The embryo now has a distinctly human appearance. (Courtesy of Dr. Kazumasa Hoshino, former Professor of Anatomy and Director of the Congenital Anomaly Center, Faculty of Medicine, Kyoto University, Kyoto, Japan.)

ment of CRL in early pregnancy. The embryonic CRL was determined as early as 25 days after follicle aspiration in pregnancies resulting from *in vitro* fertilization (Schats et al., 1991). Early in the fifth week (seven weeks after LNMP), the embryo is 4 to 7 mm long (Figs. 5–13 and 5–22*A*). During the sixth and seventh weeks, discrete embryonic structures can be visualized (e.g., parts of the limbs), and crown-rump measurements are predictive of embryonic age with an accuracy of ± one to four days. Furthermore, after the sixth week (eight weeks after LNMP), dimensions of the head and trunk can be obtained and used for assessment of embryonic age (Callen, 1988; Manning, 1989; Filly, 1988; Schats et al., 1991).

SUMMARY OF THE FOURTH TO EIGHTH WEEKS

During these five weeks representing most of the embryonic period, *all major organs and systems of the body form* from the three germ layers (Fig. 5–5). At the beginning of the fourth week, folding in the median and horizontal planes converts the flat, trilaminar embryonic disc into a C-shaped, cylindrical embryo. The formation of head, tail, and lateral folds is a continuous sequence of events that results in a constriction between the embryo and yolk sac. During folding, the dorsal part of the yolk sac is incorporated into the embryo and gives rise to the primitive gut. As the head region folds ventrally, part of the yolk sac is incorporated into the developing embryonic head as the *foregut*. Folding of the head region also results in the oropharyngeal membrane and heart being carried ventrally and the developing brain becoming the most cranial part of the embryo.

As the tail region folds ventrally, part of the yolk sac is incorporated into the caudal end of the embryo as the *hindgut*. The terminal part of the hindgut expands to form the *cloaca*. Folding of the tail region also results in the cloacal membrane, allantois, and connecting stalk being carried to the ventral surface of the embryo.

Folding of the embryo in the horizontal plane incorporates part of the yolk sac into the embryo as the *midgut*. The yolk sac remains attached to the midgut

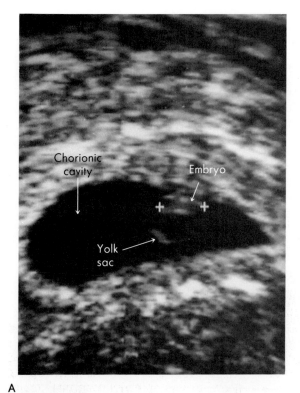

A

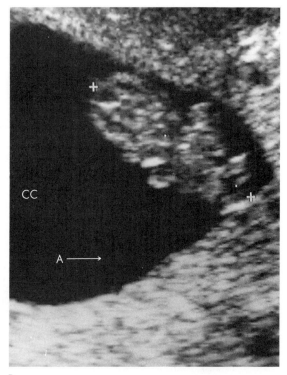

B

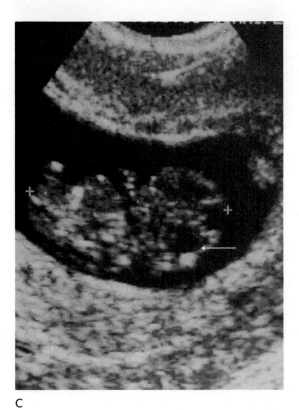

C

Figure 5–22. Ultrasound images of embryos. *A*, CRL 4.8 mm. The 4.5-week-old embryo is indicated by the measurement cursors. Ventral to the embryo is the yolk sac. The chorionic cavity appears black (see also Fig. 5–1A₂). *B*, CRL 2.09 cm. Coronal scan of 5-week-old embryo. The upper limbs are clearly shown. The embryo is surrounded by a thin amnion (*A*). The fluid in the chorionic cavity (*CC*) is more particulate than the amniotic fluid. *C*, CRL of 2.14 cm. Sagittal scan of a 7-week embryo demonstrating the eye, limbs, and the developing fourth ventricle of the brain (*arrow*). Courtesy of Dr. E.A. Lyons, Professor of Radiology and Obstetrics & Gynecology, and Head of Radiology, Health Sciences Centre, University of Manitoba, Winnipeg, Manitoba, Canada.

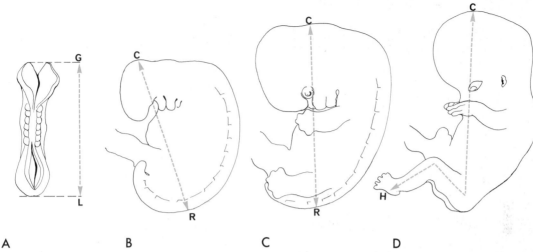

Figure 5–23. Sketches showing the methods used to measure the length of embryos. *A,* Greatest length. *B* and *C,* Crown-rump length. *D,* Crown-heel length.

by a narrow yolk stalk. During folding in the horizontal plane, the primordia of the lateral and ventral body walls are formed. As the amnion expands, it envelops the connecting stalk, yolk stalk, and allantois, thereby forming an epithelial covering for the new structure called the *umbilical cord.*

The three germ layers differentiate into various tissues and organs so that, by the end of the embryonic period, the beginnings of all the main organ systems have been established. The external appearance of the embryo is greatly affected by the formation of the brain, heart, liver, somites, limbs, ears, nose, and eyes. As these structures develop, the appearance of the embryo changes so that it has unquestionably human characteristics. Because the beginnings of all essential external and internal structures are formed during the fourth to eighth weeks, this is the most critical period of development. Developmental disturbances during this period may give rise to major congenital anomalies of the embryo (see Chapter 8).

Reasonable estimates of the age of embryos can be determined from: (1) the day of onset of the last normal menstrual period (LNMP), (2) the estimated time of fertilization, (3) measurements of the chorionic sac and embryo, and (4) study of the external characteristics of the embryo.

CLINICALLY ORIENTED QUESTIONS FOR PROBLEM-BASED LEARNING SESSIONS

1. A 28-year-old woman, who has been a heavy cigarette smoker since her teens, was informed that she was in the second month of pregnancy. What would the doctor likely tell the patient about her smoking habit and the use of other drugs (e.g., alcohol)?
2. Why is the embryonic period such a critical stage of development?
3. Can one predict the possible harmful effects of drugs on the human embryo from studies performed in experimental animals? Discuss germ layer formation and organogenesis.
4. Why may information about the starting date of a pregnancy provided by a patient be unreliable? What techniques are now available for evaluating embryonic (gestational) age?
5. Would a drug known to cause severe limb defects be likely to cause these abnormalities if it was administered during the eighth week? Discuss the mechanism of the action of these teratogens (see Chapter 8).

The answers to these questions are given on page 460.

References and Suggested Reading

Barnea ER, Hustin J, Jauniaux E (eds): *The First Twelve Weeks of Gestation.* Berlin, Springer-Verlag, 1992.

Benson PF, McCance RA (eds): *The Biochemistry of Development.* Philadelphia, JB Lippincott, 1971.

Biggers JD: Arbitrary Partitions of Prenatal Life. *Human Reprod* 5:1, 1990.

Callen PW (ed): *Ultrasonography in Obstetrics and Gynecology,* 2nd ed. Philadelphia, WB Saunders, 1988.

Chapman MG, Grudzinskas JG, Chard T (eds): *The Embryo. Normal and Abnormal Development and Growth.* New York, Springer Verlag, 1990.

Cooke J: The early embryo and the formation of body pattern. *American Scientist* 76:35, 1988.

De Haan R, Ursprung H: *Organogenesis.* New York, Holt, Rinehart and Winston, 1965.

Eichele G: Retinoids and vertebrate limb pattern formation. *Trends Genet* 5:246, 1990.

England MA: Cellular processes and tissue interactions in developmental pathology. *In* Harrison MR, Golbus MS, Filly RA (eds): *The Unborn Patient. Prenatal Diagnosis and Treatment,* 2nd ed. Philadelphia, WB Saunders, 1990.

Filly RA: The first trimester. *In* Callen PW (ed): *Ultrasonography in Obstetrics and Gynecology,* 2nd ed. Philadelphia, WB Saunders, 1988.

Grobstein C: Inductive tissue interactions in development. *Adv Cancer Res* 4:187, 1956.

Guthrie S: Horizontal and vertical pathways in neural induction. *Trends in Neurosciences* 14:123, 1991.

Hinrichsen KV (ed): *Humanembryologie.* Berlin, Springer-Verlag, 1990.

Iffy L, Shepard TH, Jakobovits A, Lemire RJ, Kerner P: The rate of growth in young human embryos of Streeter's horizons XIII and XXIII. *Acta Anat* 66:178, 1967.

Kalousek DK, Fitch N, Paradice BA: *Pathology of the Human Embryo and Previable Fetus. An Atlas.* New York, Springer-Verlag, 1990.

Kerner P: The rate of growth in young human embryos of Streeter's horizons XIII and XXIII. *Acta Anat* 66:178, 1967.

Khong TY: Pathology of intrauterine growth retardation. *Am J Reprod Immunol* 21:132, 1989.

Kurtz AB, Needleman L: Ultrasound assessment of fetal age. *In* Callen PW (ed): *Ultrasonography in Obstetrics and Gynecology,* 2nd ed. Philadelphia, WB Saunders, 1988.

Lyons EA, Levi CS: Ultrasound of the normal first trimester of pregnancy. Syllabus. Special Course. Ultrasound, Radiological Society of North America, 1991.

Manning FA: General principles and applications of ultrasound. *In* Creasy RK, Resnik R (eds): *Maternal-Fetal Medicine,* 2nd ed. Philadelphia, WB Saunders, 1989.

Nieuwkoop PD, Johnen AG, Albers B: *The Epigenetic Nature of Early Chordate Development. Inductive Interaction and Competence.* London, Cambridge University Press, 1985.

Nishimura H, Takano K, Tanimura T, Yasuda M: Normal and abnormal development of human embryos. *Teratology* 1:281, 1968.

Nishimura H, Tanimura T, Semba R, Uwabe C: Normal development of early human embryos: Observation of 90 specimens at Carnegie stages 7 to 13. *Teratology* 10:1, 1974.

Oppenheimer JM: The non-specificity of the germ layers. *Q Rev Biol.* 15:1–27, 1940.

O'Rahilly R: Guide to the staging of human embryos. *Anat Anz* 130:556, 1972.

O'Rahilly R, Müller F: *Developmental Stages in Human Embryos.* Washington, Carnegie Institute of Washington, 1987.

Persaud TVN: *Environmental Causes of Human Birth Defects.* Springfield, Charles C Thomas, 1990.

Ruberte E, Dolle P, Krust A, Zelent A, Morriss-Kay G, Chambon P: Specific spatial and temporal distribution of retinoic acid receptor gamma transcripts during mouse embryogenesis. *Development* 108:213, 1990.

Saxen L: Interactive mechanisms in morphogenesis. *In* Tarin D (ed): *Tissue Interactions in Carcinogenesis.* London, Academic Press, 1972.

Schats R, Van Os HC, Jansen CAM, Wladimiroff JW: The crown-rump length in early human pregnancy: a reappraisal. *Br J Obstet Gynaecol* 98:460, 1991.

Senterre J (ed): Intrauterine Growth Retardation: Nestle Nutrition Workshop Series, vol 18. New York, Raven Press, 1989.

Shepard TH: Normal and abnormal growth patterns. *In* Gardner LI (ed): *Endocrine and Genetic Diseases of Childhood and Adolescence,* 2nd ed. Philadelphia, WB Saunders, 1975.

Shiota K: Development and intrauterine fate of normal and abnormal human conceptuses. *Cong Anom* 31:67, 1991.

Streeter GL: Developmental horizons in human embryos. Description of age group XI, 13 to 20 somites, and age group XII, 21 to 29 somites. *Contrib Embryol Carnegie Inst* 30:211, 1942.

Streeter GL: Developmental horizons in human embryos: Description of age group XIII, embryos of 4 or 5 millimeters long, and age group XIV, period of identification of the lens vesicle. *Contrib Embryol Carnegie Inst* 31:27, 1945.

Streeter GL: Developmental horizons in human embryos: Description of age groups XV, XVI, XVII, and XVIII. *Contrib Embryol Carnegie Inst* 32:133, 1948.

Streeter GL, Heuser CH, Corner GW: Developmental horizons in human embryos: Description of age groups XIX, XX, XXI, XXII and XXIII. *Contrib Embryol Carnegie Inst* 34:165, 1951.

Thompson MW, McInnes RR, Willard HF: *Thompson & Thompson Genetics in Medicine,* 5th ed. Philadelphia, WB Saunders, 1991.

Torry DS, Cooper GM: Proto-oncogenes in development and cancer. *Am J Reprod Immunol* 25:129, 1991.

Villee CA: Biologic principles of growth. *In* Falkner F (ed): *Human Development.* Philadelphia, WB Saunders, 1966.

Willier, BH, Weiss PA, Hamburger V: *Analysis of Development.* New York, Hafner Publishing Co., 1971.

Yamada KM (ed): *Cell Interactions and Development.* New York, John Wiley & Sons, 1983.

The Fetal Period
THE NINTH WEEK TO BIRTH

The transformation of an embryo to a fetus is gradual, but the name change is meaningful because it signifies that the embryo has developed into a recognizable human being. Development during the fetal period is primarily concerned with rapid growth of the body and differentiation of tissues and organs that started to develop during the embryonic period. A notable change occurring during the fetal period is the relative slowdown in the growth of the head compared with the rest of the body (England, 1983; Bowie, 1988; Barnea et al., 1992).

The rate of body growth during the fetal period is very rapid (Bowie, 1988), especially between the ninth and sixteenth weeks (Figs. 6–1 and 6–7), and fetal weight gain is phenomenal during the terminal weeks (Table 6–2 and Fig. 6–13).

Fetuses weighing less than 500 gm at birth usually do not survive. If given expert postnatal care, some fetuses weighing 500 to 1000 gm may survive; they are referred to as *immature infants*. Most fetuses weighing between 1500 and 2500 gm survive but face difficulties; they are called *premature infants*. Prematurity is one of the most common causes of morbidity and perinatal death (Behrman, 1992). Many full-term *low-birth-weight babies* result from intrauterine growth retardation (IUGR).

ESTIMATION OF FETAL AGE

If doubt arises about the age of a fetus, ultrasonic measurements can be taken to determine its size and probable age and to provide a reliable prediction of the *expected date of confinement* (EDC) for delivery of the fetus (Kurtz and Needleman, 1988). The intrauterine period may be divided into days, weeks, or months (Table 6–1), but confusion arises if it is not stated whether the age is calculated from: (1) the onset of the last normal menstrual period (LNMP), or (2) the estimated day of fertilization. Most uncertainty arises when months are used, particularly when it is not stated whether calendar months (28 to 31 days) or lunar months (28 days) are meant. Unless otherwise stated, fetal age in this book is calculated from the estimated time of fertilization, and months refer to calendar months. It is best to express fetal age in weeks and to state whether the beginning or end of a week is meant because statements such as "in the tenth week" are nonspecific.

Clinically, gestation is divided into three periods or **trimesters**, each lasting three calendar months. By the end of the first trimester, all major systems are developed and the crown-rump length (CRL) of the fetus is about the width of one's palm (Fig. 6–8). At the end of the second trimester (26 weeks after LNMP; 24 weeks after the estimated day of fertilization), the fetus is usually too immature to survive if born prematurely even though its length is nearly equal to the span of one's hand.

External Characteristics of Fetuses

Various measurements and external characteristics are useful for estimating fetal age (Table 6–2). CRL is usually the most reliable measurement (see Fig. 5–23), but the length of fetuses, like that of infants, varies considerably for a given age. *Foot length* correlates well with CRL and is particularly useful for estimating the age of incomplete or macerated fetuses. *Fetal weight* is often a useful criterion for estimating age, but there may be a discrepancy between the fertilization age and the weight of a fetus, particularly when the mother has had metabolic disturbances during pregnancy; e.g., diabetes mellitus. In these cases, fetal weight often exceeds values considered normal for CRL.

Freshly expelled fetuses have a shiny translucent appearance (Fig. 6–9), whereas those that have been dead for several days prior to abortion or delivery have a tanned appearance and lack normal resilience (Fig. 6–10). Fetal dimensions obtained from ultrasound measurements of fetuses closely approximate CRL measurements obtained from aborted fetuses (Fig. 6–2; Table 6–2). *Ultrasound CRL measurements* are now predictive of fetal age with an accuracy of ± one to two days. In addition, the biparietal

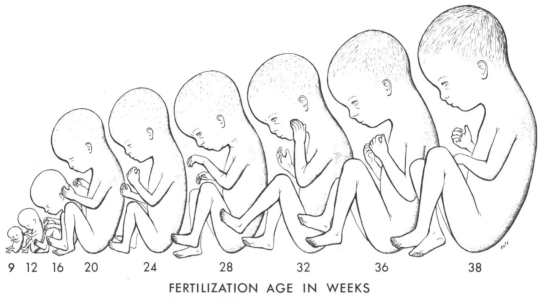

9   12   16   20   24   28   32   36   38

FERTILIZATION AGE IN WEEKS

Figure 6–1. Drawings of fetuses, about one-fifth actual size. Head hair begins to appear at about 20 weeks, and eyebrows and eyelashes are usually recognizable by 24 weeks. The eyes are open by 26 weeks.

diameter of the head and the dimension of the trunk may be obtained (Kurtz and Needleman, 1988). At 9 to 10 weeks, the head is still slightly larger than the trunk. Assessment of fetal size and age is enhanced when head and trunk dimensions are considered along with the CRL measurements. Recently, cheek-to-cheek (Abramowicz et al., 1991) and transverse cerebellar measurements (Lee et al., 1991) have been used for the assessment of fetal growth and gestational age, respectively. Determination of the size of a fetus, especially of its head, is of great value to the obstetrician for the management of patients; e.g., women with small pelves and/or those fetuses with IUGR and/or congenital anomalies (Filly, 1991a).

HIGHLIGHTS OF THE FETAL PERIOD

No formal system of staging is used for the fetal period, but it is helpful to consider the distinctive changes that occur in periods of four to five weeks.

Table 6–1. COMPARISON OF GESTATIONAL TIME UNITS

Reference Point	Days	Weeks	Calendar Months	Lunar Months
Fertilization*	266	38	8¾	9½
LNMP	280	40	9¼	10

* The date of birth is calculated as 266 days after the estimated day of fertilization, or 280 days after the onset of the last normal menstrual period (*LNMP*). From fertilization to the end of the embryonic period (8 weeks), age is best expressed in days; thereafter age is often given in weeks.

Nine to Twelve Weeks

At the beginning of the ninth week, the head constitutes one half the CRL of the fetus (Figs. 6–2 and 6–3). Subsequently, growth in body length accelerates rapidly so that, by the end of 12 weeks, the CRL has more than doubled (Table 6–2). Although growth of the head slows down considerably, it is still disproportionately large compared with the rest of the body (Figs. 6–2 to 6–6). At nine weeks the face is broad, the eyes widely separated, the ears low-set, and the eyelids fused. By the end of 12 weeks, *primary ossification centers* appear in the skeleton, especially in the skull and long bones (see Fig. 15–14).

Early in the ninth week, the legs are short and the thighs are relatively small. By the end of 12 weeks, the upper limbs have almost reached their final relative lengths, but the lower limbs are still not so well developed and are slightly shorter than their final relative lengths. The external genitalia of males and females appear similar until the end of the ninth week. Their mature fetal form is not established until the twelfth week.

Intestinal coils are clearly visible in the proximal end of the umbilical cord until the middle of the tenth week (Figs. 6–4*B*; see also Fig. 12–12). By the eleventh week the intestines have usually returned to the abdomen (Fig. 6–6). At the beginning of the fetal period, the liver is the major site of *erythropoiesis* (formation of red blood cells). By the end of the twelfth week, this activity has decreased in the liver

Table 6-2. CRITERIA FOR ESTIMATING FERTILIZATION AGE DURING THE FETAL PERIOD

Age (weeks)	CR Length (mm)*	Foot Length (mm)*	Fetal Weight (gm)†	Main External Characteristics
Previable Fetuses				
9	50	7	8	*Eyes closing or closed.* Head large and more rounded. External genitalia still not distinguishable as male or female. Intestines in proximal part of umbilical cord. Ears are low-set.
10	61	9	14	*Intestines in the abdomen.* Early fingernail development.
12	87	14	45	*Sex distinguishable externally.* Well-defined neck.
14	120	20	110	*Head erect.* Eyes face anteriorly. Ears are close to their definitive position. Lower limbs well-developed. Early toenail development.
16	140	27	200	*External ears stand out* from head.
18	160	33	320	*Vernix caseosa covers skin.* Quickening (signs of life) felt by mother.
20	190	39	460	*Head and body hair (lanugo) visible.*
Viable Fetuses‡				
22	210	45	630	*Skin wrinkled,* translucent, and pink to red.
24	230	50	820	*Fingernails present.* Lean body.
26	250	55	1000	*Eyes partially open.* Eyelashes present.
28	270	59	1300	*Eyes wide open.* Good head of hair often present. Skin slightly wrinkled.
30	280	63	1700	*Toenails present.* Body filling out. Testes descending.
32	300	68	2100	*Fingernails reach finger tips.* Skin pink and smooth.
36	340	79	2900	*Body usually plump.* Lanugo hairs almost absent. Toenails reach toe tips. Flexed limbs; firm grasp.
38	360	83	3400	*Prominent chest*; breasts protrude. Testes in scrotum or palpable in inguinal canals. Fingernails extend beyond finger tips.

* These measurements are averages and so may not apply to specific cases; dimensional variations increase with age. The method for taking CR (crown-rump) measurements is illustrated in Figure 5–23.

† These weights refer to fetuses that have been fixed for about two weeks in ten per cent formalin. Fresh specimens usually weigh about five per cent less.

‡ There is no sharp limit of development, age, or weight at which a fetus automatically becomes viable or beyond which survival is assured, but experience has shown that it is rare for a baby to survive whose weight is less than 500 gm or whose fertilization age is less than 22 weeks. Even fetuses born between 26 and 28 weeks have difficulty surviving, mainly because the respiratory system and the central nervous system are not completely differentiated. The term *abortion* refers to all pregnancies that terminate before the period of viability. Thereafter, terminations are referred to as *premature births* (miscarriages).

and has begun in the spleen. *Urine formation* begins between the ninth and twelfth weeks, and urine is discharged into the amniotic fluid. The fetus reabsorbs some of this fluid after swallowing it (p. 128). Fetal waste products are transferred to the maternal circulation by passing across the placental membrane (see Fig. 7–8 and p. 119).

Thirteen to Sixteen Weeks

Growth is very rapid during this period (Figs. 6–7 and 6–8; Table 6–2). By 16 weeks the head is relatively small compared with that of the 12-week fetus (Fig. 6–3), and the lower limbs have lengthened. Limb movements, which first occur at the end of the embryonic period (eight weeks), become coordinated by the fourteenth week but are too slight to be felt by the mother (Drife, 1985). *Ossification of the skeleton* is active during this period, and the bones are clearly

visible on radiographs of the mother's abdomen by the beginning of the sixteenth week.

Birnholz (1981) revealed by ultrasonography that slow *eye movements occur at 14 weeks* (16 weeks after LNMP). Scalp hair patterning is also determined during this period. By 16 weeks the ovaries are differentiated and contain primordial follicles that have oogonia (see Fig. 13–21). At this time the appearance of the fetus is even more human because its eyes face anteriorly rather than anterolaterally. In addition, the external ears are close to their definitive position on the sides of the head.

Seventeen to Twenty Weeks

Growth slows down during this period, but the fetus still increases its CRL by about 50 mm (Table 6–2). The lower limbs reach their final relative proportions (Fig. 6–9) and fetal movements known as

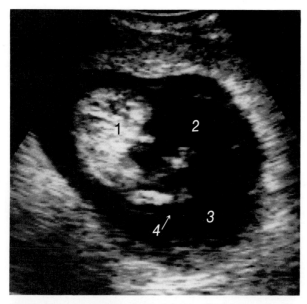

Figure 6-2. Transvaginal ultrasound scan of a fetus early in the ninth week (1), showing its relationship to the amniotic cavity (2), the extrafetal or chorionic cavity (3), and amnion (4). (From Wathen NC, Cass PL, Kitan MJ, Chard T: *Prenatal Diagnosis 11:*145, Reprinted by permission of John Wiley & Sons, Ltd. 1991).

quickening are commonly felt by the mother. The mean time that intervenes between a mother's first detection of fetal movements and delivery is 147 days, with a standard deviation of ± 15 days (Page et al., 1981).

The skin is now covered with a greasy, cheeselike material known as *vernix caseosa*. It consists of a mixture of a fatty secretion from the fetal sebaceous glands of the skin and dead epidermal cells. The vernix caseosa protects the delicate fetal skin from abrasions, chapping, and hardening that could result from its exposure to the amniotic fluid. The bodies of 20-week fetuses are usually completely covered with fine downy hair called *lanugo*; this hair helps to hold the vernix caseosa on the skin. Eyebrows and head hair are also visible at 20 weeks.

Brown fat forms during the seventeenth through twentieth weeks and is the site of heat production, particularly in the newborn infant. This specialized adipose tissue produces heat by oxidizing fatty acids. Brown fat is chiefly found at the root of the neck, posterior to the sternum, and in the perirenal area (England, 1983). Brown fat has a high content of mitochondria, giving it a definite brown hue.

By 18 weeks the uterus is formed and canalization of the vagina has begun. By this time many *primordial ovarian follicles* containing oogonia have formed (see Chapter 13). By 20 weeks the *testes* have begun to descend but are still located on the posterior abdominal wall, as are the *ovaries* in female fetuses.

Twenty-one to Twenty-five Weeks

There is a *substantial weight gain* during this period. Although still somewhat lean, the fetus is better proportioned (Fig. 6-10). The skin is usually wrinkled, particularly during the early part of this period, and is more translucent. The skin is pink to red in fresh specimens because blood is visible in the capillaries. At 21 weeks rapid eye movements begin, and *blink-startle responses* have been reported at 22 to 23 weeks following application of a vibroacoustic noise source to the mother's abdomen (Birnholz and Benaceraff, 1983).

By 24 weeks the secretory epithelial cells (type II pneumocytes) in the interalveolar walls of the lung have begun to secrete *surfactant*, a surface-active lipid that maintains the patency of the developing alveoli of the lungs (see Chapter 11). *Fingernails* are also present by 24 weeks. Although a 22- to 25-week fetus born prematurely may survive if given intensive care, it may die during early infancy because its respiratory system is still immature.

Twenty-six to Twenty-nine Weeks

During this period a fetus often survives if born prematurely and given intensive care because its *lungs are now capable of breathing air.* The lungs and pulmonary vasculature have developed sufficiently to provide adequate gas exchange (see Fig. 11-8). In addition, the central nervous system has matured to the stage where it can direct rhythmic breathing movements and control body temperature. The greatest neonatal losses occur in infants who weigh less than 2000 gm (Bowie, 1988).

The *eyes reopen* at 26 weeks, and lanugo and head hair are well developed (Fig. 6-11). Toenails become visible, and considerable subcutaneous fat is now present under the skin, smoothing out many of the wrinkles. During this period the quantity of white fat increases to about 3.5 per cent of body weight. *The fetal spleen is now an important site of hematopoiesis.*[1] Erythropoiesis in the spleen ends by 28 weeks, by which time bone marrow has become the major site of formation of erythrocytes (Boles Jr., 1991).

---

[1] The process of formation and development of various types of blood cells and other formed elements.

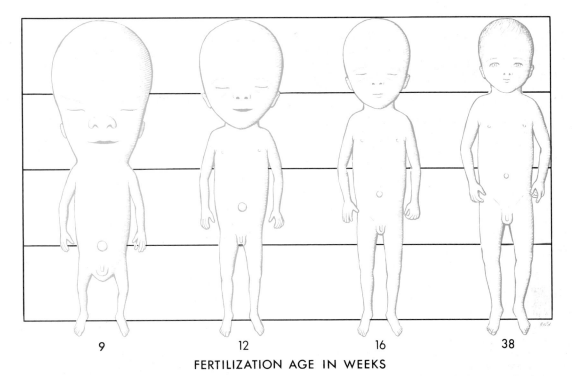

FERTILIZATION AGE IN WEEKS

Figure 6-3. Diagram illustrating the changing proportions of the body during the fetal period. At nine weeks the head is about half the crown-rump length of the fetus. By 36 weeks the circumferences of the head and the abdomen are approximately equal. After this, the circumference of the abdomen may be greater. All stages are drawn to the same total height.

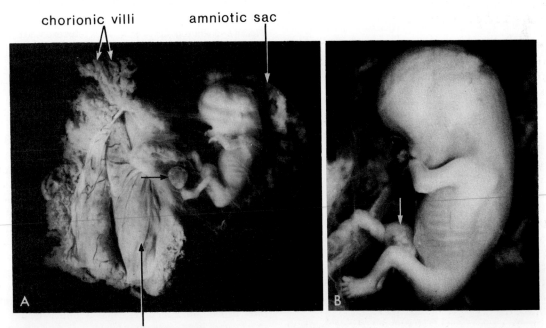

chorionic villi   amniotic sac

chorionic sac

Figure 6-4. Photographs of a nine-week fetus in the amniotic sac exposed by removal from its chorionic sac. *A*, Actual size. The remnant of the yolk sac is indicated by an arrow. *B*, Enlarged photograph of the fetus (× 2). Note the following features: (1) large head, (2) cartilaginous ribs, and (3) intestines in the proximal part of the umbilical cord (arrow). (Courtesy of Professor Jean Hay, Department of Anatomy, University of Manitoba, Winnipeg, Canada.)

Thirty to Thirty-four Weeks

The *pupillary light reflex* of the eyes can be elicited by 30 weeks. Usually by the end of this period, the skin is pink and smooth, and the upper and lower limbs have a chubby appearance. At this stage the quantity of white fat is about 8 per cent of body weight. Fetuses 32 weeks and older usually survive if born prematurely. If a normal-weight fetus is born during this period, it is "premature by date" as opposed to being "premature by weight."

Thirty-five to Thirty-eight Weeks

Fetuses at 35 weeks have a firm grasp and exhibit a spontaneous orientation to light. As term approaches (37 to 38 weeks), the nervous system is sufficiently mature to carry out some integrative functions (Drife, 1985). Most fetuses during this "finishing period" are plump (Fig. 6–12). By 36 weeks the circumferences of the head and abdomen are approximately equal. After this, the circumference of the abdomen may be greater than that of the head. There is a *slowing of growth* as the time of birth approaches (Fig. 6–13). Normal fetuses usually reach a CRL of 360 mm and weigh about 3400 gm. By full term the amount of white fat is about 16 per cent of body weight. A fetus adds about 14 gm of fat a day during these last weeks of gestation. In general, male fetuses are longer and weigh more at birth than females.

By full term (38 weeks after fertilization; 40 weeks after LNMP), the skin is normally bluish-pink. The chest is prominent and the breasts protrude slightly in both sexes. The testes are usually in the scrotum in

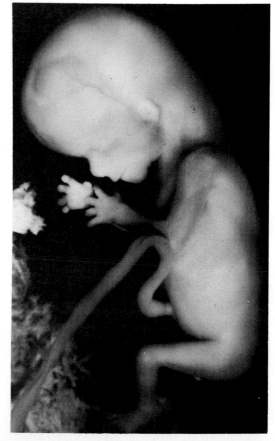

Figure 6–6. Photograph of an 11-week fetus exposed by removal from its chorionic and amniotic sacs (× 1.5). Note the relatively large head and that the intestines are no longer in the umbilical cord. (Courtesy of Professor Jean Hay, Department of Anatomy, University of Manitoba, Winnipeg, Canada.)

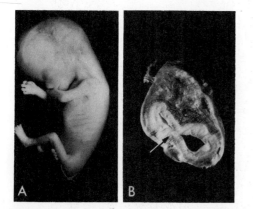

Figure 6–5. Photographs of: (A) 10-week fetus, and (B) section of the mother's ovary showing the corpus luteum of pregnancy (*arrow*). The corpus luteum secretes both estrogen and progesterone, important hormones for the maintenance of pregnancy. Actual size.

full-term male infants; their descent begins at 28 to 32 weeks. Thus, premature male infants commonly have undescended testes. Although the head at full term is smaller in relation to the rest of the body than it was earlier in fetal life, it still is one of the largest regions of the fetus. This is an important consideration related to its passage through the birth canal (cervix and vagina; see Figures 7–10 and 7–11).

Not all low-weight babies are premature. About one third of those with a birth weight of 2500 gm or less are actually small or undergrown for their gestational age. These infants, often called "small for dates," may be underweight because of *placental insufficiency* (see Chapter 7). The placentas are often small and/or poorly attached. Placental insufficiency often results from degenerative changes in the placenta that progressively reduce the oxygen supply and nourishment to the fetus (Behrman, 1992).

Text continued on page 104

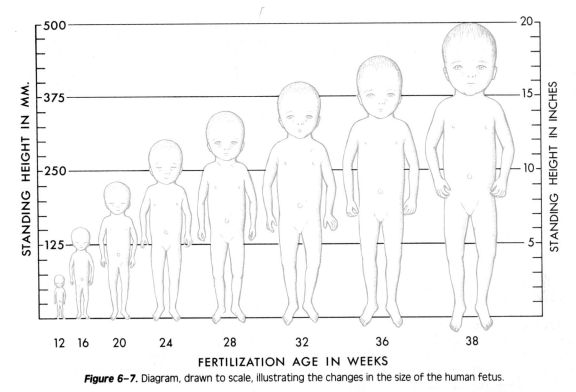

Figure 6–7. Diagram, drawn to scale, illustrating the changes in the size of the human fetus.

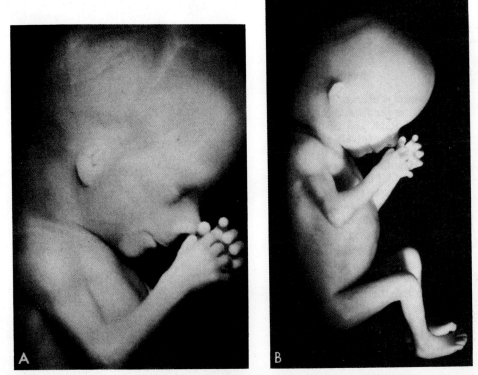

Figure 6–8. Photographs of a 13-week fetus. *A,* Enlarged photograph of its head and shoulders (× 2). Note that its eyes are closed. *B,* Actual size. Note that its CRL is about the same as the width of your palm. (Courtesy of Professor Jean Hay, Department of Anatomy, University of Manitoba, Winnipeg, Canada.)

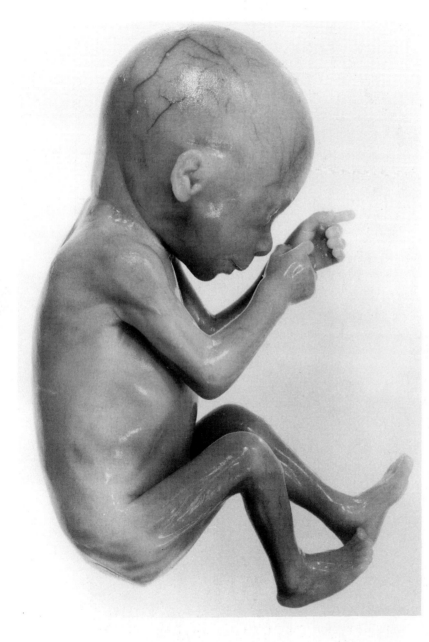

Figure 6–9. Photograph of a 17-week fetus. Actual size. Because there is very little subcutaneous fat and the skin is thin, the blood vessels of the scalp are visible. Fetuses at this age are unable to survive if born prematurely, mainly because their respiratory systems are immature.

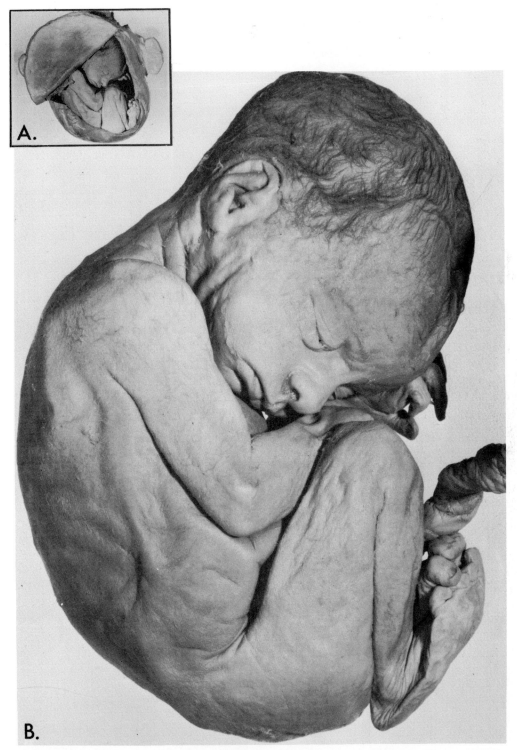

Figure 6–10. Photographs of a 25-week fetus. *A*, In the uterus. *B*, Actual size. Note the wrinkled skin and rather lean body caused by the scarcity of subcutaneous fat. Observe that the eyes are beginning to open. A fetus at this age might survive if born prematurely; hence, it is a viable fetus. The mother of this fetus was killed in an automobile accident.

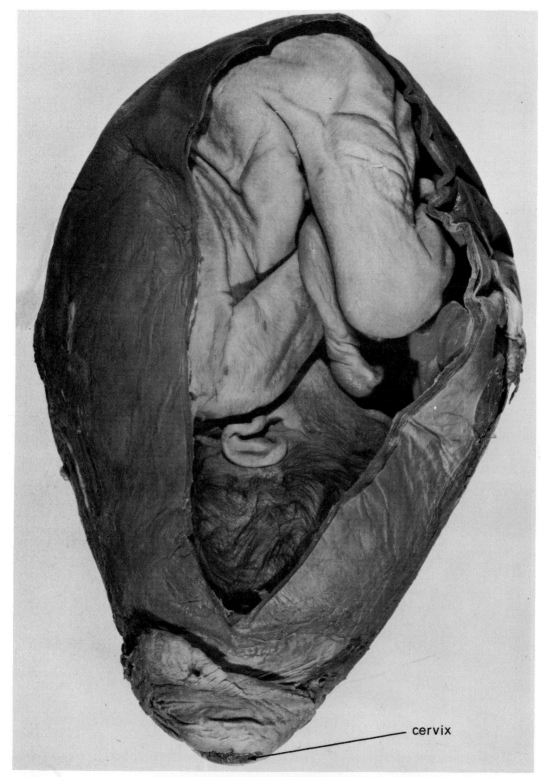

Figure 6–11. Photograph of a 29-week fetus in the uterus. Actual size. Note that the fetus is upside down; this is the normal presentation at this period of gestation. A portion of the wall of the uterus and parts of the chorion and amnion have been removed to show the fetus. This fetus and its mother died as the result of injuries sustained in an automobile accident.

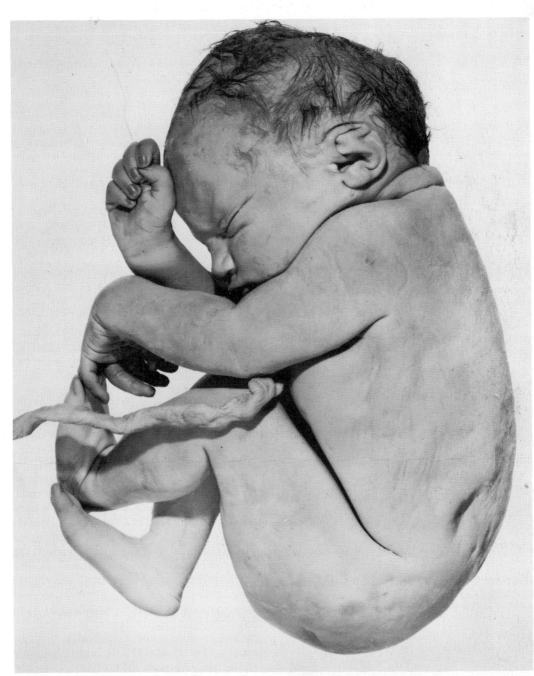

Figure 6–12. Photograph of a 36-week fetus. Half actual size. Fetuses at this size and age usually survive. Note the plump body resulting from the deposition of subcutaneous fat. This fetus's mother was killed in an automobile accident, and the fetus died before it could be delivered by Cesarean section.

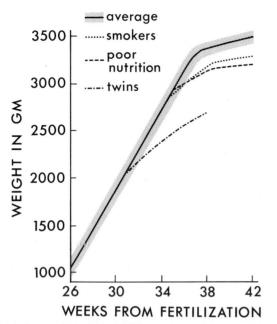

Figure 6–13. Graph showing the rate of fetal growth during the last trimester. Average refers to babies born in the United States. After 36 weeks the growth rate deviates from the straight line. The decline, particularly after full term (38 weeks), probably reflects inadequate fetal nutrition caused by degenerative, placental changes. (Adapted from Gruenwald P: *Am J Obstet Gynecol* 94:1112, 1966.)

It is important to distinguish between *full-term infants* who have a low birth weight because of IUGR and *preterm infants* who are underweight because of a shortened gestation (i.e., "premature by date"). IUGR may be caused by placental insufficiency, multiple gestations (e.g., triplets), infectious diseases, cardiovascular malformations, inadequate maternal nutrition, and maternal and fetal hormones. Teratogens (drugs, chemicals, and viruses) and genetic factors are also known to cause *IUGR* (see Table 8–6). Infants with IUGR show a characteristic lack of subcutaneous fat and their skin is wrinkled, suggesting that white fat has actually been lost. Brown fat is also reduced or absent.

The Time of Birth

The expected time of birth is 266 days or 38 weeks after fertilization; i.e., 280 days or 40 weeks after LNMP (Table 6–1). About 12 per cent of babies, however, are born one to two weeks after the expected date of confinement (*EDC*). Prolongation of pregnancy for three or more weeks beyond the EDC occurs in 5 to 6 per cent of women.

Some infants in prolonged pregnancies develop the *postmaturity syndrome*. They are thin and have dry, parchmentlike skin, but they are often overweight and character-

ized by absence of lanugo hair, decreased or absent vernix caseosa, long nails, and increased alertness. "When delivery is delayed three weeks or more beyond term, there is a significant increase in mortality" (Behrman, 1992). Because of this, labor is often induced (Chapter 7, p. 53).

The common clinical method of determining EDC is to count back three calendar months from the first day of the LNMP and then add a year and seven days (*Naegele's rule*). In women with regular menstrual cycles, this method gives a reasonably accurate EDC. If the woman's cycles were irregular, however, miscalculations of two to three weeks may occur. In addition, *implantation bleeding* (p. 53) occurs in some pregnant women at the time of the first missed period (about two weeks after fertilization). Should the woman interpret this bleeding as a normal menstruation, the estimated time of birth could be miscalculated by two or more weeks. Ultrasonographic examinations of the fetus, in particular CRL measurements between 9 and 12 weeks of gestation (7 to 10 weeks after fertilization), are commonly used now for a more reliable prediction of the EDC (Resnik, 1990; Lyons and Levi, 1991).

FACTORS INFLUENCING FETAL GROWTH

The fetus requires substrates for the production of energy and growth. Gases and nutrients pass freely to the fetus from the mother via the placental membrane (see Fig. 7–8). **Glucose** is a primary source of energy for fetal metabolism and growth; *amino acids* are also required. These substances pass from the mother's blood to the fetus via the placental membrane (p. 119). The **insulin** required for the metabolism of glucose is secreted by the fetal pancreas; no significant quantities of maternal insulin reach the fetus because the placental membrane is relatively impermeable to this hormone. Insulin, human growth hormone, and some small polypeptides (such as somatomedin C) are believed to stimulate fetal growth. For a comprehensive account of human fetal growth, see Miller and Merritt (1979); Page et al. (1981), and Bowie (1988).

Many factors may affect fetal growth: maternal, fetal, and environmental. In general, factors operating throughout pregnancy (e.g., *cigarette smoking* and *consumption of alcohol*) tend to produce IUGR and small infants (p. 105), whereas factors operating during the last trimester (e.g., maternal malnutrition) usually produce underweight infants with normal length and head size. IUGR is usually defined as infant weight within the lowest tenth percentile for gestational age (Bowie, 1988; Behrman, 1992).

Maternal Malnutrition. Severe malnutrition resulting from a poor-quality diet is known to cause reduced fetal growth (Fig. 6–13). Poor nutrition and faulty food habits are common during pregnancy and are not restricted to mothers belonging to poverty groups (Illsley and Mitchell, 1984; Creasy and Resnik, 1989).

Cigarette Smoking. Smoking is a well-established cause of IUGR (Nash and Persaud, 1988). The growth rate for fetuses of mothers who smoke cigarettes is less than normal during the last six to eight weeks of pregnancy (Fig. 6–13). On average, the birth weight of infants whose mothers smoke heavily during pregnancy is 200 gm less than normal, and *perinatal morbidity* is increased when adequate medical care is unavailable (Behrman, 1992). The effect of maternal smoking is greater on fetuses whose mothers also receive inadequate nutrition. Presumably, there is an additive effect of heavy smoking and poor-quality diet.

Multiple Pregnancy. Individuals of twin, triplet, and other multiple births usually weigh considerably less than infants resulting from a single pregnancy (Fig. 6–13). It is evident that the total requirements of two or more fetuses exceed the nutritional supply available from the placenta during the third trimester.

Social Drugs. Infants born to alcoholic mothers often exhibit IUGR as part of the *fetal alcohol syndrome* (see Chapter 8). Similarly, the use of *marijuana* and narcotic drugs (e.g., *heroin*) can cause IUGR and other obstetrical complications (Persaud, 1988, 1990).

Impaired Uteroplacental Blood Flow. Maternal placental circulation may be reduced by a variety of conditions that decreases uterine blood flow (e.g., small chorionic or umbilical vessels, severe hypotension, and renal disease). Chronic reduction of uterine blood flow can cause *fetal starvation* resulting in IUGR (Rosso, 1980; Harding and Charlton, 1991).

Placental Insufficiency. Placental dysfunction or defects (e.g., infarction; see Chapter 7) can also cause IUGR. The net effect of these placental abnormalities is a reduction of the total area for exchange of nutrients between the fetal and maternal blood streams. It is very difficult to separate the effect of these placental changes from the effect of reduced maternal blood flow to the placenta. In some instances of chronic maternal disease, the maternal vascular changes in the uterus are primary and the placental defects secondary (Harding and Charlton, 1991).

Genetic Factors. It is well established that genetic factors can cause IUGR. Repeated cases of this condition in one family indicate that recessive genes may be the cause of the abnormal growth. In recent years, structural and numerical chromosomal aberrations have also been shown to be associated with cases of retarded fetal growth (Thompson et al., 1991). IUGR is pronounced in infants with Down syndrome and is characteristic of fetuses with trisomy 18 syndrome (Chapter 8, p. 146).

PERINATOLOGY

By accepting the shelter of the uterus, the fetus also takes the risk of maternal disease or malnutrition and of biochemical, immunological and hormonal adjustment.
    —*George W. Corner,*
    American embryologist, 1888–1981.

Perinatology is the branch of medicine concerned with the well-being of the fetus and newborn infant, generally covering the period from about 26 weeks after fertilization to four weeks after birth. The subspecialty of *perinatal medicine* combines certain aspects of obstetrics and pediatrics. A third-trimester fetus is now commonly regarded as an *unborn patient* on whom diagnostic and therapeutic procedures may be performed (Harrison et al., 1991). Several techniques are now available for assessing the status of the fetus and providing prenatal treatment if required.

PROCEDURES FOR ASSESSING THE STATUS OF THE FETUS

Fetal activity felt by the mother or palpated by the physician were the first clues for assessing fetal well-being. Then the fetal heartbeat was detected, first by auscultation and later by electronic monitors. These techniques indicated fetal stress and distress. Later, gonadotrophic hormones were detected in maternal blood. Many new procedures for assessing the status of the fetus have been developed in the last two decades. It is now possible to treat many fetuses whose lives are in jeopardy (Harrison, 1991; Behrman, 1992).

Diagnostic Amniocentesis. This is the most common invasive prenatal diagnostic procedure (Wilson, 1991). For prenatal diagnosis, amniotic fluid is sampled by inserting a hollow needle through the mother's anterior abdominal and uterine walls into the amniotic cavity by piercing the chorion and amnion (Fig. 6–14*A*). A syringe is attached and amniotic fluid withdrawn. Bevis (1952) introduced diagnostic amniocentesis with his report on the antenatal prediction of hemolytic disease in the newborn (HDN). Because there is relatively little amniotic fluid prior to the fourteenth week after LNMP (p. 128), amniocentesis is difficult to perform prior to this time. Thus, amniocentesis is usually performed during the fourteenth to sixteenth weeks after LNMP (twelfth to fourteenth week after fertilization). The procedure is relatively devoid of risk, especially when the procedure is performed by an experienced physician who is guided by ultrasonography for outlining the position of the fetus and placenta.

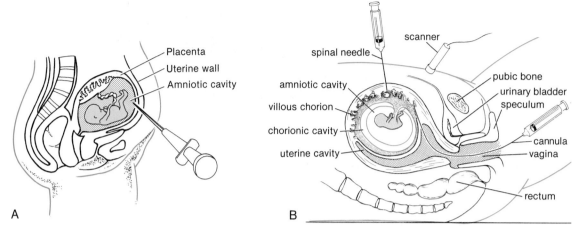

Figure 6–14. *A,* Drawing illustrating the technique of amniocentesis. A needle is inserted through the lower abdominal wall and uterine wall into the amniotic cavity. A syringe is attached and amniotic fluid withdrawn for diagnostic purposes (e.g., for cell cultures or alpha-fetoprotein studies). The technique is usually performed during the fourteenth to sixteenth week after the last normal menstrual period (*LNMP*). *B,* Drawing illustrating chorionic villus sampling (CVS). This technique is usually performed around the ninth week after LNMP. Two sampling approaches are illustrated: via the maternal anterior abdominal wall with a spinal needle, and via the vagina and cervical canal using a malleable cannula. Success and safety in both approaches depend upon use of a scanner (ultrasound imaging).

Amniocentesis is a common technique for detecting genetic disorders (e.g., Down syndrome). Complications associated with amniocentesis are relatively uncommon. There is a small risk of inducing an abortion, estimated to be about 0.5 per cent by Thompson et al. (1991). The common *indications for amniocentesis* are: (1) advanced maternal age (e.g., 38 years or older); (2) previous birth of a trisomic child (e.g., Down syndrome); (3) a chromosome abnormality in either parent (e.g., a chromosome translocation; see Chapter 8, p. 149); (4) women who are carriers of X-linked recessive disorders (e.g., *hemophilia*); (5) a history of neural tube defects (NTDs) in the family (e.g., spina bifida cystica; see Chapter 18), and (6) carriers of inborn errors of metabolism (Anon, 1991; Hobbins, 1991).

Alpha-fetoprotein (AFP) Assay. AFP escapes from the circulation into the amniotic fluid from fetuses with open *neural tube defects* (NTDs), such as spina bifida with myeloschisis or meroanencephaly (see Chapter 18). The term "open" refers to lesions that are not covered with skin. AFP also enters the amniotic fluid from open ventral wall defects (VWDs), such as gastroschisis and omphalocele (see Chapter 12).

The concentration of AFP in the amniotic fluid surrounding fetuses with open NTDs and VWDs is remarkably high. It is therefore possible to detect the presence of these severe abnormalities of the central nervous system and ventral wall by measuring the concentration of AFP in amniotic fluid (Haddow, 1991). *Amniotic fluid AFP* concentration is measured by immunoassay; and, when used with ultrasonographic scanning, about 99 per cent of fetuses with these severe defects can be diagnosed prenatally. When a fetus has an open NTD, the concentration of AFP is also likely to be higher than normal in the maternal serum. *Maternal serum AFP* concentration is low when the fetus has Down syndrome and other chromosome defects (Merkatz et al., 1984; Thompson et al., 1991).

Spectrophotometric Studies. Examination of amniotic fluid by this method may be used for assessing the degree of *erythroblastosis fetalis* (also called HDN). This condition results from destruction of fetal red blood cells by maternal antibodies (see Chapter 7, p. 121).

Sex Chromatin Patterns. Fetal sex can be diagnosed by noting the presence or absence of sex chromatin in the nuclei of cells recovered from amniotic fluid (Fig. 6–15*A* and *B*). By use of a special staining technique, the Y chromosome can also be identified in cells recovered from the amniotic fluid surrounding male fetuses (Fig. 6–15*C*). Knowledge of *fetal sex* can be useful in diagnosing the presence of severe, sex-linked, hereditary diseases, such as *hemophilia* and muscular dystrophy (Simpson and Elias, 1989; Thompson et al., 1991). These tests are not routine and are not performed to satisfy the parents' curiosity about the sex of a fetus.

Cell Cultures. Fetal sex and chromosomal aberrations can also be determined by studying the sex chromosomes in cultured fetal cells obtained during amniocentesis. These cultures are commonly done when an autosomal abnormality is suspected, such as

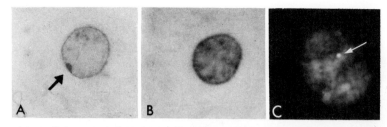

Figure 6-15. Nuclei of cells in amniotic fluid obtained by amniocentesis. *A*, Chromatin-positive nucleus indicating the presence of a female fetus; the sex chromatin is indicated by an arrow. *B*, Chromatin-negative nucleus indicating the presence of a male fetus. No sex chromatin is visible. Cresylecht violet stain (× 1000). *C*, Y-chromatin-positive nucleus indicating the presence of a male fetus. The arrow indicates the Y chromatin as an intensely fluorescent body obtained after staining the cell in quinacrine mustard.(*A* and *B*, From Riis M, Fuchs F: *In* Moore KL [ed]: *The Sex Chromatin.* Philadelphia, WB Saunders, 1966. *C*, Courtesy of Dr. M. Ray, Department of Medical Genetics and Department of Anatomy, University of Manitoba and Health Sciences Centre, Winnipeg, Canada.)

occurs in the Down syndrome. *Inborn errors of metabolism* in fetuses can also be detected by studying cell cultures. Enzyme deficiencies can be determined by incubating cells recovered from amniotic fluid and then detecting the specific enzyme deficiency in the cells (Polin and Mennuti, 1987; Weaver, 1989).

Chorionic Villus Sampling (CVS). Biopsies of chorionic villi (mostly trophoblast) may be obtained by inserting a needle, guided by ultrasonography, through the mother's abdominal and uterine walls into the uterine cavity. To understand how such a biopsy can be obtained, see Figure 6–14*B*. Chorionic villi sampling is more commonly performed transcervically using real-time ultrasound guidance (Young et al., 1991; Hogge, 1991).

Biopsies of chorionic villi are used for detecting chromosomal abnormalities, inborn errors of metabolism, and X-linked disorders (Verma and Babu, 1989; Thompson et al., 1991). CVS can be performed as early as the ninth week of gestation (seven weeks after fertilization). The rate of fetal loss is about one per cent, slightly more than the risk from amniocentesis (Thompson et al., 1991). The major advantage of CVS over amniocentesis is that it allows the results of chromosomal analysis to be available several weeks earlier than when performed by amniocentesis.

Intrauterine Fetal Transfusion. Some fetuses with *hemolytic disease of the newborn* (HDN) can be saved by receiving intrauterine blood transfusions (Liley, 1965). The blood is injected through a needle inserted into the fetal peritoneal cavity (Bowman, 1989). Over a period of five to six days, most of the injected cells pass into the fetal circulation via the diaphragmatic lymphatics (Pritchard and Weisman, 1957). With recent advances in percutaneous *umbilical cord puncture,* blood can be transfused directly into the fetal vascular system (Harrison, 1991).

The need for fetal blood transfusions is reduced nowadays due to the treatment of Rh-negative mothers of Rh-positive fetuses with anti-Rh immunoglobulin. Consequently, *HDN is relatively uncommon now* because Rh immunoglobulin usually prevents development of this disease of the Rh system (Thompson et al., 1991).

Fetoscopy. Using fiberoptic lighting instruments, parts of the fetal body may be directly observed. It is possible to scan the entire fetus looking for congenital anomalies, such as cleft lip and limb defects. The fetoscope is usually introduced through the anterior abdominal and uterine walls into the amniotic cavity similar to the way the needle is inserted during amniocentesis (Fig. 6–14*A*). Because of the risk to the fetus (estimated to be about five per cent by Behrman, 1992) compared to other prenatal diagnostic procedures as well as the poorer detail of the fetal anatomy that can be visualized, fetoscopy now has few indications for routine prenatal diagnosis or treatment of the fetus.

Cordocentesis or Percutaneous Umbilical Cord Blood Sampling (PUBS). Fetal blood samples may be obtained from umbilical vessels for chromosome analysis. Ultrasonographic scanning facilitates the procedure by outlining the location of the vessels. PUBS is often used about 20 weeks after LNMP for chromosome analysis when ultrasonographic or other examinations have shown a fetal anomaly.

Ultrasonography. The chorionic (gestational) sac and its contents may be visualized during the embryonic and fetal periods by using ultrasound techniques. Placental and fetal size, multiple births, and abnormal presentations can also be determined (Jeantry and Romero, 1984; Callen, 1988b; Wathen et al., 1991). *Ultrasonic scans* give accurate measurements of the biparietal diameter of the fetal skull from which close estimates of fetal age and length can be made

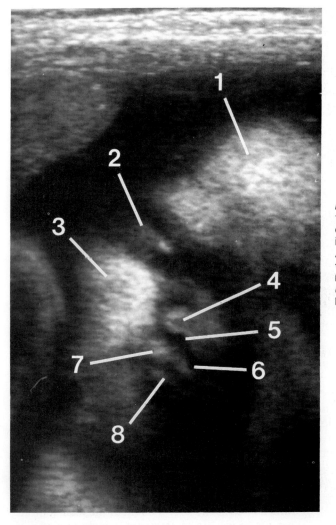

Figure 6–16. Sonogram of a third trimester fetus showing that the face can be viewed with considerable clarity (*1*, brow; *2*, eyelid; *3*, cheek; *4*, ala, i.e., side of nose; *5*, nostril; *6*, philtrum, i.e., depression in upper lip; *7*, right side of lip; *8*, lower lip). Amniotic fluid surrounding the face provides the "contrast" for visualization. (From Filly RA: Sonographic anatomy of the normal fetus. *In* Harrison MR, Globus MS, Filly RA [eds]: *The Unborn Patient: Prenatal Diagnosis and Treatment.* 2nd ed. Philadelphia, WB Saunders, 1991.)

(Kurtz and Needleman, 1988). In most cases the male genitalia can be visualized by ultrasound.

Figure 6–16 illustrates how details of the fetus can be observed in ultrasound scans. Ultrasound examinations are also helpful for diagnosing abnormal pregnancies at a very early stage (Filly, 1991a); e.g., the so-called "blighted embryo". Rapid advances in ultrasonography have made this technique a major tool for prenatal diagnosis of fetal abnormalities, i.e., meroanencephaly (anencephaly), hydrocephaly, microcephaly, fetal ascites, and renal agenesis (Spirt et al., 1987; Callen, 1988b; Pilling, 1990; Harrison et al., 1991).

Computed Tomography (CT) and Magnetic Resonance Imaging (MRI). When planning fetal treatment, (e.g., surgery [Filly, 1991a and b]), CT and MRI may be used to provide more information about an abnormality that has been detected in an ultrasonic scan. The disadvantages of current MRI include high cost, fixed planes of section, and limited fetal resolution.

Amniography and Fetography. When performing these techniques, a radiopaque substance is injected into the amniotic cavity to outline the amniotic sac and the external features of the fetus. A water-soluble contrast medium is used in amniography, and an oil-soluble contrast medium is injected during fetography. The latter medium is apparently absorbed by the vernix caseosa (p. 96). These procedures increase the risk of premature rupture of the membranes and preterm labor (p. 118). Like fetoscopy, these procedures have been more or less replaced by noninvasive, high resolution, ultrasonic imaging techniques, which

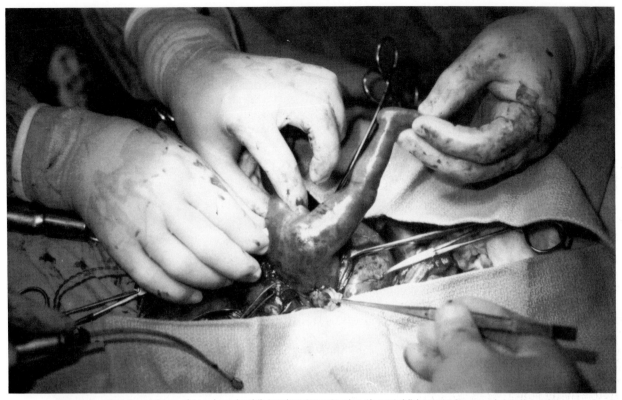

Figure 6–17. Fetus at 21 weeks undergoing bilateral ureterostomies, the establishment of external openings of the ureters into the bladder. (From Harrison MR, Globus MS, Filly RA [eds]: *The Unborn Patient: Prenatal Diagnosis and Treatment.* 2nd ed. Philadelphia, WB Saunders, 1991.)

give an even more accurate delineation of fetal structures (Fig. 6–16).

Fetal Monitoring. Continuous fetal heart rate monitoring in high-risk pregnancies is routine and provides information about the oxygenation of the fetus. **Fetal distress** (e.g., indicated by an abnormal heart rate or rhythm) suggests that the fetus is in jeopardy.

There are various causes of prenatal antepartum fetal distress, such as maternal diseases that reduce oxygen transport to the fetus (e.g., cyanotic heart disease). The external mode of monitoring uses transducers placed on the mother's abdomen; for example, an ultrasound transducer picks up high-frequency sound waves that reflect the mechanical action of the fetal heart. For more information on fetal distress and continuous fetal heart monitoring, see Behrman (1992) and Rosen (1991).

SUMMARY OF THE FETAL PERIOD

The fetal period begins nine weeks after fertilization (11 weeks after LNMP) and ends at birth. It is characterized by rapid body growth and differentiation of tissues and organ systems. An obvious change is the relative slowing of head growth compared with that of the rest of the body. By the beginning of the twentieth week, lanugo and head hair appear, and the skin is coated with vernix caseosa. The eyelids are closed during most of the fetal period but begin to reopen at about 26 weeks. Until this time, the fetus is usually incapable of extrauterine existence, mainly because of the immaturity of its respiratory system.

Until about 30 weeks, the fetus appears reddish and wizened because of the thinness of its skin and the relative absence of subcutaneous fat. Fat usually develops rapidly during the last six to eight weeks, giving the fetus a smooth, plump appearance. This terminal ("finishing") period is devoted mainly to building up of tissues and to preparing systems involved in the transition from intrauterine to extrauterine environments, primarily the respiratory and cardiovascular systems. Fetuses born prematurely during the 26- to 36-week period usually survive, but full-term fetuses have the best chance of survival.

Changes occurring during the fetal period are not so dramatic as those appearing in the embryonic period, but they are very important. The fetus is less vulnerable to the teratogenic effects of drugs, viruses, and radiation, but these agents may interfere with growth and normal functional development, especially of the brain and eyes (see Chapter 8).

Various techniques are available for assessing the status of the fetus and for diagnosing certain diseases (e.g., HDN) and developmental abnormalities (e.g., limb defects) before birth. The physician can now determine whether or not a fetus has a particular disease or a congenital defect by using various diagnostic techniques; e.g., amniocentesis and ultrasonography.

Prenatal diagnosis can be made early enough to allow early termination of the pregnancy if elected; e.g., when serious anomalies incompatible with postnatal life are diagnosed. In selected cases, various treatments can be given to the fetus; e.g., the administration of drugs to correct cardiac arrhythmia (Harrison, 1991). Surgical correction of congenital anomalies in utero is also possible; e.g., ureterostomies on fetuses that have ureters that do not have openings into the bladder (Fig. 6–17).

CLINICALLY ORIENTED QUESTIONS FOR PROBLEM-BASED LEARNING SESSIONS

1. A woman in the twentieth week of a high-risk pregnancy was scheduled for a repeat Cesarean section. Her physician wanted to establish an estimated date of confinement (EDC). How would an estimate of EDC be established? When would labor likely be induced? How could this be accomplished?
2. A 42-year-old pregnant woman was worried that she might be carrying a fetus with major congenital anomalies. How could the status of her fetus be obtained? What chromosomal abnormality would most likely be found? What other chromosomal aberrations might be detected? If this was of clinical interest, how could the sex of the fetus be determined in a family known to have hemophilia or muscular dystrophy?
3. A 19-year-old woman in the second trimester of pregnancy asked a physician whether her fetus was vulnerable to "over-the-counter drugs" and street drugs. She also wondered about the effect of her heavy drinking and cigarette smoking on her fetus. What would the physician likely tell her?
4. What factors may cause IUGR. Discuss them. Which factors can the mother eliminate?
5. A woman in the first trimester of her pregnancy who was to undergo amniocentesis expressed concerns about a miscarriage and the possibility of injury to her fetus. What is the risk of these complications? What procedures are used to minimize these risks? What other technique might be used for obtaining cells for chromosome study? What does the acronym "PUBS" mean? Describe how this technique is performed and how it is used to assess the status of a fetus.
6. What types of fetal anomaly can be indicated by an alpha-fetoprotein (AFP) assay of maternal serum? Explain. What is the significance of high and low levels of AFP?

The answers to these questions are given on page 460.

References and Suggested Reading

Abramowicz JS, Sherer DM, Bar-Tov E, Woods Jr, JR: The cheek-to-cheek diameter in the ultrasonographic assessment of fetal growth. *Am J Obstet Gynecol 165*:846, 1991.

Anon: Canadian Guidelines for Prenatal Diagnosis of Genetic Disorders: An Update. A Joint Document of the Canadian College of Medical Geneticists and the Society of Obstetricians and Gynaecologists of Canada. *Journal SOGC 13*:13, 1991.

Barnea ER, Hustin J, Jauniaux E (eds): *The First Twelve Weeks of Gestation.* Berlin, Springer-Verlag, 1992.

Beck F, Moffat DB, Davies DP: *Human Embryology.* 2nd ed. Oxford, Blackwell Scientific Publications, 1985.

Behrman RE: *Nelson Textbook of Pediatrics.* 14th ed. Philadelphia, WB Saunders, 1992.

Benson CB, Doubilet PM: Sonographic prediction of gestational age '91–Accuracy of second-trimester and third-trimester fetal measurements. *Amer J Roentgenol 157*:1275, 1991.

Bevis DCA: The antenatal prediction of hemolytic disease of the newborn. *Lancet 1*:395, 1952.

Biggers JD: Arbitrary partitions of prenatal life. *Human Reprod 5*:1, 1990.

Birnholz JC: The development of human fetal eye movement patterns. *Science 213*:679, 1981.

Birnholz JC, Benaceraff BR: The development of human fetal hearing. *Science 222*:516, 1983.

Boehm CD, Kazazian Jr, HH: Prenatal diagnosis by DNA analysis. *In* Harrison MR, Golbus MS, Filly RA (eds): *The Unborn Patient: Prenatal Diagnosis and Treatment.* 2nd ed. Philadelphia, WB Saunders, 1991.

Boles Jr, ET: The spleen. *In* Schiller M (ed): *Pediatric Surgery of the Liver, Pancreas and Spleen*. Philadelphia, WB Saunders, 1991.

Bowie JD: Fetal growth. *In* Callen PW (ed): *Ultrasonography in Obstetrics and Gynecology*. Philadelphia, WB Saunders, 1988.

Bowman JM: Hemolytic disease (Erythroblastosis fetalis). *In* Creasy RK, Resnik R (eds): *Maternal-Fetal Medicine. Principles and Practice*. 2nd ed. Philadelphia, WB Saunders, 1989.

Callen PW: *Ultrasonography in Obstetrics and Gynecology*. 2nd ed. Philadelphia, WB Saunders, 1988a.

Callen PW: The obstetric ultrasound examination. *In* Callen PW (ed): *Ultrasonography in Obstetrics and Gynecology*. 2nd ed. Philadelphia, WB Saunders, 1988b.

Cooke RWI: The low birth weight baby. *In* Lister J, Irving IM (eds): *Neonatal Surgery*, 3rd ed. London, Butterworth, 1990.

Creasy RK, Resnik R: Intrauterine growth retardation. *In* Creasy RK, Resnik R (eds): *Maternal-Fetal Medicine: Principles and Practice*. 2nd ed. Philadelphia, WB Saunders, 1989.

Drife JO: Can the fetus listen and learn? *Brit J Obstet Gynecol 92*:777, 1985.

England MA: *Color Atlas of Life Before Birth*. Chicago, Year Book Medical Publishers, 1983.

Filly RA: The first trimester. *In* Callen PW (ed): *Ultrasonography in Obstetrics and Gynecology*. 2nd ed. Philadelphia, WB Saunders, 1988.

Filly RA: Sonographic anatomy of the normal fetus. *In* Harrison MR, Golbus MS, Filly RA (eds): *The Unborn Patient: Prenatal Diagnosis and Treatment*. 2nd ed. Philadelphia, WB Saunders, 1991a.

Filly RA: Alternative imaging techniques: computed tomography and magnetic resonance imaging. *In* Harrison MR, Golbus MS, Filly RA (eds): *The Unborn Patient. Prenatal Diagnosis and Treatment*. 2nd ed. Philadelphia, WB Saunders, 1991b.

Haddow JE: α-Fetoprotein. *In* Harrison MR, Golbus MS, Filly RA (eds): *The Unborn Patient: Prenatal Diagnosis and Treatment*. 2nd ed. Philadelphia, WB Saunders, 1991.

Harding JE, Charlton V: Experimental nutritional supplementation for intrauterine growth retardation. *In* Harrison MR, Golbus MS, Filly RA (eds): *The Unborn Patient: Prenatal Diagnosis and Treatment*. 2nd ed. Philadelphia, WB Saunders, 1991.

Harrison MR: Selection for treatment: Which defects are correctable. *In* Harrison MR, Golbus MS, Filly RA (eds): *The Unborn Patient: Prenatal Diagnosis and Treatment*. 2nd ed. Philadelphia, WB Saunders, 1991.

Harrison MR, Golbus MS, Filly RA (eds): *The Unborn Patient. Prenatal Diagnosis and Treatment*. 2nd ed. Philadelphia, WB Saunders, 1991.

Hinrichsen KV (ed): *Humanembryologie*. Berlin, Springer-Verlag, 1990.

Hobbins JC: Amniocentesis. *In* Harrison MR, Golbus MS, Filly RA (eds): *The Unborn Patient: Prenatal Diagnosis and Treatment*. 2nd ed. Philadelphia, WB Saunders, 1991.

Hogge WA: Chorionic villus sampling. *In* Harrison MR, Golbus MS, Filly RA (eds): *The Unborn Patient: Prenatal Diagnosis and Treatment*. 2nd ed. Philadelphia, WB Saunders, 1991.

Hull D: Brown adipose tissue in the newborn. *In* Philipp EE, Barnes J, Newton M (eds): *Scientific Foundations of Obstetrics and Gynecology*. London, William Heinemann, 1970.

Illingworth RS: *The Development of the Infant and Young Child*. 9th ed. New York, Churchill Livingstone, 1987.

Illsley R, Mitchell RG: The developing concept of low birth weight and the present state of knowledge. *In* Illsley R, Mitchell RGF (eds): *Low Birth Weight: A Medical, Psychological and Social Study*. New York, John Wiley & Sons, 1984.

Jeantry P, Romero R: *Obstetrical Ultrasound*. New York, McGraw-Hill, 1984.

Kalousek DK, Fitch N, Paradice BA: *Pathology of the Human Embryo and Previable Fetus. An Atlas*. New York, Springer-Verlag, 1990.

Kolata G: Finding biological clocks in fetuses. *Science 230*:929, 1985.

Kurtz AB, Needleman L: Ultrasound assessment of fetal age. *In* Callen PW (ed): *Ultrasonography in Obstetrics and Gynecology*. Philadelphia, WB Saunders, 1988.

Lee W, Barton S, Comstock CH, Bajorek S, Batton D, Kirk JS: Transverse cerebellar diameter: A useful predictor of gestational age for fetuses with asymmetric growth retardation. *Am J Obstet Gynecol 165*:1044, 1991.

Liley AW: The use of amniocentesis and fetal transfusion in erythroblastosis fetalis. *Pediatrics 35*:876, 1965.

Lucey JF: Conditions and diseases of the newborn. *In* Reid DE, Ryan KJ, Benirschke K (eds): *Principles and Management of Human Reproduction*. Philadelphia, WB Saunders, 1972.

Lyons EA, Levi CS: *Ultrasound of the normal first trimester of pregnancy*. Syllabus: Special Course Ultrasound. Radiological Society of North America, 1991.

MacIntyre M: Chromosomal problems of intrauterine diagnosis. *In* Bergsma D, Motulsky AG, Jackson C, Sitter J (eds): *Symposium on Intrauterine Diagnosis. Birth Defects 7*:10, 1971.

Manning F: Fetal assessment. *Manitoba Medicine 61*:63, 1991.

Merkatz IR, Nitowsky HM, Macri JN: An association between low maternal serum alpha-fetoprotein and fetal chromosome abnormalities. *Am J Obstet Gynecol 148*:886, 1984.

Miller HC, Merritt TA: *Fetal Growth in Humans*. Chicago, Year Book Medical Publishers, 1979.

Moore KL (ed): *The Sex Chromatin*. Philadelphia, WB Saunders, 1966.

Nash JE, Persaud TVN: Embryopathic risks of cigarette smoking. *Exp Pathol 33*:65, 1988.

O'Rahilly R, Müller F: *Developmental Stages in Human Embryos*. Publication 637. Washington, Carnegie Institution of Washington, 1987.

Page EW, Villee CA, Villee DB: *Human Reproduction: Essentials of Reproductive and Perinatal Medicine*. 3rd ed. Philadelphia, WB Saunders, 1981.

Persaud TVN: *Prenatal Pathology. Fetal Medicine*. Springfield, Illinois, Charles C Thomas, 1979.

Persaud TVN: Fetal alcohol syndrome. *CRC Critical Rev. in Anatomy & Cell Biology 1*:277, 1988.

Persaud TVN: *Environmental Causes of Human Birth Defects*. Springfield, Charles C Thomas, 1990.

Pilling DW: Antenatal diagnosis and its relevance to pediatric surgeons. *In* Lister J, Irving IM (eds): *Neonatal Surgery*. 3rd ed. London, Butterworth, 1990.

Platek DN, Divon MY, Anyaegbunam A, Merkatz IR: Intrapartum ultrasonographic estimates of fetal weight by the house staff. *Am J Obstet Gynecol 165*:842, 1991.

Polin RA, Mennuti MTP: Genetic disease and chromosomal abnormalities. *In* Fanaroff AA, Martin RJ (eds): *Neonatal-Perinatal Medicine. Diseases of the Fetus and Infant*. St Louis, CV Mosby, 1987.

Pritchard JA, Weisman R: The absorption of labelled erythrocytes from the peritoneal cavity of humans. *J Lab Clin Med 49*:756, 1957.

Quilligan EJ, Zuspan FP (eds): *Current Therapy in Obstetrics and Gynecology*. vol 3. Philadelphia, WB Saunders, 1990.

Resnik R: Post-term pregnancy. *In* Quilligan EJ, Zuspan FP (eds): *Current Therapy in Obstetrics and Gynecology*. vol 3. Philadelphia, WB Saunders, 1990.

Riis P, Fuchs F: Sex chromatin and antenatal sex diagnosis.

In Moore KL (ed): *The Sex Chromatin*. Philadelphia, WB Saunders, 1966.

Roberts L: Fishing cuts the angst in amniocentesis. *Science 254*:378, 1991.

Rosen M: Anesthesia and monitoring for fetal intervention. *In* Harrison MR, Golbus MS, Filly RA (eds): *The Unborn Patient: Prenatal Diagnosis and Treatment*. 2nd ed. Philadelphia, WB Saunders, 1991.

Rosso P: Placental growth, development, and function in relation to maternal nutrition. *Fed Proc 39*:250, 1980.

Scammon RE, Calkins HA: *Development and Growth of the External Dimensions of the Human Body in the Fetal Period*. Minneapolis, University of Minnesota Press, 1929.

Schats R, Van Os HC, Jansen CAM, Wladimiroff JW: The crown-rump length in early human pregnancy: A reappraisal. *Br J Obstet Gynaecol 98*:460, 1991.

Senterre J (ed): *Intrauterine Growth Retardation*. Nestle Nutrition Workshop Series. Vol 18. New York, Raven Press, 1989.

Shepard TH: Normal and abnormal growth patterns. *In* Gardner LI (ed): *Endocrine and Genetic Diseases of Childhood and Adolescence*. 2nd ed. Philadelphia, WB Saunders, 1975.

Shiota K: Development and intrauterine fate of normal and abnormal human conceptuses. *Cong Anom 31*:67, 1991.

Simpson JL, Elias S: Prenatal diagnosis of genetic disorders. *In* Creasy RK, Resnik R (eds): *Maternal-Fetal Medicine. Principles and Practice*. 2nd ed. Philadelphia, WB Saunders, 1989.

Sinclair D: *Human Growth After Birth*. Oxford, Oxford University Press, 1985.

Smith DW, Gong BT: Scalp hair patterning as a clue to early fetal brain development. *J Pediatr 83*:379, 1973.

Spirt BA, Gordon LP, Oliphant M: *Prenatal Ultrasound: A Color Atlas with Anatomic and Pathologic Correlation*. New York, Churchill Livingstone, 1987.

Stevenson RE: *The Fetus and Newly Born Infant. Influences of the Prenatal Environment*. St Louis, CV Mosby, 1973.

Streeter GL: Weight, sitting height, head size, foot length and menstrual age of the human embryo. *Contrib Embryol Carnegie Inst 11*:143, 1920.

Thompson MW, McInnes RR, Willard HF: *Thompson & Thompson: Genetics in Medicine*. 5th ed. Philadelphia, WB Saunders, 1991.

Tulchinsky D, Ryan KJ: *Maternal-Fetal Endocrinology*. Philadelphia, WB Saunders, 1980.

Usher RH, McLean FH: Normal fetal growth and the significance of fetal growth retardation. *In* Davis JA, Dobbing J (eds): *Scientific Foundation of Paediatrics*. Philadelphia, WB Saunders, 1974.

Verma RS, Babu A: *Human Chromosomes*. New York, Pergamon Press, 1989.

Wald NJ, Cuckle HS: AFP screening in early pregnancy. *In* Spencer JAD (ed): *Fetal Monitoring*. Oxford, Oxford University Press, 1991.

Wald NJ, Cuckle HS, Densem JW, et al: Maternal serum screening for Down's syndrome in early pregnancy. *Br Med J 297*:883, 1988.

Wathen NC, Cass PL, Kitau MJ, Chard T: Human chorionic gonadotrophin and alpha-fetoprotein levels in matched samples of amniotic fluid, extraembryonic coelomic fluid, and maternal serum in the first trimester of pregnancy. *Prenatal Diagnosis 11*:145, 1991.

Weaver DD: Inborn errors of metabolism. *In* Weaver DD (ed): *Catalogue of Prenatally Diagnosed Conditions*. Baltimore, The Johns Hopkins University Press, 1989.

Wilson RD: How to perform genetic amniocentesis. *Journal SOGC 13*:61, 1991.

Yen SSC, Jaffe RB: *Reproductive Endocrinology: Physiology, Pathophysiology and Clinical Management*. 3rd ed. Philadelphia, WB Saunders, 1991.

Young SR, Shipley CF, Wade RV, Edwards JG, Waters MB, Cantu ML, Best RG, Dennis EJ: Single-center comparison of results of 1000 prenatal diagnoses with chorionic villus sampling and 1000 diagnoses with amniocentesis. *Am J Obstet Gynecol 165*:255, 1991.

The Placenta and Fetal Membranes

The fetal part of the placenta and the fetal membranes separate the fetus from the endometrium of the uterus. There is an interchange of substances (e.g., nutrients and oxygen) between the maternal and fetal blood streams via the placenta. The vessels in the umbilical cord connect the placental circulation with the fetal circulation. The chorion, amnion, yolk sac, and allantois constitute the fetal membranes, which develop from the zygote, but do not form parts of the embryo or fetus except for parts of the yolk sac and allantois. Part of the yolk sac is incorporated into the embryo as the primordium of the primitive gut (see Fig. 5–1). The allantois forms a fibrous cord that is known as the urachus in the fetus and the median umbilical ligament in the adult (see Fig. 7–20). It extends from the apex of the urinary bladder to the umbilicus.

THE PLACENTA

The human placenta is a **fetomaternal organ** that has two components: (1) a large *fetal portion* that develops from the chorionic sac, and (2) a small *maternal portion* that is derived from the endometrium (Fig. 7–1). The placenta and umbilical cord function as a *transport mechanism* between the mother and the fetus. Nutrients pass from the maternal blood through the placenta to the fetal blood, and waste materials pass from the fetus to the mother. The fetal membranes and placenta perform the following functions and activities: protection, nutrition, respiration, excretion, and hormone production. At birth the placenta and fetal membranes are expelled from the uterus as the "afterbirth" (Figs. 7–10F and 7–12).

The Decidua

The term decidua (L. *deciduus*, a falling off) is applied to the *gravid endometrium* (the functional layer of the endometrium in a pregnant woman). The name indicates that this part of the endometrium separates ("falls away") from the remainder of the uterus at *parturition* (childbirth). In response to increasing progesterone levels, the connective tissue (stromal) cells of the endometrium enlarge to form pale-staining *decidual cells*. The endometrial cellular and vascular changes resulting from pregnancy are referred to as the **decidual reaction**. Decidual cells are a characteristic feature of the decidua that contain large amounts of glycogen and lipids (Fig. 7–2B). Many decidual cells degenerate near the fetus in the region of the *syncytiotrophoblast* (see Fig. 3–6) and, together with maternal blood and uterine secretions, provide a rich source of fetal nutrition. The full significance of decidual cells is not understood, but it has also been suggested that they protect the maternal tissue against uncontrolled invasion by the syncytiotrophoblast and that they may be involved in hormone production.

Three regions of the decidua are named according to their relation to the implantation site (Fig. 7–1): (1) The part of the decidua deep to the conceptus that forms the maternal component of the placenta is called the *decidua basalis*; (2) the superficial portion overlying the conceptus is known as the *decidua capsularis*; and (3) all the remaining endometrium is referred to as the *decidua parietalis* (decidua vera). These decidual regions, clearly recognizable during *ultrasonography*, are important in diagnosing early pregnancy (Filly, 1988; Lyons and Levi, 1991).

Development of the Placenta

Previous descriptions of early placental development traced the rapid proliferation of the trophoblast and the development of the chorionic sac and its villi (see Chapters 3 and 4). By the end of the third week, the anatomical arrangements necessary for physiological exchanges between the mother and embryo are established (see Fig. 4–11).

Up to the eighth week, chorionic villi cover the entire chorionic sac (Figs. 7–1C and 7–3A). As this

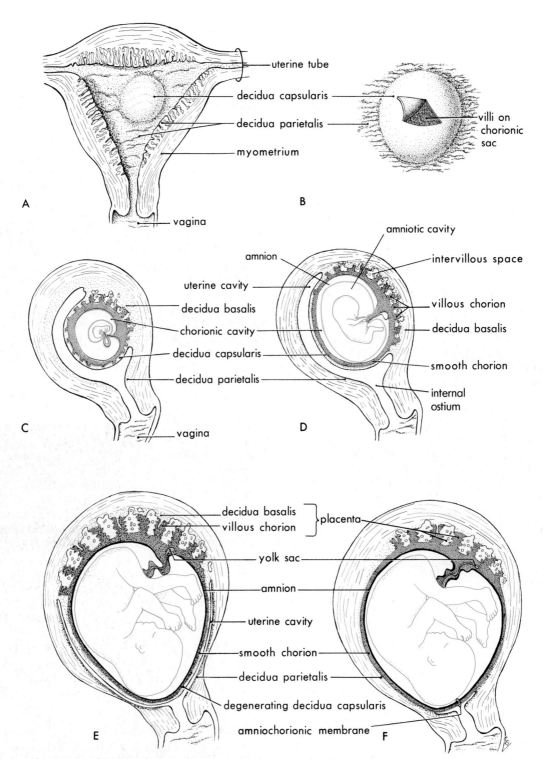

Figure 7-1. Drawings illustrating development of the human placenta and fetal membranes. *A,* Frontal section of the uterus showing elevation of the decidua capsularis caused by the expanding chorionic sac of a four-week embryo, implanted in the endometrium on the posterior wall. *B,* Enlarged drawing of the implantation site. The chorionic villi have been exposed by cutting an opening in the decidua capsularis. *C to F,* Sagittal sections of the gravid uterus from the fifth to twenty-second weeks, showing the changing relations of the fetal membranes to the decidua. In *F,* the amnion and chorion are fused with each other and the decidua parietalis, thereby obliterating the uterine cavity. Note in *D to F* that chorionic villi persist only where the chorion is associated with the decidua basalis, i.e., where the placenta forms.

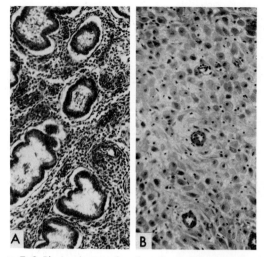

Figure 7–2. Photomicrographs of sections of the endometrium. *A,* During the secretory phase of the menstrual cycle (p. 27). Note the appearance of the stromal (connective tissue) cells around the uterine glands. *B,* The decidua during the second month of pregnancy showing the characteristic, pale-staining decidual cells. These glycogen- and lipid-laden cells are highly modified stromal cells (× 80). (Courtesy of Professor Jean Hay, Department of Anatomy, University of Manitoba, Winnipeg, Canada.)

sac grows, the villi associated with the decidua capsularis are compressed and the blood supply to them is reduced. These villi soon degenerate (Figs. 7–1*D* and 7–3*B*), producing a relatively avascular bare area known as the *smooth chorion* or chorion laeve (L. *levis,* smooth). As these villi disappear, those associated with the decidua basalis rapidly increase in number, branch profusely, and enlarge (Fig. 7–4). This bushy portion of the chorionic sac is known as the *villous chorion* or chorion frondosum (L. *frondosus,* leafy). The increase in the thickness of the placenta results from the branching of the stem villi (Figs. 7–5 and 7–6).

> The size of the chorionic sac is useful in determining *gestational age* (time elapsed since LNMP) in patients with uncertain menstrual histories (Filly, 1988; Lyons and Levi, 1991). Growth of the chorionic sac is extremely rapid between the fifth and tenth weeks. Modern ultrasound equipment, especially instruments equipped with intravaginal transducers, enables ultrasonographers to detect the chorionic (gestational) sac when it has a *median sac diameter* (MSD) of 2 to 3 mm. Chorionic sacs with this MSD indicate that the gestational age is about 31 days (i.e., 16 to 17 days after fertilization).

As the fetus grows, the uterus and placenta enlarge. Growth in the thickness of the placenta continues until the fetus is about 18 weeks old (20 weeks gestation). The fully developed placenta covers 15 to 30 per cent of the decidua. The **fetal component of the pla-**

centa is formed by the *villous chorion.* The stem villi that arise from it project into the intervillous space containing maternal blood (Figs. 7–1*D* and 7–6). The **maternal component of the placenta** is formed by the *decidua basalis* (Figs. 7–1*E,* 7–5, and 7–6). This

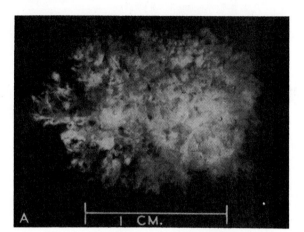

smooth chorion   villous chorion

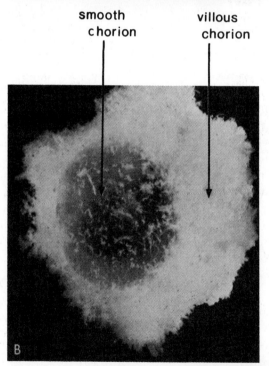

Figure 7–3. Photographs of spontaneously aborted human chorionic sacs. *A,* 21 days. The entire sac is covered with chorionic villi (× 4). *B,* Eight weeks (actual size). As the decidua capsularis becomes stretched and thin, the chorionic villi on the corresponding part of the chorionic sac gradually degenerate and disappear, leaving a smooth chorion (see Fig. 7–1*C* and *D*). The remaining villous chorion (Fig. 7–1*E* and *F*) forms the fetal contribution to the placenta. (From Potter EL, Craig JM: *Pathology of the Fetus and the Infant.* 3rd ed. Copyright 1975 by Year Book Medical Publishers, Chicago.)

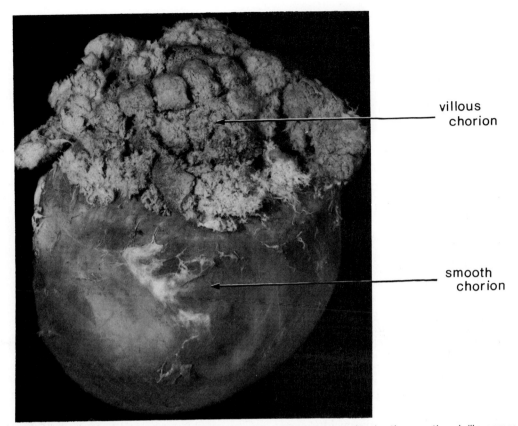

villous chorion

smooth chorion

Figure 7–4. Photograph of a human chorionic sac containing a 13-week fetus, showing the smooth and villous areas of the chorion. Actual size. To visualize how this chorionic sac was related to the uterus prior to its spontaneous abortion, see Figs. 7–1*E* and 7–5.

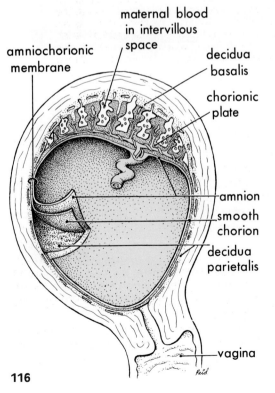

maternal blood
in intervillous
space

amniochorionic
membrane

decidua
basalis

chorionic
plate

amnion

smooth
chorion

decidua
parietalis

vagina

Figure 7–5. Drawing of a sagittal section of a gravid uterus at 22 weeks, showing the relation of the placenta and fetal membranes to each other and to the regions of the decidua. The fetus has been removed, and the amnion and smooth chorion have been cut and reflected to show their relationship to each other and the decidus parietalis.

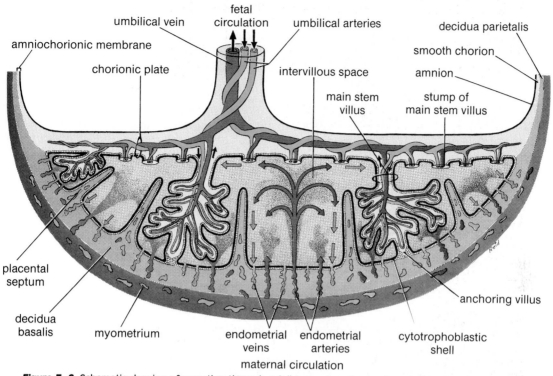

Figure 7–6. Schematic drawing of a section through a full-term placenta showing: (1) the relation of the villous chorion (fetal part of placenta) to the decidua basalis (maternal part of placenta), (2) the fetal placental circulation, and (3) the maternal placental circulation. Maternal blood flows into the intervillous space in funnel-shaped spurts, and exchanges occur with the fetal blood as the maternal blood flows around the branch villi (branches of stem villi). It is through the branch villi that the main exchange of material between the mother and embryo/fetus occurs. The inflowing arterial blood pushes venous blood out into the endometrial veins, which are scattered over the entire surface of the decidua basalis. Note that the umbilical arteries carry poorly oxygenated fetal blood (blue) to the placenta and that the umbilical vein carries oxygenated blood (red) to the fetus. Note that the cotyledons are separated from each other by decidual septa, projections of the maternal portion of the placenta (decidua basalis). Each cotyledon consists of two or more main stem villi and their many branches. In this drawing, only one stem villus is shown in each cotyledon, but the stumps of those that have been removed are indicated. See Figure 14–42 for a drawing of the fetal circulation and its relationship to the placenta.

is the endometrium that is related to the fetal component of the placenta. By the end of the fourth month, the decidua basalis is almost entirely replaced by the fetal component of the placenta.

The Fetomaternal Junction. The fetal portion of the placenta (villous chorion) is attached to the maternal portion of the placenta (decidua basalis) by the *cytotrophoblastic shell* (see Figs. 4–11 and 7–6). Stem chorionic villi ("anchoring villi") are attached firmly to the decidua basalis through the cytotrophoblastic shell. The stem villi anchor the *chorionic sac* and placenta to the decidua basalis. Maternal arteries and veins pass freely through gaps in the cytotrophoblastic shell and open into the intervillous space (Fig. 7–6).

The *shape of the placenta* is determined by the form of the persistent area of the chorionic villi (Fig. 7–1*F*). Usually, this is a circular area, giving the pla-

centa a discoid shape (Figs. 7–4 and 7–12). As the chorionic villi invade the decidua basalis during placental formation, endometrial tissue is eroded ("scooped out") to enlarge the intervillous space. This process produces several wedge-shaped areas of decidual tissue called *placental septa* that project toward the *chorionic plate* (Fig. 7–6). The placental septa divide the fetal part of the placenta into irregular convex areas called *cotyledons* (Fig. 7–12*A*). Each cotyledon, visible on the maternal surface of the placenta (Figs. 7–4 and 7–12*A*), consists of two or more stem villi and their many branch villi. By the end of the fourth month, the decidua basalis is almost entirely replaced by the cotyledons.

The **decidua capsularis**, the part of the decidua superficial to the conceptus, forms a capsule over its external surface (Fig. 7–1*A*). As the conceptus enlarges, the decidua capsularis bulges into the uterine cavity and becomes greatly attenuated. Eventually it contacts and fuses with the decidua parietalis, thereby obliterating the uterine cavity (Fig. 7–1*E*). By about 22 weeks, reduced blood supply to the decidua capsularis causes it to degenerate and disappear (Fig. 7–1*F*).

The Intervillous Space (Figs. 7–1*D*, 7–5, and 7–6). The intervillous space, *filled with maternal blood*, is derived from the lacunae that developed in the syncytiotrophoblast during the second week (see Fig. 3–1*C*). This large, blood-filled space results from the enlargement and coalescence of the lacunae. The intervillous space is divided into compartments by *placental septa*, but there is free communication between these compartments because the placental septa do not reach the *chorionic plate* (Fig. 7–6).

Maternal blood enters the intervillous space from the *spiral arteries* in the decidua basalis. These endometrial arteries pass through gaps in the cytotrophoblastic shell and discharge their blood into the intervillous space (see Figs. 4–11 and 7–6). This large space is drained by endometrial veins that also penetrate the cytotrophoblastic shell. They are found over the entire surface of the decidua basalis. The *branch villi*[1] are continuously showered with maternal blood that circulates through the intervillous space. The blood carries nutritional materials and oxygen that are necessary for fetal growth and development. It also takes away fetal waste products (e.g., carbon dioxide and excess water, salts, and products of protein metabolism).

The Amniochorionic Membrane (Figs. 7–1, 7–5, 7–6, and 7–17). The amniotic sac enlarges faster than the chorionic sac. As a result, the amnion and smooth chorion soon fuse to form the amniochorionic membrane. This composite membrane fuses with the decidua capsularis and, after disappearance of this part of the decidua, adheres to the decidua parietalis. It is the amniochorionic membrane that ruptures during labor (Fig. 7–10). Preterm rupture of this membrane ("bag of waters") is the most common event leading to premature labor. When the amniochorionic membrane ruptures, the amniotic fluid escapes through the cervix and vagina to the exterior.

Placental Circulation

The many branch villi of the placenta provide a large surface area where materials may be exchanged across the *placental membrane* (barrier) interposed between the fetal and maternal circulations (Figs. 7–6 to 7–8). It is through the numerous *branch villi* which

---

[1] Branches of the stem villi (Fig. 7–6).

arise from the sides of the *stem villi* that the main exchange of material between the mother and fetus takes place. The circulations of the fetus and the mother are separated by the very thin placental membrane consisting of extrafetal tissues (Figs. 7–7 and 7–8).

Fetal Placental Circulation (Figs. 7–6 and 7–7; see also Fig. 14–43). Poorly oxygenated blood leaves the fetus and passes through the *umbilical arteries* to the placenta. At the site of attachment of the cord to the placenta, these arteries divide into a number of radially disposed vessels that branch freely in the *chorionic plate* before entering the villi (Figs. 7–6 and 7–12*B*). The blood vessels form an extensive *arteriocapillary-venous system* within the villi (Fig. 7–7*A*), which brings the fetal blood extremely close to the maternal blood (Fig. 7–8). This system provides a very large area for the exchange of metabolic and gaseous products between the maternal and fetal blood streams. There is normally *no intermingling of fetal and maternal blood*, but very small amounts of fetal blood may enter the maternal circulation through minute defects that sometimes develop in the placental membrane (Fig. 7–7).

The well-oxygenated fetal blood passes into thin-walled veins that follow the placental arteries to the site of attachment of the umbilical cord where they converge to form the *umbilical vein*. This large vessel carries the oxygen-rich blood to the fetus (Fig. 7–6). For details about fetal circulation, see Chapter 14 (p. 341), Figure 14–43.

Maternal Placental Circulation (see Figs. 2–5*B* and 7–6). The blood in the intervillous space is temporarily outside the maternal circulatory system. It enters the intervillous space through 80 to 100 *spiral arteries* in the decidua basalis. These vessels discharge into the intervillous space through gaps in the cytotrophoblastic shell. The blood flow from the spiral arteries is pulsatile and is propelled in jetlike fountains by the maternal blood pressure. The entering blood is at a considerably higher pressure than that in the intervillous space; hence, it spurts toward the *chorionic plate*, forming the "roof" of the intervillous space. As the pressure dissipates, the blood flows slowly around the branch villi, allowing an exchange of metabolic and gaseous products with the fetal blood. The blood eventually returns to the endometrial veins and the maternal circulation.

The welfare of the embryo and fetus depends more on the adequate bathing of the branch villi with maternal blood than on any other factor. Reductions of uteroplacental circulation (e.g., caused by the effects of nicotine in cigarette smoke [p. 105]) result in fetal hypoxia and IUGR (Werler et al., 1986). Severe reductions of uteroplacental circulation can result in

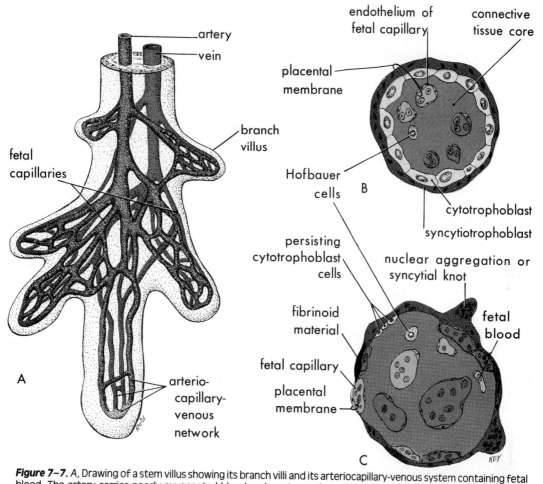

Figure 7–7. *A*, Drawing of a stem villus showing its branch villi and its arteriocapillary-venous system containing fetal blood. The artery carries poorly oxygenated blood and waste products from the fetus, whereas the vein carries oxygenated blood and nutrients to the fetus. *B* and *C*, Drawings of sections through a branch villus at ten weeks and full term, respectively. The branch villi (branches of stem villi) are bathed externally in maternal blood. The placental membrane, composed of extrafetal tissues, separates the maternal blood from the fetal blood. Note that this membrane becomes very thin at full term. These changes suggest that the permeability of the placental membrane increases during the later stages of pregnancy. Hofbauer cells are thought to be phagocytic cells.

fetal death. The intervillous space of the mature placenta contains about 150 ml of blood that is replenished three or four times per minute. The intermittent contractions of the uterus during pregnancy decrease uteroplacental blood flow slightly, but they do not force significant amounts of blood out of the intervillous space. Consequently, oxygen transfer to the fetus is decreased during uterine contractions, but the process does not stop.

The Placental Membrane (Barrier)

This composite membrane *consists of extrafetal tissues* separating the maternal and fetal blood (Figs. 7–7 and 7–8). Until about 20 weeks, it consists of four layers: (1) syncytiotrophoblast, (2) cytotrophoblast, (3) connective tissue in the chorionic villus, and (4) endothelium of the fetal capillaries. After the twentieth week, histological changes occur in the villi that result in the cytotrophoblast in many of the branch villi becoming attenuated. Eventually it disappears over large areas of the villi, leaving only thin patches of syncytiotrophoblast (Fig. 7–7C). As a result, in most places, the placental membrane consists of three layers only.

Although the placental membrane is often called the *placental barrier*, this term is inappropriate because there are only a few compounds, endogenous or

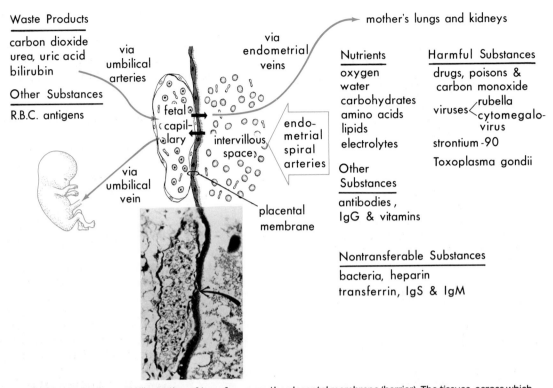

Figure 7-8. Diagrammatic illustration of transfer across the placental membrane (barrier). The tissues, across which transport of substances between the mother and fetus occurs collectively, constitute the placental membrane. This composite membrane is composed entirely of tissues of extrafetal origin: cytotrophoblast, syncytiotrophoblast, stroma in the villus, and endothelium of the fetus capillary; see also Fig. 7-7. (Inset photomicrograph from Javert CT: *Spontaneous and Habitual Abortion.* 1957. Courtesy of The Blakiston Division, McGraw-Hill Copyright 1957 by McGraw-Hill. Used by permission of McGraw-Hill Book Company.)

exogenous, that are unable to pass through the placental membrane in detectable amounts. The placental membrane acts as a true barrier only when the molecule has a certain size, configuration, and charge (e.g., heparin). Some metabolites, toxins, and hormones, though present in the maternal circulation, do not pass through the placental membrane in sufficient concentrations to affect the embryo/fetus.

Most drugs and other substances present in the maternal plasma pass through the placental membrane and are found in the fetal plasma. Electron micrographs of the syncytiotrophoblast show that its free surface has many *microvilli* that increase the surface area for exchange between the maternal and fetal circulations. As pregnancy advances, the placental membrane becomes progressively thinner, and the blood in many fetal capillaries is extremely close to the maternal blood in the intervillous space (Fig. 7-7C).

At some sites nuclei in the syncytiotrophoblast assemble to form nuclear aggregations or *syncytial knots* (Fig. 7-7C). These aggregations continually break off and are carried from the intervillous space into the maternal circulation. Some of them lodge in capillaries of the maternal lung where they are rapidly destroyed by local enzyme action. Toward the end of pregnancy, *fibrinoid material* forms on the surfaces of villi (Fig. 7-7C). It consists of fibrin and other unidentified substances that stain intensely with eosin. Fibrinoid material results mainly from aging and appears to reduce placental functions.

Functions of the Placenta

The placenta has *three main functions*: (1) metabolism, (2) transport of substances (e.g., oxygen and carbon dioxide), and (3) endocrine secretion. These comprehensive activities are essential for maintaining pregnancy and promoting normal fetal development.

Placental Metabolism. The placenta, particularly during early pregnancy, synthesizes glycogen, cholesterol, and fatty acids, which serve as sources of nutrients and energy for the embryo/fetus. Many of its metabolic activities are undoubtedly critical for its other two major placental activities (transport and endocrine secretion).

Placental Transport of Substances. Almost all materials are transported across the placental membrane by one of the following *four main transport mechanisms*: (1) simple diffusion, (2) facilitated diffusion, (3) active transport, and (4) pinocytosis. Passive transport by *simple diffusion* is usually characteristic of substances moving from areas of higher to lower concentration until equilibrium is established. In *facilitated diffusion* there is transport through electrical charges. *Active transport* against a concentration gradient requires energy. Such systems may involve enzymes that temporarily combine with the substances concerned. *Pinocytosis* (Gr. *pinein*, to drink) is a form of endocytosis in which the material being engulfed is a small sample of extracellular fluid (Cormack, 1987). This method of transport is usually reserved for large molecules.

There are three other methods that substances use to cross the placental membrane. In the first one, fetal red blood cells pass into the maternal circulation, particularly during parturition, presumably through microscopic breaks in the placental membrane. Labeled maternal red blood cells have also been found in the fetal circulation (Page et al., 1981). Thus, red blood cells may pass in either direction through very small defects or breaks in the placental membrane. In the second method, cells cross the placental membrane under their own power, e.g., maternal leukocytes and *Treponema pallidum*, the organism that causes syphilis. In the third method, some bacteria and protozoa (e.g., *Toxoplasma gondii*, see Chapter 8) infect the placenta by creating lesions and then cross the placental membrane through the defects that are created.

Gases. Oxygen, carbon dioxide, and carbon monoxide cross the placental membrane by simple diffusion. *Interruption of oxygen transport for even a few minutes will endanger fetal survival.* The placental membrane approaches the efficiency of the lungs for gas exchange. The quantity of oxygen reaching the fetus is primarily flow-limited rather than diffusion-limited; hence, fetal hypoxia results primarily from factors that diminish either the uterine blood flow or the fetal blood flow.

Nutritional Substances. Water is rapidly and freely exchanged by simple diffusion between the mother and her fetus and in increasing amounts as pregnancy advances. There is little or no transfer of maternal cholesterol, triglycerides, or phospholipids. Although there is transport of free fatty acids, the amount transferred appears to be relatively small. *Vitamins* cross the placenta and are essential for normal development. Water-soluble vitamins cross the placental membrane more quickly than fat-soluble ones. *Glucose* from the mother, and produced by the pla-

centa, is quickly transferred to the embryo or fetus by diffusion.

Hormones. Protein hormones do not reach the embryo or fetus in significant amounts except for a slow transfer of thyroxine and triiodothyronine. Unconjugated steroid hormones pass the placental membrane rather freely. Testosterone and certain synthetic progestins cross the placenta and may cause masculinization of female fetuses (see Fig. 8–15 and Table 8–6).

Electrolytes. These compounds are freely exchanged across the placental membrane in significant quantities, each at its own rate. When a mother receives *intravenous fluids*, they also pass to the fetus and affect its water and electrolyte status.

Antibodies. Some passive immunity is conferred upon the fetus by the placental transfer of maternal antibodies. The alpha and beta globulins reach the fetus in very small quantities; but many of the gamma globulins, notably the IgG (7S) class, are readily transported to the fetus. *Maternal antibodies confer fetal immunity* to such diseases as diphtheria, smallpox, and measles, but no immunity is acquired to pertussis (whooping cough) or chickenpox. The fetus has a poor capacity to produce antibodies until well after birth (Beck et al., 1985).

Other Substances. As previously stated small amounts of blood may pass from the fetus to the mother through microscopic breaks in the placental membrane. If the fetus is Rh-positive and the mother Rh-negative, the fetal cells may stimulate the formation of anti-Rh antibody by the mother. This passes to the fetal blood stream and causes hemolysis of fetal Rh-positive blood cells and anemia in the fetus. Some fetuses with this condition, known as *hemolytic disease of the newborn* (HDN), fail to make a satisfactory intrauterine adjustment and may die unless delivered early or given intrauterine blood transfusions (discussed in Chapter 6, p. 107). HDN is relatively uncommon now because Rh immune globulin given to the mother usually prevents development of this disease in the fetus (Thompson et al., 1991).

Waste Products. The major waste product, carbon dioxide, diffuses through the placental membrane even more rapidly than oxygen. Urea and uric acid pass the placental membrane by simple diffusion, and bilirubin is quickly cleared.

Drugs. Most drugs and their metabolites cross the placenta by simple diffusion, the exception being those with a structural similarity to amino acids (e.g., methyldopa and antimetabolites). As pregnancy advances, *thinning of the placental membrane facilitates drug passage.* Some drugs (e.g., thalidomide) cause major congenital anomalies (see Fig. 8–19). *Fetal drug addiction* may occur after maternal use of drugs such as heroin, and newborns may experience withdrawal symptoms. Because psychic dependence on these drugs is not developed during the fetal period, no liability to subsequent narcotic addiction exists in the infant after withdrawal is complete.

Except for muscle relaxants, such as succinylcholine and curare, most agents used for the management of labor readily cross the placental membrane. Depending on the dose and its timing in relation to delivery, these drugs may cause respiratory depression of the newborn infant. All sedatives and analgesics affect the fetus to some degree. Drugs taken by the mother can affect the embryo/fetus directly or indirectly by interfering with maternal or placental metabolism (Gill and Davis, 1974). The amount of drug or metabolite reaching the placenta is controlled by the maternal blood level and by the blood flow through the placenta from both the maternal and fetal circulations.

Infectious Agents. Cytomegalovirus, rubella, Coxsackie viruses, and those viruses associated with variola, varicella, measles, and poliomyelitis may pass through the placental membrane and cause *fetal infection.* In some cases (e.g., rubella virus), severe congenital anomalies may be produced (see Fig. 8–20). Microorganisms, such as *Treponema pallidum* that cause syphilis and *Toxoplasma gondii* that produces destructive changes in the brain and eyes (p. 166), also cross the placental membrane. These organisms enter the fetal blood, often causing anomalies and/or death (Chapter 8).

Placental Endocrine Secretion

Using precursors derived from the fetus and/or the mother, the *syncytiotrophoblast synthesizes various hormones.*

Protein Hormones. The well-documented protein hormone products synthesized by the placenta are: (1) *human chorionic gonadotropin* (hCG), and (2) *human chorionic somatomammotropin* (hCS), also known as *human placental lactogen* (hPL). The glycoprotein hCG, similar to luteinizing hormone (LH), is first secreted by the syncytiotrophoblast during the second week. HCG maintains the corpus luteum, preventing the onset of the next menstrual period (p. 40). The concentration of hCG in the maternal blood and urine rises to a maximum by the eighth week and then declines. In addition to hCG and hPL, *human chorionic thyrotropin* (hCT) and *human chorionic adreno-corticotropin* (hCACTH) are formed by the placenta.

Steroid Hormones. The placenta plays a major role in the production of *progestins* and *estrogens.* Progesterone can be obtained from the placenta at all stages

of gestation, indicating that it is essential for the maintenance of pregnancy. The placenta forms progesterone from maternal cholesterol or pregnenolone. The ovaries of a pregnant woman can be removed after the first trimester without causing an abortion because large amounts of progesterone are produced during the first weeks of pregnancy by the corpus luteum of pregnancy in the ovary (see Fig. 6–5B), but the placenta soon takes over production of this hormone. Estrogens are also produced in large quantities by the syncytiotrophoblast. The placenta forms them from 19 carbon precursors, many of which are supplied by the fetus (Villee, 1975).

Uterine Growth During Pregnancy

The uterus of a nonpregnant woman lies in the pelvis minor or true pelvis (Fig. 7–9A). It increases in size during pregnancy to accommodate the growing conceptus (Fig. 7–9B and C). While the uterus is enlarging, it increases in weight and its walls become thinner. During the first trimester, the uterus rises out of the pelvic cavity and usually reaches the level of the umbilicus by 20 weeks (Fig. 7–9B). By 28 to 30 weeks, it reaches the epigastric region[2] (Fig. 7–9C). The increase in size of the uterus largely results from hypertrophy of preexisting smooth muscle fibers, and partly from the development of new fibers.

PARTURITION (CHILDBIRTH)

Parturition (L. *parturitio*, childbirth) is the *birth process* during which the fetus, placenta, and fetal membranes are expelled from the mother's reproductive tract (Fig. 7–10). **Labor** is the sequence of involuntary *uterine contractions* that result in dilation of the cervix and delivery of the fetus and placenta from the uterus. The factors that trigger these contractions are not completely understood, but several hormones are related to the initiation of labor. Peristaltic contractions of uterine smooth muscle are elicited by **oxytocin** which is released by the posterior cerebral hypophysis (pituitary gland). This hormone is administered clinically if it is necessary to induce labor. Oxytocin also stimulates release of *prostaglandins* from the musculature which stimulate myometrial contractility by sensitizing the myometrial cells to oxytocin. *Estrogens* also increase myometrial

---

[2] The area inferior to the xiphoid process of the sternum and superior to the umbilicus.

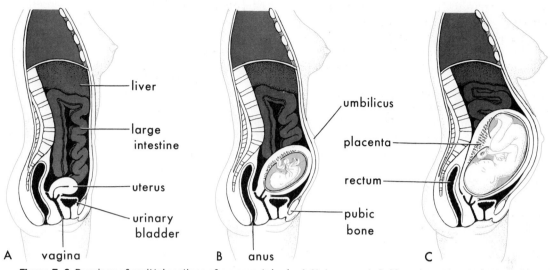

Figure 7–9. Drawings of sagittal sections of a woman's body. *A,* Not pregnant. *B,* 20 weeks pregnant. *C,* 30 weeks pregnant. Note that, as the fetus enlarges, the uterus increases in size to accommodate the rapidly growing fetus. By 20 weeks the uterus and fetus reach the level of the umbilicus; by 30 weeks they reach the epigastric region. The mother's abdominal viscera are displaced, and the skin and muscle of her anterior abdominal wall are greatly stretched.

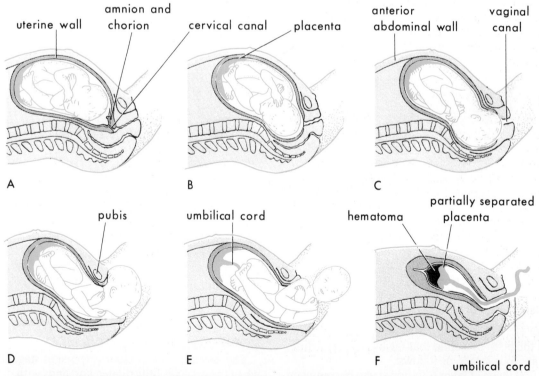

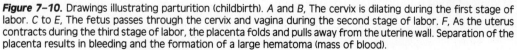

Figure 7–10. Drawings illustrating parturition (childbirth). *A* and *B,* The cervix is dilating during the first stage of labor. *C* to *E,* The fetus passes through the cervix and vagina during the second stage of labor. *F,* As the uterus contracts during the third stage of labor, the placenta folds and pulls away from the uterine wall. Separation of the placenta results in bleeding and the formation of a large hematoma (mass of blood).

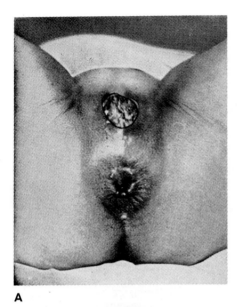

A

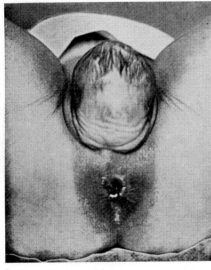

B

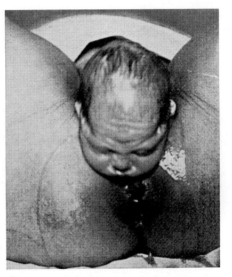

C

Figure 7–11. Photographs illustrating delivery of the baby's head during the second stage of labor. *A*, The head distends the mother's perineum, and its crown is visible. *B*, The perineum slips back over the head and face. *C*, The head is delivered; subsequently, the body of the fetus is expelled. (From Greenhill JB, Friedman EA: *Biological Principles and Modern Practice of Obstetrics*. Philadelphia, WB Saunders, 1974.)

activity and stimulate the release of oxytocin and prostaglandins.

The Stages of Labor

Labor (L. toil or suffering) is the process involved during the birth of a child that facilitates parturition. There are four stages, as follows:

The first stage of labor (dilation stage) begins when there is objective evidence of progressive dilation of the cervix. This happens when the onset of *regular contractions of the uterus occurs* (less than 10 minutes apart and painful). The first stage ends with complete dilation of the cervix. This stage is by far the most time-consuming part of the labor process. The average duration is about 12 hours for first pregnancies (nulliparous patients or *primigravidas*) and about 7 hours for women who have had a child previously (multiparous patients or *multigravidas*). There are, however, wide variations.

The second stage of labor (expulsion stage) begins when the cervix is fully dilated and ends with delivery of the baby (Figs. 7–10 and 7–11). During this stage the *fetus descends through the vagina* and is delivered. As soon as the fetus is outside the mother, it is called a newborn infant (baby). The average duration of this stage for primigravidas is 50 minutes, and 20 minutes for multigravidas. Uterine contractions begin again shortly after the baby is born.

The third stage of labor (placental stage) begins as soon as the baby is born and ends when the placenta and membranes are expelled (Fig. 7–10). The duration of this stage is 15 minutes in about 90 per cent of pregnancies. *Retraction of the uterus reduces the area of placental attachment*; thus, the placenta and fetal membranes separate from the uterine wall and are expelled through the vagina and pudendal cleft.[3] The placenta separates through the spongy layer of the decidua basalis (p. 20). After delivery of the baby, the uterus continues to contract. A *hematoma* soon forms deep to the placenta and separates it from the uterine wall (Fig. 7–10*F*).

The fourth stage of labor (recovery stage) begins as soon as the placenta and fetal membranes are expelled. This stage lasts about two hours. The myometrial contractions constrict the spiral endometrial arteries that formerly supplied blood to the intervillous space (Fig. 7–6). These contractions prevent excessive uterine bleeding.

THE PLACENTA, UMBILICAL CORD, AND FETAL MEMBRANES AFTER BIRTH

The placenta (Gr. *plakuos*, a flat cake) commonly has a discoid shape (Fig. 7–12), with a diameter of 15 to 20 cm and a thickness of 2 to 3 cm. It weighs 500 to 600 gm, usually about one sixth the weight of the fetus. The margins of the placenta are continuous with the ruptured amniotic and chorionic sacs (Figs. 7–6 and 7–12*A* and *C*).

Variations in Placental Shape. As the placenta develops (p. 115), chorionic villi usually persist only where the villous chorion is in contact with the decidua basalis (Figs. 7–1*D* and 7–4). This results in the usual discoid placenta (Fig. 7–12). When villi persist elsewhere, several variations in placental shape occur: *accessory placenta* (Fig. 7–13), bidiscoid placenta, diffuse placenta, and horseshoe placenta. Although there are innumerable variations in the size and shape of the placenta, most of them are of little physiological or clinical significance. Examination of the placenta, however, may provide information about the causes of: (1) placental dysfunction, (2) IUGR, (3) neonatal illness, and (4) infant death. Placental studies can also determine whether the placenta is complete. Reten-

---

[3] The slit between the labia majora into which the vestibule of the vagina opens.

tion of a cotyledon or an accessory placenta in the uterus may lead to *uterine hemorrhage*.

Choriocarcinoma. In some pregnancies abnormal proliferation of the cytotrophoblast and syncytiotrophoblast results in *malignant tumors*. They invade the decidua basalis, penetrate its blood vessels and lymphatics, and metastasize to the lungs, bone marrow, liver, and other organs. *Gestational choriocarcinomas* are highly sensitive to chemotherapy and cures are usually achieved (Cotran et al., 1989).

The Maternal Surface of the Placenta

The characteristic cobblestone appearance of this surface is produced by the *cotyledons*, which are separated by grooves that were formerly occupied by *placental septa* (Fig. 7–6 and Fig. 7–12*A*). The surface of the cotyledons is covered by thin, grayish shreds of decidua basalis that separated with the placenta. These are recognizable in sections of the placenta examined under a microscope. Most of the decidua is temporarily retained in the uterus and shed with subsequent uterine bleeding.

The Fetal Surface of the Placenta

The umbilical cord usually attaches to the fetal surface, and its amniotic covering is continuous with the amnion adherent to the chorionic plate of the placenta (Figs. 7–6 and 7–12*B*). The chorionic vessels radiating to and from the umbilical cord are clearly visible through the smooth, transparent amnion. The *umbilical vessels* branch on the fetal surface to form *chorionic vessels*, which enter the stem villi (Figs. 7–6 and 7–7).

THE UMBILICAL CORD

The attachment of the umbilical cord, which connects the embryo/fetus to the placenta, is usually near the center of the fetal surface of this organ (Fig. 7–12*B*), but it may be found at any point; for example, insertion of it at the placental margin produces a *battledore placenta* (Fig. 7–12*D*), and its attachment to the membranes is called a *velamentous insertion of the cord* (Fig. 7–14). As the amniotic cavity enlarges, the amnion enfolds the umbilical cord, forming its epithelial covering (Figs. 7–16 and 7–17).

The umbilical cord is usually 1 to 2 cm in diameter and 30 to 90 cm in length (average 55 cm). Excessively long or short cords are uncommon. Long cords have a tendency to prolapse and/or to coil around the fetus (Fig. 7–18). Prompt recognition of *prolapse of the cord* is important because the cord may be compressed between the presenting body part of the

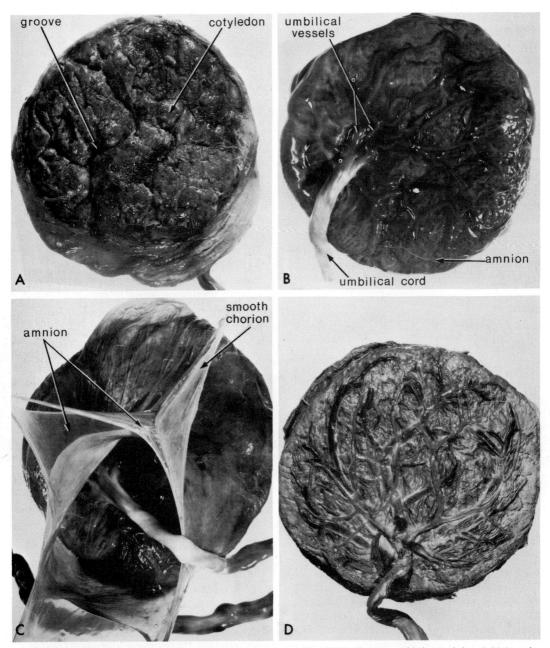

Figure 7–12. Photographs of placentas and fetal membranes after birth, about one third actual size. *A*, Maternal surface showing cotyledons and grooves around them. Each convex cotyledon consists of a number of stem villi with their many branch villi (Fig. 7–6). The grooves were occupied by the placental septa when the maternal and fetal parts of the placenta were together (see Fig. 7–6). *B*, Fetal surface showing the blood vessels running in the chorionic plate deep to the amnion and converging to form the umbilical vessels at the attachment of the umbilical cord. *C*, The amnion and smooth chorion are arranged to show that they are (1) fused and (2) continuous with the margins of the placenta. See Figures 7–5 and 7–6 also for visualizing the relationship between the amnion and smooth chorion. *D*, Placenta with a marginal attachment of the cord, often called a battledore placenta because of its resemblance to the bat used in the medieval game of battledore and shuttlecock.

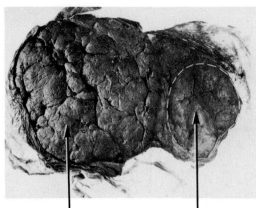

main
placenta

accessory
placenta

Figure 7–13. Photograph of the maternal surface of a full-term placenta with an accessory placenta; about one quarter actual size. The accessory placental tissue developed from a patch of chorionic villi that persisted a short distance from the main placenta (Fig. 7–1).

margin of placenta

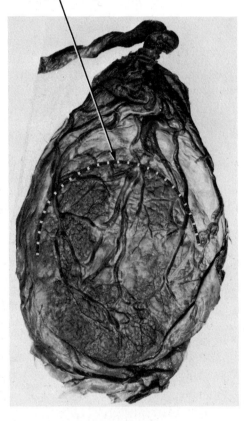

Figure 7–14. Photograph of a placenta with a velamentous insertion of the umbilical cord. The cord is attached to the membranes (amnion and chorion), not to the placenta. The umbilical vessels leave the cord and run between the amnion and chorion before spreading over the placenta. The vessels are easily torn in this location, especially when they course over the inferior (lower) uterine segment; this latter condition is known as vasa previa. If the vessels rupture before birth, the fetus loses blood and could be near exsanguination at birth.

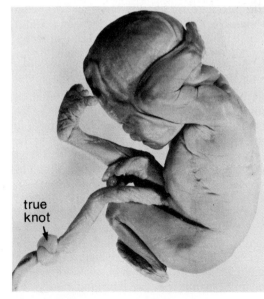

true
knot

Figure 7–15. Photograph of a 20-week fetus with a true knot (arrow) in its umbilical cord. Half actual size. The diameter of the cord is greater in the portion closest to the fetus, indicating that there was an obstruction of blood flow from the fetus in the umbilical arteries. Undoubtedly, this knot caused severe anoxia (decreased amount of oxygen in the tissues and organs) and was a major cause of the fetus's death.

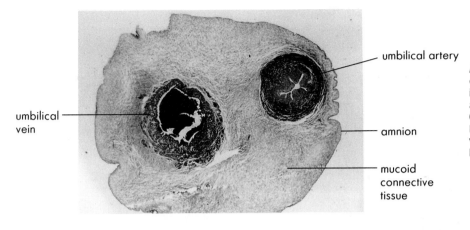

Figure 7-16. Transverse section of a full-term umbilical cord showing only one artery. Usually there are two arteries and one vein. (Courtesy of Professor V. Becker, Pathologisches Institut der Universität, Erlangen, Federal Republic of Germany).

fetus and the mother's bony pelvis. This causes *fetal hypoxia* or anoxia; and, if it persists for more than five minutes, the baby's brain may be damaged, producing mental retardation.

The umbilical cord usually has two arteries and one vein that are surrounded by mucoid connective tissue *(Wharton's jelly)*. Because the umbilical vessels are longer than the cord, twisting and bending of the vessels is common. They frequently form loops, producing *false knots* that are of no significance; however, in about one per cent of deliveries, *true knots* in the cord are formed that may tighten and cause fetal death due to *fetal anoxia* (Fig. 7-15). In most cases the knots form during labor as a result of the fetus passing through a loop of the cord. Because these knots are usually loose, they have no clinical significance. Simple *looping of the cord around the fetus* occasionally occurs (Fig. 7-18). In about one fifth of all deliveries, the cord is loosely looped once around the neck without increased fetal risk (Page et al., 1981).

In about one in 200 newborns, only *one umbilical artery* is present (Fig. 7-16), a condition that may be associated with fetal abnormalities, particularly of the cardiovascular system. *Absence of an umbilical artery* is accompanied by a 15 to 20 per cent incidence of cardiovascular anomalies in the fetus. Absence of an artery results from either agenesis or degeneration of this vessel early in development.

THE AMNION AND AMNIOTIC FLUID

The amnion forms a fluid-filled, membranous, *amniotic sac* that surrounds the embryo (Fig. 7-17A and B) and, later, the fetus (Figs. 7-4, 7-17C and D and 7-18). Because the amnion is attached to the margins of the embryonic disc (Fig. 7-17A), its junction with the embryo (future umbilicus) is located on the ventral surface after embryonic folding (Fig. 7-17B). As the amnion enlarges, it gradually obliter-

ates the chorionic cavity and enfolds the umbilical cord (Fig. 7-17C and D).

Origin of Amniotic Fluid. Initially some fluid may be secreted by amniotic cells, but most amniotic fluid is derived from the *maternal tissue (interstitial) fluid* by diffusion across the amniochorionic membrane from the decidua parietalis (Fig. 7-1F). Later, there is diffusion of fluid through the chorionic plate from blood in the intervillous space of the placenta (Fig. 7-6). Before keratinization of the skin occurs, a major pathway for the passage of water and solutes in tissue fluid from the fetus to the amniotic cavity is through the skin (Callen and Filly, 1990); thus, amniotic fluid is similar to fetal tissue fluid. Fluid is also secreted by the fetal respiratory tract and enters the amniotic cavity. Bisonnette (1986) estimated that the daily rate of contribution of fluid to the amniotic cavity from the respiratory tract was 300 to 400 ml. Beginning in the eleventh week, the fetus also makes a contribution to the amniotic fluid by expelling urine into the amniotic cavity. By late pregnancy about a half liter of urine is added daily. The volume of amniotic fluid normally increases slowly, reaching *about* 30 ml at 10 weeks, 350 ml at 20 weeks, and 700 to 1000 ml by 37 weeks.

Circulation of Amniotic Fluid. The water content of amniotic fluid changes every three hours. Large amounts of water pass through the amniochorionic membrane into the maternal tissue fluid and enter the uterine capillaries. An exchange of fluid with fetal blood also occurs through the umbilical cord and where the amnion adheres to the chorionic plate on the fetal surface of the placenta (Figs. 7-6 and 7-12B); thus, amniotic fluid is in balance with the fetal circulation. *Amniotic fluid is swallowed by the fetus* and absorbed by the fetus's respiratory and digestive tracts. It has been estimated that, during the final stages of pregnancy, the fetus swallows up to 400 ml of amniotic fluid per day. The fluid passes into the fetal blood stream, and the waste products in it cross the placental membrane and enter the maternal blood in the intervillous space. Excess water in the fetal blood is excreted by the fetal kidneys and returned to the amniotic sac through the fetal urinary tract.

Low volumes of amniotic fluid (e.g., 400 ml in the third trimester), a condition called *oligohydramnios*, results in most cases from placental insufficiency with diminished placental blood flow. Preterm rupture of the amniochorionic membrane (Fig. 7–1*F*) occurs in approximately 10 per cent of pregnancies and is the most common cause of oligohydramnios (Callen and Filly, 1990). When there is *renal agenesis* (failure of kidney formation), the absence of the fetal urine contribution to the amniotic fluid is the main cause of oligohydramnios. A similar situation arises when there is *obstructive uropathy* (urinary tract obstruction).

High volumes of amniotic fluid (e.g., in excess of 2000 ml), a condition called *polyhydramnios*, results when the fetus does not swallow the usual amount of amniotic fluid. This condition is often associated with severe anomalies of the central nervous system (e.g., *meroanencephaly* [see Fig. 18–17]). In other anomalies, such as *esophageal atresia* (see Fig. 11–5*A*), the fetus is unable to swallow amniotic fluid, which accumulates because it is unable to pass to the fetal stomach and intestines for absorption. *Ultrasonography* has become the technique of choice for diagnosing polyhydramnios (Callen and Filly, 1990).

Exchange of Amniotic Fluid. Large volumes of fluid move in both directions between the fetal and maternal circulations, mainly via the placental membrane. Fetal swallowing of amniotic fluid is also a normal occurrence. Most of the fluid passes into the gastrointestinal tract, but some of it also enters the lungs. In either case, the fluid is absorbed and enters the fetal circulation. It then passes into the maternal circulation via the placental membrane.

Composition of Amniotic Fluid. About 99 per cent of the fluid in the amniotic cavity is water. Amniotic fluid is a solution in which undissolved material is suspended (e.g., desquamated fetal epithelial cells and approximately equal portions of organic and inorganic salts). Half the organic constituents are protein; the other half consists of carbohydrates, fats, enzymes, hormones, and pigments. As pregnancy advances, the composition of the amniotic fluid changes as fetal excreta (*meconium* [fetal feces] and urine) are added. Because urine is added to amniotic fluid, studies of fetal enzyme systems, amino acids, hormones,

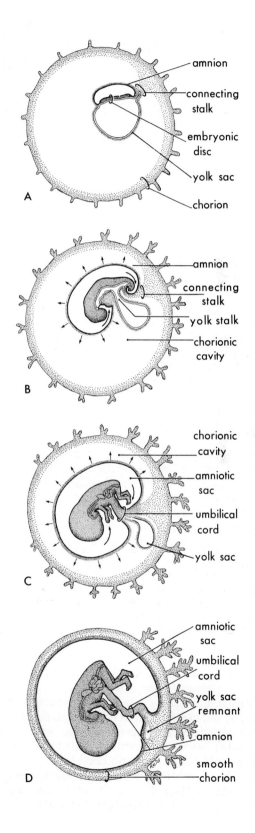

Figure 7–17. Drawings illustrating how the amnion enlarges and fills the chorionic sac. Also shown is how the amnion enfolds on the umbilical cord and becomes its epithelial covering (Fig. 7–16) and how the yolk sac is partially incorporated into the embryo as the primitive gut. Formation of the fetal part of the placenta and degeneration of chorionic villi are also shown. *A,* Three weeks. *B,* Four weeks. *C,* Ten weeks. *D,* 20 weeks.

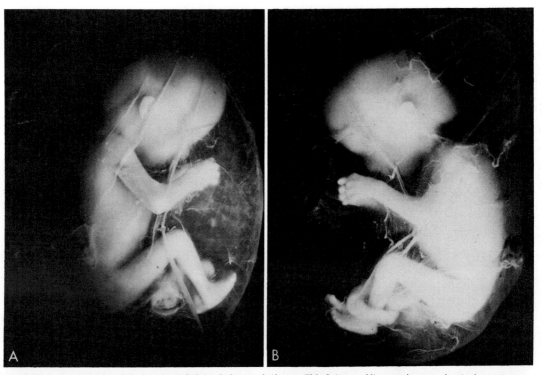

Figure 7–18. Photographs of a 12-week fetus in its amniotic sac. This fetus and its membranes aborted spontaneously. It was then removed from its chorionic sac with its amniotic sac intact. Actual size. In *B*, note that the umbilical cord is looped around the left ankle of the fetus. Coiling of the cord around parts of the fetus affects their development when the coils are so tight that the circulation to those parts is affected.

and other substances can be conducted on fluid removed by amniocentesis (see Fig. 6–14*A*). Studies of cells in amniotic fluid permit diagnosis of the sex of the fetus and detection of fetuses with chromosomal abnormalities (e.g., trisomy 21 resulting in the Down syndrome). High levels of *alpha-fetoprotein* (AFP) in the amniotic fluid usually indicate the presence of a severe neural tube defect (e.g., meroanencephaly). Low levels of AFP may indicate chromosomal aberrations, such as trisomy 21 that produces Down syndrome (p. 146).

The Significance of Amniotic Fluid. The embryo, suspended in amniotic fluid by the umbilical cord, floats freely. Amniotic fluid has critical functions in the normal development of the fetus (Callen and Filly, 1990). This buoyant medium: (1) permits symmetrical external growth of the embryo, (2) acts as a barrier to infection, (3) permits normal fetal lung development, (4) prevents adherence of the amnion to the embryo, (5) cushions the embryo against injuries by distributing impacts the mother may receive, (6) helps control the embryo's body temperature by maintaining a relatively constant temperature, and (7) enables the fetus to move freely, thereby aiding muscular development (e.g., in the limbs).

Premature Rupture of the Membranes. As previously stated (p. 118), preterm rupture of the amniochorionic membrane occurs in about 10 per cent of pregnancies. It is the most common event leading to premature labor and delivery and the most common complication resulting in oligohydramnios (p. 129). The absence of amniotic fluid also removes the major protection the fetus has against infection (Callen and Filly, 1990).

Rupture of the amnion may cause various fetal anomalies that constitute the *amniotic band disruption complex* (ABDC). These anomalies vary from digital constriction to major scalp, craniofacial, and visceral defects (Callen and Filly, 1990). The cause of these anomalies is probably related to constriction by encircling amniotic bands (Fig. 7–19). The incidence of the *amniotic band syndrome* (ABS) is about 1 in every 1200 live births (Seed et al., 1982). Prenatal ultrasound diagnosis of ABS is now possible (Filly and Golbus, 1990).

THE YOLK SAC

Early development of the yolk sac was described in Chapters 3 and 5 (pp. 43 and 71). By nine weeks the yolk sac has shrunk to a pear-shaped remnant, about 5 mm in diameter. It is connected to the midgut by a

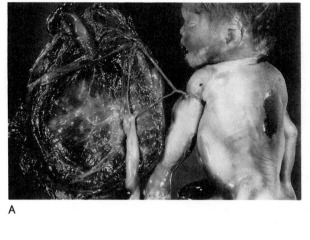

A

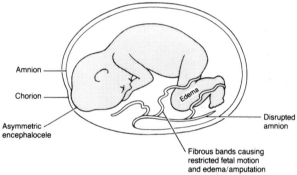

B

Figure 7–19. *A,* Photograph of a fetus with the amniotic band syndrome, showing amniotic bands constricting its left arm. (Courtesy of Professor V. Becker, Pathologisches Institut der Universität, Erlangen, Federal Republic of Germany). *B,* Diagram illustrating the essential features of the amniotic band syndrome. Observe the entrapment of the fetal limbs and that the head is adherent to the amnion and chorion which has produced herniation of the brain (encephalocele). (From Nyberg MD, Mack LA: *Abdominal wall defects. In* Callen PW: *Ultrasonography In Obstetrics and Gynecology.* 2nd ed. Philadelphia, WB Saunders, 1988.)

narrow *yolk stalk* (see Figs. 6–4*A* and 7–17*C*). By 20 weeks the yolk sac is very small (Fig. 7 – 17*D*); thereafter, it is usually not visible. The yolk sac can be observed sonographically early in the fifth week (see Fig. 5–22*A*). The amnion is also visible at this time (Lyons and Levi, 1991). The presence of the amnion and yolk sac enable early recognition and measurement of the embryo. The yolk sac is recognizable in ultrasound examinations until the end of the first trimester (Filly, 1988; Lyons and Levi, 1991).

Significance of the Yolk Sac. Although this sac is nonfunctional as far as yolk storage is concerned, its presence is essential for several reasons:

1. It has a role in the *transfer of nutrients* to the embryo during the second and third weeks (fourth to

fifth weeks of gestation), during the period when the uteroplacental circulation is being established.

2. *Blood development* first occurs in the wall of the yolk sac beginning in the third week (see Fig. 4–9) and continues to form there until hemopoietic activity begins in the liver during the sixth week.

3. During the fourth week the dorsal part of the yolk sac is incorporated into the embryo as the *primitive gut* (see Fig. 5–1). Its endoderm gives rise to the epithelium of the trachea, bronchi, and lungs (see Chapter 11) and of the digestive tract (see Chapter 12).

4. *Primordial germ cells* appear in the wall of the yolk sac in the third week and subsequently migrate to the developing sex glands or gonads (see Fig. 13–20). They differentiate into the germ cells (spermatogonia in males and oogonia in females).

Fate of the Yolk Sac. At 10 weeks the small yolk sac lies in the chorionic cavity between the amnion and chorionic sac (Fig. 7–17*C*). It atrophies as pregnancy advances, eventually becoming very small (Fig. 7–17*D*). In very unusual cases, the yolk sac persists throughout pregnancy and appears as a small structure on the fetal surface of the placenta, deep to the amnion near the attachment of the umbilical cord. Persistence of the yolk sac is of no clinical significance. The *yolk stalk* usually detaches from the midgut loop by the end of the sixth week (see Fig. 12–11). In about 2 per cent of adults, the proximal intraabdominal part of the yolk stalk persists as an *ileal diverticulum* known clinically as *Meckel's diverticulum* (see Figs. 12–17 and 12–18).

THE ALLANTOIS

The early development of the allantois was described in Chapter 4,(p. 61). During the second month the extraembryonic umbilical portion of the allantois degenerates (Fig. 7–20*B*). Although the allantois is not functional in human embryos, it is important for four reasons: (1) blood formation occurs in its wall during the third to fifth weeks, (2) its blood vessels become the umbilical vein and arteries (Fig. 7–20 *A* and *B*), (3) fluid from the amniotic cavity diffuses into the umbilical vein and enters the fetal circulation for transfer to the maternal blood through the placental membrane, (4) the intraembryonic portion of the allantois runs from the umbilicus to the urinary bladder, with which it is continuous (Fig. 7–20*B*). As the bladder enlarges, the allantois involutes to form a thick tube called the urachus (Fig. 7–20*C*). After birth, the *urachus* becomes a fibrous cord, called the *median umbilical ligament*, that extends from the apex of the urinary bladder to the

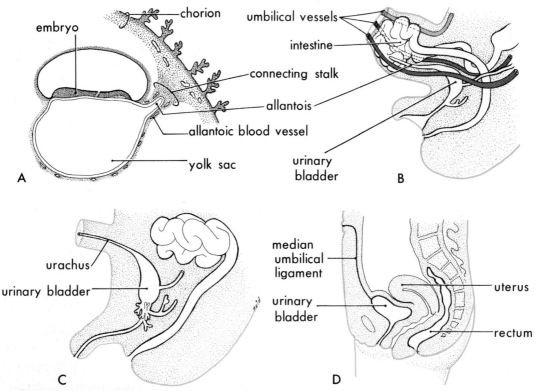

Figure 7–20. Drawings illustrating the development and usual fate of the allantois. *A*, Three weeks. *B*, Nine weeks. *C*, Three months. *D*, Adult. This nonfunctional structure forms the urachus, which is represented in adults by the median umbilical ligament.

umbilicus (Fig. 7–20*D*). For a discussion of urachal anomalies and their clinical significance, see Chapter 13 (p. 277).

TWIN AND OTHER MULTIPLE PREGNANCIES

Multiple births are more common now due to the stimulation of ovulation that occurs when exogenous gonadotropins are administered to women with ovulatory failure and to those being treated for infertility by in vitro fertilization and embryo transfer (p. 33). In North America, *twins* normally occur about once in every 90 pregnancies, *triplets* about once in 90^2 pregnancies, *quadruplets* about once in 90^3 pregnancies, and *quintuplets* about once in 90^4 pregnancies. These estimates increase when ovulations have been primed with hormones, a technique that is in general use for women who are sterile because of tubal occlusion (p. 25).

Twins (MZ and DZ)

Twins may originate from two zygotes (Fig. 7–21), in which case they are called *dizygotic* (DZ) *twins* or fraternal twins, or from one zygote (Fig. 7–22), i.e., *monozygotic* (MZ) *twins* or identical twins. The fetal membranes and placenta(s) vary according to the origin of the twins (Table 7–1) and, in the case of MZ twins, the type of placenta and membranes formed depends on when the twinning process occurs. If division of the embryoblast occurs after the amniotic cavity forms (about eight days), which is uncommon, the MZ embryos will be within the same amniotic and chorionic sacs (Figs. 7–26*A*; Table 7–1).

About two thirds of twins are DZ. The frequency of DZ twinning shows marked racial differences, but *the incidence of MZ twinning is about the same in all populations* (Thompson et al., 1991). In addition, the rate of MZ twinning shows little variation with the mother's age, whereas *the rate of DZ twinning increases with maternal age*. The study of twins is important in human genetics because it is useful for comparing the effects of genes and environment on development. If an abnormal condition does not show a simple genetic pattern, comparison of its incidence in MZ and DZ twins may reveal that heredity is involved. For more information, see Thompson et al. (1991).

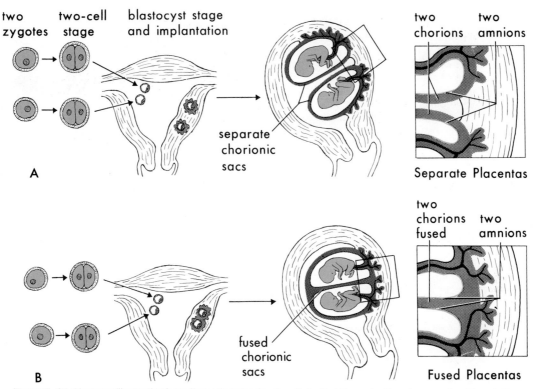

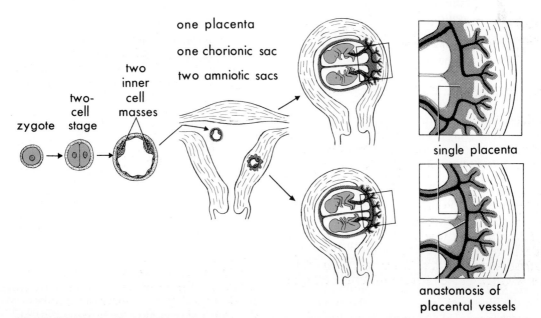

Figure 7–21. Diagrams illustrating how dizygotic twins develop. Note that they arise from two zygotes. The relations of the fetal membranes and placentas are shown for instances in which, A, the blastocysts implant separately, and B, the blastocysts implant close together. In both cases there are two amnions and two chorions, and the placentas are usually fused when they implant close together.

Figure 7–22. Diagrams illustrating how about 65 per cent of monozygotic twins develop from one zygote by division of the inner cell mass (embryoblast) of the blastocyst. If there is anastomosis of the placental vessels, one twin may receive most of the nutrition from the placenta (see Figs. 7–23 and 7–24). Such twins always have separate amnions, a single chorionic sac, and a common placenta.

The tendency for DZ but not MZ twins to repeat in families is evidence of hereditary influence. Studies in a Mormon population showed that the genotype of the mother affects the frequency of DZ twins, but the genotype of the father has no effect (Page et al., 1981). It has also been found that, if the firstborn are twins, a repetition of twinning or some other form of multiple birth is about five times more likely to occur at the next pregnancy than it is in the general population. Anastomoses between blood vessels of fused placentas of human DZ twins occasionally occur and result in *erythrocyte mosaicism* (Figs. 7-22 and 7-23). The members of these DZ twins have red cells of two different types because red cells were exchanged between the two fetal placental circulations.

Anastomosis of placental blood vessels commonly occurs in cattle and causes *freemartinism* (Moore, 1966). Freemartins are intersexual female calves born as twins with male calves. They are intersexual because of male hormones that reach them through anastomosed fetal placental vessels. When placental vascular anastomoses occur in *human* DZ twins in cases in which one fetus is a male and the other is female, masculinization of the female fetus does not occur, but the anastomotic condition may give rise to *blood group chimeras;* i.e., persons with populations of blood cells of two genotypes that are from different zygotes (Thompson et al., 1991).

Dizygotic (DZ) Twins. Because they result from the fertilization of two ova by two different sperms, DZ twins develop from two zygotes and may be of the same sex or different sexes (Fig. 7-21). For the same reason, they are no more alike genetically than brothers or sisters born at different times. The only thing they have in common is that they were in the mother's uterus at the same time (i.e., "they were womb mates"). DZ twins always have two amnions and two chorions, but the chorions and placentas may be fused (Table 7-1).

DZ twinning shows a hereditary tendency. The recurrence risk in families is about triple the general population risk. The incidence of DZ twinning shows considerable variation, being about 1 in 500 in Asians, 1 in 125 in Caucasians, and as high as 1 in 20 in some African populations (Thompson et al., 1991).

Monozygotic (MZ) Twins. Because they result from the fertilization of one ovum (Fig. 7-22), MZ twins are of the same sex, genetically identical, and very similar in physical appearance. Physical differences between newborn MZ twins are environmentally induced; e.g., anastomosis of placental vessels resulting in differences in blood supply from the placenta (Figs. 7-23 and 7-24). MZ twinning usually begins in the blastocyst stage around the end of the first week (see Fig. 2-16) and results from division of the inner cell mass or embryoblast into two embryonic primordia. Subsequently, two embryos, each in

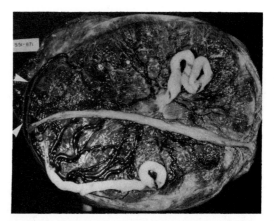

Figure 7-23. Photograph of the fetal surface of a placenta from monozygotic twins. The separate amnions are rolled at the center. There are several vascular communications between the circulations of the placentas (also see Fig. 7-22). A large arteriovenous shunt is visible at the left (arrows), and a direct, artery-to-artery anastomosis crosses the midline (deep to the amnions) from one placental half to the other. (Courtesy of Dr. K. Benirschke, University of California, San Diego.)

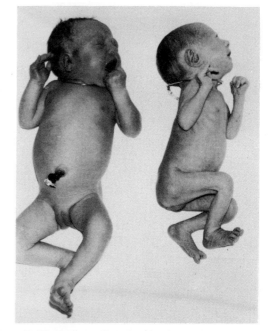

Figure 7-24. Monozygotic twins showing a wide discrepancy in size resulting from an uncompensated arteriovenous anastomosis of placental vessels. Blood was shunted from the smaller twin to the larger one, producing the so-called fetal transfusion syndrome. (Courtesy of Dr. Harry Medovy, Children's Centre, Winnipeg, Canada.)

Table 7-1. FREQUENCY OF TYPES OF PLACENTAS AND FETAL MEMBRANES IN MONOZYGOTIC (MZ) AND DIZYGOTIC (DZ) TWINS[1]

Zygosity	Single Chorion		Two Chorions	
	Single Amnion	Two Amnions	Fused Placenta[2]	Two Placentas
MZ	Uncommon	65%	25%	10%
DZ	—	—	40%[3]	60%

[1] Modified slightly from Thompson MW, McInnes RR, Willard HF: *Thompson & Thompson Genetics in Medicine.* 5th ed. Philadelphia, WB Saunders, 1991.
[2] Results from secondary fusion.
[3] DZ twins, the most common type, have their own amniotic and chorionic sacs, but the placentas may be fused (see Fig. 7-21).

its own amniotic sac, develop within one chorionic sac and have a *common placenta* (Fig. 7-22; Table 7-1).

Uncommonly early separation of embryonic blastomeres (e.g., during the two- to eight-cell stages) results in MZ twins with two amnions, two chorions, and two placentas that may or may not be fused (Fig.

7-25). In such cases it is impossible to determine from the membranes alone whether the twins are MZ or DZ. To determine the relationship of twins of the same sex with similar blood groups, one must wait until other characteristics develop, e.g., eye color, fingerprints, and so forth.

Establishment of the zygosity of twins has become important, particularly since the introduction of organ transplantation (e.g., bone marrow transplants). The determination of twin zygosity is now done by *molecular diagnosis* because any two people who are not MZ twins are virtually certain to show differences in some of the large number of DNA markers that can be studied (Thompson et al., 1991).

About 35 per cent of MZ twins result from early separation of the embryonic blastomeres (i.e., during the first three days of development). The other 65 per cent of MZ twins originate at the end of the first week of development, i.e., right after the blastocyst has formed (Fig. 7-22). Late division of pre-embryonic cells (i.e., division of the embryonic disc during the second week) results in MZ twins that are in one amniotic sac and one chorionic sac (Fig. 7-26A). Such twins are rarely delivered alive because the umbilical cords are frequently so entangled that circulation of the

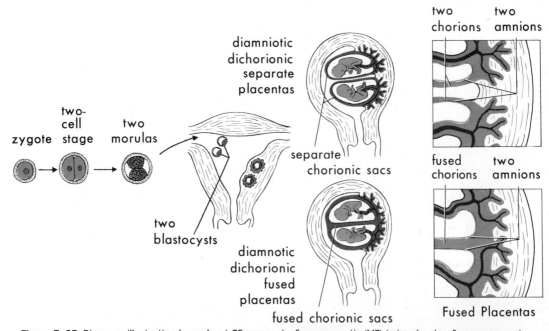

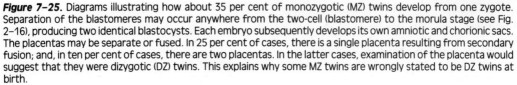

Figure 7-25. Diagrams illustrating how about 35 per cent of monozygotic (MZ) twins develop from one zygote. Separation of the blastomeres may occur anywhere from the two-cell (blastomere) to the morula stage (see Fig. 2-16), producing two identical blastocysts. Each embryo subsequently develops its own amniotic and chorionic sacs. The placentas may be separate or fused. In 25 per cent of cases, there is a single placenta resulting from secondary fusion; and, in ten per cent of cases, there are two placentas. In the latter cases, examination of the placenta would suggest that they were dizygotic (DZ) twins. This explains why some MZ twins are wrongly stated to be DZ twins at birth.

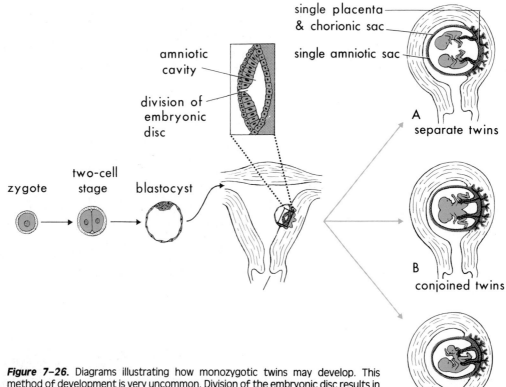

Figure 7–26. Diagrams illustrating how monozygotic twins may develop. This method of development is very uncommon. Division of the embryonic disc results in two embryos within one amniotic sac. *A*, Complete division of the disc gives rise to separate twins. Such twins rarely survive because their umbilical cords are often so entangled that interruption of the blood supply to the fetuses occurs. *B* and *C*, Incomplete division of the disc results in various types of conjoined twins.

blood through their vessels ceases and one or both fetuses die. It has been estimated that the frequency of monoamniotic twins among MZ twins is about four per cent (Bulmer, 1970).

MZ twins may sometimes be discordant for a variety of birth defects and genetic disorders despite their origin from a single zygote. In addition to environmental differences and chance variation, the following reasons for discordance given by Thompson et al. (1991) are recognized:

1. Mechanisms of embryological development, such as *vascular abnormalities*, that can lead to discordance for anomalies.

2. Postzygotic changes, such as *somatic mutation*, leading to discordance for cancer, or somatic rearrangement of immunoglobulin or T-cell receptor genes.

3. *Chromosome aberrations* originating in one blastocyst after the twinning event.

4. Uneven *X chromosome inactivation* between female MZ twins with the result that one twin preferentially expresses the paternal X, the other the maternal X.

Early Death of a Twin. Since ultrasonographic studies have become a common part of prenatal care, it is known that early death and resorption of one

member of a twin pair is fairly common (Filly, 1988). Awareness of this possibility must be considered when discrepancies occur between prenatal cytogenetic findings and the karyotype of an infant. Errors in prenatal diagnosis may arise if extraembryonic tissues (e.g., part of a chorionic villus; see Fig. 6–14*B*) from the resorbed twin are examined.

Conjoined Twins. If the embryoblast or embryonic disc does not divide completely, various types of conjoined twins may form (Figs. 7–26*B* and *C*, 7–27 and 7–28). These are named according to the regions that are attached; e.g., *thoracopagus* indicates that there is anterior union of the thoracic regions (Fig. 7–27). It has been estimated that, about once in every 40 MZ twin pregnancies, the twinning is incomplete and conjoined (*Siamese*) twins result. In some cases, the twins are connected to each other by skin only or by cutaneous and other tissues, e.g., fused livers (Fig. 7–27*A*). These conjoined twins can be successfully separated by surgical procedures (Fig. 7–27*B*). For a discussion of the theoretical basis of conjoined twins, see Spencer (1992).

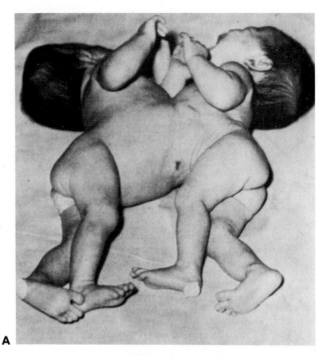

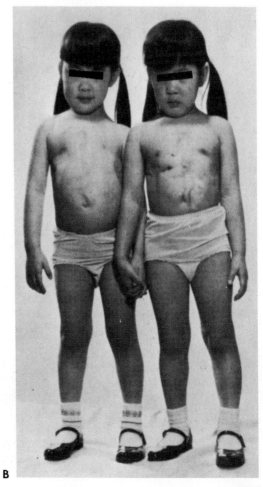

Figure 7–27. *A*, Photograph of newborn monozygotic conjoined twins show-ing union in the thoracic regions (thoracopagus). *B*, The twins about four years after separation. (From deVries PA: The San Francisco twins. *In* Bergsma D. (ed): "Conjoined twins." New York: Alan R. Liss for the National Foundation-March of Dimes, BD:OAS III(1), 141–142, 1967, with permission of the copyright holder.

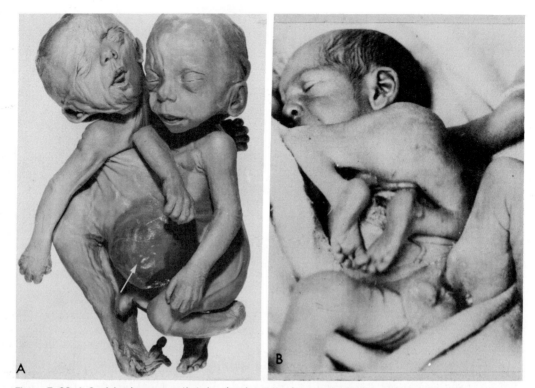

Figure 7–28. *A,* Conjoined monozygotic twins showing extensive anterior fusion and an omphalocele (arrow). This hernia contained intestines from both fetuses. These fetuses died before they could be delivered. The lower limbs of the left fetus are fused, a condition known as sirenomelia. *B,* Parasitic fetus with its lower limbs and pelvis attached to the thorax of an otherwise normal male infant.

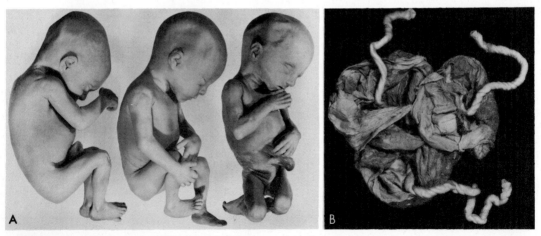

Figure 7–29. *A,* Photograph of 20-week-old triplets: monozygotic male twins (left) and a single female (right). *B,* Photograph of their fused placentas shows the twin placenta with two amnions (left) and the single placenta (upper right). These twins obviously developed from two zygotes.

diamniotic dichorionic placenta

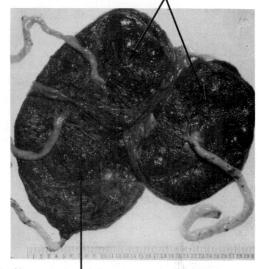

diamniotic monochorionic placenta

Figure 7–30. Photograph of the placentas from quadruplets. The upper two placentas (and the dizygotic fetuses associated with them) were derived from two zygotes; whereas, the lower fused placenta was attached to monozygotic twins. Reprinted with permission from The American College of Obstetricians and Gynecologists (Obstetrics and Gynecology, 1961, 18:309).

Other Types of Multiple Birth

Triplets may be derived from: (1) one zygote and be identical, (2) two zygotes and consist of identical twins and a different infant (Fig. 7–29), or (3) three zygotes and be of the same sex or of different sexes. In the last case, the infants are no more similar than infants from three separate pregnancies. Similar combinations occur in quadruplets (Fig. 7–30), quintuplets, sextuplets, and septuplets.

Superfecundation is the fertilization of two or more ova around the same time by sperms from different men. This phenomenon commonly occurs in some mammals (e.g., cats and dogs). DZ human twins with different fathers have been confirmed by genetic markers (Terasaki et al., 1978).

SUMMARY OF THE PLACENTA AND FETAL MEMBRANES

In addition to the embryo, the fetal membranes and most of the placenta originate from the zygote. The placenta consists of two parts: (1) a larger fetal portion derived from the villous chorion, and (2) a maternal portion formed by the decidua basalis. The two parts are held together by stem villi that are attached to the cytotrophoblastic shell which adheres to the decidua basalis (see Figs. 4–11B and 7–6). The principal ac-

tivities of the placenta are (1) metabolism, (2) transfer, and (3) endocrine secretion. All three activities are essential to maintaining pregnancy and promoting normal fetal development.

The fetal circulation is separated from the maternal circulation by a thin layer of extrafetal tissues known as the **placental membrane** (barrier). It is a permeable membrane that allows water, oxygen, nutritive substances, hormones, and noxious agents to pass from the mother to the embryo or fetus (Fig. 7–8). Excretory products pass through the placental membrane from the fetus to the mother.

The fetal membranes and placenta(s) in *multiple pregnancies* vary considerably depending on the derivation of the embryos and the time when division of embryonic cells occurs. The common type of twins is *dizygotic twins* (DZ), with two amnions, two chorions, and two placentas that may or may not be fused. *Monozygotic twins* (MZ), the less common type, represent about a third of all twins; they are derived from one zygote. MZ twins commonly have two amnions, one chorion, and one placenta. Twins with one amnion, one chorion, and one placenta are always monozygotic, and their umbilical cords are often entangled. Other types of multiple birth (triplets, etc.) may be derived from one or more zygotes.

The yolk sac and allantois are vestigial, human structures, but their presence is essential to normal embryonic development. Both are early sites of blood formation and are incorporated into the embryo. Primordial germ cells also originate in the yolk sac. The amnion forms a sac for amniotic fluid and provides a covering for the umbilical cord. The amniotic fluid has three main functions: (1) to provide a protective buffer for the embryo or fetus, (2) to allow room for fetal movements, and (3) to assist in the regulation of fetal body temperature.

CLINICALLY ORIENTED QUESTIONS FOR PROBLEM-BASED LEARNING SESSIONS

1. How does a physician calculate the estimated date of confinement (EDC) or estimated delivery date (EDD) of a baby? How could this EDD be confirmed in a high-risk obstetrical patient?
2. A pregnant woman was told that she had *polyhydramnios* and asks you to explain what the term means. What would be your answer? What conditions are often associated with polyhydramnios? Explain why it occurs.
3. Does twinning "run" in families? Is maternal age a factor? If uncertainty arose, how would you determine whether twins were monozygotic or dizygotic?
4. During the examination of a section of an umbilical cord, you noticed that there was only one umbilical artery. How often does this anomaly occur? What kind of fetal abnormalities might be associated with this condition?
5. An ultrasonographic examination revealed a twin pregnancy with a single placenta. Chorionic villus sampling and chromosome analysis revealed that the twins were female. At birth the twins were not identical. How could this error have occurred?
6. An ultrasound examination of a pregnant woman during the second trimester revealed multiple amniotic bands. What produces these bands? What congenital defects may result from them?

The answers to these questions are given on page 461.

References and Suggested Reading

Aplin JD: Implantation, trophoblast differentiation and haemochorial placentation: mechanistic evidence *in vivo* and *in vitro*. *J Cell Sci* 99:681, 1991.

Bassett JM: Current perspectives on placental development and its integration with fetal growth. *Proc Nutr Soc* 50:311, 1991.

Beck F, Moffat DB, Davies DP: *Human Embryology*. 2nd ed. Oxford, Blackwell Scientific Publications, 1985.

Beck T: Placental morphometry using a computer assisted measuring programme. Reference values for normal pregnancies at term. *Arch Gynecol Obstet* 249:135, 1991.

Behrman RE (ed): *Nelson Textbook of Pediatrics*. 14th ed. Philadelphia, WB Saunders, 1992.

Benirschke K: Incidence and prognostic implication of congenital absence of one umbilical artery. *Am J Obstet Gynecol* 79:251, 1960.

Benirschke K: Implantation, placental development, uteroplacental blood flow. *In* Reid DE, Ryan KJ, Benirschke K (eds): *Principles and Management of Human Reproduction*. Philadelphia, WB Saunders, 1992.

Benirschke K, Driscoll SG: *The Pathology of the Human Placenta*. New York, Springer-Verlag, 1967.

Benirschke K, Kaufman P: *The Pathology of the Human Placenta*. Berlin, Springer-Verlag, 1990.

Bergsma D (ed): *Conjoined Twins. Birth Defects III* (1):1–147, 1967.

Billington WB: Trophoblast. *In* Philipp EE, Barnes J, Newton M, (eds): *Scientific Foundations of Obstetrics and Gynecology*. London, William Heinemann, 1970.

Bisonnette J: Placental and fetal physiology. *In* Gabbe SG, Neibyl JR, Simpson JL (eds): *Obstetrics, Normal and Problem Pregnancies*. New York, Churchill Livingstone, 1986.

Bohn H, Winckler W, Grundmann U: Immunochemically detected placental proteins and their biological functions. *Arch Gynecol Obstet* 249:107, 1991.

Boura ALA, Walters WAW: Autocoids and the control of vascular tone in the human umbilical-placental circulation. *Placenta* 12:453, 1991.

Brock DJH: Prenatal diagnosis–chemical methods. *In* Berry CL (ed): *Human Malformations. Br Med Bull* 32:16, 1976.

Bulmer MG: *The Biology of Twinning in Man*. Oxford, Clarendon Press, 1970.

Callen PW, Filly RA: Amniotic fluid evaluation. *In* Harrison MR, Golbus MS, Filly RA (eds): *The Unborn Patient. Prenatal Diagnosis and Treatment* 2nd ed. Philadelphia, WB Saunders, 1990.

Carr BR: Fertilization, implantation, and endocrinology of pregnancy. *In* Griffin JE, Ojeda SR (eds): *Textbook of Endocrine Physiology*. New York and Oxford, Oxford University Press, 1988.

Chamberlain G, Wilkinson A (eds): *Placental Transfer*. Baltimore, University Park Press, 1979.

Cormack DH: *Ham's Histology*. 9th ed. Philadelphia, JB Lippincott, 1987.

Cotran RS, Kumar V, Robbins SL: *Robbins Pathologic Basis of Disease*. 4th ed. Philadelphia, WB Saunders, 1989.

Cunningham FG, MacDonald PC, Grant NF (eds): *Williams Obstetrics*. 18th ed. Norwalk, Appleton & Lange, 1990.

Demir R, Kaufmann P, Castellucci M, Erbengi T, Kotowski A: Fetal vasculogenesis and angiogenesis in human placenta villi. *Acta Anat* 136:190, 1989.

deVries PA: Case history–the San Francisco twins. *In* Bergsma D (ed): *Conjoined Twins. Birth Defects III (1)*:141, 1967.

Dungy LJ, Siddigi TA, Khan S: Transforming growth factor-expression during placental development. *Am J Obstet Gynecol* 165:853, 1991.

Enders AC: Structural responses of the primate endometrium to implantation. *Placenta* 12:309, 1991.

Filly RA: The first trimester. *In* Callen PW (ed): *Ultrasonography in Obstetrics and Gynecology.* 2nd ed. Philadelphia, WB Saunders, 1988.

Filly RA, Golbus MS: The fetus with amniotic band syndrome. *In* Harrison MR, Golbus MS, Filly RA (eds): *The Unborn Patient. Prenatal Diagnosis and Treatment.* 2nd ed. Philadelphia, WB Saunders, 1990.

Fox H: *Pathology of the Placenta.* Philadelphia, WB Saunders, 1978.

Fox H: Trophoblastic pathology. *Placenta* 12:479, 1991.

Gadd RL: The liquor amnii. *In* Philipp EE, Barnes J, Newton M (eds): *Scientific Foundations of Obstetrics and Gynecology.* London, William Heinemann, Ltd., 1970.

Gill S, Davis JA: The pharmacology of the fetus, baby, and growing child. *In* Davis JA, Dobbing J (eds): *Scientific Foundations of Paediatrics.* Philadelphia, WB Saunders, 1974.

Glasser SR, Bullock DW (eds): *Cellular and Molecular Aspects of Implantation.* New York, Plenum Press, 1981.

Green JR: Placenta previa and abruptio placentae. *In* Creasy RK, Resnik R (eds): *Maternal-Fetal Medicine. Principles and Practice.* 2nd ed. Philadelphia, WB Saunders, 1989.

Haugen G, Stray-Pedersen S, Bjøro K: Prostanoid production in umbilical arteries from preterm and term deliveries perfused in vitro. *Early Hum Develop* 24:153, 1990.

Hay WW: In vivo measurements of placental transport and metabolism. *Proc Nutr Soc* 50:355, 1991.

Jauniaux E, Jurkovic D, Henriet Y, Rodesch F, Hustin: Development of the secondary human yolk sac–correlation of sonographic and anatomical features. *Hum Reprod* 6:309, 1991.

Javert, CT: *Spontaneous and Habitual Abortion.* New York, The Blakiston Division, McGraw-Hill, 1957.

Johnson MH, Everitt B: *Essential Reproduction.* Oxford, Blackwell Scientific Publications, 1984.

Jollie WP: Development, morphology and function of the yolk-sac placenta of laboratory rodents. *Teratology* 41:361, 1990.

Kennedy LA, Persaud TVN: Pathogenesis of developmental defects induced in the rat by amniotic sac puncture. *Acta Anat* 97:23, 1977.

Klopper A, Chard T (eds): *Placental Proteins.* Berlin, Springer-Verlag, 1978.

Lichnovsky V, Lojda Z, Bocek M, Vlkova M: Histochemistry of some enzymes in human embryonic and fetal placentae. *Acta Univ Palacki Olomuc Fac Med* 126:11, 1990.

Lyons EA, Levi CS: Ultrasound of the normal first trimester of pregnancy. Syllabus. Special Course. Ultrasound, Radiological Society of North America, 1991.

Mäkilä U-M, Jouppila P, Kirkinen P, Viinikka L, Ylikorkala O: Placental thromboxane and prostacyclin in the regulation of placental blood flow. *Obstet Gynecol* 68:537, 1986.

Martin CB: The anatomy and circulation of the placenta. *In* Barnes AC (ed): *Intra-Uterine Development.* Philadelphia, Lea & Febiger, 1968.

Moore KL: The sex chromatin of freemartins and other animal intersexes. *In* Moore KL (ed): *The Sex Chromatin.* Philadelphia, WB Saunders, 1966.

Mossman HW: Classics revisited: comparative morphogenesis of fetal membranes and accessory uterine structures. *Placenta* 12:1, 1991.

Naeye RL: *Disorders of the Placenta, Fetus, and Neonate.* St. Louis, Mosby-Year Book, 1992.

Nash JE, Persaud TVN: Embryopathic risks of cigarette smoking. *Exp Pathol* 33:65, 1988.

Nyberg DA, Callen PW: Ultrasound evaluation of the placenta. *In* Callen PW (ed): *Ultrasonography in Obstetrics and Gynecology.* 2nd ed. Philadelphia, WB Saunders, 1988.

Oxorn H: *Human Labor and Birth.* 5th ed. Norwalk, Appleton-Century-Crofts, 1989.

Page EW, Villee CA, Villee DB: *Human Reproduction. Essentials of Reproductive and Perinatal Medicine.* 3rd ed. Philadelphia, WB Saunders, 1981.

Peipert JF, Donnenfeld AE: Oligohydramnios: a review. *Obstet Gynecol* 46:325, 1991.

Persaud TVN, Tiess D: Plazentare Übertragung von Aethylbarbital *Naturwissenschaften* 53:385, 1966.

Petraglia F, Angioni S, Coukos G, Uccelli E, Didomenica P, Deramundo BM, Genazzani AD, Garuti GC, Segre A: Neuroendocrine mechanisms regulating placental hormone production. *Contr Gynecol Obstet* 18:147, 1991.

Rosso P: Placental growth, development, and function in relation to maternal nutrition. *Fed Proc* 39:250, 1980.

Schnaufer L: Conjoined twins. *In* Raffensperger JG (ed): *Swenson's Pediatric Surgery.* 5th ed. Norwalk, Appleton & Lange, 1990.

Schneider H: Placental transport function. *Reprod Fert Develop* 3:345, 1991.

Schumacher GH, Gill H, Persaud TVN, Gill H: Historical documents concerning craniopagi and conjoined twins. *Gegenbaurs morphol Jahrb* 134:541, 1988.

Scott JR, DiSaia PJ, Hammond CB, Spellacy WN (eds): *Danforth's Obstetrics and Gynecology.* 6th ed. Philadelphia, JB Lippincott, 1990.

Seed JW, Cefalo RC, Herbert WNP: Amniotic band syndrome. *Am J Obstet Gynecol* 144:243, 1982.

Seeds AE, Jr: Amniotic fluid and fetal water metabolism. *In* Barnes AC (ed): *Intra-Uterine Development.* Philadelphia, Lea & Febiger, 1968.

Spencer R: Conjoined twins: theoretical embryologic basis. *Teratology* 45:591, 1992.

Terasaki PI, Gjertson D, Bernoco D, et al: Twins with two different fathers identified by HLA. *N Engl J Med* 299:590, 1978.

Thompson MW, McInnes RR, Willard HF: *Thompson & Thompson Genetics in Medicine.* 5th ed. Philadelphia, WB Saunders, 1991.

Turksoy RN, Toy BL, Rogers J, Papageorge W: Birth of septuplets following human gonadotropin administration in Chiari-Frommel syndrome. *Obstet Gynecol* 30:692, 1967.

Villee DB: *Human Endocrinology. A Developmental Approach.* Philadelphia, WB Saunders, 1975.

Waisman HA, Kerr G: *Fetal Growth and Development.* New York, McGraw-Hill, 1970.

Wald NJ, Cuckle HS: AFP screening in early pregnancy. *In* Spencer JAD (ed): *Fetal Monitoring.* Oxford, Oxford University Press, 1991.

Watson WJ, Chescheir NC, Katz VL, Seeds JW: The role of ultrasound in evaluation of patients with elevated maternal serum alpha-fetoprotein: a review. *Obstet Gynecol* 78:123, 1991.

Werler MM, Pober BR, Holmes LB: Smoking and pregnancy. *In* Sever JL, Brent RL (eds): *Teratogen Update. Environmentally Induced Birth Defect Risks.* New York, Alan R. Liss, 1986.

8

Human Birth Defects

We ought not to set them aside with idle thoughts or idle words about "curiosities" or "chances." Not one of them is without meaning; not one that might not become the beginning of excellent knowledge, if only we could answer the question—why is it rare, or being rare, why did it in this instance happen?

—James Paget, Lancet 2:1017, 1882.

Birth defects, congenital malformations, and congenital anomalies are all-encompassing terms currently used to describe developmental defects present at birth (L. *congenitus*, born with). Birth defects may be structural, functional, metabolic, behavioral, or hereditary. The most widely used reference guide for classifying birth defects is the *International Statistical Classification of Diseases*, published by the World Health Organization in 1975. It is recognized, however, that no single classification and nomenclature has universal appeal. Each is limited, having been designed for a particular purpose. Attempts to classify birth defects, especially those resulting from errors of morphogenesis, reveal the frustration and obvious difficulties in the formulation of concrete proposals that could be used in medical practice (Persaud et al., 1985). Spranger et al (1982) proposed a practical classification system for developmental defects which is widely accepted among clinicians. It should be emphasized, however, that with an increase in our understanding of normal and abnormal embryogenesis, further revisions may be necessary. The terminology currently used to describe birth defects can be confusing; therefore a **glossary of the terms**[1] used in this chapter and in current research and clinical literature follows.

Anomaly: A structural abnormality of any type. It is, however, important to keep in mind that *not all variants are anomalies*. Anatomical variations are common; e.g., bones vary among themselves, not only in their basic shape but in lesser details of surface structure (Moore, 1992). There are four clinically significant *types of anomaly*:

1. Malformation: A morphologic defect of an organ, part of an organ, or larger region of the body that *results from an intrinsically abnormal developmental process*. Reference is made to "intrinsic" and "abnormality of an organ." *Intrinsic* implies that the developmental potential of the primordium (anlage) is abnormal from the beginning, e.g., chromosome abnormalities at fertilization. Most malformations are considered to be a *defect of a morphogenetic or developmental field* "which responds as a coordinated unit to embryonic interaction and results in complex or multiple malformations."

2. Disruption: A morphological defect of an organ, part of an organ, or a larger region of the body that *results from the extrinsic breakdown of, or an interference with, an originally normal developmental process*. Thus, morphological alterations following exposure to **teratogens**, such as drugs and viruses (p. 155), should be considered as disruptions. *A disruption cannot be inherited*, but "inherited factors can predispose to and influence the development of a disruption."

3. Deformation: An abnormal form, shape, or position of a part of the body that *results from mechanical forces*. Intrauterine compression, resulting from oligohydramnios (p. 129) that produces an equinovarus foot or *clubfoot* (see Fig. 17–9 *C*), is an example of a deformation produced by extrinsic forces. Some central nervous system defects, such as *meningomyelocele* (p. 395), produce intrinsic functional disturbances that also cause fetal deformation (Graham, 1988).

4. Dysplasia: An abnormal organization of cells into tissue(s) and its morphological result(s). In other words, dysplasia is the process (and the consequence) of *dyshistogenesis* (abnormal tissue formation). All abnormalities relating to histogenesis are therefore classified as dysplasias, e.g., *congenital ectodermal dysplasia* (p. 445) and Marfan syndrome. Dysplasia is causally nonspecific and often affects several organs because of the nature of the underlying cellular disturbances.

Other Descriptive Terms: To describe infants with multiple anomalies, other terms have evolved to express causation and pathogenesis. These include: *polytopic field defect*, a pattern of anomalies derived from the disturbance of a *single* developmental field; *sequence*, a pattern of multiple anomalies derived from a single known or presumed struc-

---

[1] The glossary is set in smaller type because it is material that will not be referred to frequently.

tural defect or mechanical factor; *syndrome*, a pattern of multiple anomalies thought to be pathogenetically related and not known to represent a single sequence or a polytopic field defect; and *association*, a nonrandom occurrence in two or more individuals of multiple anomalies not known to be a polytopic field defect, sequence, or syndrome.

Whereas a sequence (anomalad or complex in older literature) is a pathogenetic and not a causal concept, *syndrome* often implies a single cause, e.g., trisomy 21 in Down syndrome (p. 146). In both cases, however, the pattern of anomalies is known or considered to be pathogenetically related. In the case of a sequence, the primary initiating factor and cascade of secondary developmental complications are known; e.g., the Potter sequence that is attributed to oligohydramnios (p. 129) results from either renal agenesis or leakage of amniotic fluid. An *association*, in contrast, refers to statistically, not pathogenetically or causally, related defects. One or more sequences, syndromes, or field defects may very well constitute an *association* (Spranger et al., 1982).

Dysmorphology is the area of clinical genetics that is concerned with the diagnosis and interpretation of patterns of structural defects. "The diagnosis of a malformation syndrome is made on the basis of the overall pattern of anomalies in a patient; however, problems in interpretation may arise because the characteristic abnormalities of any syndrome vary to some extent from patient to patient" (Thompson et al., 1991). For clinical examples and a detailed discussion of the above nomenclature, see Cohen Jr. (1982).

Teratology is the branch of science concerned with all aspects of abnormal prenatal development including the *study of the causes and pathogenesis of congenital defects*. A fundamental concept in teratology is that certain stages of embryonic development are more vulnerable than others (p. 154). Until the 1940s it was generally believed that human embryos were protected from environmental agents (e.g., drugs and viruses) by their extraembryonic/fetal membranes (amnion and chorion) and their mothers' abdominal and uterine walls. Gregg (1941) presented the first well-documented evidence that an environmental agent (rubella virus) could produce severe developmental disruptions (congenital cataracts) if present during the critical periods of human development (p. 154). It was, however, the sagacious observations of Lenz (1961) and McBride (1961) that focused attention on the role of drugs in the etiology of human birth defects. They described severe limb anomalies and other developmental disruptions that were caused by *thalidomide* during early pregnancy (see Newman, 1986a; Brent and Holmes, 1988; Holmes, 1992). It is estimated that between seven and ten per cent of human birth defects result from the disruptive actions of drugs, viruses, and other environmental factors (Persaud et al., 1985; Persaud, 1990; Thompson et al., 1991; Tables 8–1 and 8–6).

Table 8–1. ESTIMATED INCIDENCE OF CAUSES OF MAJOR CONGENITAL ANOMALIES[1]

Causes	Incidence (%)
Chromosome abnormalities (p. 144)	6–7
Mutant genes (p. 152)	7–8
Environmental factors (p. 157)	7–10
Multifactorial inheritance (p. 168)	20–25
Unknown etiology[2]	50–60

[1] Based on data, combined with reasoning, from Connor and Ferguson-Smith (1987), Persaud et al. (1990), and Thompson et al. (1991)
[2] It is likely that the majority of infants with congenital anomalies of unknown cause has a genetic disorder. Molecular biological techniques are likely to reduce the number of anomalies of unknown etiology.

According to data from the *U.S. Centers for Disease Control* in 1989, the leading cause of death for white infants was birth defects. In Canada the situation is the same. *More than 20 per cent of infant deaths in North America are attributed to birth defects*. Major structural anomalies (e.g., spina bifida cystica; see Fig. 18–14) are observed in about three per cent of newborn infants. Additional anomalies can be detected after birth; thus, the incidence reaches about six per cent in 2-year-olds and eight per cent in 5-year-olds (Connor and Ferguson-Smith, 1987; Nelson and Holmes, 1989: Thompson et al, 1991).

The **causes of congenital anomalies** are often divided into *genetic factors* (e.g., chromosome abnormalities) and *environmental factors*, such as drugs. Many common congenital anomalies, however, are caused by genetic and environmental factors acting together. This is called *multifactorial inheritance* (p. 168). For 50 to 60 per cent of congenital anomalies, the causes are unknown (Table 8–1).

Anomalies may be single or multiple and of major or minor clinical significance. Single *minor anomalies* are present in about 14 per cent of newborns (Jones, 1988). These anomalies (e.g., of the external ear) are of no serious medical or cosmetic significance, but they indicate to the clinician the possible presence of associated major anomalies; for example, a single umbilical artery (see Fig. 7–16) alerts the clinician to the possible presence of cardiovascular and renal anomalies (p. 128).

Ninety per cent of infants with three or more minor anomalies also have one or more major defects (Connor and Ferguson-Smith, 1987; Jones, 1988). Of the three per cent born with clinically significant congenital anomalies, 0.7 per cent have multiple major anomalies. Most of these infants die during infancy (e.g., those with trisomy 18 [Figs. 8–3 and 8–4]). Major developmental defects are much more common in early embryos (10 to 15 per cent), but most of them abort spontaneously. Chromosome abnormalities are present in 50 to 60 per cent of spontaneously aborted conceptuses (Shiota et al., 1987; Shepard et al., 1989; Kaufman, 1991).

ANOMALIES CAUSED BY GENETIC FACTORS[2]

Numerically, *genetic factors are the most important causes of congenital anomalies*. It has been estimated that they cause about a third of all birth defects (Table 8–1) and nearly 85 per cent of all those with known causes. Any mechanism as complex as mitosis or meiosis may occasionally malfunction; thus, *chromosomal aberrations are common* and are present in *about* six per cent of zygotes. Many of these primordial cells never undergo normal cleavage (mitosis) and become blastocysts. *In vitro studies* of cleaving human zygotes (pre-embryos) less than five days old have revealed a high incidence of abnormalities. More than 60 per cent of day two cleaving zygotes were found to be abnormal (Winston et al., 1991). Many defective zygotes, blastocysts and early embryos abort spontaneously during the first three weeks, and the overall frequency of chromosome abnormalities in them is at least 50 per cent (Thompson et al, 1991).

Two kinds of change occur in chromosome complements: numerical and structural, and they may affect the sex chromosomes and/or the autosomes.[3] In some cases, both kinds of chromosome are affected. Persons with chromosome abnormalities usually have characteristic phenotypes (e.g., the physical characteristics of infants with Down syndrome [Fig. 8–3]). They often look more like other persons with the same chromosome abnormality than like their own siblings (brothers or sisters). This characteristic appearance results from genetic imbalance. Genetic factors initiate anomalies by biochemical or other means at the subcellular, cellular, or tissue level. The abnormal mechanism initiated by the genetic factor may be identical or similar to the causal mechanism initiated by a teratogen (e.g., a drug). For a discussion of human teratogens, see page 157.

---

[2] We are grateful to Dr. A.E. Chudley, M.D., F.R.C.P.C., F.C.C.M.G., Professor of Pediatrics and Child Health; Director of Clinical Genetics, Health Sciences Centre, University of Manitoba, Winnipeg, Manitoba for assistance with the preparation of this section. We also relied heavily on the commendable work of Thompson et al, 1991.

[3] Autosomes are any chromosomes other than sex chromosomes. There are 22 pairs in the human karyotype.

Numerical Chromosome Abnormalities

Numerical aberrations of chromosomes usually result from **nondisjunction**, an error in cell division in which there is failure of a chromosomes pair or two chromatids of a chromosome to disjoin during mitosis or meiosis. As a result, the chromosome pair or chromatids pass to one daughter cell and the other daughter cell receives neither (Fig. 8–1; see also Fig. 2–3). Nondisjunction may occur during maternal or paternal gametogenesis (p. 141).

The chromosomes in somatic cells normally exist in pairs; the homologous chromosomes making up a pair are called *homologs*. Normal human females have 22 pairs of autosomes plus two X chromosomes; whereas, normal males have 22 pairs of autosomes plus one X and one Y chromosome. During embryogenesis, one of the two X chromosomes in female somatic cells is randomly inactivated and appears as a mass of *sex chromatin* (Fig. 8–7B). This mass is not present in cells of normal males or in females lacking a sex chromosome (Fig. 8–2). Although sex chromatin studies are useful in diagnosing errors of sex development (see Fig. 13–28), they provide no information about the presence or absence of the Y chromosome; however, Pearson et al. (1970) demonstrated that the Y chromosome can be detected in interphase cells by means of quinacrine fluorescence staining (Fig. 8–7D).

Inactivation of genes on one X chromosome in somatic cells of female pre-embryos occurs at about the time of implantation (Thompson et al, 1991). *X-inactivation is important clinically* because it means that each cell from a carrier of an X-linked disease has the mutant gene causing the disease, either on the active X chromosome or on the inactivated X chromosome that is represented by sex chromatin. Uneven X-inactivation in MZ twins (p. 136) is one reason given for discordance for a variety of congenital anomalies (Thompson et al., 1991). The genetic basis of this discordance is that one twin preferentially expresses the paternal X, the other the maternal X.

Changes in chromosome number represent either aneuploidy or polyploidy.

Aneuploidy. Any deviation from the human diploid number of 46 chromosomes is called aneuploidy. An *aneuploid* is an individual or a cell that has a chromosome number that is not an exact multiple of the haploid number of 23 (e.g., 45 or 47). The principal cause of aneuploidy is nondisjunction during cell division (Fig. 8–1). This results in an unequal distribution of one pair of homologous chromosomes to the daughter cells. One cell has two chromosomes and the other has neither chromosome of the pair. As a result, the embryo's cells may be *hypodiploid* (45,X as in Turner syndrome [Fig. 8–2]), or *hyperdiploid* (usually 47, as in trisomy 21 or Down syndrome [Fig. 8–3]).

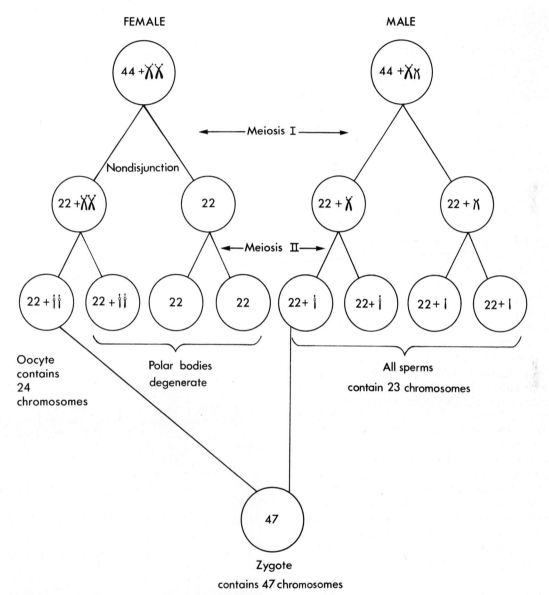

Figure 8–1. Diagram showing nondisjunction of chromosomes during the first meiotic division of a primary oocyte resulting in an abnormal oocyte (ovum) with 24 chromosomes. Subsequent fertilization by a normal sperm produces a zygote with 47 chromosomes, a condition called aneuploidy (p. 144).

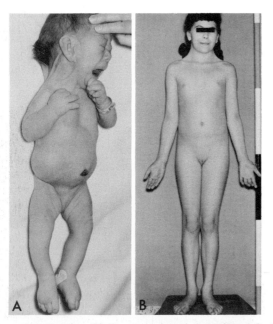

Figure 8–2. Females with Turner syndrome. *A*, Newborn infant. Note the webbed neck and lymphedema of the hands and feet. *B*, 13-year-old girl showing the classic features: short stature, webbed neck, absence of sexual maturation, and broad, shieldlike chest with widely spaced nipples. (From Moore KL: *The Sex Chromatin*, Philadelphia, WB Saunders, 1966.)

Monosomy. Embryos missing a chromosome usually die. Monosomy of an autosome is extremely uncommon, and about 99 per cent of embryos lacking a sex chromosome spontaneously abort (Connor and Ferguson-Smith, 1987). About one per cent of monosomy X female embryos survive and develop characteristics of **Turner syndrome** (Fig. 8–2). The incidence of *45,X*, or Turner syndrome, in newborn females is approximately one in 5000 live female births (Thompson et al, 1991).

The *phenotype*[4] of Turner syndrome is illustrated in Figure 8–2. The *monosomy X chromosome abnormality* is the most common cytogenetic abnormality observed in fetuses that abort spontaneously, and it accounts for about 18 per cent of all abortions caused by chromosome abnormalities. The error in gametogenesis (nondisjunction) that causes monosomy X, when it can be traced, is usually (about 75 per cent) in the paternal gamete (i.e., it is the paternal X chromosome that is missing). The most frequent chromosome constitution in Turner syndrome is 45,X (also written as 45,XO); however, nearly 50 per cent of these people have other karyotypes (Hook and Warburton, 1983). For the clinical significance of these

---

[4] The observed morphological characteristics of an individual as determined by his or her genotype and the environment in which it is expressed (Thompson et al, 1991).

chromosome constitutions (e.g., a mosaic karyotype of 45,X/46,XX), see Thompson et al. (1991).

Trisomy. If three chromosomes are present instead of the usual pair, the disorder is called trisomy. The usual cause of this error is *nondisjunction of chromosomes* (Fig. 8–1; see also Fig. 2–3), resulting in a germ cell with 24 instead of 23 chromosomes and subsequently in a zygote with 47 chromosomes.

Trisomy of the autosomes compatible with postnatal survival is associated with three syndromes (Table 8–2). The most common condition is *trisomy 21 or Down syndrome* (Fig. 8–3), in which three number 21 chromosomes are present. Trisomy 18 (Fig. 8–4) and trisomy 13 (Fig. 8–5) are much less common; infants with these chromosome disorders are severely malformed and mentally retarded, and they usually die early in infancy. *Autosomal trisomies occur with increasing frequency as maternal age increases*; for example, trisomy 21 (Down syndrome) occurs once in about 1400 births in mothers aged 20 to 24 years, but once in about 25 births in mothers 45 years and over (Table 8–3). Because of the current trend of increasing maternal age, it has been estimated that, by the

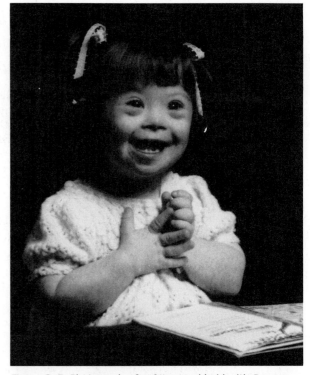

Figure 8–3. Photograph of a 2½-year-old girl with Down syndrome (trisomy 21). Note the round face, upslanted palpebral fissures, epicanthic folds, cupped ear, short digits with incurving of the fifth digit, a condition known as clinodactyly. (Courtesy of Dr. A.E. Chudley, Children's Centre, Winnipeg, Canada).

Table 8–2. TRISOMY OF THE AUTOSOMES

Chromosomal Aberration/Syndrome	Incidence	Usual Characteristics	Figures
Trisomy 21 or Down syndrome*	1:800	Mental deficiency; brachycephaly, flat nasal bridge; upward slant to palpebral fissures; protruding tongue; simian crease, clinodactyly of 5th digit; congenital heart defects.	8–3
Trisomy 18 syndrome†	1:8000	Mental deficiency; growth retardation; prominent occiput; short sternum; ventricular septal defect; micrognathia; low-set malformed ears; flexed digits, hypoplastic nails; rocker-bottom feet.	8–4
Trisomy 13 syndrome†	1:25000	Mental deficiency; severe central nervous system malformations; sloping forehead; malformed ears, scalp defects; microphthalmia; bilateral cleft lip and/or palate; polydactyly; posterior prominence of the heels	8–5

* The importance of this disorder in the overall problem of mental retardation is indicated by the fact that persons with Down syndrome represent ten to 15 per cent of institutionalized mental defectives (Breg, 1975). *The incidence of trisomy 21 at fertilization is greater than at birth,* but 75 per cent of the embryos are spontaneously aborted and at least 20 per cent are stillborn.

† Infants with this syndrome rarely survive beyond six months.

end of this decade, children born to women older than 34 years will account for 39 per cent of trisomy 21 cases (Goodwin and Huether, 1987).

Trisomy of the sex chromosomes is a common condition (Table 8–4); however, because there are no characteristic physical findings in infants or children, this disorder is not usually detected until adolescence (Fig. 8–6). *Sex chromatin studies* are useful in detecting some types of trisomy of the sex chromosomes because two masses of sex chromatin are present in nuclei of XXX females (Fig. 8–7C), and nuclei of XXY males contain a mass of sex chromatin.

Tetrasomy and pentasomy of the sex chromosomes also occurs. These persons have four or five sex chromosomes; the following chromosome complexes have been reported: *in females,* 48,XXXX and 49,XXXXX; and *in males,* 48,XXXY, 48,XXYY, 49,XXXYY, and 49,XXXXY. The extra sex chromosomes do not accentuate sexual characteristics; however, usually the greater the number of sex chromosomes present, the greater the severity of the mental retardation and physical impairment (Neu and Gardner, 1975; Thompson et al, 1991).

Mosaicism. A person who has at least two cell lines with *two or more different genotypes* (genetic constitutions) is

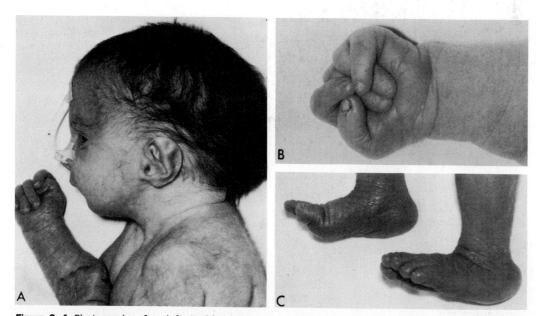

Figure 8–4. Photographs of an infant with trisomy 18 syndrome. *A,* Prominent occiput and malformed ears. *B,* Typical flexed fingers. *C,* Rocker-bottom feet showing posterior prominences of the heels. Most trisomy 18 fetuses abort spontaneously. For those that are born, the mean survival is only two months. (Courtesy of Dr. H. Medovy, Children's Centre, Winnipeg, Canada.)

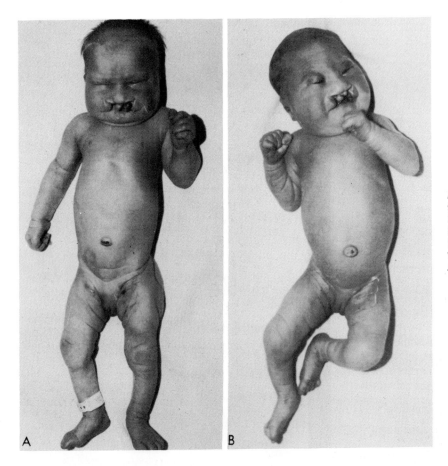

Figure 8–5. Female infants with trisomy 13 syndrome. Note bilateral cleft lip, sloping forehead, and rocker-bottom feet. This severe condition is lethal in about half the live-born infants within the first month. (From Smith DW: *Am J Obstet Gynecol 90*:1055, 1964.)

called a *mosaic*. Either the autosomes or sex chromosomes may be involved. Usually the anomalies are less serious than in persons with monosomy or trisomy; e.g., the features of Turner syndrome are not as evident in 45,X/46,XX mosaic females as in the usual 45,X females (Thompson et al, 1991). Mosaicism usually results from nondisjunction during early cleavage of the zygote (see Fig. 2–3). Mosaicism due to loss of a chromosome by *anaphase lagging* also occurs; the chromosomes separate normally, but one of them is delayed in its migration and is eventually lost.

Polyploidy. Polyploid cells contain multiples of the haploid number of chromosomes (e.g., 69 and 92). Polyploidy is a significant cause of spontaneous abortion (Carr et al., 1972; Kaufman, 1991). The most common type of polyploidy is **triploidy** (69 chromosomes). This could result from the second polar body failing to separate from the oocyte during the second meiotic division (see Chapter 2); but, more likely, triploidy results when an ovum is fertilized by two sperms almost simultaneously (dispermy). Connor and Ferguson-Smith (1987) estimated that 66 per cent of triploid embryos result from *dispermy*. Triploidy occurs in about two per cent of embryos, but most of them abort spontaneously. Although *triploid fetuses* have been born alive, this occurrence is exceptional. These infants all died within a few days because of multiple anomalies and low birth weight (Connor and Ferguson-Smith, 1987).

Doubling of the diploid chromosome number to 92 (*tetraploidy*) probably occurs during the first cleavage division (p. 33). Division of this abnormal zygote would subsequently result in an embryo with cells containing 92 chromosomes. *Tetraploid embryos* abort very early, and often all that is recovered is an empty chorionic sac (Carr, 1971; Kaufman, 1991). This is often referred to as a "blighted embryo".

Structural Chromosome Abnormalities

Most aberrations of chromosome structure result from chromosome breakage followed by reconstitution in an abnormal combination (Fig. 8–8). *Chromosome breaks* are induced by various environmental factors; e.g., radiation, drugs, chemicals, and viruses (Connor and Ferguson-Smith, 1987). The type of abnormality of chromosome structure that results depends upon what happens to the broken pieces (Fig. 8–8). The only two aberrations of chromosome structure that are likely to be transmitted from

Table 8-3. INCIDENCE OF DOWN SYNDROME IN NEWBORN INFANTS*

Maternal Age* (Years)	Incidence
20-24	1:1400
25-29	1:1100
30-34	1:700
35	1:350
37	1:225
39	1:140
41	1:85
43	1:50
45+	1:25

* Based on data from Hook et al. (1983, 1988). Figures have been rounded and are approximate.

parent to child are structural rearrangements, such as inversion and translocation (Thompson et al., 1991).

Translocation. This is the transfer of a piece of one chromosome to a nonhomologous chromosome. If two nonhomologous chromosomes exchange pieces, it is called a *reciprocal translocation* (Fig. 8-8A and G). Translocation does not necessarily cause abnormal development. A person with a translocation, for example, between a number 21 chromosome and a number 14 (Fig. 8-8G), is phenotypically normal. Such persons are called *balanced translocation carriers*. They have a tendency, independent of age, to produce germ cells with an abnormal translocation chromosome. Three to four per cent of persons with Down syndrome have translocation trisomies, i.e., the extra 21 chromosome is attached to another chromosome.

Deletion. When a chromosome breaks, a portion of the chromosome may be lost (Fig. 8-8B). A partial terminal deletion from the short arm of chromosome 5 causes the **cri du chat syndrome** (Fig. 8-9). Affected infants have a weak, catlike cry, microcephaly, severe mental retardation, and congenital heart disease. A *ring chromosome* is a type of deletion chromosome from which both ends have been lost, and the broken ends have rejoined to form a ring-shaped chromosome (Fig. 8-8C). These abnormal chromosomes

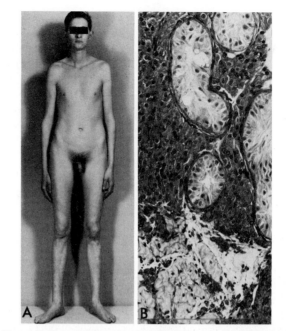

Figure 8-6. *A,* Adult male with Klinefelter syndrome (XXY trisomy). Note the long lower limbs and normal trunk length. About 40 per cent of persons with this syndrome have gynecomastia (excessive development of the male mammary glands). *B,* Section of a testicular biopsy showing some seminiferous tubules without germ cells and others that are hyalinized. (From Ferguson-Smith MA: *In* Moore KL [ed]: *The Sex Chromatin.* Philadelphia, WB Saunders, 1966.)

have been described in persons with Turner syndrome, trisomy 18, and other abnormalities (Hirschhorn, 1992). For a full description of *autosomal deletion syndromes,* see Thompson et al. (1991).

Microdeletions. High-resolution banding techniques have allowed detection of very small interstitial and terminal deletions in a number of disorders. Normal resolution chromosome banding reveals 350 bands per haploid set; whereas, *high-resolution chromosome banding* reveals up to 1300 bands per haploid set. Because the deletions span several contiguous genes, these disorders have been referred to as **contiguous gene syndromes.** Two examples are: (1) the

Table 8-4. TRISOMY OF THE SEX CHROMOSOMES

Chromosome Complement*	Sex	Incidence†	Usual Characteristics
47,XXX	Female	1:960	Normal in appearance; usually fertile; 15-25 per cent are mildly mentally retarded.
47,XXY	Male	1:1080	Klinefelter syndrome: small testes, hyalinization of seminiferous tubules; aspermatogenesis; often tall with disproportionately long lower limbs. Intelligence is less than in normal siblings.
47,XYY	Male	1:1080	Normal in appearance; often tall; often exhibits aggressive behavior.

* The numbers designate the total number of chromosomes including the sex chromosomes shown after the comma.
† Data from Hook EB, Hamerton JL (1977)

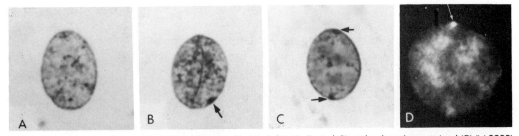

Figure 8-7. Oral epithelial nuclei stained with cresyl echt violet (*A*, *B*, and *C*) and quinacrine mustard (*D*) (× 2000). *A*, From normal male. No sex chromatin is visible (chromatin negative). *B*, From normal female. The arrow indicates a typical mass of sex chromatin (chromatin positive). *C*, From female with XXX trisomy. The arrows indicate two masses of sex chromatin. *D*, From normal male. The arrow indicates a mass of Y-chromatin as an intensely fluorescent body. (*A* and *B* are from Moore KL, Barr ML: *Lancet 2*:57, 1955. *D*, Courtesy of Dr. M. Ray, Department of Human Genetics, University of Manitoba, Winnipeg, Canada.)

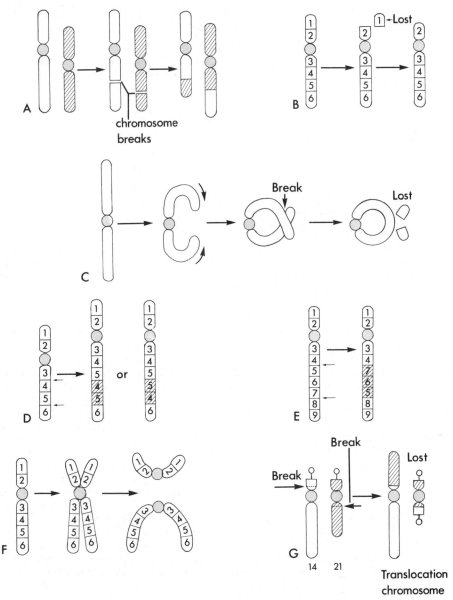

Figure 8-8. Diagrams illustrating various structural abnormalities of chromosomes. *A*, Reciprocal translocation. *B*, Terminal deletion. *C*, Ring. *D*, Duplication. *E*, Paracentric inversion. *F*, Isochromosome. *G*, Robertsonian translocation.

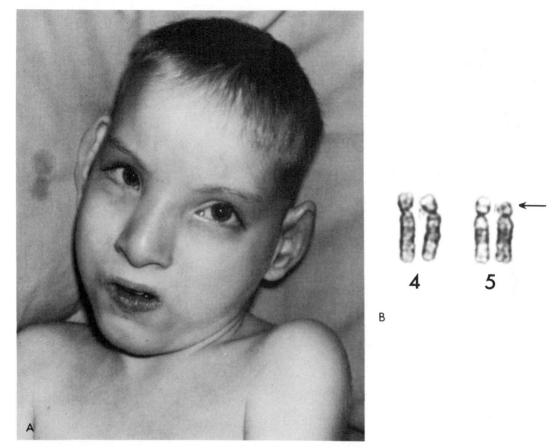

Figure 8–9. *A*, Male child with cri du chat syndrome. (From Gardner EJ: *Principles of Genetics.* 5th ed. New York, John Wiley & Sons, Inc., 1975.) *B*, A partial karyotype of this child showing a terminal deletion of the short arm end of the chromosome number 5. The arrow indicates the abnormal short arm. (Courtesy of Dr. M. Ray, Department of Human Genetics, University of Manitoba, Winnipeg, Canada.)

Prader-Willi syndrome, a sporadically occurring disorder associated with short stature, mild mental retardation, obesity, hyperphagia (overeating) and hypogonadism, and (2) the *Angelman syndrome*, characterized by severe mental retardation, microcephaly, brachycephaly, seizures, and ataxic (jerky) movements of limbs and trunk. Both disorders are often associated with a visible deletion of band q12 on chromosome 15. The clinical phenotype is determined by the parental origin of the deleted chromosome 15. If the deletion arises in the mother, Angelman syndrome will occur; if passed on by the father, the child will exhibit the Prader-Willi phenotype. This suggests the phenomenon of genetic imprinting whereby differential expression of genetic material is dependent on the sex of the transmitting parent (Knoll et al., 1989; Kirkilionis et al., 1991).

Molecular Cytogenetics. Several new methods for merging classical cytogenetics with DNA technology have facilitated a more precise definition of chromosome abnormalities, location or origins, including unbalanced translocations, accessory or marker chromosomes, as well as *gene mapping.* One new approach to chromosome iden-

tification is based on *fluorescent in situ hybridization* (FISH) whereby chromosome-specific DNA probes can adhere to complementary regions located on specific chromosomes (Pinkel et al., 1986). This allows improved identification of chromosome location and number in metaphase spreads or even in interphase cells (Manuelidis, 1985). FISH techniques using interphase cells may soon obviate the need to culture cells for specific chromosome analysis, such as in the case of prenatal diagnosis of fetal trisomies.

Duplication. This abnormality may be represented as a duplicated portion of a chromosome: within a chromosome (Fig. 8–8*D*); attached to a chromosome; or as a separate fragment. *Duplications are more common than deletions, and they are less harmful* because there is no loss of genetic material. Duplication may involve part of a gene, whole genes, or a series of genes (Thompson et al., 1991).

Inversion. This is a chromosomal aberration in which a segment of a chromosome is reversed. Paracentric inversion (Fig. 8–8*E*) is confined to a single arm of the chromosome, whereas pericentric inversion involves both arms and includes the centromere. Carriers of pericentric inversions are at risk of having offspring with abnormalities as a result of unequal crossing over and malsegregation at meiosis (Allderice et al, 1975; Thompson et al, 1991).

Isochromosomes. The abnormality resulting in these chromosomes occurs when the centromere divides transversely instead of longitudinally (Fig. 8–8F). An isochromosome is a chromosome in which one arm is missing and the other duplicated. It appears to be the *most common structural abnormality of the X chromosome.* Patients with this chromosomal abnormality are often short in stature and have other stigmata of Turner syndrome (Fig. 8–2). These characteristics are related to the loss of an arm of an X chromosome (Neu and Gardner, 1975; Thompson et al, 1991).

Anomalies Caused by Mutant Genes

Seven to eight per cent of congenital anomalies are caused by gene defects (Table 8–1). A mutation usually involves a loss or a change in the function of a gene and is any permanent, heritable change in the sequence of genomic DNA (Thompson et al, 1991). Because a random change is unlikely to lead to an improvement in development, most mutations are deleterious and some are lethal. The mutation rate can be increased by a number of environmental agents; e.g., large doses of radiation and some chemicals, especially carcinogenic (cancer-inducing) ones. Anomalies resulting from gene mutation are inherited according to mendelian laws; consequently, predictions can be made about the probability of their occurrence in the affected person's children and in other relatives.

Examples of *dominantly inherited congenital anomalies* are **achondroplasia** (Fig. 8–10) and polydactyly, or extra digits (see Chapter 17). Other anomalies are attributed to *autosomal recessive inheritance;* e.g., congenital adrenal hyperplasia (Fig. 8–12) and microcephaly (see Fig. 18–33). Autosomal recessive genes manifest themselves only when homozygous; as a consequence, many carriers of these genes (heterozygous persons) remain undetected.

The fragile X syndrome is the most common inherited cause of moderate mental retardation (Fig. 8–11), and is *second only to Down syndrome among all causes of moderate mental retardation in males* (Chudley and Hagerman, 1987; Thompson et al., 1991). This syndrome has a frequency of 1 in 1500 male births and may account for much of the excess of males in the mentally retarded population (Thompson et al, 1991). The diagnosis can be confirmed by chromosome analysis demonstrating the fragile X chromosome[5] or by DNA studies of the fragile X gene. X-linked recessive genes are usually manifest in

---

[5] The area at the end of the long arm of the chromosome looks like it is breaking off.

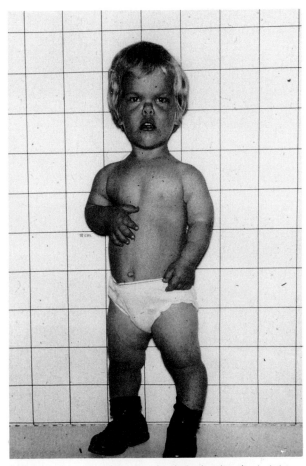

Figure 8–10. A boy with achondroplasia showing short stature, short limbs and fingers, normal length of the trunk, bowed legs, a relatively large head, prominent forehead, and depressed nasal bridge. (Courtesy of Dr. A.E. Chudley, Children's Centre, Winnipeg, Canada.)

affected (hemizygous) males and occasionally in carrier (heterozygous) females, e.g., fragile X syndrome (Chudley and Hagerman, 1987; Heitz et al., 1991).

The human genome contains an estimated 50,000 to 100,000 structural genes per haploid set. The fact that, up to 1992, fewer than 5000 gene mutations have been identified suggests that the majority of gene mutations have yet to be discovered. It is plausible that the majority of infants with congenital anomalies of unknown cause likely have a genetic disorder. Molecular biological techniques will accelerate gene discoveries over the next few decades.

ANOMALIES CAUSED BY ENVIRONMENTAL FACTORS

Although the human embryo is well protected in the uterus, certain environmental agents called

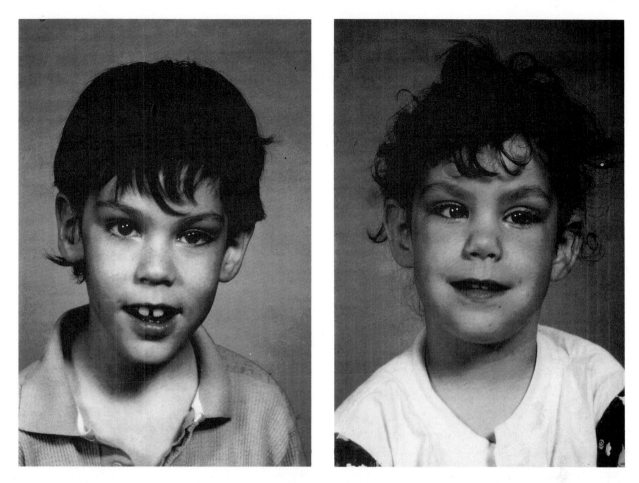

Figure 8–11. *A,* This 8-year-old, mentally retarded boy has the fragile X syndrome. Note the relatively normal appearance with a long face and prominent ears. *B,* His 6-year-old sister also has this syndrome. She has a mild learning disability and similar features of long face and prominent ears. Note the strabismus of the right eye. Although an X-linked disorder, sometimes female carriers will have expression of the disease (Courtesy of Dr. A.E. Chudley, Children's Centre, Winnipeg, Canada.)

teratogens may cause developmental disruptions following maternal exposure to them (Table 8–5). A teratogen is any agent that can produce a congenital anomaly or raise the incidence of an anomaly in the population (Johnson, 1986; Persaud, 1990). Environmental factors, such as infection and drugs, may simulate genetic conditions; e.g., when two or more children of normal parents are affected (Holmes, 1992). The important principle here is that "not everything that is familial is genetic." The organs and parts of an embryo are most sensitive to teratogenic agents during periods of rapid differentiation (Fig. 8–13).

Environmental factors cause 7 to 10 per cent of congenital anomalies (Tables 8–1 and 8–5). Because biochemical differentiation precedes morphological differentiation, the period during which structures are sensitive to interference often precedes the stage of their visible development by a few days (Fig. 8–13). Teratogens do not appear to be effective in causing anomalies until cellular differentiation has begun; however, their early actions may cause the death of the embryo (Fig. 8–13).

The exact *mechanisms* by which drugs, chemicals, and other environmental factors interfere with embryonic development and induce abnormalities still remain obscure. Even thalidomide's (one of the best known and most studied teratogens) mechanisms of action on the embryo are a "mystery," and more than 20 hypotheses have been postulated to explain how it disrupts development of the embryo (Stephens, 1988). Many studies have shown that certain hereditary and environmental influences may adversely affect embryonic development by altering such fundamental processes as the intracellular compartment,

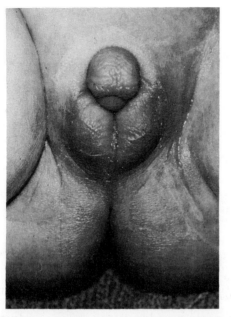

Figure 8–12. Masculinized external genitalia of a female infant caused by congenital virilizing adrenal hyperplasia. The virilization was caused by excessive androgens produced by the suprarenal (adrenal) glands during the fetal period.

the surface of the cell, extracellular matrix, and the fetal environment; but, as yet, there is no fundamental hypothesis to explain the underlying mechanisms (Saxén 1976; Persaud, 1979; and Persaud et al, 1985).

It has been suggested that the initial cellular response may take more than one form (genetic, molecular, biochemical, biophysical), resulting in different sequences of cellular changes (cell death, faulty cellular interaction-induction, reduced biosynthesis of substrates, impaired morphogenetic movements, and mechanical disruption). Eventually these different types of pathological lesion could possibly lead to the final defect (intrauterine death, developmental anomalies, fetal growth retardation or functional disturbances) via a common pathway (Wilson, 1973; and Beckman and Brent, 1984).

Rapid progress in the field of **molecular biology** is now providing more information on the genetic control of differentiation as well as the cascade of events involved in the expression of homeobox genes and pattern formation. It is reasonable to speculate that disruption of gene activity at any critical stage could lead to a developmental defect. This view is supported by recent experimental studies which showed that exposure of mouse and amphibian embryos to the teratogen *retinoic acid* altered the domain of gene expression and disrupted normal morphogenesis. Researchers are now directing increasing attention to the

molecular mechanisms of abnormal development in an attempt to understand the pathogenesis of congenital anomalies better (De Luca 1991).

Basic Principles in Teratogenesis

When considering the possible teratogenicity of an agent (e.g., drug or chemical), *three important principles* must be considered: *critical periods* of development, the *dosage* of the drug or chemical, and the *genotype*[6] of the embryo.

Critical Periods in Human Development. (Fig. 8–13). The stage of development of an embryo when an agent is present determines its susceptibility to a teratogen. The most critical period in development is when cell division, cell differentiation, and morphogenesis are at their peak. Table 8–6 indicates the relative frequencies of anomalies for certain organs.

The most *critical period for brain development* is from three to 16 weeks (Fig. 8–13), but its development may be disrupted after this because the brain is differentiating and growing rapidly at birth and continues to do so throughout the first two years after birth. Teratogens (e.g., alcohol) may produce mental retardation during the embryonic and fetal periods. *Tooth development* also continues long after birth (see Chapter 20); hence, the development of permanent teeth may be disrupted by *tetracyclines* (p. 159) from 18 weeks (prenatal) to 16 years. The *skeletal system* has a prolonged critical period of development extending into childhood; hence, the growth of skeletal tissues provides a good gauge of general growth.

Environmental disturbances during the first two weeks after fertilization may interfere with cleavage of the zygote and implantation of the blastocyst and/or cause early death and spontaneous abortion of the embryo, but they are not known to cause congenital anomalies in human embryos (Fig. 8–13). Most development during this period is concerned with the formation of extraembryonic structures (e.g., the amnion, yolk sac, and chorionic sac; see Chapter 3).

Development of the embryo is most easily disrupted when the tissues and organs are forming (i.e., during the **organogenetic period**). During this period (Fig. 8–13), teratogenic agents may induce major congenital anomalies. Physiological defects, minor morphological anomalies (e.g., of the external ear), and functional disturbances (e.g., mental retardation) are likely to result from disruptions of development during the fetal period. Some microorganisms, however (e.g., *Toxoplasma gondii*), are known to cause serious congenital anomalies, particularly of

---

[6] The genetic constitution (genome). More specifically, the alleles present at one location (Thompson et al, 1991).

Table 8-5. TERATOGENS KNOWN TO CAUSE HUMAN BIRTH DEFECTS*

Agents	Most Common Congenital Anomalies
DRUGS	
Alcohol	*Fetal alcohol syndrome (FAS):* intrauterine growth retardation *(IUGR);* mental retardation, microcephaly; ocular anomalies; joint abnormalities; short palpebral fissures (Fig. 8-14).
Androgens and high doses of progestogens	Varying degrees of masculinization of female fetuses: ambiguous external genitalia resulting in labial fusion and clitoral hypertrophy (Fig. 8-15).
Aminopterin	IUGR; skeletal defects (Fig. 8-17); malformations of the central nervous system, notably meroanencephaly (most of the brain is absent).
Busulfan	Stunted growth; skeletal abnormalities; corneal opacities; cleft palate; hypoplasia of various organs.
Cocaine	IGUR; microcephaly; cerebral infarction; urogenital anomalies; neurobehavioral disturbances.
Diethystilbesterol	Abnormalities of the uterus and vagina; cervical erosion and ridges.
Isotretinoin (13-cis-retinoic acid)	Craniofacial abnormalities; neural tube defects *(NTDs),* such as spina bifida cystica; cardiovascular defects.
Lithium carbonate	Various anomalies usually involving the heart and great vessels.
Methotrexate	Multiple malformations, especially skeletal, involving the face, skull, limbs, and vertebral column.
Phenytoin (Dilantin)	*Fetal hydantoin syndrome (FHS):* IUGR; microcephaly; mental retardation; ridged metopic suture; inner epicanthal folds; eyelid ptosis; broad depressed nasal bridge; phalangeal hypoplasia (Fig. 8-16).
Tetracycline	Stained teeth; hypoplasia of enamel.
Thalidomide	Abnormal development of the limbs (Fig. 8-19), e.g., meromelia (partial absence) and amelia (complete absence); facial anomalies; systemic anomalies, e.g., cardiac and kidney defects.
Trimethadione	Development delay; V-shaped eyebrows; low-set ears; cleft lip and/or palate.
Valproic acid	Craniofacial anomalies; NTDs; often hydrocephalus; heart and skeletal defects.
Warfarin	Nasal hypoplasia; stippled epiphyses; hypoplastic phalanges; eye anomalies; mental retardation.
CHEMICALS	
Methylmercury	Cerebral atrophy; spasticity; seizures; mental retardation.
PCBs	IGUR; skin discolorization.
INFECTIONS	
Cytomegalovirus	Microcephaly; chorioretinitis; sensorineural loss; delayed psychomotor/mental development; hepatosplenomegaly; hydrocephaly; cerebral palsy; brain (periventricular) calcification.
Herpes simplex virus	Skin vesicles and scarring; chorioretinitis; hepatomegaly; thrombocytopenia; petechiae; hemolytic anemia; hydranencephaly.
Human immunodeficiency virus (HIV)	Growth failure; microcephaly; prominent boxlike forehead; flattened nasal bridge; hypertelorism; triangular philtrum and patulous lips.
Human parvovirus B19	Eye defects; degenerative changes in fetal tissues.
Rubella virus	IUGR; postnatal growth retardation; cardiac and great vessel malformations; microcephaly; sensorineural deafness; cataract; microphthalmos; glaucoma (Fig. 8-20); pigmented retinopathy; mental retardation; newborn bleeding; hepatosplenomegaly; osteopathy.
Toxoplasma gondii	Microcephaly; mental retardation; microphthalmia; hydrocephaly; chorioretinitis; cerebral calcifications.
Treponema pallidum	Hydrocephalus; congenital deafness; mental retardation; abnormal teeth and bones.
Venezuelan equine encephalitis virus	Microcephaly; microphthalmia; cerebral agenesis; CNS necrosis; hydrocephalus.
Varicella virus	Cutaneous scars (dermatome distribution); neurological anomalies (limb paresis, hydrocephaly, seizures, etc.); cataracts; microphthalmia; Horner syndrome; optic atrophy; nystagmus; chorioretinitis; microcephaly; mental retardation; skeletal anomalies (hypoplasia of limbs, fingers, and toes, etc.); urogenital anomalies.
HIGH LEVELS OF IONIZING RADIATION	Microcephaly; mental retardation; skeletal anomalies.

* The spectrum and severity of congenital anomalies may vary from one case to another. For more information see Gibbs and Sweet, 1989; Holmes, 1992; Persaud, 1990; Remington and Klein, 1990; Shepard, 1992.

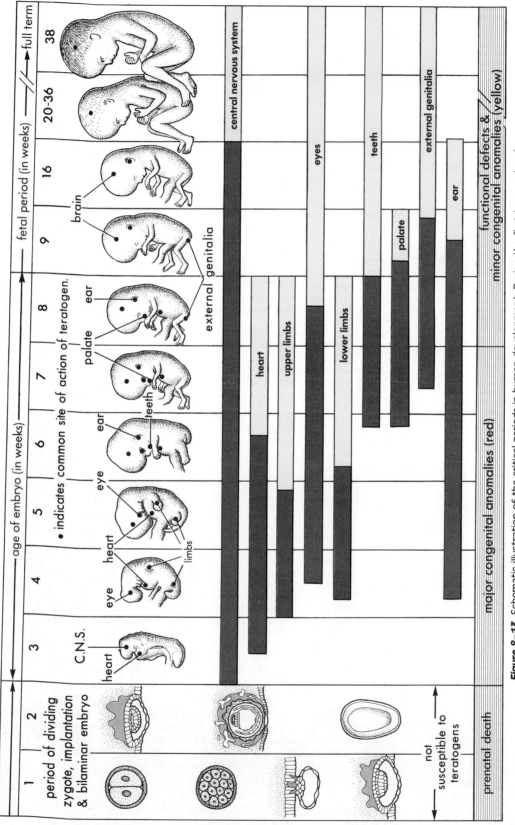

Figure 8–13. Schematic illustration of the critical periods in human development. During the first two weeks of development, the embryo is usually not susceptible to teratogens. During these pre-embryonic stages, a teratogen either damages all or most of the cells, resulting in its death, or damages only a few cells, allowing the conceptus to recover and the embryo to develop without birth defects. *Red denotes highly sensitive periods* when major defects may be produced (e.g., amelia, absence of limbs). Yellow indicates stages that are less sensitive to teratogens when minor defects may be induced (e.g., hypoplastic thumbs).

156

Table 8-6. INCIDENCE OF MAJOR MALFORMATIONS IN HUMAN ORGANS AT BIRTH*

Organ	Incidence of Malformations
Brain	10:1000
Heart	8:1000
Kidneys	4:1000
Limbs	2:1000
All other	6:1000
Total	30:1000

* Data from Connor and Ferguson-Smith (1987).

the brain and eyes, when they infect the fetus (see Table 8-5). If present during the embryonic period, they often kill the embryo.

Each part and organ of an embryo has a critical period during which its development may be disrupted (Fig. 8-13). The type of congenital anomalies produced depends upon which parts and organs are most susceptible at the time the teratogen is active. The following examples illustrate that teratogens may affect different organ systems that are developing at the same time:

1. High levels of radiation produce abnormalities of the central nervous system and eyes, as well as mental retardation (p. 167). The period of greatest sensitivity for *radiation damage to the brain* leading to severe mental retardation is from eight to 16 weeks after fertilization.

2. The rubella virus causes eye defects (glaucoma and cataracts), deafness, and cardiac anomalies.

3. Thalidomide induces limb defects and several other anomalies (e.g., of the ear). Early in the sensitive period, it causes severe limb defects; e.g., *amelia* (absent upper and/or lower limbs). Later in the sensitive period, it causes mild to moderate limb defects; e.g., hypoplasia of radius and ulna, and *meromelia* (absence of parts of limbs, such as the hands). There is no clinical evidence that thalidomide was capable of damaging the embryo when it was administered after the critical period of development (Newman, 1986a).

Embryological timetables, such as Figure 8-13, are helpful when considering the cause of human birth defects, but it is wrong to assume that anomalies always result from a single event occurring during the critical period or that one can determine from these tables the day on which the anomaly was produced. All one can state is that the teratogen would have had to disrupt development before the end of the critical period of the part or organ concerned. The *critical period for limb development*, for example, is 24 to 36 days after fertilization (Fig. 8-13).

The Dosage of the Drug or Chemical. Animal research has shown that there is a dose-response rela-

tionship for teratogens. One must be aware, however, that the dose used in animals to produce anomalies is often at levels much higher than human exposures. For this reason, *animal studies are not readily applicable to human pregnancies.* For a drug to be considered a teratogen, a dose-response relationship has to be observed; i.e., the greater the exposure during pregnancy, the more severe the phenotypic effect.

Genotype of the Embryo. There are numerous examples in experimental animals and several suspected human cases which show that there are genetic differences in response to a teratogen; for example, *phenytoin* is a well-known human teratogen (Table 8-5). Five to ten per cent of embryos exposed to this anticonvulsant medication develop the fetal dilantin (phenytoin) syndrome (p. 160). About one third of exposed embryos, however, have only some congenital anomalies, and more than half of them are unaffected. It appears, therefore, that the genotype of the embryo determines whether an agent will disrupt its development.

Human Teratogens and Congenital Anomalies

Awareness that certain agents can disrupt development offers the opportunity to prevent some congenital anomalies (Tables 8-1 and 8-5); for example, if women are made aware of the harmful effects of drugs (e.g., alcohol), environmental chemicals (e.g., PCBs) and viruses, most of them will not expose their embryos to these teratogenic agents. The general objective of teratogenicity testing of drugs, chemicals, food additives, and pesticides is to identify agents that may be teratogenic during human development and to alert pregnant women of their possible danger to the embryo/fetus (Shepard, 1992).

To prove that an agent is a teratogen, one must show either that the frequency of anomalies is increased above the spontaneous rate in pregnancies in which the mother is exposed to the agent (*the prospective approach*) or that malformed infants have a history of maternal exposure to the agent more often than normal children (*the retrospective approach*). Both types of data are difficult to obtain in an unbiased form. *Case reports are not convincing* unless both the agent and type of anomaly are so uncommon that their association in several cases can be judged not coincidental (e.g., thalidomide).

Drug Testing in Animals. Although the testing of drugs in pregnant animals is important, it should be emphasized that the results are of limited value for predicting drug effects on human embryos. *Animal experiments can only suggest that similar effects may occur in humans.* If a drug or chemical produces teratogenic effects in two or more species, the probability of potential human hazard must be considered to be high; however, the dosage of the drug has to be considered.

Drugs as Teratogens

Drugs vary considerably in their teratogenicity. Some of them cause severe disruptions of development if administered during the organogenetic period (e.g., thalidomide). Others produce mental and growth retardation and other anomalies if used excessively throughout development (e.g., alcohol). *The use of prescription and nonprescription drugs during pregnancy is surprisingly high.* From 40 to 90 per cent of pregnant women consume at least one drug. Several studies have indicated that some pregnant women take an average of four drugs, excluding nutritional supplements, and about half of these women take them during the first trimester of pregnancy.

Drug consumption also tends to be higher during the critical period of development among heavy smokers and heavy drinkers (Persaud, 1990). Despite this, *less than two per cent of congenital anomalies are caused by drugs and chemicals* (Brent, 1986a). Only a few drugs have been positively implicated as human teratogenic agents (Table 8–5).

It is best for women to avoid using all medication during the first trimester, especially during the first eight weeks after conception (ten weeks after LNMP), unless there is a strong medical reason for its use, and then only if it is recognized as reasonably safe for the human embryo. The reason for this caution is that, even though well-controlled studies of certain drugs (e.g., *marijuana*) have failed to demonstrate a teratogenic risk to human embryos (p. 164), it does harm the embryo (i.e., it causes a decrease in birthweight [Holmes, 1992]).

Cigarette Smoking. Despite warnings that cigarette smoking is harmful to the fetus, more than 25 per cent of women continue to smoke during their pregnancies. *Maternal smoking is a well-established cause of intrauterine growth retardation* (IUGR). In heavy cigarette smokers (20 or more cigarettes per day), premature delivery is twice as frequent as in mothers who do not smoke, and their infants weigh less than normal (see Fig. 6–13). *Low birth weight* (below 2000 gm) is the chief predictor of infant death. Epidemiological studies have not indicated a strong association between maternal smoking and the overall occurrence of congenital anomalies. There is, however, some evidence that maternal smoking may cause behavioral problems and decreased physical growth.

Infants of mothers who stop smoking during pregnancy show an improvement in their birth weights. The benefit is greatest in those mothers who quit smoking before 16 weeks of gestation. *Nicotine constricts uterine blood vessels, causing a decrease in uterine blood flow.* This lowers the supply of oxygen and nutrients available to the embryo in the intervillous space. The resulting deficiency in the embryo impairs cell growth and may also have an adverse effect on mental development. High levels of *carboxyhemoglobin*, resulting from cigarette smoking, appear in the maternal and fetal blood and may alter the capacity of the blood to transport oxygen. As a result, chronic fetal hypoxia may occur and affect fetal growth and development.

Caffeine. Caffeine is the most popular drug in North America because it is present in several widely consumed beverages (e.g., coffee, tea, and cola drinks), chocolate products, and in some drugs. It is *not known to be a human teratogen*, but there is no assurance that heavy maternal consumption of it is safe for the embryo. For this reason, excessive drinking of coffee, tea, and colas containing caffeine should be avoided.

Alcohol. Severe alcoholism is a common drug abuse problem that affects one to two per cent of women of childbearing age. Infants born to chronic alcoholic mothers exhibit a specific pattern of defects (Golbus, 1980; Persaud, 1988, 1990 and Holmes 1992), including prenatal and postnatal growth deficiency, mental retardation, and other anomalies (Fig. 8–14; Table 8–5). Microcephaly, short palpebral fissures, epicanthal folds, maxillary hypoplasia, short nose, thin upper lip, abnormal palmar creases, joint anomalies, and congenital heart disease are also present in most infants (Jones et al., 1974; Mulvihill, 1986). This set of symptoms is known as the **fetal alcohol syndrome (FAS)**. The incidence of FAS, estimated to be about 2 per 1000 live births, is related to the population studied.

Maternal alcohol abuse is now thought to be the most common cause of mental retardation. Even moderate maternal alcohol consumption (e.g., 1 to 2 ounces per day) may produce *fetal alcohol effects* (FAE); i.e., children with behavioral and learning difficulties, especially if the drinking is associated with malnutrition. *Binge drinking* (heavy consumption of alcohol for one to three days during pregnancy) is very likely to produce FAE. The susceptible period of brain development spans the major part of gestation (Fig. 8–13); therefore, the safest advice is total abstinence from alcohol during pregnancy.

Androgens and Progestogens[7]. Any hormone that has androgenic or masculinizing activities may affect the female fetus, producing masculinization of the

---

[7] The terms "progestogens" and "progestins" are used for substances, natural or synthetic, that produce some or all the biological changes produced by progesterone, a hormone produced by the corpus luteum that promotes and maintains a gravid endometrium or decidua (p. 27). Some of these substances have androgenic or masculinizing properties.

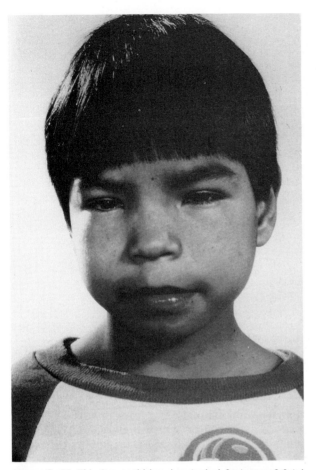

Figure 8-14. This 9-year-old boy has typical features of fetal alcohol syndrome (FAS). Note the widely spaced eyes, short palpebral fissures, long philtrum, and thin upper lip. He has an attention deficit disorder with hyperactivity and is mildly mentally retarded. His mother drank heavily throughout her pregnancy. (Courtesy of Dr. A.E. Chudley, Children's Centre, Winnipeg, Canada).

external genitalia (Fig. 8-15). The incidence of anomalies varies with the drug and the dosage. The preparations that should be avoided are the progestins, ethisterone and norethisterone. From a practical standpoint, the teratogenic risk of these hormones is low (Jones 1989; Persaud, 1990). Progestin exposure during the critical period of development is also associated with an increased prevalence of cardiovascular abnormalities (Heinonen et al, 1977), and exposure of male fetuses during this period may double the incidence of *hypospadias* (p. 294) in the offspring. Obviously, the administration of *testosterone* will also produce similar masculinizing effects in female fetuses.

More than 13 million women use contraceptive hormones ("birth control pills") in the United States (Forrest and Fordyce, 1988). *Oral contraceptives* containing progestogens and estrogens, taken during the early stages of an unrecognized pregnancy, are suspected of being teratogenic agents, but the results of several recent epidemiological studies are conflicting (Persaud, 1990). The infants of 13 of 19 mothers who had taken progestogen-estrogen *birth control pills* during the critical period of development exhibited the VACTERL syndrome (Nora and Nora, 1975). The acronym VACTERL stands for *v*ertebral, *a*nal, *c*ardiac, *t*racheo*e*sophageal, *r*enal, and *l*imb anomalies. As a precaution, use of oral contraceptives should be stopped as soon as pregnancy is detected because of these possible teratogenic effects (Kelsey, 1980).

Diethylstilbestrol (stilbestrol) is recognized as a human teratogen. Both gross and microscopic congenital abnormalities of the uterus and vagina have been detected in women who were exposed to diethylstilbestrol *in utero* (Ulfelder, 1986). Three types of lesion were observed: vaginal adenosis, cervical erosions, and ridges. A number of young women aged 16 to 22 years have developed *adenocarcinoma of the vagina* after a common history of exposure to the synthetic estrogen *in utero* (Herbst et al., 1974; Hart et al., 1976); however, the probability of cancers developing at this early age in females exposed to diethylstilbestrol (DES) *in utero* now appears to be low. The risk of cancer from DES exposure in utero is estimated to be less than 1 in 1000 (Ulfelder, 1986); for more information, see Noller (1990).

Antibiotics. Tetracyclines cross the placental membrane (see Fig. 7-8) and are deposited in the embryo's bones and teeth at sites of active calcification (Kalant et al, 1990). As little as 1 g per day of *tetracycline* during the third trimester of pregnancy can produce yellow staining of the primary or deciduous teeth (Cohlan, 1986). Tetracycline therapy during the second and third trimesters of pregnancy may cause tooth defects (e.g., hypoplasia of enamel), yellow to brown discoloration of the teeth, and diminished growth of long bones. Calcification of the secondary or permanent teeth begins at birth and, except for the third molars, is complete by seven to eight years of age; hence, long-term tetracycline therapy during early childhood can affect the permanent teeth. Tetracyclines should, therefore, not be administered to pregnant women or during early childhood if adequate antibiotic alternatives are available (Cohlan, 1986).

Deafness has been reported in infants of mothers who have been treated with high doses of streptomycin and dihydrostreptomycin as *antituberculosis agents* (Golbus, 1980). More than 30 cases of hearing deficit and eighth cranial nerve damage have been reported in infants exposed to streptomycin derivatives *in utero* (Rasmussen, 1969; Ganguin and Rempt, 1970; Warkany, 1986). *Penicillin* has been

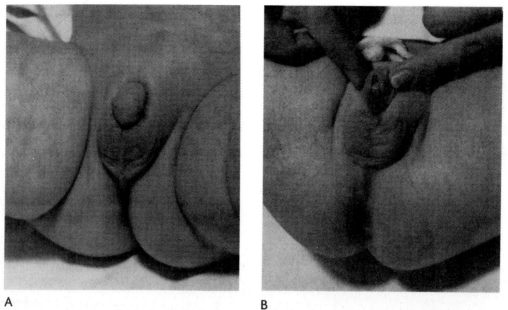

A   B

Figure 8-15. The external genitalia of a newborn female infant showing labial fusion and enlargement of the clitoris. This masculinization was caused by an androgenic agent given to the infant's mother during the first trimester. The 17-ketosteroid output was normal. (From Jones HW, Scott WW: *Hermaphroditism, Genital Anomalies and Related Endocrine Disorders.* 1958. Copyright © 1958 by Williams & Wilkins, Baltimore.)

used extensively during pregnancy and appears to be harmless to the human embryo and fetus.

Anticoagulants. All anticoagulants except heparin cross the placental membrane (see Fig. 7-8) and may cause hemorrhage in the fetus. Warfarin and other coumarin derivatives are antagonists of vitamin K. Warfarin is used for the treatment of thromboembolitic disease and for patients with artificial heart valves.

Warfarin is definitely a teratogen. There are reports of infants with hypoplasia of the nasal cartilage, stippled epiphyses, and various central nervous system defects whose mothers took this anticoagulant during the critical period of their embryo's development (Holzgreve et al., 1976). The period of greatest sensitivity is between six and 12 weeks after fertilization (8 to 14 weeks after LNMP). Second- and third-trimester exposure may result in mental retardation, optic atrophy, and microcephaly (Golbus, 1980).

Heparin is not a teratogen. Furthermore, it does not cross the placental membrane and so is the drug of choice for pregnant women requiring anticoagulant therapy (Ginsberg and Hirsh, 1988).

Anticonvulsants. Approximately one of 200 pregnant women is epileptic and requires treatment with an anticonvulsant. Of the anticonvulsant drugs available, there is strong evidence that *trimethadione* (Tridione) is a teratogen (Goldman et al., 1986). The main features of the *fetal trimethadione syndrome* are prenatal and postnatal growth retardation, developmental delay, V-shaped eyebrows, low-set ears, and cleft lip and/or palate, and cardiac and genitourinary as well as limb defects. Use of this drug is contraindicated during pregnancy (Paulson and Paulson, 1990).

Phenytoin. (Dilantin, Novophenytoin) is definitely a teratogen (Fig. 8-16). The *fetal hydantoin syndrome* occurs in five to ten per cent of children born to mothers treated with phenytoins or hydantoin anticonvulsants. The pattern of anomalies consists of: intrauterine growth retardation (IUGR), microcephaly, mental retardation, ridged metopic (frontal) suture, inner epicanthal folds, eyelid ptosis, broad depressed nasal bridge, nail and/or distal phalangeal hypoplasia, and hernias (Hanson, 1986; Chodirker et al., 1987; Behrman, 1992).

Valproic acid had been the drug of choice for the management of different types of epilepsy; however, its use by pregnant women has led to a *pattern of anomalies* consisting of craniofacial, heart, and limb defects. There is also an increased risk of neural tube defects (Sever and Brent, 1986; Paulson and Paulson, 1990; Holmes, 1992).

Phenobarbital is considered to be a safe, antiepileptic drug for use during pregnancy (Persaud, 1990).

Antinauseants. There has been extensive debate in the lay press and in the courts as to whether *Bendectin*

(Debendox, Lenotan) is a human teratogenic drug (Brent, 1986a; Holmes, 1986). Teratologists consider Bendectin to be nonteratogenic in humans because large-scale epidemiologic studies of infants have failed to show an increased risk of birth defects after its administration to pregnant women (Holmes, 1986). In addition, there is no convincing evidence that it is a teratogenic agent in animals.

Antineoplastic Agents. About 20 cytotoxic agents are currently available for clinical use. With the exception of the folic antagonist *aminopterin*, few well-documented reports of teratogenic effects are available for assessment. Because the data available on the possible teratogenicity of antineoplastic drugs are in-adequate, it is recommended that they should be avoided, especially during the first trimester of pregnancy.

Tumor-inhibiting chemicals are highly teratogenic. This is not surprising because these agents inhibit mitosis in rapidly dividing cells. The use of aminopterin during the embryonic period often results in intra-uterine death of the embryos, but the 20 to 30 per cent of those that survive are severely malformed (Fig. 8–17). *Busulfan and 6-mercaptopurine* administered in alternating courses throughout pregnancy have produced multiple severe abnormalities, but neither drug alone appears to cause major anomalies. (For information on the long-term development of

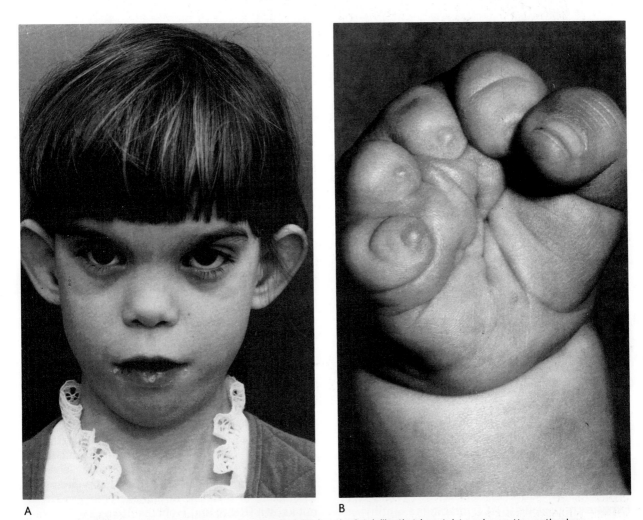

A　　　　　　　　　　　　　　　　　　　　　B

Figure 8–16. *A*, This young girl with a learning disability has the fetal dilantin (phenytoin) syndrome. Her mother has epilepsy and took dilantin throughout her pregnancy. Note the unusual ears, wide space between the eyes, epicanthal folds, short nose, and long philtrum. (Courtesy of Dr. A.E. Chudley, Children's Centre, Winnipeg, Canada). *B*, Right hand of infant with severe digital hypoplasia (short fingers) born to a mother who took dilantin throughout her pregnancy. (From Chodirker et al.: *Am J Med Genet* 27:373, copyright © 1987. Reprinted by permission of Wiley-Liss, a division of John Wiley and Sons, Inc.).

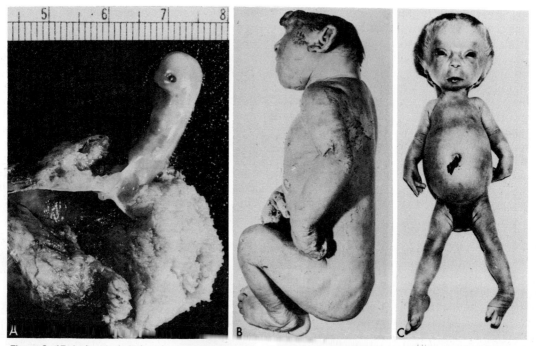

Figure 8–17. Aminopterin-induced congenital anomalies. *A,* Grossly malformed embryo and its membranes. (Courtesy of Dr. J.B. Thiersch, Seattle, Washington.) *B,* Newborn infant with meroanencephaly or partial absence of the brain. (From Thiersch JB: *In* Wolstenholme GEW, O'Connor CM [eds]: Ciba Foundation Symposium on Congenital Malformations. London, J. & A. Churchill, Ltd., 1960, pp. 152–154) *C,* Newborn infant showing marked intrauterine growth retardation, a large head, a small mandible, deformed ears, clubhands, and clubfeet. (From Warkany J, Beaudry PH, Hornstein S: *Am J Dis Child* 97:274–281, 1959.)

children exposed *in utero* to antineoplastic drugs, see Garber, 1989).

Aminopterin is a potent teratogen that produces major congenital anomalies (Fig. 8–17), especially of the skeletal and central nervous systems (Thiersch, 1952; Warkany et al., 1960; Sever and Brent, 1986; Holmes, 1992). Aminopterin, an antimetabolite, is a *folic acid antagonist.* Milunsky et al. (1968) described multiple skeletal and other congenital anomalies in an infant born to a mother who attempted to terminate her pregnancy by taking *methotrexate,* a derivative of aminopterin that is also a folic acid antagonist.

Corticosteroids. Cortisone causes cleft palate and cardiac defects in susceptible strains of mice and rabbits, but *cortisone does not induce cleft palate* or any other anomaly in human embryos (Shepard, 1989; Fraser, 1990).

Angiotensin-Converting Enzyme (ACE) Inhibitors. Exposure of the fetus to ACE inhibitors as antihypertensive agents causes oligohydramnios (p. 129), fetal death, long-lasting hypoplasia, and renal dysfunction (Holmes, 1992). During early pregnancy the risk to the embryo is apparently less, and there is no indication in such a case to terminate a wanted pregnancy. It

is recommended that, because of the high incidence of serious perinatal complications, ACE inhibitors should not be prescribed during pregnancy (Hanssens et al., 1991; Brent and Beckman, 1991).

Insulin and Hypoglycemic Drugs. Insulin is not teratogenic in human embryos except possibly in maternal insulin coma therapy. Hypoglycemic drugs (e.g., tolbutamide) have been implicated, but evidence for their teratogenicity is very weak; consequently, despite their marked teratogenicity in rodents, there is no convincing evidence that oral hypoglycemic agents (particularly sulfonylureas) are teratogenic in human embryos. The incidence of congenital anomalies (e.g., *sacral agenesis*) is increased two to three times in the offspring of diabetic mothers, and about 40 per cent of all perinatal deaths among diabetic infants are the result of congenital anomalies. The teratogenic mechanism of diabetic embryopathy is not known (Reece and Hobbins, 1986).

Retinoic Acid (Vitamin A). This is a well-established teratogen in animals, and its teratogenicity in humans was recognized a decade ago (Rosa et al., 1986). *Isotretinoin (13-cis-retinoic acid),* used for the oral treatment of severe cystic acne, *is teratogenic* *at very low doses in humans.* The critical period for exposure appears to be from the third week to the fifth week (five to seven weeks after LNMP). The risk of spontaneous abortion and birth defects following *in utero* exposure to retinoic acid is high. The most common major anomalies observed are craniofacial dysmorphism (microtia, micrognathia), cleft palate and/or thymic aplasia defects, cardiovascular anomalies, and neural tube defects. Postnatal longitudinal follow-up of children exposed *in utero* to isotretinoin revealed significant neuropsychological impairment (Persaud, 1990) Vitamin A is a valuable and necessary nutrient during pregnancy, but long-term exposure to large doses (25,000 units/day) is unwise.

Salicylates. There is some evidence that *acetylsalicylic acid* (ASA) *or aspirin,* the most commonly ingested drug during pregnancy, is potentially harmful to the embryo or fetus when administered to pregnant women in *large doses* (Corby, 1978; Kalant et al, 1990). Epidemiological studies indicate that *aspirin is not a teratogenic agent,* but large doses of the drug should be avoided, especially during early pregnancy.

Thyroid Drugs. *Potassium iodide* in cough mixtures and large doses of *radioactive iodine* may cause congenital goiter (Shepard, 1992). Iodides readily cross the placental membrane and interfere with thyroxin production, and they may cause thyroid enlargement and *cretinism* (arrested physical and mental development and dystrophy of bones and soft parts). Pregnant women have been advised to avoid using douches or creams containing povidone-iodine because it is absorbed by the vagina and may be teratogenic (Vorherr et al., 1980). *Propylthiouracil* interferes with thyroxin formation in the fetus and may cause goiter. The administration of *antithyroid substances* for the treatment of maternal thyroid disorders may cause congenital goiter in an infant (Fig. 8–18) if the mother is given the substance in excess of requirements to control the disease (Reid et al., 1972). Warkany (1954, 1986) warned that maternal iodine deficiency may cause congenital cretinism.

Tranquilizers. *Thalidomide is a potent teratogen.* This hypnotic agent was once widely used in Europe as a tranquilizer and sedative. The *thalidomide epidemic* started in 1959 (Newman, 1986a,b). It has been estimated that nearly 12,000 infants were born with defects caused by thalidomide (Randall, 1990). The characteristic feature of the *thalidomide syndrome* is meromelia (e.g., phocomelia or seallike limbs, Fig. 8–19), but the anomalies ranged from *amelia* (absence of limbs) through intermediate stages of development (rudimentary limbs) to *micromelia* (abnormally small and/or short limbs). Thalidomide also caused *anomalies of other organs*; e.g., absence of the external and internal ears, hemangioma on the fore-

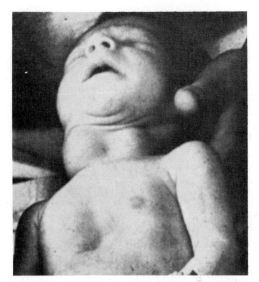

Figure 8–18. Newborn infant with congenital enlargement of the thyroid gland (goiter). The condition resulted from the administration of antithyroid drugs to the mother in excess of the amount needed to control the disease. (From Reid DF, Ryan KJ, Benirschke K: *Principles and Management of Human Reproduction.* Philadelphia, WB Saunders, 1972. Courtesy of Dr. Keith Russell.)

head, heart defects, and anomalies of the urinary and alimentary systems (Persaud, 1990). It is well-established clinically that the period when thalidomide caused congenital anomalies was from 24 to 36 days after fertilization (38 to 50 days after LNMP). This sensitive period coincides with the critical periods for the development of the affected parts and organs (Fig. 8–13).

Lithium is the drug of choice for the long-term maintenance of patients with manic-depressive psychosis; however, it has caused congenital anomalies, mainly of the heart and great vessels, in infants born to mothers given the drug early in pregnancy. Although lithium carbonate is a known human teratogen (Warkany, 1988), the United States Food and Drug Administration (FDA) has stated that the agent may be used during pregnancy if "in the opinion of the physician the potential benefits outweigh the possible hazards."

Benzodiazepine derivatives are psychoactive drugs frequently used by pregnant women. These include *diazepam* and *ozazepam* that readily cross the placental membrane (see Fig. 7–8). The use of these drugs during the first trimester of pregnancy is associated with transient withdrawal symptoms and *craniofacial deformities* in the newborn. Patients are warned not to take these drugs during pregnancy

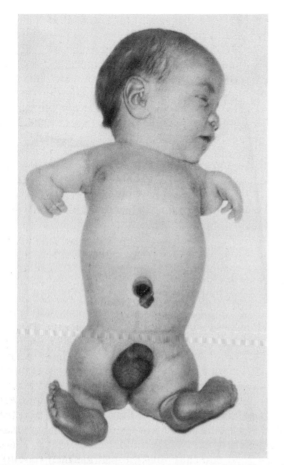

Figure 8-19. Newborn male infant showing typically malformed limbs (meromelia [limb reduction]) caused by thalidomide ingested by his mother during the critical period of limb development; see Fig. 8-13. (From Moore KL: *Manit Med Rev 43*:306, 1963.)

because of their possible teratogenic effects (Laegreid et al., 1989).

Illicit (Street) Drugs. Several currently popular drugs are used for their hallucinogenic properties. *Lysergic acid diethylamide* (LSD) is not known to be a teratogen. Long (1972) reviewed the literature on 161 infants born to women who ingested LSD before conception and/or during pregnancy. Five infants had limb defects similar to those previously reported by Zellweger and associates (1967). Jacobson and Berlin (1972) also reported limb defects and noted a 9.6 per cent incidence of nervous system defects. There is no strong evidence to indicate that LSD is teratogenic; but, in view of the reported cases, it should be avoided during pregnancy (Persaud, 1990).

Marijuana. There is no evidence that this drug is a human teratogen (Nahas, 1986). There is some indication that marijuana use during the first two months of pregnancy affects fetal length, but not birth weight.

In addition, sleep and EEG patterns in newborns exposed prenatally to marijuana were altered. For these reasons, pregnant women should not use marijuana during pregnancy (Day et al., 1991).

Phencyclidine (PCP, Angel Dust). Golden and colleagues (1980) reported a case of an infant with several birth defects and behavioral disturbances whose mother used PCP throughout her pregnancy. This suggests, but does not prove, a causal association.

Cocaine is now one of the most commonly abused illicit drugs in North America, and of concern is its increasing use by women of child-bearing age (Behrman, 1992). There have been many reports dealing with the prenatal effects of cocaine. These include spontaneous abortion, prematurity, intrauterine growth retardation, microcephaly, cerebral infarction, urogenital anomalies, and neurobehavioral disturbances. The use of cocaine during pregnancy should be avoided because of its teratogenic effects (Rosenak et al., 1990; Behrman, 1992).

Methadone, used for the treatment of heroin addiction, is considered to be a "behavioral teratogen," as is heroin (Persaud, 1990). Infants born to narcotic-dependent women maintained on methadone therapy were found to have central nervous system dysfunction and smaller birth weights and head circumferences than nonexposed infants. There is also concern about the long-term, postnatal developmental effects of methadone. The problem, however, is difficult to resolve because other drugs are often used in combination with methadone, and heavy use of alcohol and cigarettes is prevalent among narcotic-dependent women (Kaltenbach and Finnegan, 1989).

Environmental Chemicals as Teratogens

In recent years there has been increasing concern about the possible teratogenicity of environmental chemicals, including industrial pollutants and food additives. Most of these chemicals have not been positively implicated as teratogens in humans (Persaud, 1990).

Organic Mercury. Infants of mothers whose main diet during pregnancy consists of fish containing abnormally high levels of organic mercury acquire fetal *Minamata disease* and exhibit neurological and behavioral disturbances resembling cerebral palsy (Matsumoto et al., 1965; Bakir et al., 1973). In some cases, severe *brain damage*, mental retardation, and blindness have been present in the infants of mothers who received *methylmercury* in their food (Amin-Zaki et al., 1974). Similar observations have been made in infants of mothers who ate pork that became contaminated when the pigs ate corn grown from seeds sprayed with a mercury-containing fungicide

(Snyder, 1971). Methylmercury is considered to be a teratogen that causes cerebral atrophy, spasticity, seizures, and *mental retardation* (Sever and Brent, 1986; Melkonian and Baker, 1988; Burbacher et al., 1990).

Lead. Abundantly present in the workplace and environment, lead is transferred across the placental membrane and accumulates in fetal tissues. Prenatal exposure to lead has been associated with increased abortions, fetal anomalies, intrauterine growth retardation, and functional deficits. Recent studies have indicated that children born to mothers who were exposed to subclinical levels of lead revealed neurobehavioral and psychomotor disturbances (Persaud, 1990; Davis et al., 1990).

Polychlorinated Biphenyls (PCBs). These are teratogenic chemicals that produce *intrauterine growth retardation* (IUGR) and skin discoloration. The main dietary source of PCBs in North America is probably sport fish caught in contaminated waters (Rogan, 1986). In Japan and Taiwan, the teratogenic chemical was found in contaminated cooking oil.

Infectious Agents as Teratogens

Throughout prenatal life the embryo and fetus are endangered by a variety of microorganisms. In most cases the assault is resisted; in some cases, an abortion or stillbirth occurs, and in others the infants are born with growth retardation, congenital anomalies or neonatal diseases (Table 8–5). Many of these congenital defects can be detected *in utero* by sonography (Drose et al., 1991). The microorganisms cross the placental membrane and enter the fetal blood stream (see Fig. 7–8). The fetal blood-brain barrier also appears to offer little resistance to microorganisms because there is a propensity for the central nervous system to be affected.

Rubella (German or Three-Day Measles). The rubella virus that causes this communicable disease is the prime example of an *infective teratogen* (Korones, 1986). In cases of primary maternal infection during the first trimester of pregnancy, the overall risk of embryonic/fetal infection is about 20 per cent (Gibbs and Sweet, 1989). The virus crosses the placental membrane and infects the embryo/fetus. The usual features of **congenital rubella syndrome (CRS)** are *cataract, cardiac defects,* and *deafness,* but the following abnormalities are occasionally observed: mental deficiency, chorioretinitis, glaucoma (Fig. 8–20), microphthalmia, and tooth defects (Cooper, 1975).

The earlier in pregnancy the maternal rubella infection occurs, the greater the danger that the embryo will be malformed (Isada et al., 1990; Behrman, 1992). Most infants have congenital anomalies if the disease occurs during the first four to five weeks after fertilization. This is understandable because this period includes the most susceptible organogenetic periods of the eye, internal ear, heart, and brain (Fig. 8–13). The risk of anomalies from rubella infection during the second and third trimesters is low (about 10 per cent), but functional defects of the central nervous system (mental retardation) and the internal ear (hearing loss) may result if infection occurs during the late fetal period. There is no evidence of fetal anomalies after the fifth gestational month (Korones, 1986; Isada et al., 1990); however, infections may produce chronic disease and dysfunction of the eye, ear, and central nervous system (Behrman, 1992).

Cytomegalovirus (CMV). Infection with CMV is the most common viral infection of the human fetus. Because the disease seems to be fatal when it affects

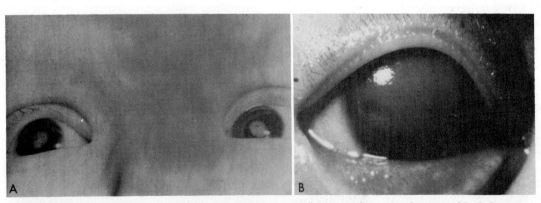

Figure 8–20. Congenital anomalies of the eye caused by the rubella virus. *A,* Cataracts. (Courtesy of Dr. R. Baragry, Department of Ophthalmology, Cornell, New York Hospital) *B,* Glaucoma. (Courtesy of Dr. D.I. Weiss, Department of Ophthalmology, New York University School of Medicine) (Photos from Cooper LA et al.: *Am J Dis Child* 110:416–427, 1965. Copyright 1965, American Medical Association.)

the embryo, it is believed that most pregnancies end in spontaneous abortion when the infection occurs during the first trimester. Newborn infants infected during the early fetal period usually show no clinical signs and are identified through screening programs (Williamson et al, 1990). Later in pregnancy, infection may result in IUGR, microphthalmia, chorioretinitis, blindness, microcephaly, cerebral calcification, mental retardation, deafness, cerebral palsy, and hepatosplenomegaly (Reynolds et al., 1986; Persaud, 1990; Behrman, 1992). Of particular concern are cases of *asymptomatic CMV infection,* which are often associated with audiologic, neuroradiological, and neurobehavioral disturbances in infancy (Williamson et al, 1990).

Herpes Simplex Virus (HSV). It has been reported that maternal infection with HSV in early pregnancy increases the abortion rate by threefold, and infection after the twentieth week is associated with a higher rate of prematurity. Infection of the fetus with HSV usually occurs very late in pregnancy, probably most often during delivery. The congenital abnormalities that have been observed in the offspring included typical cutaneous lesions and, in some cases, microcephaly, microphthalmia, spasticity, retinal dysplasia, and mental retardation (Gibbs and Sweet, 1989; Persaud, 1990; Behrman, 1992).

Varicella (Chickenpox). Varicella and herpes zoster (shingles) are caused by the same virus, *varicella-zoster virus* (Fuccillo, 1986). There is convincing evidence that maternal varicella infection during the first four months of pregnancy causes congenital anomalies (skin scarring, muscle atrophy, hypoplasia of the limb, rudimentary digits, and mental retardation; Gibbs and Sweet, 1989). There is about a 20 per cent chance of these or other abnormalities when the infection occurs during the critical period of development (Fig. 8–13).

Human Immunodeficiency Virus (HIV). This retrovirus causes acquired immunodeficiency syndrome (AIDS), a major public health problem worldwide. As yet, there is no treatment for this disease which is increasing in prevalence among women of childbearing age (Gwinn et al., 1991). There is conflicting information on the fetal effects of *in utero* infection with HIV (Embree et al., 1989). Some of the congenital anomalies reported are growth failure, microcephaly, and specific craniofacial features (Evans, 1992). Preventing the transmission of the virus to women and their infants is of obvious importance because of any potential embryopathic effects (Persaud, 1990; Blanche et al. 1990; Evans, 1992).

Toxoplasma gondii. This widespread protozoan is an *intracellular parasite.* It was named after the gondi, a North African rodent in which the organism was first detected. This parasite may be found in the blood stream, in the tissues, or reticuloendothelial cells, leukocytes, and epithelial cells. Maternal infection is usually acquired by eating raw or *poorly cooked meat* (usually pork or lamb) containing *toxoplasma cysts,* through close contact with infected domestic animals (usually *cats*), or from the soil (McLeod and Remington, 1992). It is thought that the soil or garden vegetables may become contaminated with infected cat feces carrying oocysts (Walpole et al., 1991). Oocytes can also be transported to food by flies and cockroaches.

The *Toxoplasma gondii organism* crosses the placental membrane (see Fig. 7–8) and infects the fetus, causing destructive changes in the brain and eyes that result in *mental deficiency,* microcephaly, microphthalmia, and hydrocephaly (Larson, 1986; Persaud, 1990; McLeod and Remington, 1992). The mothers of congenitally defective infants are often unaware of having had **toxoplasmosis,** the disease caused by the parasitic organism. Because animals (cats, dogs, rabbits, and other domestic and wild animals) may be infected with this parasite, pregnant women should avoid them and the eating of raw or poorly cooked meat from them (e.g., rabbits). In addition, eggs should be well cooked and unpasteurized milk should be avoided (McLeod and Remington, 1992).

Syphilis. The incidence of congenital syphilis is steadily increasing with more cases now than in any of the past two decades. One in 10,000 live-born infants in the United States is infected (Ricci et al., 1989). *Treponema pallidum,* the small, spiral microorganism that causes syphilis, rapidly crosses the placental membrane after the twentieth week of gestation. The fetus can become infected at any stage of the disease or at any stage of pregnancy. Untreated *primary maternal infections* (acquired during pregnancy) nearly always cause serious fetal infection and congenital anomalies; however, adequate treatment of the mother before the sixteenth week of pregnancy kills the organism, thereby preventing it from crossing the placental membrane and infecting the fetus (Holmes, 1977). *Secondary maternal infections* (acquired before pregnancy) seldom result in fetal disease and anomalies. If the mother is untreated, stillbirths occur in about one fourth of the cases.

Early manifestations of untreated maternal syphilis are congenital deafness, abnormal teeth and bones, hydrocephalus, and mental retardation (Ingall and Musher, 1983; Sever and Brent, 1986; Persaud, 1990). Late manifestations of untreated congenital syphilis are destructive lesions of the palate and nasal septum, dental abnormalities (centrally notched, widely spaced, peg-shaped upper central incisors called *Hutchinson's teeth*), and abnormal facies (frontal bossing, saddlenose, and poorly developed maxilla).

Radiation as a Teratogen

Exposure to *ionizing radiation* may injure embryonic cells, resulting in cell death, chromosome injury, and retardation of mental development and physical growth. The severity of the embryonic damage is related to the absorbed dose, the dose rate, and the stage of embryonic or fetal development during which the exposure occurs (For more information, see Kriegel et al, 1982, 1986 and Brent, 1986b). In the past, large amounts of ionizing radiation (hundreds to several thousand rads) were given inadvertently to embryos and fetuses of pregnant women who had cancer of the cervix. In all cases their embryos were severely malformed or killed.

Growth retardation, microcephaly, spina bifida cystica (see Fig. 18–14), pigment changes in the retina, cataracts, cleft palate, skeletal and visceral abnormalities, and mental retardation have been observed in infants who survived after receiving high levels of ionizing radiation. Development of the central nervous system was nearly always affected (Kriegel et al, 1986).

Observations of Japanese atomic bomb survivors suggest that eight to 16 weeks after fertilization (ten to 18 weeks after LNMP) is the period of greatest sensitivity for radiation damage to the brain leading to *severe mental retardation*. By the end of the 16th week, most neuronal proliferation is completed, after which the risk of mental retardation decreases. It is generally accepted that large doses of radiation (over 25,000 millirads) are harmful to the developing central nervous system (Kriegel et al., 1982; 1986).

Accidental exposure of pregnant women to radiation is a common cause for anxiety (Holmes, 1992). There is no proof that human congenital anomalies have been caused by diagnostic levels of radiation. Scattered radiation from an x-ray examination of a part of the body that is not near the uterus (e.g., the chest, sinuses, teeth) produces a dose of only a few millirads, which is not teratogenic to the embryo. As an example: a radiograph of the chest of a pregnant woman in the first trimester results in a whole-body dose to her embryo or fetus of approximately 1 millirad. If the embryonic radiation exposure is 5 rads or less, the radiation risks to the embryo are minuscule (Brent, 1986b; Bentur et al., 1991; Holmes, 1992).

It is prudent, however, to be cautious during diagnostic examinations of the pelvic region in pregnant women (x-ray examinations and medical diagnostic tests using radioisotopes) because they result in exposure of the embryo to 0.3 to 2 rads. The recommended limit of maternal exposure of the whole body to radiation from all sources is 500 millirads for the entire gestational period (Holmes, 1992).

Maternal Factors as Teratogens

Maternal diseases can sometimes lead to a higher risk of abnormalities in the offspring. Poorly controlled *diabetes mellitus* in the mother with persisting hyperglycemia and ketosis, particularly during embryogenesis, is associated with a two- to three-fold higher incidence of birth defects (Miller et al, 1981). No specific diabetic embryopathic syndrome exists, but common abnormalities include holoprosencephaly, meroencephaly, sacral agenesis, vertebral anomalies, congenital heart defects and limb abnormalities (Holmes, 1992).

If untreated, women who are homozygous for phenylalanine hydroxylase deficiency (*phenylketonuria* [PKU]) and those with hyperphenylalaninemia are at a high risk of having an offspring with microcephaly, septal cardiac defects, and mental retardation. The congenital anomalies can be prevented if the PKU mother is placed on a phenylalanine-restricted diet prior to and during the pregnancy (Lenke and Levy, 1980).

Mechanical Factors as Teratogens

The significance of mechanical influences in the uterus on congenital postural deformities is still an open question (McKeown, 1976). The amniotic fluid absorbs mechanical pressures, thereby protecting the embryo from most external trauma. It is generally accepted that congenital abnormalities caused by external injury to the mother are extremely rare, but possible (Hinden, 1965, and Warkany, 1971). *Congenital dislocation of the hip and clubfoot* may be caused by mechanical forces (p. 381), particularly in a malformed uterus. Such deformations may be caused by any factor that restricts the mobility of the fetus, thereby causing prolonged compression in an abnormal posture (Connor and Ferguson-Smith, 1987).

A significantly reduced quantity of amniotic fluid (*oligohydramnios*) may result in mechanically induced deformation of the limbs; e.g., hyperextension of the knee (Dunn, 1976). Intrauterine amputations or other anomalies caused by local constriction during fetal growth may result from *amniotic bands* rings (see Fig. 7–19) formed as a result of rupture of the amnion during early pregnancy (Behrman, 1992). For information on the pathogenesis of *amniotic band syndrome* (p. 130), see Lockwood et al. (1989).

ANOMALIES CAUSED BY MULTIFACTORIAL INHERITANCE

Many common congenital anomalies (e.g., cleft lip with/without cleft palate) have familial distributions consistent with multifactorial inheritance (Table 8–1). For a list of the characteristics of multifactorial inheritance (MFI), see Thompson et al. (1991). MFI may be represented by a model in which "liability" to a disorder is a continuous variable determined by a combination of genetic and environmental factors, with a developmental threshold dividing individuals with the anomaly from those without it (Fig. 8–21).

Multifactorial traits are often single major anomalies, such as cleft lip, isolated cleft palate, neural tube defects (e.g., meroanencephaly and spina bifida cystica), pyloric stenosis, and congenital dislocation of the hip. Some of these anomalies may also occur as part of the phenotype in syndromes determined by single-gene inheritance, chromosome abnormality, or an environmental teratogen.

The recurrence risks used for genetic counseling of families having congenital anomalies determined by MFI are *empirical risks* based on the frequency of the anomaly in the general population and in different categories of relatives. In individual families, such estimates may be inaccurate because they are usually averages for the population rather than precise probabilities for the individual family. For further discussion of MFI and genetic counseling of families of patients with multifactorial traits, see Thompson et al (1991).

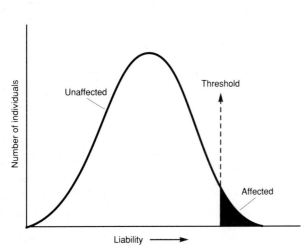

Figure 8–21. The multifactorial threshold model. Liability to a trait is distributed normally, with a threshold dividing the population into unaffected and affected classes. (From Thompson MW et al.: *Genetics in Medicine.* 5th ed. Philadelphia, WB Saunders, 1991.)

SUMMARY

A congenital anomaly is a structural abnormality of any type that is present at birth. It may be macroscopic or microscopic, on the surface or within the body. There are *four clinically significant types of anomaly*: malformation, disruption, deformation, and dysplasia (p. 142). Congenital anomalies may be caused by genetic factors or by environmental factors that cause disruptions during prenatal development, but most common congenital anomalies show the family patterns expected of *multifactorial inheritance* with a threshold and are determined by a combination of genetic and environmental factors (Table 8–1).

About three per cent of all live born infants have an obvious major anomaly. Additional anomalies are detected after birth; thus, the incidence is about six per cent in 2-year-olds and eight per cent in 5-year-olds. Other anomalies (about two per cent) are detected later in life (e.g., during surgery or autopsy). Congenital anomalies may be single or multiple and of minor or major clinical significance. *Single minor anomalies are present in about 14 per cent of newborns.* These anomalies (e.g., cutaneous ear tags, Fig. 19–18) are of no serious medical consequence, but they alert the clinician to the possible presence of an associated major anomaly. Ninety per cent of infants with multiple minor anomalies have one or more associated major anomalies. Of the three per cent of infants born with a major congenital anomaly, 0.7 per cent have multiple major anomalies (Tables 8–2 and 8–4).

Major anomalies are more common in early embryos (up to 15 per cent) than they are in newborn infants (up to three per cent), but most severely malformed embryos are usually spontaneously aborted during the first six to eight weeks. Some congenital anomalies are caused by *genetic factors* (chromosome abnormalities and mutant genes). A few congenital abnormalities are caused by *environmental factors* (infectious agents, environmental chemicals, and drugs), but most common anomalies result from a complex *interaction between genetic and environmental factors.* The cause of most congenital anomalies is unknown (Table 8–1).

During the first two weeks of development, teratogenic agents usually kill the embryo rather than cause congenital anomalies. During the *organogenetic period*, teratogenic agents disrupt development and may cause *major congenital anomalies.* During the fetal period teratogens may produce morphological and functional abnormalities, particularly of the brain and eyes. *Mental retardation* may result from high levels of radiation and infectious agents.

CLINICALLY ORIENTED QUESTIONS FOR PROBLEM-BASED LEARNING SESSIONS

1. Women take an average of four drugs, excluding nutritional supplements, during the first trimester of pregnancy. What percentage of congenital anomalies are caused by drugs, environmental chemicals, and infectious agents? Why may it be difficult for doctors to attribute specific congenital anomalies to specific drugs? What should pregnant women know about the use of drugs during pregnancy?

2. Do women over the age of 35 have an increased risk of bearing abnormal children? If a 40-year-old woman becomes pregnant, what prenatal diagnostic test would likely be performed? What abnormality might be detected? Can a 44-year-old woman have a normal baby?

3. Are any drugs considered safe during early pregnancy? If so, name some commonly prescribed ones. What commonly used drugs should be avoided?

4. A 12-year-old girl contracted German measles, and her mother was worried that the child might develop cataracts. What would the doctor likely tell the mother?

5. A pregnant woman with two cats that often "spent the night out" was told by a friend that she should avoid them during her pregnancy. She was also told to avoid flies and cockroaches. When she consulted her physician, what would she likely be told?

The answers to these questions are given on page 461.

References

Allderice PW, Browne N, Murphy DP: Chromosome 3 duplication q21-qter deletion p25-pter syndrome in children of carriers of a pericentric inversion inv (3) (p25 q21). *Am J Hum Genet* 27:699, 1975.

Amin-Zaki L, Elhassani S, Majeed MA, et al: Intrauterine methylmercury poisoning in Iraq. *Pediatrics* 54:587, 1974.

Anders GJ: Congenital malformations: genetic background and genetic counselling. *In* Huffstadt AJ (ed): *Congenital Malformations.* Amsterdam, Excerpta Medica, 1980.

Bakir F, Damluji SF, Amin-Zaki L, et al: Methylmercury poisoning in Iraq. *Science 181*:320, 1973.

Beckman DA, Brent RL: Mechanisms of teratogenesis. *Annual Rev Pharmacol Toxicol 24*:483, 1984.

Behrman RE (ed): *Nelson Textbook of Pediatrics.* 14th ed. Philadelphia, WB Saunders, 1992.

Bennett R, Persaud TVN, Moore KL: Experimental studies on the effects of aluminum on pregnancy and fetal development. *Anat Anz 138*:365, 1975.

Bentur Y, Horlatsch N, Koren G: Exposure to ionizing radiation during pregnancy: Perception of teratogenic risk and outcome. *Teratology 43*:109, 1991.

Bergsma D (ed): *Birth Defects Atlas and Compendium.* The National Foundation–March of Dimes. Birth Defects: Original Article Series. Baltimore, Williams & Wilkins, 1973.

Berlin CM, Jacobson CB: Congenital anomalies associated with parental LSD ingestion. *Society for Pediatric Research Abstracts, Second Plenary Session,* 1970.

Blanche S, Tardieu M, Duliege A-M, et al: Longitudinal study of 94 symptomatic infants with perinatally acquired human immunodeficiency virus infection. *Am J Dis Chld 144*:1210, 1990.

Breg WR: Autosomal abnormalities. *In* Gardner LI (ed): *Endocrine and Genetic Diseases of Childhood and Adolescence.* 2nd ed. Philadelphia, WB Saunders, 1975.

Brent RL: Radiation teratogenesis. *In* Sever JL, Brent RL (eds):

Teratogen Update: Environmentally Induced Birth Defect Risks. New York, Alan R. Liss, 1986b.

Brent RL: The complexities of solving the problem of human malformation. *In* Sever JL, Brent RL (eds): *Teratogen Update Environmental Induced Birth Defect Risks.* New York, Alan R. Liss, 1986a.

Brent RL, Beckman DA: Angiotensin-converting enzyme inhibitors, an embryopathic class of drugs with unique properties: Information for clinical teratology counselors. *Teratology 43*:543, 1991.

Brent RL, Harris MI: *Prevention of Embryonic, Fetal, and Perinatal Disease.* Fogarty International Center Series on Preventive Medicine, vol 3, 1976.

Brent RL, Holmes LB: Clinical and basic science from the thalidomide tragedy: what have we learned about the causes of limb defects? *Teratology 38*:241, 1988.

Briggs GG, Freeman RK, Yaffe SJ: *Drugs in Pregnancy and Lactation.* 3rd ed. Baltimore, Williams & Wilkins, 1990.

Brown RT, Coles CD, Smith IE, Platzman KA, Silverstein J, Erickson S, Falek A: Effects of prenatal alcohol exposure at school age. II. Attention and behavior. *Neurotoxicol Teratol 13*:369, 1991.

Browne D: Congenital deformity. *Br Med J 2*:1450, 1960.

Buitendijk S, Bracken MB: Medication in early pregnancy—Prevalence of use and relationship to maternal characteristics. *Am J Obstet Gynecol 165*:33, 1991.

Burbacher TM, Rodier PM, Weiss B: Methylmercury developmental neurotoxicity: A comparison of effects in humans and animals. *Neurotoxicol Teratol 12*:191, 1990.

Carakushansky G, Neu RL, Gardner LI: Lysergide and cannabis as possible teratogens in man. *Lancet 1*:150, 1969.

Carr DH: Chromosome studies in selected spontaneous abortions: Polyploidy in man. *J Med Genet 8*:164, 1971.

Carr DH: Heredity and the embryo. *Science J (London) 6*:75, 1970.

Carr DH, Law EM, Ekins JG: Chromosome studies in selected spontaneous abortions. IV. Unusual cytogenetic disorders. *Teratology 5*:49, 1972.

Caspersson T, Zech L, Johansson C, Modest EJ: Identification of human chromosomes by DNA-binding fluorescent agents. *Chromosoma 30*:215, 1970.

Chodirker BN, Chudley AE, Reed MH, Persaud TVN: Possible prenatal hydantoin effect in a child born to a nonepileptic mother. *Am J Med Genet 27*:373, 1987.

Chudley AE, Hagerman RJ: The fragile X syndrome. *J Pediatr 110*:821, 1987.

Cohen Jr, MM: *The Child with Multiple Birth Defects.* New York, Raven Press, 1982.

Cohlan SQ: Tetracycline staining of teeth. *In* Sever JL, Brent RL (eds): *Teratogen Update: Environmentally Induced Birth Defect Risks.* New York, Alan R. Liss, 1986.

Connor JM, Ferguson-Smith MA: *Essential Medical Genetics.* 2nd ed. Oxford, Blackwell Scientific Publications, 1987.

Cooper LZ: Congenital rubella in the United States. *In* Krugman S, Gershon AA (eds): *Infections of the Fetus and Newborn Infant.* Progress in Clinical and Biological Research, vol 3. New York, Alan R. Liss, 1975.

Corby DG: Aspirin in pregnancy: Maternal and fetal effects. *Pediatrics 62*:930, 1978.

Cummings MR: *Human Heredity. Principles and Issues.* 2nd ed. New York, West Publishing, 1991.

Dansky LV, Finnell RH: Parental epilepsy, anticonvulsant drugs, and reproductive outcome–epidemiologic and experimental findings spanning 3 decades. 2. Human studies. *Reprod Toxicol 5*:301, 1991.

Davis JM, Otto DA, Weil DE, Grant LD: The comparative developmental neurotoxicity of lead in humans and animals. *Neurotoxicol Teratol 12*:215, 1990.

Day N, Sambamoorthi V, Taylor P, Richardson G, Robles N, Jhon Y, Scher M, Stoffer D, Cornelius M, Jasperse D: Prenatal marijuana use and neonatal outcome. *Neurotoxicol Teratol 13*:329, 1991.

De Luca LM: Retinoids and their receptors in differentiation, embryogenesis, and neoplasia. *FASEB J 5*:2924, 1991.

di Maria H, Courpotin C, Rouzioux C, Cohen D, Rio D, Bousin F: Transplacental transmission of human immunodeficiency virus. *Lancet 2*:215, 1986.

Dishotsky NI, Loughman WD, Mogar RE, Lipscomb WR: LSD and genetic damage. *Science 172*:431–440, 1971.

Drose JA, Dennis MA, Thickman D: Infection in utero: US findings in 19 cases. *Radiology 178*:369, 1991.

Dudgeon JA: Infective causes of human malformations. *Br Med Bull 32*:77, 1976.

Dunn PM: Congenital postural deformities. *Br Med Bull 32*:71, 1976.

Embree JE, Braddick M, Datta P, et al: Lack of correlation of maternal human immunodeficiency virus infection with neonatal malformations. *Pediatr Infect Dis J 8*:700, 1989.

Epstein SS: Environmental pathology. *Am J Pathol 66*:352, 1972.

Evans HE: Human immunodeficiency virus (HIV) infection. *In* Behrman RD: *Nelson Textbook of Pediatrics.* 14th ed. Philadelphia, WB Saunders, 1992.

Fantel AG, Shepard TH: Prenatal cocaine exposure. *Reprod Toxicol 4*:83, 1990.

Ferguson-Smith MA: Sex chromatin, Klinefelter's syndrome and mental deficiency. *In* Moore KL (ed): *The Sex Chromatin.* Philadelphia, WB Saunders, 1966.

Forrest DD, Fordyce RR: *Fam Plan Perspect 20*:112, 1988. (Cited in Djerassi C: The bitter pill. *Science 245*:356, 1989).

Fraser FC: Of mice and children: reminiscences of a teratogeneticist. *In* Kalter H (ed): *Issues and Reviews in Teratology.* Vol 5. New York, Plenum Press, 1990.

Fuccillo D: Congenital varicella. *In* Sever JL, Brent RL (eds): *Teratogen Update: Environmentally Induced Birth Defect Risks.* New York, Alan R. Liss, 1986.

Ganguin G, Rempt E: Streptomycinbehandlung in der Schwangerschaft und ihre Answirkung auf des Gehör des Kindes. *Z Laryngol Rhinol Otol 49*:496, 1970.

Garber JE: Long-term follow-up of children exposed *in utero* to antineoplastic agents. *Seminar in Oncology 16*:437, 1989.

Gardner EJ, Simons MJ, Snustad DP: *Principles of Genetics.* 8th ed. New York, John Wiley & Sons, 1991.

Gardner LI: *Endocrine and Genetic Diseases of Childhood and Adolescence.* 2nd ed. Philadelphia, WB Saunders, 1975.

Garza A, Cordero JF, Mulinare J: Epidemiology of the early amnion rupture spectrum of defects. *Am J Dis Chld 142*:541, 1988.

Giacola GP, Wood BP: Radiological case of the month—Congenital syphilis. *Amer J Dis Child 145*:1045, 1991.

Gibbs RS, Sweet RL: Maternal and fetal infections—Clinical disorders. *In* Creasy RK, Resnik R (eds): *Maternal-Fetal Medicine: Principles and Practice.* 2nd ed. Philadelphia, WB Saunders, 1989.

Ginsberg JS, Hirsh J: Optimum use of anticoagulants in pregnancy. *Drugs 36*:505, 1988.

Ginsburg KA, Blacker CM, Abel EL, Sokol RJ: Fetal alcohol exposure and adverse pregnancy outcome. *Contr Gynecol Obstet 18*:115, 1991.

Golbus MS: Teratology for the obstetrician: Current status. *Obstet Gynecol 55*:269, 1980.

Golden NL, Sokol RJ, Rubin I: Angel dust: Possible effects on the fetus. *Pediatrics 65*:18, 1980.

Goldman AS, Zackai EH, Yaffe SJ: Fetal trimethadione syndrome. *In* Sever JL, Brent RL (eds): *Teratogen Update: Environmentally Induced Birth Defect Risks.* New York, Alan R. Liss, 1986.

Goodwin BA, Huether CA: Revised estimates and projections of Down syndrome births in the United States, and the effects of prenatal diagnosis utilization, 1970–2002. *Prenat Diagn 7*:261, 1987.

Graham JM: *Smith's Recognizable Patterns of Human Deformation.* 2nd ed. Philadelphia, WB Saunders, 1988.

Greenough A, Osborne J, Sutherland S (eds): *Congenital, Perinatal and Neonatal Infections.* Edinburgh, Churchill Livingstone, 1992.

Gregg NM: Congenital cataract following German measles in the mother. *Trans Ophthalmol Soc Aust 3*:35, 1941.

Gwinn M, Pappaioanou M, George JR, et al: Prevalence of HIV infection in childbearing women in the United States. *JAMA 265*:1704, 1991.

Hall JG, Pauli RM, Wilson KM: Maternal and fetal sequelae of anticoagulation during pregnancy. *Am J Med 68*:122, 1980.

Hansen N, Coury DL: Congenital anomalies of the neonate. *In* Quilligan EJ, Zuspan FP (eds): *Current Therapy in Obstetrics and Gynecology.* Vol 3. Philadelphia, WB Saunders, 1990.

Hanson JW: Fetal hydantoin effects. *In* Sever JL, Brent RL (eds): *Teratogen Update: Environmentally Induced Birth Defect Risks.* New York, Alan R. Liss, 1986.

Hanssens M, Keirse MJNC, Vankelecom F, Van Assche FA: Fetal and neonatal effects of treatment with angiotensin-converting enzyme inhibitors in pregnancy. *Obstet Gynecol 78*:128, 1991.

Harris LE, Stayura LA, Ramirez-Talavera PF, Annegers JF: Congenital and acquired abnormalities observed in live-born and stillborn neonates. *Mayo Clin Proc 50*:85, 1975.

Hart WR, Zaharrow I, Kaplan BJ, et al: Cytologic findings in stilbestrol-exposed females with emphasis on detection of vaginal adenosis. *Acta Cytol (Baltimore) 20*:7, 1976.

Hegge FN: *A Practical Guide to Ultrasound of Fetal Anomalies.* New York, Raven Press, 1992.

Heinonen OP, Slone D, Shapiro S: *Birth Defects and Drugs in Pregnancy.* Littleton, Massachusetts, Publishing Sciences Group, 1977.

Heitz D, Rousseau F, Devys D, et al: Isolation of sequences that span the fragile X and identification of a fragile X-related CpG island. *Science 251*:1236, 1991.

Herbst AL, Robboy SJ, Scully RE, Poskanzer DC: Clear-cell adenocarcinoma of the vagina and cervix in girls. Analysis of 170 registry cases. *Am J Obstet Gynecol 119*:713, 1974.

Herbst ALH, Ulfelder H, Poskanzer DC: Adenocarcinoma of the vagina. *N Engl J Med 284*:878, 1971.

Hill RM, Craig JP, Chaney MD, et al: Utilization of over-the-counter drugs during pregnancy. *Clin Obstet Gynecol 20*:381, 1977.

Hinden E: External injury causing fetal deformity. *Arch Dis Child 40*: 80, 1965.

Hirschhorn K: Chromosomes and their abnormalities. *In* Behrman RE: *Nelson Textbook of Pediatrics.* 14th ed. Philadelphia, WB Saunders, 1992.

Holmes KK: Syphilis. *In* Thor GW, Adams RD, Braunwald E, et al. (eds): *Harrison's Principles of Internal Medicine.* 8th ed. New York, McGraw-Hill, 1977.

Holmes LB: Bendectin. *In* Sever JL, Brent RL (eds): *Teratogen Update: Environmentally Induced Birth Defect Risks.* New York, Alan R. Liss, 1986.

Holmes LB: Teratogens. *In* Behrman RE (ed): *Nelson Textbook of Pediatrics.* 14th ed. Philadelphia, WB Saunders, 1992.

Holzgreve W, Carey JC, Hall BD: Warfarin-induced fetal abnormalities. *Lancet 2*:914, 1976.

Hook EB: Rates of chromosomal abnormalities at different maternal ages. *Obstet Gynecol 58*:282, 1981.

Hook EB: Rates of Down's syndrome in live births and at midtrimester amniocentesis. *Lancet 1*:1053, 1978.

Hook EB, Cross PK, Jackson L, et al.: Maternal age-specific rates of 47, +21 and other cytogenetic abnormalities diagnosed in the first trimester of pregnancy in chorionic villus biopsy specimens: Comparison with rates expected from observations at amniocentesis. *Am J Hum Genet 42*:797, 1988.

Hook EB, Cross PK, Schreinemachers DM: Chromosomal abnormality rates at amniocentesis and in live-born infants. *JAMA 249*:2034, 1983.

Hook EB, Hamerton JL: The frequency of chromosome abnormalities detected in consecutive newborn studies — Differences between studies — Results by sex and by severity of phenotypic involvement. *In* Hook EB, Porter IH (eds): *Population Cytogenetics: Studies in Humans.* New York, Academic Press, 1977.

Hook EB, Warburton D: The distribution of chromosomal genotypes associated with Turner syndrome: Livebirth prevalence rates and evidence for diminished fetal mortality and severity in genotypes associated with structural X abnormalities or mosaicism. *Hum Genet 64*:24, 1983.

Ingall D, Musher D: Syphilis. *In* Remington JS, Klein JO (eds): *Diseases of the Fetus and Newborn Infant.* 2nd ed. Philadelphia, WB Saunders, 1983.

Isada N, Sever J, Larsen J: Rubella. *In* Quilligan EJ, Zuspan FP (eds): *Current Therapy in Obstetrics and Gynecology.* vol 3. Philadelphia, WB Saunders, 1990.

Jacobson CB, Berlin CM: Possible reproductive detriment in LSD users. *JAMA 222*:1367, 1972.

Johnson EM: False positives/false negatives in developmental toxicology and teratology. *Teratology 34*:361, 1986.

Jones KL: Effects of chemical and environmental agents. *In* Creasy RK, Resnik R (eds): *Maternal-Fetal Medicine: Principles and Practice.* 2nd ed. Philadelphia, WB Saunders, 1989.

Jones KL: *Smith's Recognizable Patterns of Human Malformation.* 4th ed. Philadelphia, WB Saunders, 1988.

Jones KL, Smith DW, Streissguth AP, Myrianthopoulos NC: Outcome in offspring of chronic alcoholic women. *Lancet 1*:1076, 1974.

Kalant H, Roschlau HE, Hickie RA (eds): *Essentials of Medical Pharmacology.* Toronto, BC Decker, 1990.

Kaltenbach KA, Finnegan LP: Prenatal narcotic exposure: Perinatal and developmental effects. *Neurotoxicol 10*:597, 1989.

Kaufman MH: New insights into triploidy and tetraploidy, from an analysis of model systems for these conditions. *Human Reprod 6*:8, 1991.

Kelsey FO: The importance of epidemiology in identifying drugs which may cause malformations — with particular reference to drugs containing sex hormones. *Acta Morphol Acad Sci Hung 28*:189, 1980.

Kirkilionis AJ, Chudley AE, Gregory CA, Hamerton JL: Molecular and clinical overlap of Angelman and Prader-Willi syndrome phenotypes. *Am J Med Genet 40*:454, 1991.

Knoll JHM, Nicholls RD, Magenis RE, Graham Jr JM, Lalande M, Latt SA: Angelman and Prader-Willi syndrome share a common chromosome 15 deletion but differ in parental origin of the deletion. *Am J Med Genet 32*:285, 1989.

Koren G (ed): *Maternal-Fetal Toxicology: A Clinicians Guide.* New York, Marcel Dekker, 1990.

Korones SB: Congenital rubella — An encapsulated review. *In* Sever JL, Brent RL (eds): *Teratogen Update: Environmentally Induced Birth Defect Risks.* New York, Alan R. Liss, 1986.

Kriegel H, Schmahl W, Gerber GB, Stieve FE: *Radiation Risks to the Developing Nervous System.* Stuttgart, Gustav Fischer, 1986.

Kriegel H, Schmahl W, Kistner G, Stieve FE (eds): *Developmental Effects of Prenatal Irradiation.* Stuttgart, Gustav Fischer, 1982.

Laegreid L, Olegard R, Walstrom J, Conradi N: Teratogenic effects of benzodiazepine use during pregnancy. *J Pediatr 114*:126, 1989.

Lammer EJ, Chen ET, Hoar RM, Agnish ND, Benke PJ, Braun JT, Curry CJ, Fernhoff PM, Grix Jr AW, Lott IT, Richard JM, Sun SC: Retinoic acid embryopathy. *New Engl J Med 313*:837, 1985.

Larson JW, Jr: Congenital toxoplasmosis. *In* Sever JL, Brent RL (eds): *Teratogen Update: Environmentally Induced Birth Defect Risks.* New York, Alan R. Liss, 1986.

Lenke RR, Levy HL: Maternal phenylketonuria and hyperphenylalaninemia. An international survey of untreated and treated pregnancies. *N Engl J Med 303*:1202, 1980.

Lenz W: A short history of thalidomide embryopathy. *Teratology 38*:203, 1988.

Lenz W: Kindliche Missbildungen nach Medikament während der Gravidität? *Dtsch Med Wochenschr 86*:2555, 1961.

Leviton A: Caffeine consumption and the risk of reproductive hazards. *J Reprod Med 33*:175, 1988.

Lockwood C, Ghidini A, Romero R, Hobbins JC: Amniotic band syndrome: reevaluation of its pathogenesis. *Am J Obstet Gynecol 160*:1030, 1989.

Long SY: Does LSD induce chromosomal damage and malformations? A review of the literature. *Teratology 6*:75, 1972.

Longo LD: Environmental pollution and pregnancy: Risks and uncertainties for the fetus and infant. *Am J Obstet Gynecol 137*:162, 1980.

Manuelidis L: Individual interphase chromosome domains revealed by *in situ* hybridization. *Hum Genet 71*:288, 1985.

Matsumoto HG, Goyo L, Takevchi T: Fetal minamata disease. A neuropathological study of two cases of intrauterine intoxication by a methyl mercury compound. *J Neuropathol Exp Neurol 24*:563, 1965.

Mattos TC, Giugliani R, Haase HB: Congenital malformations detected in 731 autopsies of children aged 0 to 14 years. *Teratology 35*:305, 1987.

McBride WG: Thalidomide and congenital abnormalities. *Lancet 2*:1358, 1961.

McKeown T: Human malformations: Introduction. *Br Med Bull 32*:1, 1976.

McKusick VA: Mendelian Inheritance in Man. Catalogs of Autosomal Dominant, Autosomal Recessive, and X-linked Phenotypes. Baltimore, The Johns Hopkins University Press, 1975.

McLachlan JA, Pratt RM, Market CL (eds): *Developmental Toxicology: Mechanisms and Risk.* (Banbury Report vol 26). New York, Cold Spring Harbor Laboratory, 1987.

McLeod R, Remington JS: Toxoplasmosis. *In* Behrman RE: *Nelson's Textbook of Pediatrics.* 14th ed. Philadelphia, WB Saunders, 1992.

Melkonian R, Baker D: Risks of industrial mercury exposure in pregnancy. *Obstet Gynecol Surv 43*:637, 1988.

Miller E, Hare JW, Cloherty JP, Dunn PJ, Gleason RE, Soeldner, JS, Kitzmiller JL: Elevated maternal hemoglobin A,C in early pregnancy and major congenital anomalies in infants of diabetic mothers. *N Engl J Med 304*:1331, 1981.

Milunsky A, Graef JW, Gaynor MF, Jr: Methotrexate-induced congenital malformations. *J Pediatr 72*:790, 1968.

Mole RH: Consequences of pre-natal radiation exposure for postnatal development. *Int J Radiol Biol 42*:1, 1982.

Mole RH: Radiation effects on prenatal development and the radiological significance. *Br J Radiol 52*:89, 1979.

Moore KL (ed): *The Sex Chromatin.* Philadelphia, WB Saunders, 1966.

Moore KL: *Clinically Oriented Anatomy.* 3rd ed. Williams & Wilkins, 1992.

Moore KL, Barr ML: Smears from the oral mucosa in the detection of chromosomal sex. *Lancet 2*:57, 1955.

Mulvihill JL: Fetal alcohol syndrome. *In* Sever JL, Brent RL, (eds): *Teratogen Update: Environmentally Induced Birth Defect Risks.* New York, Alan R. Liss, 1986.

Nahas GG: Cannabis: Toxicological properties and epidemiological aspects. *MJ Australia 145*:82, 1986.

Nahmias AJ, Visintine AM, Reimer CB, et al.: Herpes simplex virus infection of the fetus and newborn. *In* Krugman S, Gershon AA (eds): *Infections of the Fetus and Newborn.* Progress in Clinical and Biological Research. vol 3. New York, Alan R. Liss, 1975.

Nelson K, Holmes LB: Malformations due to presumed spontaneous mutations in newborn infants. *N Engl J Med 320*:19, 1989.

Nelson MM, Fofar JL: Associations between drugs administered during pregnancy and congenital abnormalities of the fetus. *Br Med J 1*:523, 1971.

Neu RL, Gardner LI: Abnormalities of the sex chromosomes. *In* Gardner LL (ed): *Endocrine and Genetic Diseases of Childhood and Adolescence.* 2nd ed. Philadelphia, WB Saunders, 1975.

Newman CGH: Clinical aspects of thalidomide embryopathy — A continuing preoccupation. *In* Sever JL, Brent RL (eds): *Teratogen Update: Environmentally Induced Birth Defect Risks.* New York, Alan R. Liss, 1986a.

Newman CGH: The thalidomide syndrome: risks of exposure and spectrum of malformations. *Clin Perinatol 13*:555, 1986b.

Noller KL: In utero DES exposure. *In* Quilligan EJ, Zuspan FP (eds): *Current Therapy in Obstetrics and Gynecology.* vol 3. Philadelphia, WB Saunders, 1990.

Nora AH, Nora JJ: A syndrome of multiple congenital anomalies associated with teratogenic exposure. *Arch Environ Health 30*:17, 1975.

Nyberg DA, Mahony BS, Pretorius DH (eds): *Diagnostic Ultrasound of Fetal Anomalies.* Chicago, Year Book Medical Publishers, 1990.

Oppenheim BE, Griem ML, Meier P: The effects of diagnostic x-ray on the human fetus: An examination of evidence. *Radiology 114*:529, 1975.

Otake M, Schull WJ, Yoshimaru H: Brain damage among the prenatally exposed. *J Rad Res 32(Suppl.)*:249, 1991.

Page EW, Villee CA, Villee DB: *Human Reproduction: Essentials of Reproductive and Perinatal Medicine.* 3rd ed. Philadelphia, WB Saunders, 1981.

Patterson RM: Seizure disorders in pregnancy. *Med Clin NA 73*:661, 1989.

Paulson G, Paulson RB: Seizure disorders in pregnancy. *In* Quilligan EJ, Zuspan FP (eds): *Current Therapy in Obstetrics and Gynecology.* vol 3. Philadelphia, WB Saunders, 1990.

Pearson PL, Bobrow M, Vosa CG: Technique for identifying Y chromosomes in human interphase nuclei. *Nature 226*:78, 1970.

Persaud TVN: *Environmental Causes of Human Birth Defects.* Springfield, Charles C Thomas, 1990.

Persaud TVN: Fetal alcohol syndrome. *Critical Rev Anat Cell Biol 1*:277, 1988.

Persaud TVN: Meromelia and other developmental abnormalities in experimental oligohydramnios. *Anat Anz 133*:499, 1973.

Persaud TVN: *Problems of Birth Defects. From Hippocrates to Thalidomide and After.* Baltimore, University Park Press, 1977.

Persaud TVN: *Teratogenesis. Experimental Aspects and Clinical Implications.* Jena, Gustav Fischer Verlag, 1979.

Persaud TVN, Chudley AE, Skalko RG: *Basic Concepts in Teratology.* New York, Alan R. Liss, 1985.

Persaud TVN, Ellington AC: Teratogenic activity of cannabis resin. *Lancet 2*:406, 1968.

Persaud TVN, Moore KL: Causes and prenatal diagnosis of congenital abnormalities. *J Obstet Gynecol Nursing 3*:40, 1974.

Pinkel D, Straume T, Gray JW: Cytogenetic analysis using quantitative, high sensitivity, fluorescence hybridization. *Proc Natl Acad Sci USA 83*:2934, 1986.

Randall T: Thalidomide's back in the news, but in more favorable circumstances. *JAMA 263*:1467, 1990.

Rasmussen F: The oto-toxic effect of streptomycin and dihydrostreptomycin on the foetus. *Scand J Respi. Dis 50*:61, 1969.

Reece EA, Hobbins JC: Diabetic embryopathy: pathogenesis, prenatal diagnosis and prevention. *Obstet. Gynecol. Surv. 41*:325, 1986.

Reid DE, Ryan KJ, Benirschke K (eds): *Principles and Management of Human Reproduction.* Philadelphia, WB Saunders, 1972.

Remington JS, Klein JO (eds): *Infectious Diseases of the Fetus and Newborn Infant.* 3rd ed. Philadelphia, WB Saunders, 1990.

Rendle-Short TJ: Tetracycline in teeth and bone. *Lancet 1*:118, 1962.

Reynolds DW, Stagno S, Alford CA: Congenital cytomegalovirus infection. *In* Sever JL, Brent RL (eds): *Teratogen Update: Environmentally Induced Birth Defect Risks.* New York, Alan R. Liss, 1986.

Ricci JM, Fojaco RM, O'Sullivan MJ: Congenital syphilis: The University of Miami/Jackson Memorial Medical Centre Experience, 1986–1988. *Obstet Gynecol 74*:687, 1989.

Rogan WJ: PCBs and cola colored babies: Japan 1968 and Taiwan, 1979. *In* Sever JL, Brent RL (eds): *Teratogen Update: Environmentally Induced Birth Defect Risks.* New York, Alan R. Liss, 1986.

Rosa FW, Wilk AL, Kelsey FO: Vitamin A congeners. *In* Sever JL, Brent RL (eds): *Teratogen Update: Environmentally Induced Birth Defect Risks.* New York, Alan R. Liss, 1986.

Rosenak D, Diamant YZ, Yaffe H, Hornstein E: Cocaine: Maternal use during pregnancy and its effect on the mother, the fetus, and the infant. *Obstet Gynecol Surv 45*:348, 1990.

Saxén L: Mechanisms of teratogenesis. *J Embryol Exp Morph 36*:1, 1976.

Saxén L, Rapola J: *Congenital Defects*. New York, Holt, Rinehart and Winston, 1969.

Sever JL, Nelson KB, Gilkeson MR: Rubella epidemic 1964: Effect on 6000 pregnancies. *Am J Dis Child 110*:395, 1964.

Shaw EB, Steinbach HL: Aminopterin-induced fetal malformations: Survival of infant after attempted abortion. *Am J Dis Child 115*:477, 1968.

Shepard TH: *Catalog of Teratogenic Agents*. 7th ed. Baltimore, The Johns Hopkins University Press, 1992.

Shepard TH, Fantel AG, Fitzsimmons J: Congenital defect rates among spontaneous abortuses. Twenty years of monitoring. *Teratology 39*:325, 1989.

Shiota K, Uwabe C, Nishimura H: High prevalence of defective human embryos at the early postimplantation period. *Teratology 35*:309, 1987.

Smith DW: Autosomal abnormalities. *Am J Obstet Gynec 90*: 1055, 1964.

Snyder RD: Congenital mercury poisoning. *N Engl J Med 284*:1014, 1971.

Sobell JL, Heston LL, Sommer SS: Delineation of genetic predisposition to multifactorial disease—A general approach on the threshold of feasibility. *Genomics 12*:1, 1992.

South MA, Tompkins WAF, Morris CR, Rawls WE: Congenital malformations of the central nervous system associated with genital type (type 2) herpesvirus. *J Pediatr 75*:13, 1969.

Speidel BD, Meadow SR: Maternal epilepsy and abnormalities of the fetus and newborn. *Lancet 2*:839, 1972.

Spranger J, Benirschke K, Hall JG, Lenz W, Lowry RB, Opitz JM, Pinsky L, Schwarzacher HG, Smith DW: Errors of morphogenesis: Concepts and terms. *J Pediatr 100*:160, 1982.

Stephens TD: Proposed mechanisms of action in thalidomide embryopathy. *Teratology 38*:229, 1988.

Taeusch HW, Ballard RA, Avery ME (eds): *Schaffer and Avery's Diseases of the Newborn*. 6th ed. Philadelphia, WB Saunders, 1991.

Thiersch JB: Therapeutic abortions with a folic acid antagonist, 4-aminopteroylglutamic acid (4-amino-PGA), administered by the oral route. *Am J Obstet Gynecol 63*:1298, 1952.

Thompson MW, McInnes RR, Willard HF: *Thompson and Thompson Genetics in Medicine*. 5th ed. Philadelphia, WB Saunders, 1991.

Uchida IA: Radiation-induced nondisjunction. *Environ. Health Perspect. 31*:13, 1979.

Ulfelder H: DES—Transplacental teratogen—and possible carcinogen. *In* Sever JL, Brent RL (eds): *Teratogen Update: Environmentally Induced Birth Defect Risks*. New York, Alan R. Liss, 1986.

Venning GR: The problem of human foetal abnormalities with special reference to sex hormones. *In* Robson JM, Sullivan FM, Smith RL (eds): *Embryopathic Activity of Drugs*. London, J. & A. Churchill, 1965.

Vorherr H, Vorherr UF, Mehta P, Ulrich JA, Messer RH: Vaginal absorption of povidone-iodine. *JAMA 244*:2628, 1980.

Wald NJ, Cuckle HS: AFP screening in early pregnancy. *In* Spencer, J.A.D. (ed.): *Fetal Monitoring*. Oxford, Oxford University Press, 1991.

Walpole IR, Hodgen N, Bower C: Congenital toxoplasmosis: A large survey in Western Australia. *Med J Aust 154*:720, 1991.

Warkany J: Anti-tuberculous drugs. *In* Sever JL, Brent RL (eds): *Teratogen Update: Environmentally Induced Birth Defect Risks*. New York, Alan R. Liss, 1986.

Warkany J: Congenital malformations induced by maternal dietary deficiency; Experiments and their interpretations. *Harvey Lect 48*:383, 1954.

Warkany J: *Congenital Malformations: Notes and Comments*. Chicago, Year Book Medical Publishers, 1971.

Warkany J: Teratogen update: lithium. *Teratology 38*:593, 1988.

Warkany J: Warfarin embryopathy. *Teratology 14*:205, 1976.

Warkany J, Beaudry PH, Hornstein S: Attempted abortion with 4-aminopterolyglutamic acid (Aminopterin): Malformations of the child. *Am J Dis Child 97*:274, 1960.

Weiss B, Doherty RA: Methylmercury poisoning. *Teratology. 12*:311, 1975.

Werler MM, Pober BR, Holmes LB: Smoking and Pregnancy. *In* Sever JL, Brent RL (eds): *Teratogen Update: Environmentally Induced Birth Defect Risks*. New York, Alan R. Liss, 1986.

Wilkins L, Jones HW, Jr, Holman GH, Stempfel RS, Jr: Masculinization of the female fetus in association with administration of oral and intramuscular progestins during gestation; nonadrenal female pseudohermaphroditism. *J Clin Endocrinol Metab 18*:559, 1958.

Williamson WD, Percy AK, Yow MD, Gerson P, Catlin FI, Koppelman ML, Thurber S: Asymptomatic congenital cytomegalovirus infection. *Am J Dis Chld 144*:1365, 1990.

Wilson JG: *Environment and Birth Defects*. New York, Academic Press, 1973a.

Wilson JG: Mechanisms of teratogenesis. *Am J Anat 136*:129, 1973b.

Winston NJ, Braude PR, Pickering SJ, George MA, Cant A, Currie J, Johnson MH: The incidence of abnormal morphology and nucleocytoplasmic ratios in 2-, 3- and 5-day human pre-embryos. *Human Reprod 6*:17, 1991.

Wynter HH, Persaud TVN: Results of a three-year study of birth defects in Jamaica. *Environ Child Health 18*:293, 1972.

Zellweger H, McDonald JS, Abbo G: Is lysergic acid diethylamide a teratogen? *Lancet 2*:1066, 1967.

9

Body Cavities, Primitive Mesenteries, and the Diaphragm

Early development of the **intraembryonic coelom** (primordium of the embryonic body cavities) during the third week is described in Chapter 4 (p. 63). By the fourth week, the coelom appears as a horseshoe-shaped cavity in the cardiogenic and lateral mesoderm (Fig. 9–1). The curve or bend in this cavity represents the future *pericardial cavity*, and its limbs (lateral parts) indicate the future *pleural and peritoneal cavities*.

The distal part of each limb of the intraembryonic coelom opens into the *extraembryonic coelom* at the lateral edges of the embryonic disc (see Figs. 5–3 and 9–1). This communication is important because most of the midgut normally herniates through this communication into the umbilical cord where it develops into most of the small intestine and part of the large intestine (see Figs. 6–4B and 12–12). In embryos of lower animal forms, the intraembryonic coelom provides short-term storage for excretory products. In human embryos, the coelom provides room for the organs to develop and move.

During embryonic folding in the horizontal plane, the limbs of the intraembryonic coelom are brought together on the ventral aspect of the embryo (see Figs. 5–1 and 9–2). The ventral mesentery degenerates in the region of the future peritoneal cavity, resulting in a large embryonic peritoneal cavity extending from the heart to the pelvic region (Figs. 9–2F and 9–3).

THE EMBRYONIC BODY CAVITY

The intraembryonic coelom gives rise to three well-defined coelomic (body) cavities in the fourth week: (1) a large *pericardial cavity* (Figs. 9–2B and 9–4), (2) two *pericardioperitoneal canals* connecting the

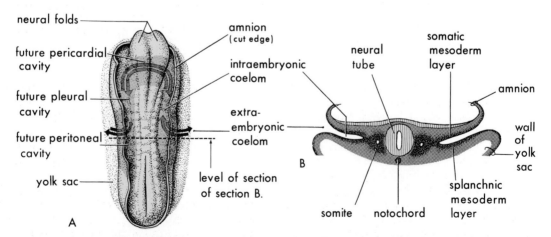

Figure 9–1. *A*, Drawing of a 22-day-old embryo showing the outline of the horseshoe-shaped intraembryonic coelom. The amnion has been removed, and the coelom is shown as if the embryo were translucent. The continuity of the intraembryonic coelom, as well as the communication of its right and left limbs with the extraembryonic coelom, are indicated by arrows. *B*, Transverse section through the embryo at the level shown in *A*.

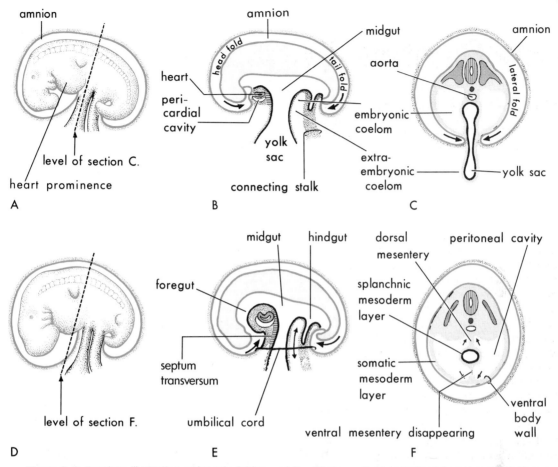

Figure 9–2. Drawings illustrating embryonic folding and its effects on the intraembryonic coelom and other structures. *A,* Lateral view of an embryo (about 26 days). *B,* Schematic sagittal section of this embryo showing the head and tail folds. *C,* Transverse section at the level shown in *A,* indicating how fusion of the lateral folds gives the embryo a cylindrical form. *D,* Lateral view of an embryo (about 28 days). *E,* Schematic sagittal section of this embryo showing the reduced communication between the intraembryonic and extraembryonic coeloms (double-headed arrow). *F,* Transverse section as indicated in *D,* illustrating formation of the ventral body wall and disappearance of the ventral mesentery. The arrows indicate the junction of the somatic and splanchnic layers of mesoderm. The somatic mesoderm will become the parietal peritoneum lining the abdominal wall, and the splanchnic mesoderm will become the visceral peritoneum covering the organs (e.g., the stomach).

pericardial and peritoneal cavities (see Figs. 5–3*B,* 9–3*B,* and 9–4), and (3) a large *peritoneal cavity* (Figs. 9–2*F,* 9–3*C* to *E* and 9–4). These cavities have a parietal wall lined by mesothelium (future peritoneum) derived from the somatic mesoderm and a visceral wall covered by mesothelium derived from the splanchnic mesoderm (Fig. 9–3*E*). The peritoneal cavity is connected with the extraembryonic coelom at the umbilicus but separates from it during the tenth week as the intestines return to the abdomen from the umbilical cord (see Fig. 12–11).

During formation of the *head fold,* the heart and pericardial cavity are carried ventrocaudally, anterior to the foregut (see Figs. 5–2 and 9–2*B*). As a result,

the pericardial cavity opens dorsally into the pericardioperitoneal canals on each side of the foregut (Fig. 9–4*B* and *D*). After embryonic folding, the caudal part of the foregut, midgut, and hindgut are suspended in the peritoneal cavity from the posterior abdominal wall by the *dorsal mesentery* (Figs. 9–2*F* and 9–3*C* to *E*).

A mesentery is a double layer of peritoneum. Transiently, the dorsal and ventral mesenteries divide the peritoneal cavity into right and left halves, but the ventral mesentery soon disappears, except where it is attached to the caudal part of the foregut (primordium of the stomach and the proximal part of the duodenum). The peritoneal cavity then becomes a

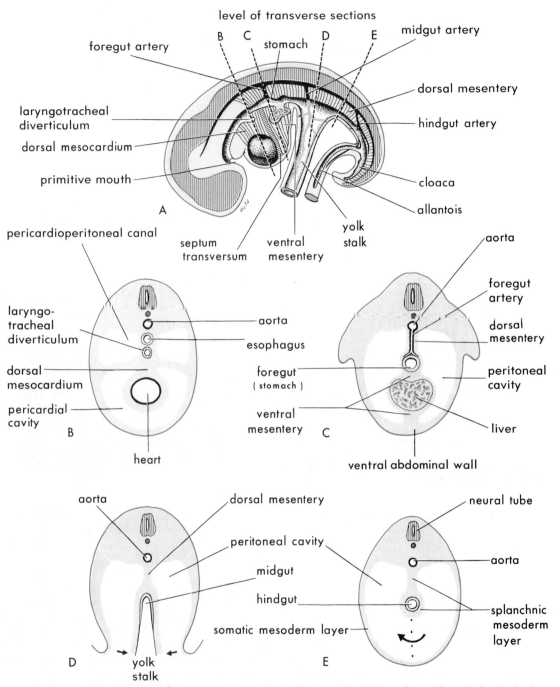

Figure 9-3. Diagrams illustrating the mesenteries at the beginning of the fifth week. *A,* Schematic longitudinal section. Note that the dorsal mesentery serves as a pathway for the arteries supplying the developing gut. Nerves and lymphatics also pass between the layers of this mesentery. *B to E,* Transverse sections through the embryo at the levels indicated in *A.* The ventral mesentery disappears, except in the region of the terminal esophagus, the stomach, and the first part of the duodenum. Note that the right and left parts of the peritoneal cavity, which are separate in *C,* are continuous in *E.*

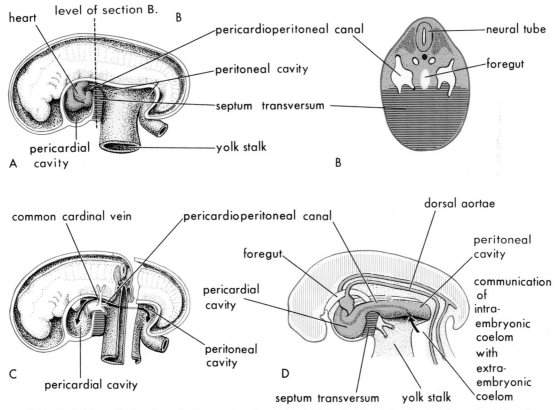

Figure 9–4. Schematic drawings of a four-week embryo (about 24 days). *A*, The lateral wall of the pericardial cavity has been removed to show the primitive heart. *B*, Transverse section of the embryo illustrating the relationship of the pericardioperitoneal canals to the septum transversum (primordium of part of the diaphragm) and the foregut. *C*, Lateral view of the embryo with the heart removed. The embryo has also been sectioned transversely to show the continuity of the intraembryonic and extraembryonic coeloms. *D*, Sketch showing the pericardioperitoneal canals arising from the dorsal wall of the pericardial cavity and passing on each side of the foregut to join the peritoneal cavity. The *arrows* show the communication of the extraembryonic coelom with the intraembryonic coelom and the continuity of the intraembryonic coelom at this stage.

continuous space (Figs. 9–3 and 9–4). The arteries supplying the primitive gut, (i.e., the celiac [foregut], the superior mesenteric [midgut], and the inferior mesenteric [hindgut]) pass between the layers of the dorsal mesentery (Figs. 9–3 and 12–1).

Division of the Embryonic Body Cavity

Each pericardioperitoneal canal lies lateral to the foregut (future esophagus) and dorsal to the *septum transversum*, which forms part of future diaphragm (Figs. 9–4*B* and 9–7*E*). Partitions form concurrently in each pericardioperitoneal canal that soon separate the pericardial cavity from the pleural cavities and the pleural cavities from the peritoneal cavity. Due to *growth of the bronchial (lung) buds* (primordia of the lungs) into the pericardioperitoneal canals (Figs. 9–5*A* and 11–7), a pair of membranous ridges is produced in the lateral wall of each canal. The cranial ridges, called *pleuropericardial membranes*, are located superior to the developing lungs; and the caudal ridges, called *pleuroperitoneal membranes*, are located inferior to them.

The Pleuropericardial Membranes (Fig. 9–5). As these cranial ridges enlarge, they form partitions that separate the pericardial cavity from the pleural cavities. Initially these membranes appear as bulges of mesenchyme that contain the *common cardinal veins* (Fig. 9–5*A*). These large veins drain the primitive venous system into the *sinus venosus* of the primitive heart (see Figs. 14–2 and 14–4).

At this stage, the *bronchial (lung) buds* are small relative to the heart and pericardial cavity. They grow laterally from the caudal end of the trachea into the corresponding pericardioperitoneal canal (pleural canal), which becomes the *primitive pleural cavity* (Fig. 9–5*B* and 11–7). As these cavities expand ventrally around the heart, they extend into the body wall

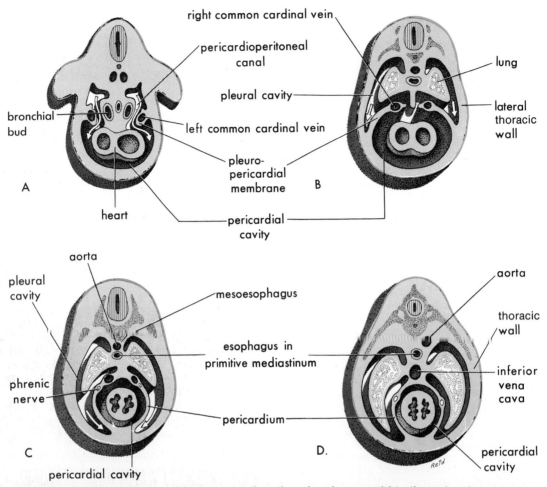

Figure 9–5. Schematic drawings of transverse sections through embryos cranial to the septum transversum, illustrating successive stages in the separation of the pleural cavities from the pericardial cavity. Growth and development of the lungs, expansion of the pleural cavities, and formation of the fibrous pericardium are also shown. A, Five weeks. The arrows indicate the communications between the pericardioperitoneal canals and the pericardial cavity. B, Six weeks. The arrows indicate development of the pleural cavities as they expand into the body wall. C, Seven weeks. Expansion of the pleural cavities ventrally around the heart is shown. The pleuropericardial membranes are now fused in the median plane with each other and with the mesoderm ventral to the esophagus. D, Eight weeks. Continued expansion of the lungs and pleural cavities and formation of the fibrous pericardium and chest wall are illustrated.

and split the mesenchyme into: (1) an external layer that becomes the thoracic wall, and (2) an internal layer (the pleuropericardial membrane) that becomes the *fibrous pericardium*, the outer fibrous layer of the pericardial sac enclosing the heart (Fig. 9–5C and D).

Initially the pleuropericardial membranes project into the cranial ends of the *pericardioperitoneal canals* (Fig. 9–5A). With subsequent growth of the common cardinal veins, descent of the heart, and expansion of the pleural cavities, these membranes become mesentery-like folds that extend from the lateral thoracic wall (Fig. 9–5B). By the seventh week the pleuropericardial membranes fuse with the meso-

derm ventral to the esophagus, which forms the *primitive mediastinum* and separates the pericardial cavity from the pleural cavities (Fig. 9–5C). The embryonic mediastinum consists of a mass of mesenchyme that extends from the sternum to the vertebral column and separates the developing lungs (Fig. 9–5D). The right pleuropericardial opening closes slightly earlier than the left one, probably because the right common cardinal vein is larger than the left one and produces a larger pleuropericardial membrane.

The Pleuroperitoneal Membranes (Figs. 9–6 and 9–7). As these caudal partitions in the pericardioperitoneal canals enlarge, they gradually separate the

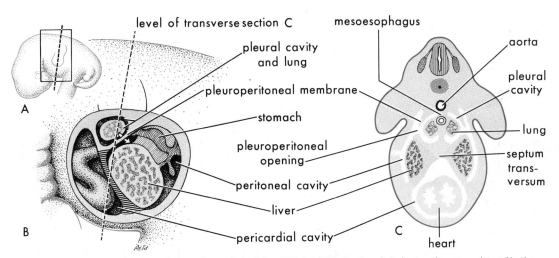

Figure 9–6. *A,* Sketch of a lateral view of an embryo (about 33 days). The rectangle indicates the area enlarged in the drawing below it. *B,* The primitive body cavities are viewed from the left side after removal of the lateral body wall. *C,* Transverse section through the embryo at the level shown in *B.*

pleural cavities from the peritoneal cavity. This pair of membranes is produced as the developing lungs and pleural cavities expand and invade the body wall. They are attached dorsolaterally to the abdominal wall, and their crescentic free edges initially project into the caudal ends of the pericardioperitoneal canals. They become relatively more prominent as the lungs enlarge cranially and the liver expands caudally.

During the sixth week the pleuroperitoneal membranes extend ventromedially until their free edges fuse with the dorsal mesentery of the esophagus and the septum transversum (Fig. 9–7C). This separates the pleural cavities from the peritoneal cavity. *Closure of the pleuroperitoneal openings* is assisted by the migration of myoblasts (primitive muscle cells) into the pleuroperitoneal membranes which form posterolateral parts of the diaphragm (Fig. 9–7E). The pleuroperitoneal opening on the right side closes slightly before the left one. The reason for this is uncertain, but it may be related to the relatively large right lobe of the liver at this stage of development (Fig. 9–6A).

DEVELOPMENT OF THE DIAPHRAGM[1]

This dome-shaped, musculotendinous partition separates the thoracic and abdominal cavities. It has a complex embryonic origin. *The diaphragm develops from four structures:* the septum transversum, the

[1] The diaphragm is a sheet of muscle with a large central tendon. For a description of its clinical anatomy, see Moore (1992).

pleuroperitoneal membranes, the dorsal mesentery of the esophagus, and the lateral body walls (Fig. 9–7).

The Septum Transversum. This transverse septum, composed of mesoderm, is the primordium of the *central tendon of the diaphragm* (Fig. 9–7E). It is located caudal to the pericardial cavity and partially separates it from the developing peritoneal cavity. The septum transversum is first identifiable at the end of the third week as a mass of mesodermal tissue cranial to the pericardial cavity (see Fig. 5–2A). After the head folds ventrally during the fourth week, the septum transversum forms a thick, incomplete partition, or partial diaphragm, between the pericardial and abdominal cavities (Fig. 9–4). The septum transversum does not separate the thoracic and abdominal cavities completely. It leaves a large opening, the *pericardioperitoneal canal*, on each side of the esophagus (Fig. 9–7A). The septum transversum soon fuses with the mesenchyme ventral to the esophagus (primitive mediastinum) and the pleuroperitoneal membranes (Fig. 9–7C).

The Pleuroperitoneal Membranes. These membranes fuse with the dorsal mesentery of the esophagus and the septum transversum (Fig. 9–7C). This completes the partition between the thoracic and abdominal cavities and forms the *primitive diaphragm.* Although the pleuroperitoneal membranes form large portions of the primitive diaphragm, they represent relatively small portions of the infant's diaphragm (Fig. 9–7E).

The Dorsal Mesentery of the Esophagus. As previously described, the septum transversum and pleuroperitoneal membranes fuse with the dorsal mesentery of the esophagus. This mesentery constitutes the

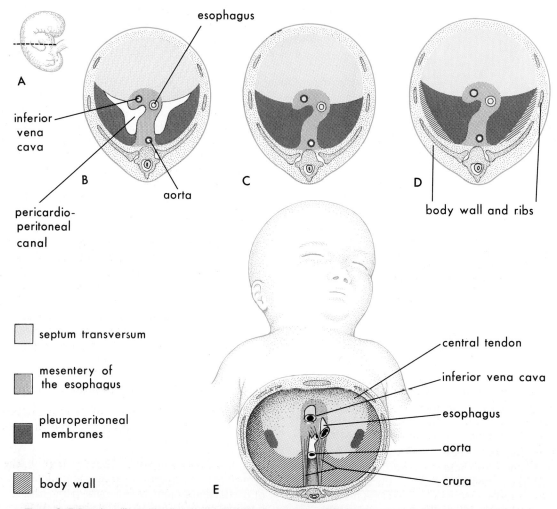

Figure 9-7. Drawings illustrating development of the diaphragm as viewed from below. *A,* Sketch of a lateral view of an embryo at the end of the fifth week (actual size), indicating the level of sections below it. *B* to *E* show the developing diaphragm as viewed inferiorly. *B,* Transverse section showing the unfused pleuroperitoneal membranes and pericardioperitoneal canals. *C,* Similar section at the end of the sixth week after fusion of the pleuroperitoneal membranes with the other two diaphragmatic components. *D,* Transverse section of a 12-week embryo after ingrowth of the fourth diaphragmatic component from the body wall. *E,* View of the diaphragm of a newborn infant, indicating the embryological origin of its components.

median portion of the diaphragm. The *crura of the diaphragm*[2] develop from myoblasts that grow into the dorsal mesentery of the esophagus (Fig. 9-7*E*).

The Lateral Body Walls. During the ninth to twelfth weeks the lungs and pleural cavities enlarge, "burrowing" into the lateral body walls (Fig. 9-5). During this "excavation" process the body-wall tissue is split into two layers: (1) an external layer that be-

comes part of the definitive abdominal wall, and (2) an internal layer that contributes muscle to peripheral portions of the diaphragm external to the parts derived from the pleuroperitoneal membranes (Fig. 9-7*D* and *E*). Further extension of the pleural cavities into the lateral body walls forms right and left *costodiaphragmatic recesses* (Fig. 9-8), establishing the characteristic, dome-shaped configuration of the diaphragm. After birth the costodiaphragmatic recesses become alternately smaller and larger as the lungs move in and out of them during inspiration and expiration (Moore, 1992).

---

[2] The crura (a leglike pair of diverging bundles of muscle) cross in the median plane anterior to the aorta (Moore, 1992).

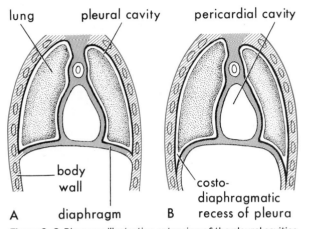

Figure 9–8. Diagrams illustrating extension of the pleural cavities into the body walls to form peripheral portions of the diaphragm, the costodiaphragmatic recesses, and the establishment of the characteristic dome-shaped configuration of the diaphragm. Note that body wall tissue is added peripherally to the diaphragm as the lungs and pleural cavities enlarge.

Positional Changes and Innervation of the Diaphragm

During the fourth week the septum transversum lies opposite the third, fourth, and fifth *cervical somites* (Fig. 9–9*A*). During the fifth week myoblasts (primitive muscle cells) from the myotome regions of these somites migrate into the developing diaphragm and bring their nerves with them; consequently, the *phrenic nerves* that supply the diaphragm come from cervical roots 3, 4, and 5. The three twigs on each side join to form a phrenic nerve. Due to the embryonic origin of the phrenic nerves, they are about 30 cm long in adults (Moore, 1992). The embryonic phrenic nerves enter the primitive diaphragm by passing through the pleuropericardial membranes. This ex-

plains why the phrenic nerves subsequently come to lie on the fibrous pericardium, the adult derivative of the pleuropericardial membranes (Fig. 9–5*C* and *D*).

Rapid growth of the dorsal part of the embryo's body results in an apparent migration or *descent of the diaphragm*. By the sixth week, the developing diaphragm is at the level of the thoracic somites (Fig. 9–9*B*). The phrenic nerves now take a descending course; and, as the diaphragm "moves" relatively farther caudally in the body, these nerves are correspondingly lengthened. By the beginning of the eighth week, the dorsal part of the diaphragm lies at the level of the first lumbar vertebra (Fig. 9–9*C*).

As the four parts of the diaphragm fuse (Fig. 9–7), mesenchyme (embryonic connective tissue) in the septum transversum extends into the other three parts. It forms myoblasts (primitive muscle cells) that differentiate into the skeletal muscle of the diaphragm; hence, the motor nerve supply to the diaphragm is from the phrenic nerves (ventral rami of C3, C4, and C5). The sensory innervation of the diaphragm is also from the phrenic nerves, but its costal rim receives sensory fibers from the lower intercostal nerves due to the origin of this peripheral part from the lateral body walls (Fig. 9–7).

Congenital Diaphragmatic Defects

Despite the rather complex embryological development of the diaphragm, congenital abnormalities are relatively uncommon.

Congenital Diaphragmatic Hernia (CDH). *Posterolateral defect of the diaphragm* is the only relatively common congenital abnormality of the diaphragm (Figs. 9–10 and 9–11). It occurs about once in 2200 newborn infants (Harrison, 1991) and is associated with CDH (herniation of abdominal contents into the thoracic cavity) and life-threatening breathing difficulties. *Polyhydramnios* is

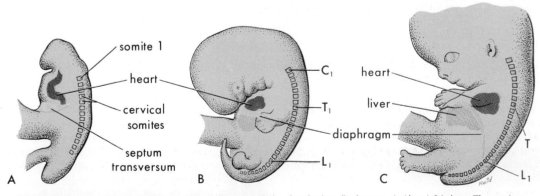

Figure 9–9. Diagrams illustrating positional changes of the developing diaphragm. *A*, About 24 days. The septum transversum (part of the primordium of the diaphragm) is at the level of the third, fourth, and fifth cervical segments. *B*, About 41 days. *C*, About 52 days.

vertebra   defect

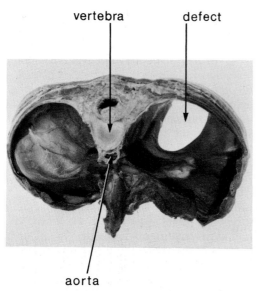

aorta

Figure 9-10. Photograph of a transverse section through the thoracic region of a stillborn infant, viewed from the thorax. Note the large, left, posterolateral defect of the diaphragm, which permitted the abdominal contents to pass into the thorax (CDH), as shown in Figure 9-11. Half actual size.

usually also present (p. 129). *Prenatal diagnosis of CDH* depends on the sonographic demonstration of abdominal organs in the thorax (Goldstein and Callen, 1988). The diagnosis can, if necessary, be confirmed by amniography (p. 108) because the fetus swallows amniotic fluid.

CDH, usually unilateral (97 per cent), results from defective formation and/or fusion of the pleuroperitoneal membrane with the other three parts of the diaphragm (Fig. 9-7). The defect commonly consists of a large opening[3] in the posterolateral region of the diaphragm (Figs. 9-10 and 9-11). The defect usually occurs on the left side (75 to 90 per cent); this preponderance is likely related to the earlier closure of the right pleuroperitoneal opening (p. 181).

The pleuroperitoneal membranes normally fuse with the other three diaphragmatic components by the end of the sixth week (Fig. 9-7C). If a pleuroperitoneal membrane is unfused when the intestines return to the abdomen from the umbilical cord in the tenth week (see Fig. 12-11C), some intestine is likely to pass into the thorax. Often the stomach, spleen, and most of the intestine herniate (Fig. 9-11). Uncommonly, the liver and kidney also pass into the thoracic cavity and displace the lungs and heart. The viscera can usually move freely through the defect; consequently, they may be in the thoracic cavity when the infant is lying down and in the abdominal cavity when the infant is upright. Most babies born with CDH die not because there is a defect in the diaphragm or viscera in the chest, but because the lung is hypoplastic due to compression during its development (Harrison, 1991).

----

[3] Sometimes referred to clinically as the foramen of Bochdalek.

The severity of pulmonary developmental abnormalities depends on when and to what extent the abdominal viscera herniate into the thorax, i.e., on the timing and degree of compression of the fetal lungs. The effect on the ipsilateral (same side) lung is greater, but the contralateral lung also shows morphological changes (Harrison, 1991). If the abdominal viscera are in the thoracic cavity at birth, the initiation of respiration is likely to be impaired. The intestines dilate with swallowed air and compromise the functioning of the heart and lungs. Because the abdominal organs are most often in the left side of the thorax, the heart and mediastinum are usually displaced to the right.

The lungs in infants with CDH are often hypoplastic and greatly reduced in size. The growth retardation of the lungs results from lack of room for them to develop normally. The lungs are often aerated and achieve their normal size after reduction (repositioning) of the herniated viscera and repair of the defect in the diaphragm; but the mortality rate is high, approximately 76 per cent (Harrison, 1991). If there is *severe lung hypoplasia*, some primitive alveoli may rupture, causing air to enter the pleural cavity, a condition known as *pneumothorax*. If necessary, CDH can be diagnosed and repaired prenatally between 22 and 28 weeks of gestation, but this intervention carries considerable risk to the fetus and mother (Harrison, 1991).

Eventration of the Diaphragm. In this uncommon condition, half the diaphragm has defective musculature and balloons into the thoracic cavity as a membranous (aponeurotic) sheet. As a result, there is superior displacement of abdominal viscera into the pocketlike outpouching of the diaphragm. This congenital anomaly mainly results from failure of muscular tissue to grow into the pleuroperitoneal membrane on the affected side. *An eventration is not a true herniation*; it is a superior displacement of viscera into a saclike part of the diaphragm. The clinical manifestations of diaphragmatic eventration, however, may simulate CDH (Behrman, 1992). During surgical repair, a muscular flap (e.g., from the latissimus dorsi muscle) or a prosthetic patch is used to strengthen the diaphragm (Beck et al., 1985).

Gastroschisis and Congenital Epigastric Hernia. This uncommon hernia occurs in the median plane between the xiphoid process and umbilicus. These defects are similar to umbilical hernias (p. 251) except for their location. Gastroschisis and epigastric hernias result from failure of the lateral body folds to fuse completely to form the anterior abdominal wall during folding in the horizontal plane in the fourth week (Fig. 9-2C and F). The small intestine herniates into the amniotic fluid and can be detected prenatally by ultrasonography (Langer and Harrison, 1991).

Congenital Hiatal Hernia. There may be herniation of part of the fetal stomach through an excessively large esophageal hiatus, but this is an uncommon congenital defect. Although hiatal hernia is usually an acquired lesion occurring during adult life (Moore, 1992), in some cases a congenitally enlarged esophageal hiatus may be the predisposing factor.

Retrosternal Hernia. Large herniations may occur through the *sternocostal hiatus* (foramen of Morgagni) for the superior epigastric vessels in the retrosternal area. Her-

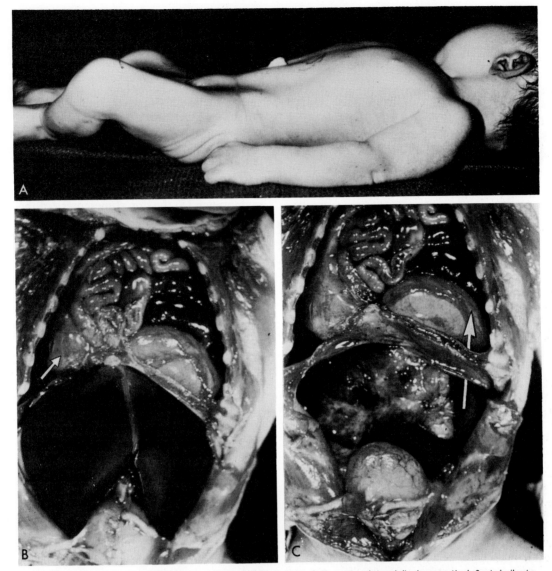

Figure 9–11. *A,* Photograph of an infant with CDH due to a large, left, posterolateral diaphragmatic defect similar to that shown in Figure 9–10. Note the relatively flat abdomen resulting from herniation of abdominal viscera into the thorax through the defect. *B,* The thoracic and abdominal cavities opened at autopsy to show the intestines and other viscera in the thoracic cavity. The *arrow* indicates the heart which has been displaced to the right. Most babies with CDH die because the lung is hypoplastic due to compression by abdominal viscera during lung development. *C,* The liver has been removed, showing that only attached parts of the large intestine have remained in the abdominal cavity. The arrow passes through the diaphragmatic defect. (Courtesy of Dr. Jan Hoogstraten, Children's Centre, Winnipeg, Canada.)

niation of the intestine into the pericardial sac may also occur (Behrman, 1992) or, conversely, part of the heart may descend into the peritoneal cavity in the epigastric region. Large defects are commonly associated with defects in the umbilical region (e.g., omphalocele; see Fig. 12–15). Radiologists and pathologists often observe *fatty herniations* through the sternocostal hiatus in the retrosternal area, but they are of no clinical significance.

Congenital Pericardial Defects. Defective formation and/or fusion of the pleuropericardial membranes that separate the pericardial and pleural cavities is an uncommon congenital anomaly. This abnormality results in a congenital defect of the pericardium, usually on the left side. The pericardial cavity communicates with the pleural cavity; and, in very unusual cases, a portion of an atrium herniates into the pleural cavity at each heartbeat.

SUMMARY

The intraembryonic coelom, the primordium of the body cavities, begins to develop near the end of the third week. By the beginning of the fourth week, it appears as a horseshoe-shaped cavity in the cardiogenic and lateral mesoderm. The curve of the "horseshoe" represents the future pericardial cavity; and its lateral parts, or limbs, represent the future pleural and peritoneal cavities.

During folding of the embryonic disc in the fourth week, the lateral parts of the intraembryonic coelom are brought together on the ventral aspect of the embryo. When the caudal part of the ventral mesentery disappears, the right and left parts of the intraembryonic coelom merge to form the peritoneal cavity. As the peritoneal portions of the intraembryonic coelom merge, the splanchnic layer of mesoderm encloses the primitive gut and suspends it from the dorsal body wall by a double-layered peritoneal membrane known as the dorsal mesentery.

Until the seventh week, the embryonic pericardial cavity communicates with the peritoneal cavity through paired *pericardioperitoneal canals*. During the fifth and sixth weeks, membranes form near the cranial and caudal ends of these canals. Fusion of the cranial *pleuropericardial membranes* with mesoderm ventral to the esophagus separates the pericardial cavity from the pleural cavities. Fusion of the caudal *pleuroperitoneal membranes* during formation of the diaphragm separates the pleural cavities from the peritoneal cavity.

The diaphragm develops from four structures: (1) the septum transversum, (2) the pleuroperitoneal membranes, (3) the dorsal mesentery of the esophagus, and (4) the lateral body walls.

A posterolateral defect of the diaphragm results in congenital diaphragmatic hernia (CDH), which is associated with herniation of abdominal viscera into the thoracic cavity. CDH occurs five times more often on the left side than on the right and results from failure of the pleuroperitoneal membrane on this side to fuse with the other diaphragmatic components and separate the pleural and peritoneal cavities.

CLINICALLY ORIENTED QUESTIONS FOR PROBLEM-BASED LEARNING SESSIONS

1. A newborn infant suffered from severe *respiratory distress*. The abdomen was unusually flat, and intestinal peristaltic movements were heard over the left side of the thorax. What congenital anomaly would you suspect? Explain the basis of the signs described above. How would the diagnosis likely be established?

2. What congenital anomaly could result in herniation of intestine into the pericardial cavity? What is the embryological basis of this defect?

3. How common is posterolateral defect of the diaphragm? How do you think a newborn infant in whom this diagnosis is suspected should be positioned? Why would this positional treatment be given? Briefly describe surgical repair of CDH. Why do most newborns with CDH die?

4. A baby was born with a hernia in the median plane between the xiphoid process and the umbilicus. Name this type of hernia. Is it common? What is the embryological basis of this congenital anomaly?

The answers to these questions are given on page 462.

References and Suggested Reading

Avery ME: Disorders of the diaphragm. *In* Avery ME, Taeusch HW (eds): *Diseases of the Newborn.* 5th ed. Philadelphia, WB Saunders, 1983.

Avery ME, Fletcher BD, Williams RG: *The Lung and Its Disorders in the Newborn Infant.* 4th ed. Philadelphia, WB Saunders, 1981.

Beck F, Moffat DB, Davies DP: *Human Embryology.* 2nd ed. Oxford, Blackwell Scientific Publications, 1985.

Behrman RE: *Nelson Textbook of Pediatrics.* 14th ed. Philadelphia, WB Saunders, 1992.

Ellis K, Leeds NE, Himmelstein A: Congenital deficiencies in the parietal pericardium. A review with two new cases including successful diagnosis by plain roentgenography. *Am J Roentgenol 82*:125, 1959.

Fosberg RG, Jakubiak JW, Delaney TB: Congenital partial absence of the pericardium. *Ann Thorac Surg 5*:171, 1968.

Goldstein RB, Callen PW: Ultrasound evaluation of the fetal thorax and abdomen. *In* Callen PW: *Ultrasonography in Ob-*

stetrics and Gynecology. 2nd ed. Philadelphia, WB Saunders, 1988.

Gray SW, Skandalakis JE: *The Embryological Basis For The Treatment of Congenital Defects.* Philadelphia, WB Saunders, 1972.

Harrison MR: The fetus with a diaphragmatic hernia: pathophysiology, natural history, and surgical management. *In* Harrison MR, Golbus MS, Filly RA (eds): *The Unborn Patient: Prenatal Diagnosis and Treatment.* 2nd ed. Philadelphia, WB Saunders, 1991.

Langer JC, Harrison MR: The fetus with an abdominal wall defect. *In* Harrison MR, Golbus MS, Filly RA (eds): *The Unborn Patient: Prenatal Diagnosis and Treatment.* 2nd ed. Philadelphia, WB Saunders, 1991.

Laxdal OE, McDougall H, Mellen GW: Congenital eventration of the diaphragm. *N Engl J Med 250*:401, 1954.

McNamara JJ, Eraklis AJ, Gross RE: Congenital posterolateral diaphragmatic hernia in the newborn. *J Thorac Cardiovasc Surg 55*:55, 1968.

Moore KL: *Clinically Oriented Anatomy.* 3rd ed. Baltimore, Williams & Wilkins, 1992.

Reynolds M: Diaphragmatic anomalies. *In* Raffensperger JG (ed): *Swenson's Pediatric Surgery.* 5th ed. Norwalk, Appleton & Lange, 1990.

Wells LJ: Development of the human diaphragm and pleural sacs. *Contr Embryol Carneg Instn 35*:107, 1954.

10

The Branchial or Pharyngeal Apparatus[1]

This apparatus consists of: (1) branchial (or pharyngeal) arches, (2) pharyngeal pouches, (3) branchial (or pharyngeal) grooves, and (4) branchial (or pharyngeal) membranes (Figs. 10–1 to 10–3). These primitive embryonic structures contribute greatly to the formation of the head and neck. Most congenital anomalies in these regions originate during transformation of the branchial (or pharyngeal) apparatus into its adult derivatives. *Branchial anomalies* (p. 196) result from persistence of parts of the branchial apparatus that normally disappear.

Study of the development of the human branchial or pharyngeal apparatus and the head and neck can be confusing if the function of the branchial apparatus in lower forms of life is not understood. In fish and larval amphibians, the branchial apparatus forms a system of gills for exchanging oxygen and carbon dioxide between the blood and the water. The branchial arches support the gills. A primitive branchial apparatus develops in human embryos, but no gills form; because of this, the term *pharyngeal arch* is often used instead of branchial arch.

BRANCHIAL OR PHARYNGEAL ARCHES

These arches begin to develop early in the fourth week as *neural crest cells* migrate into the future head and neck region (p. 71). The first pair of arches, the primordium of the jaws, appears as surface elevations lateral to the developing pharynx (Fig. 10–1). Soon, other arches appear as obliquely disposed, rounded ridges on each side of the future head and neck regions. The arches not only contribute to the formation of the neck, but the first pair plays an important role in the development of the face (Fig. 10–1E to G).

By the end of the fourth week, four well-defined pairs of arches are visible externally (Fig. 10–1D). The fifth and sixth arches are rudimentary and are not visible on the surface of the embryo. The arches are separated from each other by prominent clefts called *branchial or pharyngeal grooves* (Fig. 10–1B to D). Like the arches, they are numbered in a craniocaudal sequence.

The first branchial or pharyngeal arch, often called the mandibular arch, develops two prominences: (1) the larger *mandibular prominence* forms the mandible (lower jaw), and (2) the smaller *maxillary prominence* gives rise to the maxilla (upper jaw), the zygomatic bone, and the squamous part of the temporal bone (Fig. 10–3). As described subsequently (p. 205), the first pair of arches plays an important role in the development of the face. *The second branchial or pharyngeal arch* is often called the hyoid arch because it contributes to the formation of the hyoid bone (Fig. 10–5B). The arches caudal to the second arch are usually referred to by number only (Fig. 10–4).

The branchial or pharyngeal arches support the lateral walls of the cranial part of the foregut called the *primitive pharynx*. The primitive mouth or *stomodeum* initially appears as a slight depression of the surface ectoderm (Figs. 10–1D to G). It is separated from the primitive pharynx by a bilaminar membrane called the *oropharyngeal (buccopharyngeal) membrane*, which formed during the third week (see Fig. 4–6C). It is composed of ectoderm externally and endoderm internally. This membrane ruptures at about 26 days (Fig. 10–1F), bringing the primitive pharynx and gut (primordium of the digestive tract) into communication with the amniotic cavity (Fig. 10–2).

---

[1] The cranial region of a human embryo during the fourth week somewhat resembles a fish embryo of a comparable stage. This explains the use of the adjective *branchial*, from the Greek *branchia* meaning "gill." By the end of the embryonic period, these ancestral structures have either become rearranged and adapted to new functions or disappeared. Because the human embryo does not develop gills, these arches are often called pharyngeal arches. *Nomina Embryologica* (Warwick, 1989) recommends "pharyngeal arch," but gives "branchial arch" as the officially recognized alternative term.

Branchial or Pharyngeal Arch Components

Initially, each arch consists of a core of mesenchyme that is covered externally by ectoderm and internally by endoderm (Figs. 10–1, 10–3, and 10–4). This original mesenchyme is derived from paraxial and lateral mesoderm in the third week (p. 63). During the fourth week, mesenchyme is also derived from *neural crest cells* that migrate into the arches from the neural crests of the neural folds that will form the midbrain and hindbrain (see Fig. 4–8). It is the migration of these neural crest cells into the

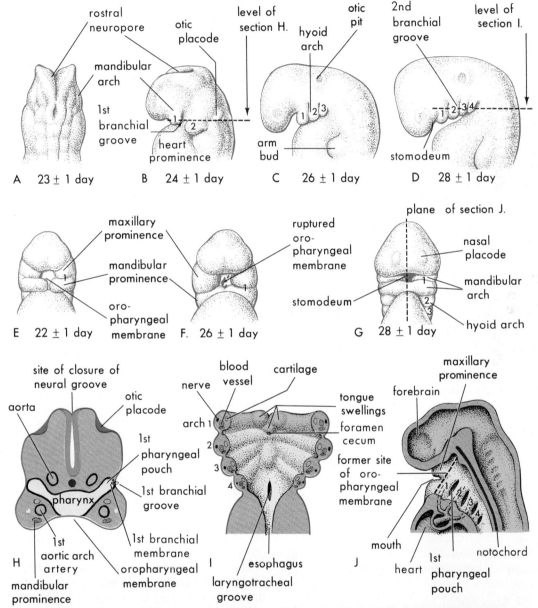

Figure 10–1. Drawings illustrating the human branchial or pharyngeal apparatus. *A,* Dorsal view of the cranial part of an early embryo. *B* to *D,* Lateral views showing later development of the branchial or pharyngeal arches. *E* to *G,* Ventral or facial views illustrating the relationship of the first arch to the stomodeum. *H,* Horizontal section through the cranial region of an embryo. *I,* Similar section illustrating the arch components and the floor of the primitive pharynx. *J,* Sagittal section of the cranial region of an embryo, illustrating the openings of the pharyngeal pouches in the lateral wall of the primitive pharynx.

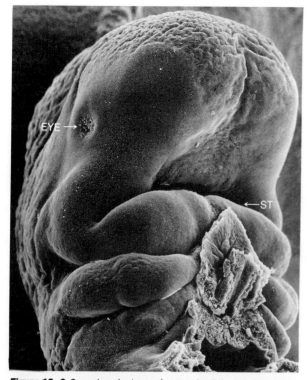

Figure 10–2. Scanning electron micrograph of the head and neck regions of a human embryo (oblique view) of about 32 days (stage 14, 6.8 mm). If necessary, see Figure 10–1A to F for identification of the parts of the head and neck. Observe the arches, eye, and large stomodeum (ST) or primitive mouth. (From Hinrichsen K: *The early development of morphology and patterns of the face in the human embryo.* In *Advances in Anatomy, Embryology and Cell Biology.* Vol. 98, New York, Springer Verlag, 1985.)

arches and proliferation of them that produce the maxillary and mandibular prominences of the first arch (Figs. 10–1 and 10–2).

Neural crest cells are unique in that, despite their neuroectodermal origin (see Fig. 4–8), they make a major contribution to mesenchyme in the head (see Fig. 5–5) as well as to many other structures (Noden, 1984; Kirby and Bockman, 1984; Hall, 1988; Sperber, 1989; Stricker et al., 1990). The literature indicates that most of the skeletal and connective tissue structures of the head and neck are derived from mesenchyme of neural crest origin. Skeletal musculature and vascular endothelia, however, are derived from the original mesoderm in the arches.

Fate of the Branchial or Pharyngeal Arches

These arches contribute extensively to the formation of the face, neck, nasal cavities, mouth, larynx, and pharynx. The *first arch* is involved with development of the face (described on p. 208). Small eleva-

tions (hillocks) develop at the dorsal ends of the first and second arches, surrounding the opening of the first branchial groove. These *auricular hillocks* gradually fuse to form the auricle of the external ear (see Figs. 10–23 and 10–27). During the fifth week, the *second arch* enlarges and overgrows the third and fourth arches, forming an ectodermal depression known as the *cervical sinus* (Fig. 10–4A to D). By the end of the seventh week, the second to fourth branchial or pharyngeal grooves and the cervical sinus have disappeared. This gives the neck a smooth contour (Fig. 10–4G).

A typical branchial arch contains: (1) an *aortic arch* (artery) that runs around the primitive pharynx to the dorsal aorta (Fig. 10–3B), (2) a *cartilaginous rod* that forms the skeleton of the arch, (3) a *muscular component* that forms muscles in the head and neck, and (4) a *nerve* that supplies the mucosa and muscles derived from the arch (Fig. 10–3). The nerves that grow into the arches are derived from neuroectoderm of the primitive brain (Fig. 10–7).

Derivatives of the Branchial or Pharyngeal Arch Arteries (Fig. 10–3B). Each arch contains an artery called an *aortic arch*. The transformation of the aortic arches into the adult arterial pattern of the head and neck is described with the cardiovascular system in Chapter 14 (p. 335). In fishes, these arteries supply blood to the capillary network of the gills. In human embryos, the blood in the aortic arch arteries supplies the arches and then enters the dorsal aorta.

Derivatives of the Branchial or Pharyngeal Arch Cartilages (Fig. 10–5; Table 10–1). The dorsal end of the *first arch cartilage* (Meckel's cartilage) is closely related to the developing ear and becomes ossified to form two middle ear bones, the *malleus* and *incus*. The intermediate portion of the cartilage regresses, but its perichondrium forms the *anterior ligament of the malleus* and the *sphenomandibular ligament*. Ventral portions of the first arch cartilage form the horseshoe-shaped primordium of the mandible and, by keeping pace with its growth (Hall, 1982), guide its early morphogenesis. Each half of the mandible forms lateral to and in close association with its cartilage. The cartilage disappears as the mandible develops around it by intramembranous ossification (Fig. 10–5B). For details on the development of the mandible, see Sperber (1989).

The dorsal end of the *second arch cartilage* (Reichert's cartilage) is also closely related to the developing ear. It ossifies to form the *stapes* of the middle ear and the *styloid process* of the temporal bone (Fig. 10–5B). The portion of cartilage between the styloid process and the hyoid bone regresses; its perichondrium forms the *stylohyoid ligament*. The ventral end of the second arch

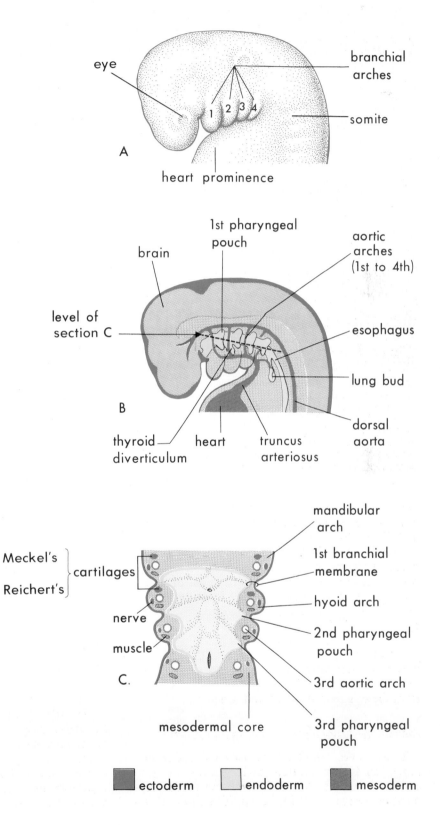

Figure 10–3. A, Drawing of the head and neck region of a human embryo (about 28 days), illustrating the branchial or pharyngeal apparatus. B, Schematic drawing showing the pharyngeal pouches and aortic arches. C, Horizontal section through the embryo showing the floor of the primitive pharynx and illustrating the germ layer of origin of the arch components.

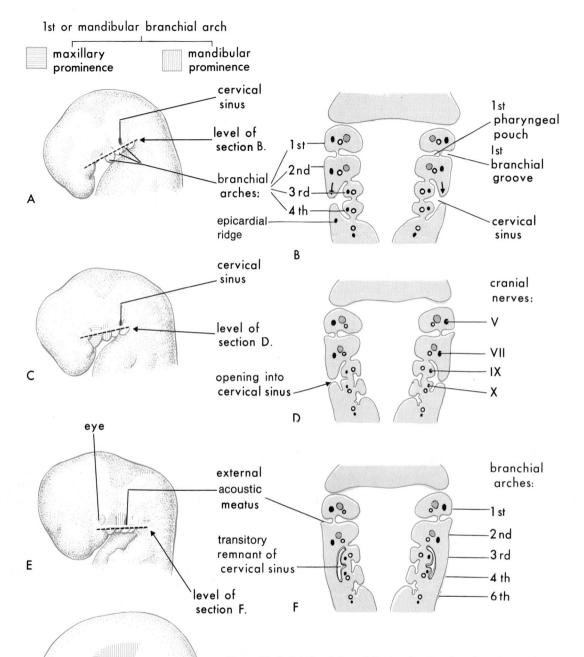

Figure 10–4. *A,* Lateral view of the head and neck region of an embryo (about 32 days; see also Fig. 10–2), showing the branchial or pharyngeal arches and the cervical sinus. *B,* Diagrammatic horizontal section through the embryo illustrating growth of the second arch over the third and fourth arches. *C,* An embryo of about 33 days. *D,* Horizontal section of the embryo illustrating early closure of the cervical sinus. *E,* An embryo of about 41 days. *F,* Horizontal section of the embryo showing the transitory cystic remnant of the cervical sinus. *G,* Twenty-week fetus illustrating the area of the face derived from the first pair of branchial or pharyngeal arches.

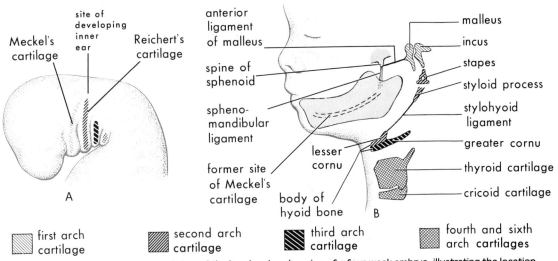

first arch cartilage

second arch cartilage

third arch cartilage

fourth and sixth arch cartilages

Figure 10–5. *A,* Schematic lateral view of the head and neck region of a four-week embryo, illustrating the location of the cartilages in the branchial or pharyngeal arches. *B,* Similar view of a 24-week fetus illustrating the adult derivatives of the arch cartilages. Note that the mandible is formed by membranous ossification of mesenchymal tissue surrounding Meckel's cartilage. This cartilage acts as a template but does not contribute directly to the formation of the mandible. Occasionally, ossification of the second arch cartilage may extend from the styloid process along the stylohyoid ligament. When this occurs, it may cause pain in the region of the palatine tonsil.

Table 10–1. STRUCTURES DERIVED FROM BRANCHIAL OR PHARYNGEAL ARCH COMPONENTS*

Arch	Nerve	Muscles	Skeletal Structures	Ligaments
First (mandibular)	Trigeminal† (V)	Muscles of mastication‡ Mylohyoid and anterior belly of digastric Tensor tympani Tensor veli palatini	Malleus Incus	Anterior ligament of malleus Sphenomandibular ligament
Second (hyoid)	Facial (VII)	Muscles of facial expressions§ Stapedius Stylohyoid Posterior belly of digastric	Stapes Styloid process Lesser cornu of hyoid Upper part of body of the hyoid bone	Stylohyoid ligament
Third	Glossopharyngeal (IX)	Stylopharyngeus	Greater cornu of hyoid Lower part of body of the hyoid bone	
Fourth and Sixth‖	Superior laryngeal branch of vagus (X) Recurrent laryngeal branch of vagus (X)	Cricothyroid Levator veli palatini Constrictors of pharynx Intrinsic muscles of larynx Striated muscles of the esophagus	Thyroid cartilage Cricoid cartilage Arytenoid cartilage Corniculate cartilage Cuneiform cartilage	

* The derivatives of the aortic arch arteries are described in Chapter 14 (see Fig. 14–35).
† The ophthalmic division does not supply any branchial components.
‡ Temporalis, masseter, medial and lateral pterygoids.
§ Buccinator, auricularis, frontalis, platysma, orbicularis oris and oculi.
‖ The fifth branchial arch is often absent. When present, it is rudimentary and usually has no recognizable cartilage bar. The cartilaginous components of the fourth and sixth arches fuse to form the cartilages of the larynx.

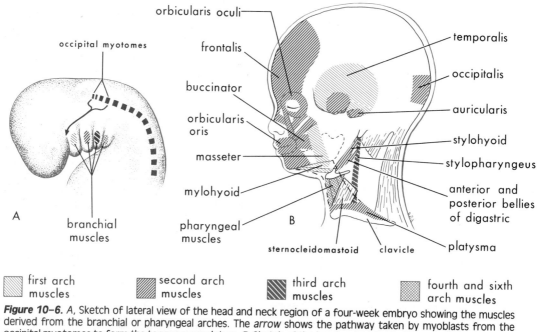

first arch muscles   second arch muscles   third arch muscles   fourth and sixth arch muscles

Figure 10-6. *A,* Sketch of lateral view of the head and neck region of a four-week embryo showing the muscles derived from the branchial or pharyngeal arches. The *arrow* shows the pathway taken by myoblasts from the occipital myotomes to form the tongue musculature. *B,* Sketch of the head and neck of a 20-week fetus, dissected to show the muscles derived from the branchial or pharyngeal arches. Parts of the platysma and sternocleidomastoid muscles have been removed to show the deeper muscles. Note that myoblasts from the second arch migrate from the neck to the head where they give rise to the muscles of facial expression. These muscles are supplied by the facial nerve (CN VII), the nerve of the second arch.

cartilage ossifies to form the lesser cornu (*L.* horn) and the superior part of the body of the *hyoid bone* (Fig. 10-5*B*).

The *third arch cartilage* is located in the ventral portion of the arch. It ossifies to form the greater cornu and the inferior part of the body of the hyoid bone. The *fourth and sixth arch cartilages* fuse to form the *laryngeal cartilages* (Fig. 10-5*B* and Table 10-1), except for the epiglottis. The cartilage of the epiglottis develops from mesenchyme in the *hypobranchial eminence* (see Fig. 10-19*A*), a prominence derived from the third and fourth branchial arches (p. 204).

Derivatives of the Branchial or Pharyngeal Arch Muscles (Fig. 10-6; Table 10-1). The muscular components of the arches form many striated muscles in the head and neck.

Derivatives of the Branchial or Pharyngeal Arch Nerves (Fig. 10-7; Table 10-1). Each arch is supplied by its own cranial nerve. The cranial nerves supplying the branchial muscles are classified as *branchial motor* or *efferent nerves.* Because mesenchyme from the branchial arches contributes to the dermis and mucous membranes of the head and neck, these areas are supplied with branchial sensory or *afferent nerves.*

The facial skin is supplied by the fifth cranial nerve (*trigeminal nerve*); however, only its caudal two branches (*maxillary* and *mandibular*) supply derivatives of the first arch (Fig. 10-7*B*). CN V is the principal sensory nerve of the head and neck, and it is the motor nerve for the muscles of mastication (Table 10-1). Its sensory branches innervate the face, teeth, and mucous membranes of the nasal cavities, palate, mouth, and tongue (Fig. 10-7*C*).

The seventh cranial nerve (*facial nerve*), the ninth cranial nerve (*glossopharyngeal nerve*), and the tenth cranial nerve (*vagus nerve*) supply the second, third, and caudal (fourth to sixth) arches, respectively. The fourth arch is supplied by the superior laryngeal branch of the vagus (CN X) and the sixth arch by its recurrent laryngeal branch. The nerves of the second to sixth arches have little cutaneous distribution, but they innervate the mucous membranes of the tongue, pharynx, and larynx, as illustrated in Fig. 10-7*C*.

PHARYNGEAL POUCHES

The *primitive pharynx,* derived from the foregut, widens cranially where it joins the primitive mouth or *stomodeum* (Fig. 10-2) and narrows caudally as it joins the esophagus (Figs. 10–1*I* and 10–3*B*). The endoderm of the pharynx lines the internal aspects of the branchial or pharyngeal arches and passes into balloonlike diverticula called *pharyngeal pouches* (Figs. 10–1*H* to *J*, 10–3*B* and *C*, and 10–8*A*). Pairs of pouches develop in a craniocaudal sequence between the arches, e.g., the first pair of pouches lies between the first and second arches.

There are four well-defined pairs of pharyngeal pouches; the fifth pair is absent or rudimentary. The endoderm of the pouches contacts the ectoderm of the branchial or pharyngeal grooves, and together they form the thin, double-layered *branchial or pharyngeal membranes* that separate the pharyngeal pouches from the branchial grooves (Figs. 10–1*H* and 10–3*C*).

Derivatives of the Pharyngeal Pouches

Because the endodermal lining of the pouches gives rise to several important organs, the fate of each pouch is discussed separately.

The First Pharyngeal Pouch (Figs. 10–8 and 10–9). This pouch expands into an elongate *tubotympanic recess*. The expanded distal part of this recess contacts the first branchial or pharyngeal groove where it later contributes to the formation of the *tympanic membrane* (eardrum). The tubotympanic recess gives rise to the *tympanic cavity* and *mastoid antrum*. The connection of the tubotympanic recess with the pharynx gradually elongates to form the *auditory tube* (eustachian tube). More details about these parts of the developing ear are given in Chapter 19.

The Second Pharyngeal Pouch (Figs. 10–8 and 10–9). Although it is largely obliterated as the *palatine tonsil* develops, part of the cavity of this pouch remains as the *intratonsillar cleft* (tonsillar fossa). The endoderm of the second pouch proliferates and grows into the surrounding mesenchyme. The central parts of these buds break down, forming crypts (pitlike depressions). The pouch endoderm forms the surface epithelium and the lining of the *crypts of the palatine tonsil*. At about 20 weeks, the mesenchyme around the crypts differentiates into lymphoid tissue, which soon organizes into the *lymphatic nodules* of the palatine tonsil (Cormack, 1984).

The Third Pharyngeal Pouch (Figs. 10–8 and 10–9). This pouch expands and develops a solid, dorsal bulbar portion and a hollow, elongate ventral

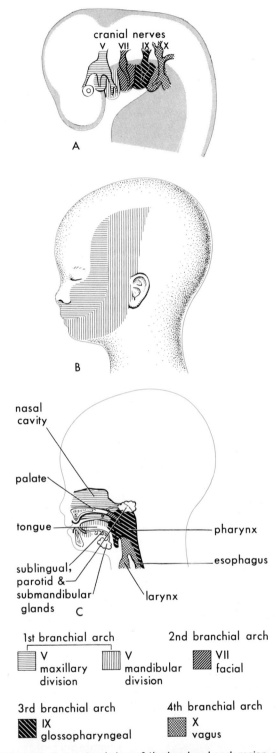

Figure 10–7. *A*, Lateral view of the head and neck region of a four-week embryo showing the nerves supplying the branchial arches. *B*, Sketch of the head and neck of a 20-week fetus showing the superficial distribution of the two caudal branches of the first arch nerve (CN V). *C*, Sagittal section of the fetal head and neck showing the deep distribution of sensory fibers of the branchial nerves to the teeth and mucosa of the tongue, pharynx, nasal cavity, palate, and larynx.

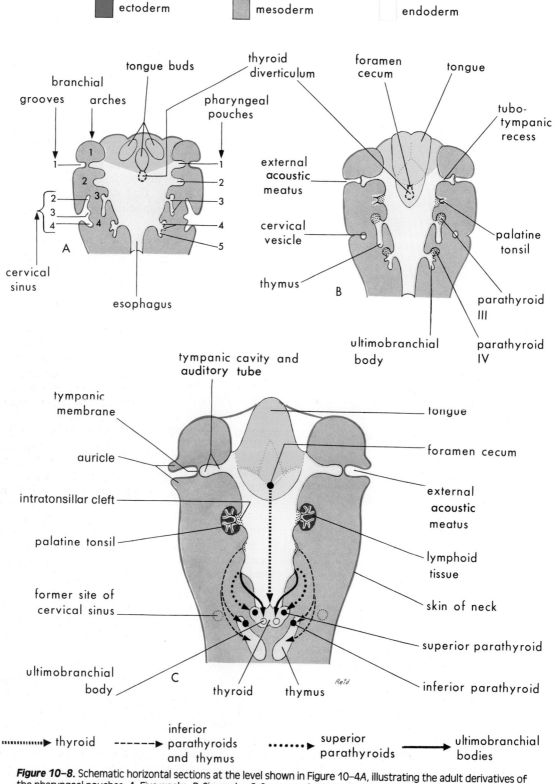

Figure 10–8. Schematic horizontal sections at the level shown in Figure 10–4A, illustrating the adult derivatives of the pharyngeal pouches. *A*, Five weeks. *B*, Six weeks. *C*, Seven weeks. Note that the second branchial or pharyngeal arch grows over the third and fourth arches, thereby burying the second to fourth branchial or pharyngeal grooves in the cervical sinus. Note the migration of the developing thymus, parathyroid, and thyroid glands into the neck.

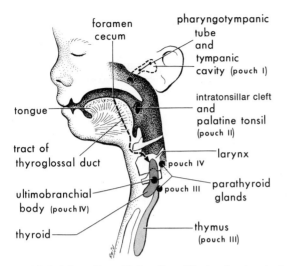

Figure 10-9. Schematic sagittal section of the head and neck of a 20-week fetus, showing the adult derivatives of the pharyngeal pouches and the descent of the thyroid gland.

portion. Its connection with the pharynx reduces to a narrow duct that soon degenerates. By the sixth week, the epithelium of each dorsal bulbar portion begins to differentiate into an *inferior parathyroid gland* (also called parathyroid III after its pouch of origin).

The epithelium of the elongate ventral portions of the two pouches proliferates, obliterating their cavities. These bilateral primordia of the thymus come together in the median plane to form the bilobed *thymus* which descends into the superior mediastinum. The bilobed form of this lymphatic organ remains throughout life, discretely encapsulated, each lobe with its own blood supply, lymphatic drainage, and nerve supply. For a discussion of its appearance in adults, see Cormack (1984) and Moore (1992). The primordia of the thymus and parathyroid glands lose their connections with the pharynx and slowly migrate caudally. Later, the parathyroid glands separate from the thymus and come to lie on the dorsal surface of the thyroid gland, which by this stage has descended from the foramen cecum of the tongue into the neck (Figs. 10-8C and 10-9).

Histogenesis of the Thymus. This gland develops from epithelial cells derived from endoderm of the third pair of pharyngeal pouches and from mesenchyme into which tubes of epithelial cells grow. The epithelial tubes soon become solid cords that proliferate and give rise to side branches. Each side branch becomes the core of a lobule of the thymus. Some cells of the epithelial cords become arranged around a central point, forming small groups of cells called *thymic (Hassall's) corpuscles* (Cormack, 1987). Other cells of the epithelial cords spread apart, but they retain connections with each other to form an *epithelial reticulum*. The mesenchyme between the epithelial cords forms thin, incomplete septa between the lobules. *Lymphocytes* soon appear and fill the interstices between the epithelial cells. The lymphocytes are derived from *hematopoietic stem cells* or a special type of immediate progeny.

The thymic primordium is surrounded by a thin layer of mesenchyme that is essential for its development. This mesenchyme, as well as certain epithelial cells in the thymus and a peculiar muscle cell in the medulla of the gland, are derived from *neural crest cells*. Extirpation of these cells in animal experiments produces a wide range of developmental defects, which also includes the thymus (Bockman and Kirby, 1984).

Growth and development of the thymus are not complete at birth. It is a relatively large organ during the perinatal period and may extend superiorly through the superior aperture of the thorax into the root of the neck. During late childhood, as puberty is reached, the thymus begins to diminish in relative size (i.e., undergoes involution). By adulthood it is often scarcely recognizable because of fat infiltrating the cortex of the gland (Steinman, 1986); however, it is still functional and important for the maintenance of health. In addition to secreting thymic hormones, the adult thymus primes thymocytes before releasing them to the periphery (Kendall, 1991).

The Fourth Pharyngeal Pouch (Figs. 10-8 and 10-9). This pouch also expands into a dorsal bulbar portion and an elongate ventral portion. Its connection with the pharynx also becomes reduced to a narrow duct that soon degenerates. By the sixth week, each dorsal portion develops into a *superior parathyroid gland* (also called parathyroid IV after its pouch of origin), which comes to lie on the dorsal surface of the thyroid gland. As described, the parathyroid glands derived from the third pouches descend with the thymus and are carried to a more inferior position than the parathyroid glands derived from the fourth pouches (Figs. 10-8 and 10-9). This explains why the parathyroid glands derived from the third pair of pouches are located inferior to those derived from the fourth pouches.

Histogenesis of the Parathyroid Glands. The epithelium of the dorsal parts of the third and fourth pouches proliferates during the fifth week and forms small nodules on the dorsal aspect of each pouch. Vascular mesenchyme soon grows into these nodules, forming a capillary network. The chief or *principal cells* differentiate during the embryonic period and are believed to become functionally active in regulating fetal calcium metabolism. The *oxyphil cells* differentiate five to seven years after birth.

The elongate ventral portion of each fourth pouch develops into an *ultimobranchial body*, which received its name because it is the last of the series of structures derived from the pharyngeal pouches. The ultimobranchial body fuses with the thyroid gland and subsequently disseminates within it to give rise to the *parafollicular cells*. They are often called *C cells* to indicate that they produce *calcitonin*, a hormone that is involved in the regulation of the normal calcium level in body fluids. The C cells differentiate from neural crest cells that migrate into these pouches from the branchial arches.

The Fifth Pharyngeal Pouch. When it develops, this rudimentary structure becomes part of the fourth pharyngeal pouch.

BRANCHIAL OR PHARYNGEAL GROOVES

The neck region of human embryos exhibits four branchial grooves (clefts) on each side from the fourth to the sixth weeks (Figs. 10–1*B* to *D*, 10–2, 10–3*A*, and 10–4). These grooves separate the branchial or pharyngeal arches externally. Only one pair of grooves contributes to adult structures. The first groove persists as the *external acoustic meatus* (Fig. 10–8 *C*). The other grooves come to lie in a slitlike depression called the *cervical sinus* and are normally obliterated with it as the neck develops (Figs. 10–4 and 10–8).

BRANCHIAL OR PHARYNGEAL MEMBRANES

These membranes appear in the bottoms of the four branchial or pharyngeal grooves on each side of the neck region of the human embryo during the fourth week (Figs. 10–1*H* and 10–3*C*). These membranes form where the epithelia of a groove and a pouch approach each other. They are temporary structures in the human embryo. The endoderm of the pouches and the ectoderm of the grooves are soon separated by mesenchyme. Only one pair of membranes contributes to the formation of adult structures. The first branchial or pharyngeal membrane, along with the intervening layer of mesenchyme, gives rise to the *tympanic membrane* (Fig. 10–8*C*).

BRANCHIAL AND PHARYNGEAL ANOMALIES

Congenital abnormalities of the head and neck mainly originate during transformation of the branchial or pharyngeal apparatus into adult structures. Most of these anomalies represent remnants of the branchial apparatus that normally disappear as the adult structures develop (Stricker et al., 1990).

Congenital Auricular Sinuses and Cysts. Small auricular sinuses (pits) and cysts are commonly found in a triangular area of skin anterior to the ear (Fig. 10–10*F*), but they may occur in other sites around the auricle or in its lobule. Although some sinuses and cysts are remnants of the first branchial or pharyngeal groove, others may represent ectodermal folds sequestered during formation of the external ear from the auricular hillocks (p. 437). These small sinuses and cysts are classified as minor malformations that are of no serious medical consequence.

Branchial Sinuses. These *lateral cervical sinuses* are uncommon, and almost all that open externally on the side of the neck result from failure of the second branchial or pharyngeal groove and the cervical sinus to obliterate (Figs. 10–10 and 10–11*B*). The blind pit, or sinus, that remains typically opens along the anterior border of the sternocleidomastoid muscle in the inferior third of the neck (Figs. 10–10*D* and *F* and 10–11*B*).

External branchial sinuses are commonly detected during infancy due to the discharge of mucous material from their orifices in the neck (Figs. 10–10*D* and 10–11*A*). These sinuses are bilateral in about ten per cent of cases and are commonly associated with auricular sinuses (described previously).

Internal branchial sinuses opening into the pharynx are very rare. Because they usually open into the intratonsillar cleft or near the palatopharyngeal arch (Fig. 10–10*D* and *F*), almost all these sinuses result from persistence of the proximal part of the second pharyngeal pouch.

Branchial Fistula (Figs. 10–10*D* and *F* and 10–11*C*). An abnormal canal that opens internally into the intratonsillar cleft and externally in the side of the neck is called a *branchial fistula*, which results from persistence of parts of the second branchial groove and second pharyngeal pouch. The fistula ascends from its cervical opening through the subcutaneous tissue, platysma muscle, and deep fascia to reach the carotid sheath (Moore, 1992). It then passes between the internal and external carotid arteries and opens into the intratonsillar cleft. In older patients there may be a disagreeable taste in the mouth due to discharge of material into the oropharynx from the fistula.

Recent studies suggest that *piriform sinus fistulae* result from persistence of remnants of the ultimobranchial body (Miyauchi et al., 1992) and that the fistulae trace the migration route of these embryonic bodies to the thyroid gland (Fig. 10–8*C*).

Branchial Cysts. The third and fourth branchial or pharyngeal arches are buried in the *cervical sinus* (Fig. 10–10*B*). Remnants of parts of the cervical sinus and/or the second branchial or pharyngeal groove may persist and form a spherical or elongate cyst (Fig. 10–10*B* and *F*). Although they may be associated with branchial sinuses and drain through them, these cysts often lie free in the neck just inferior to the angle of the mandible. They may, however, develop anywhere along the anterior border of the sternocleidomastoid muscle. Branchial cysts often do not become apparent until late childhood or early adulthood, when they produce a slowly enlarging, painless swelling in the neck (Fig. 10–12). The cysts enlarge due to an accumulation of fluid and cellular debris derived from desquamation of their

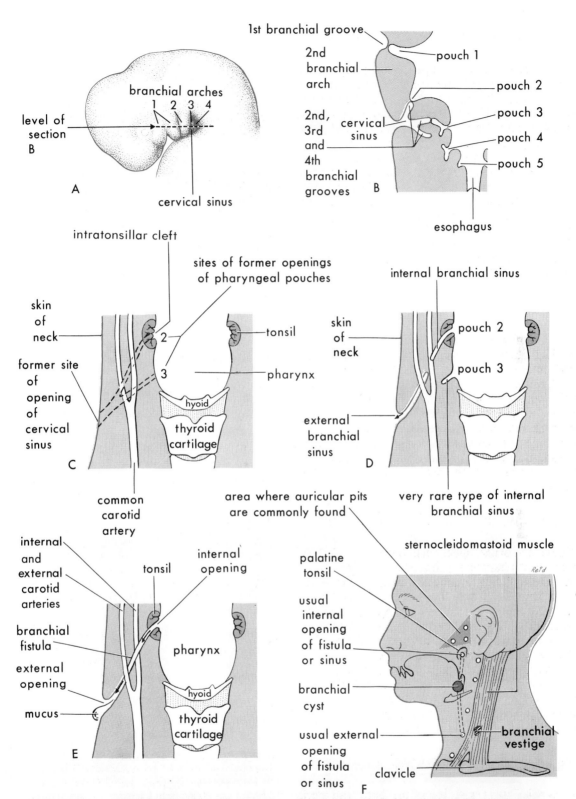

Figure 10–10. *A*, Drawing of the head and neck region of a five-week embryo showing the cervical sinus that is normally present at this stage. *B*, Horizontal section of the embryo illustrating the relationship of the cervical sinus to the branchial or pharyngeal arches and pouches. *C*, Diagrammatic sketch of the adult pharyngeal and neck regions, indicating the former sites of openings of the cervical sinus and pharyngeal pouches. The *broken lines* indicate possible courses of branchial fistulas. *D*, Similar sketch showing the embryological basis of various types of branchial sinus. *E*, Drawing of a branchial fistula resulting from persistence of parts of the second branchial or pharyngeal groove and second pharyngeal pouch. *F*, Sketch showing possible sites of branchial cysts and openings of branchial sinuses and fistulas. A branchial vestige is also illustrated (see also Fig. 10–13).

197

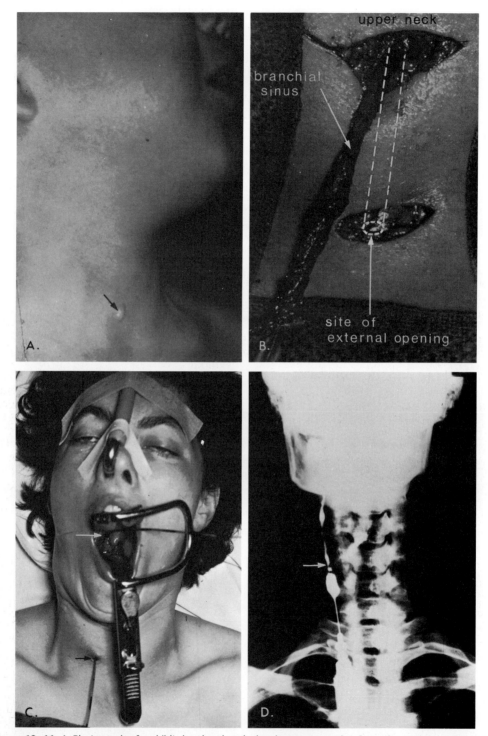

Figure 10–11. *A*, Photograph of a child's head and neck showing mucus oozing from the external opening of a branchial sinus *(arrow)*, which is located just anterior to the sternocleidomastoid muscle. *B*, Photograph of a branchial sinus taken during its excision. Its external opening in the skin of the neck and the original course of the sinus in the subcutaneous tissue are indicated by broken lines. (From Swenson O: *Pediatric Surgery*, 1958. Courtesy of Appleton-Century-Crofts). *C*, Photograph illustrating a branchial fistula in an adult female. The catheter enters the internal opening in the intratonsillar cleft *(arrow)*, passes through the fistula, and leaves through the opening in the neck *(arrow)*. *D*, Radiograph showing the course of the fistula *(arrow)* through the neck. (Courtesy of Dr. D. A. Kernahan, The Children's Memorial Hospital, Chicago.)

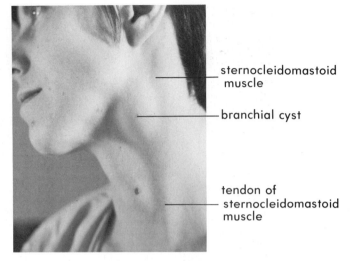

Figure 10–12. Photograph of the head and neck of a 27-year-old woman with a branchial cyst just anterior to her sternocleidomastoid muscle. The cyst was not visible at birth but developed slowly during her midtwenties. The cyst was successfully excised. (From Moore, K. L.: *Clinically Oriented Anatomy.* 3rd ed. Copyright © 1992, the Williams & Wilkins Co., Baltimore.)

sternocleidomastoid muscle

branchial cyst

tendon of sternocleidomastoid muscle

epithelial linings. These cysts have been observed in the parathyroid glands and may arise from cystic degeneration and accumulation of secretions in embryological remnants that normally disappear (Chetty and Forder, 1991).

Branchial Vestiges (Fig. 10–13). Normally the branchial cartilages disappear except for parts that form ligaments or bones (Fig. 10–5B; Table 10–1). In unusual cases, cartilaginous or bony remnants of branchial arch cartilages appear under the skin in the side of the neck. These are usually found anterior to the inferior third of the sternocleidomastoid muscle (Fig. 10–10F).

The First Arch Syndrome (Fig. 10–14). Maldevelopment of components of the *first branchial or pharyngeal arch* results in various congenital anomalies of the eyes, ears, mandible, and palate that together constitute the first arch syndrome. This set of symptoms is believed to result from insufficient migration of neural crest cells into the first arch during the fourth week. There are two main manifestations of the first arch syndrome.

In the *Treacher Collins syndrome* (mandibulofacial dysostosis), caused by an autosomal dominant gene, there is malar hypoplasia (underdevelopment of the zygomatic bones) with down-slanting palpebral fissures, defects of the lower eyelids, deformed external ears, and, sometimes, abnormalities of the middle and internal ears (van der Meulen, 1990; Gorlin et al., 1990; Behrman, 1992).

In the *Pierre Robin syndrome*, hypoplasia of the mandible, cleft palate, and defects of the eye and ear are found (van der Meulen, 1990; Gorlin et al., 1990). In the Robin morphogenetic complex, the initiating defect is a small mandible (micrognathia), which results in posterior displacement of the tongue and obstruction to the full closure of the palatine processes and a bilateral cleft palate (p. 218).

Congenital Thymic Aplasia and Absence of Parathyroid Glands (DiGeorge syndrome). Infants with these anomalies are born without thymus and parathyroid glands; but, at autopsy in some cases, ectopic glandular tissue has been found. The disease is characterized by congenital hypopara-thyroidism, increased susceptibility to infections, malformation of the mouth (shortened philtrum of lip [fish-mouth deformity]), low-set notched ears, nasal clefts, thyroid hypoplasia, and cardiac abnormalities (defects of the arch of the aorta and heart).

The *DiGeorge syndrome* occurs due to failure of the third and fourth pharyngeal pouches to differentiate into the thymus and parathyroid glands. The facial abnormalities result primarily from abnormal development of the first arch components during formation of the face and ears. There is no known genetic cause for these disturbances. The syndrome may result from a teratogen acting during the fourth to sixth weeks when the branchial arches are transforming into adult derivatives.

Accessory Thymic Tissue (Fig. 10–15). An isolated portion of thymic tissue may persist in the neck, often in close

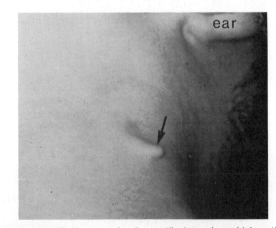

ear

Figure 10–13. Photograph of a cartilaginous branchial vestige under the skin of a child's neck. (From Raffensperger JG: Swenson's *Pediatric Surgery.* 5th ed. 1990. Courtesy of Appleton-Century-Crofts.)

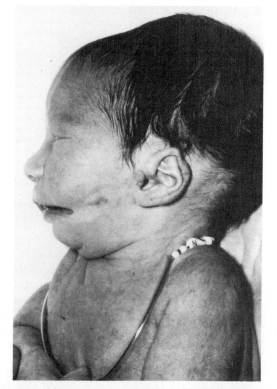

Figure 10–14. Photograph of an infant with the first arch syndrome, a pattern of anomalies resulting from insufficient migration of neural crest cells into the first branchial or pharyngeal arch. Note the following: deformed auricle of the external ear, preauricular appendage, defect in cheek between the auricle and the mouth, hypoplasia of the mandible, and macrostomia (large mouth).

association with an inferior parathyroid gland. This tissue breaks free from the thymus as it migrates caudally (Fig. 10–8*C*). Variations in the shape of the thymus occur, but they are not clinically significant. It may exhibit slender cords or prolongations into the neck on each side, anterolateral to the trachea. These processes may be connected to the inferior parathyroid glands by fibrous strands.

Ectopic Parathyroid Glands (Fig. 10–15). The parathyroids are highly variable in number (two to six) and location. They may be found anywhere near or within the thyroid gland or thymus. The superior glands are more constant in portion than the inferior ones. Occasionally, an inferior parathyroid gland fails to descend and remains near the bifurcation of the common carotid artery. In other cases, it may accompany the thymus into the thorax. Uncommonly, there are more than four parathyroid glands. *Supernumerary parathyroid glands* probably result from division of the primordia of the original glands. Absence of a parathyroid gland occurs due to failure of one of the primordia to differentiate or from atrophy of a gland early in development.

DEVELOPMENT OF THE THYROID GLAND

The thyroid is the *first endocrine gland to appear* in embryonic development. It begins to develop about 24 days after fertilization from a median endodermal thickening in the floor of the primitive pharynx (Fig. 10–16). This thickening soon forms a downgrowth or outpouching known as the **thyroid diverticulum** (Figs. 10–2*B*, 10–7*A*, and 10–15*A*). As the embryo and tongue grow, the developing thyroid gland descends

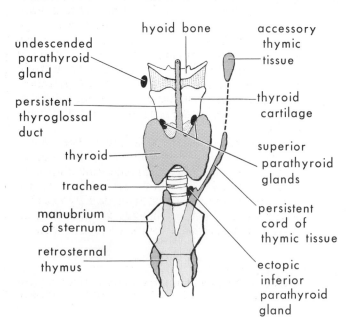

Figure 10–15. Drawing of an anterior view of the thyroid, thymus, and parathyroid glands illustrating various congenital anomalies that may occur.

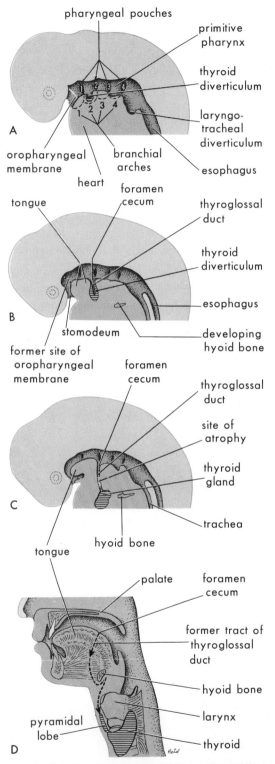

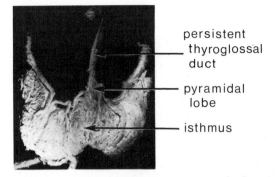

Figure 10–17. Photograph of the anterior surface of a dissected adult thyroid gland, showing persistence of the thyroglossal duct. Observe the pyramidal lobe ascending from the superior border of the isthmus. It represents a persistent portion of the inferior end of the thyroglossal duct.

in the neck, passing ventral to the developing hyoid bone and laryngeal cartilages. For a short time the developing thyroid gland is connected to the tongue by a narrow tube, the *thyroglossal duct* (Fig. 10–16*B* and *C*). The opening of this duct in the tongue is called the *foramen cecum* (see Figs. 10–20 and 10–21).

At first the thyroid diverticulum is hollow, but it soon becomes solid and divides into right and left lobes which are connected by an *isthmus* that lies anterior to the developing second and third tracheal rings. By seven weeks the thyroid gland has assumed its definitive shape and has usually reached its adult site in the anteroinferior part of the neck (Fig. 10–16*D*). By this time the thyroglossal duct has normally degenerated and disappeared. The proximal opening of the thyroglossal duct persists as a small blind pit, the *foramen cecum of the tongue* (Figs. 10–21*C* and 10–22). A *pyramidal lobe* extends superiorly from the isthmus in about 50 per cent of people (Fig. 10–16*D*). This lobe may be attached to the hyoid bone by fibrous and/or muscular tissue. A pyramidal lobe represents a persistent part of the inferior end of the thyroglossal duct (Figs. 10–16*D*, 10–17, and 10–18).

Histogenesis of the Thyroid Gland. The thyroid primordium consists of a solid mass of endodermal cells. This cellular aggregation is later broken up into a network of epithelial cords by invasion of the surrounding vascular mesenchyme (embryonic connective tissue). By the tenth week the cords have divided into small cellular groups. A lumen soon forms

Figure 10–16. *A, B,* and *C,* Schematic sagittal sections of the head and neck regions of embryos at four, five, and six weeks respectively, illustrating successive stages in the development of the thyroid gland. *D,* Drawing of a similar section of an adult head and neck showing the path taken by the thyroid gland during its embryonic descent (indicated by the former tract of the thyroglossal duct).

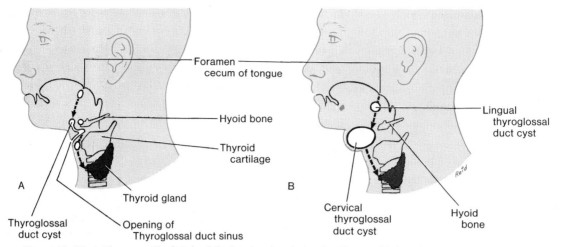

Figure 10–18. *A,* Diagrammatic sketch of the head and neck showing the possible locations of thyroglossal duct cysts. A thyroglossal duct sinus is also illustrated. The *broken line* indicates the course taken by the thyroglossal duct during descent of the developing thyroid gland from the foramen cecum in the tongue to its final position in the anterior part of the neck. *B,* Similar sketch illustrating lingual and cervical thyroglossal duct cysts. Most thyroglossal duct cysts are located just inferior to the hyoid bone (see also Fig. 10–19).

in each of these cell clusters, and the cells become arranged in a single layer around a lumen. During the eleventh week colloid begins to appear in these structures, which are now called *thyroid follicles*; thereafter, iodine concentration and the synthesis of *thyroid hormones* can be demonstrated. For a detailed account of the histogenesis of the thyroid gland, see Shepard (1975). Recent studies have shown that insulin-like growth factors, *epidermal growth factor* as well as other related factors, are involved in the replication and growth of thyroid follicular cells (Fisher and Polk, 1989).

Congenital Anomalies of the Thyroid Gland

Thyroglossal Duct Cysts and Sinuses. Cysts may form anywhere along the course followed by the thyroglossal duct during descent of the primordium of the thyroid gland from the tongue (Fig. 10–18). Normally, the thyroglossal duct atrophies and disappears, but a remnant of it may persist and form a cyst in the tongue or in the median plane of the neck, usually just inferior to the hyoid bone (Figs. 10–18*B* and 10–19). Most of these cysts are observed by the age of five years (Raffensperger, 1990). Unless the lesions become infected, most of them are asymptomatic. The swelling produced by a *thyroglossal duct cyst* usually develops as a painless, progressively enlarging, and movable mass. In some cases following infection of a cyst, a perforation of the skin occurs. This forms a *thyroglossal duct sinus* that usually opens in the median plane of the neck anterior to the laryngeal cartilages (Fig. 10–18*A*).

Ectopic Thyroid Gland. Uncommonly, the thyroid fails to descend, resulting in a *lingual thyroid* (Fig. 10–20). Incomplete descent of the thyroid results in the gland appearing high in the neck, at or just inferior to the hyoid bone. As

a rule, an ectopic thyroid gland in the median plane of the neck is the only thyroid tissue present. It is important to differentiate between this condition and a thyroglossal duct cyst (Fig. 10–19); failure to do so may result in the removal of the thyroid gland, leaving the child permanently dependent on thyroid medication (Raffensperger, 1990).

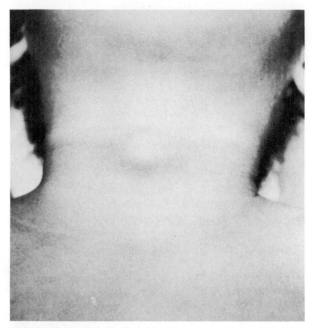

Figure 10–19. Typical thyroglossal duct cyst in a child. This rounded, firm mass was located in the median plane just inferior to the hyoid bone. From Raffensperger JG: Swenson's *Pediatric Surgery.* 5th ed. 1990, Appleton & Lange.

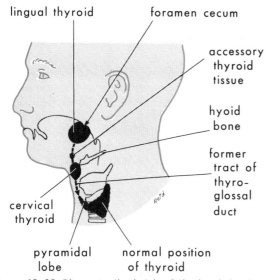

Figure 10-20. Diagrammatic sketch of the head showing the usual sites of ectopic thyroid tissue. The *broken line* indicates the path followed by the thyroid gland during its descent and the former tract of the thyroglossal duct.

Accessory thyroid tissue may appear in the tongue or in the neck superior to the thyroid gland. Although this tissue may be functional, it is often of insufficient size to maintain normal function if the thyroid gland is removed. An *accessory thyroid gland* may develop in the neck lateral to the thyroid cartilage. It usually lies on the thyrohyoid muscle (Moore, 1992). Accessory thyroid tissue and glands originate from remnants of the thyroglossal duct.

DEVELOPMENT OF THE TONGUE

Near the end of the fourth week, a median, somewhat triangular elevation appears in the floor of the primitive pharynx just rostral to the foramen cecum (Fig. 10–21*A*). This primordium of the tongue, called the *median tongue bud* (tuberculum impar), is the first indication of tongue development. Soon, two oval *distal tongue buds* (lateral lingual swellings) develop on each side of the median tongue bud. These prominences result from the proliferation of mesenchyme in the ventromedial parts of the first pair of branchial or pharyngeal arches.

The distal tongue buds rapidly increase in size, merge with each other, and overgrow the median tongue bud. The merged distal tongue buds form the anterior two thirds, or oral part, of the tongue (Fig. 10–21*C*). The plane of fusion of the distal tongue buds is indicated superficially by the *median sulcus or groove of the tongue* (Fig. 10–21*C*) and internally by the fibrous *lingual septum* (Moore, 1992). The median tongue bud forms no recognizable part of the adult tongue.

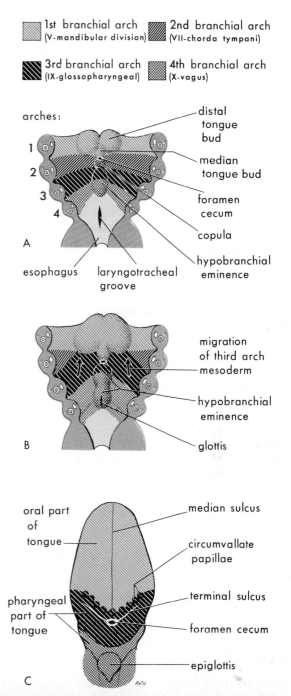

Figure 10–21. *A* and *B*, Schematic horizontal sections of the pharynx at the level shown in Figure 10–4*A*, showing successive stages in the development of the tongue during the fourth and fifth weeks. *C*, Adult tongue showing the arch derivation of the nerve supply of its mucosa.

The posterior third or *pharyngeal part of the tongue* is initially indicated by two elevations that develop caudal to the foramen cecum (Fig. 10–21*A*): (1) the *copula* (L. bond, tie), which forms by fusion of the ventromedial parts of the second pair of branchial or pharyngeal arches, and (2) the *hypobranchial eminence*, which develops caudal to the copula from mesenchyme in the ventromedial parts of the third and fourth pairs of arches. As the tongue develops, the copula is gradually overgrown by the hypobranchial eminence and disappears (Fig. 10–21*B* and *C*). As a result, the pharyngeal part of the tongue develops from the rostral part of the hypobranchial eminence, which is derived from the third pair of branchial or pharyngeal arches.

The line of fusion of the anterior and posterior parts of the tongue is roughly indicated by a V-shaped groove called the *terminal sulcus* (Figs. 10–21*C* and 10–22). Branchial arch mesenchyme forms the connective tissue and lymphatic and blood vessels of the tongue. Most of the *tongue muscles* are derived from myoblasts that migrate from the myotome regions of the *occipital somites* (Fig. 10–6*A*). The *hypoglossal nerve* (CN XII) accompanies the myoblasts during their migration and innervates the tongue muscles as they develop. The entire tongue is in the mouth at birth; its posterior third descends into the pharynx by 4 years of age (Sperber, 1989).

The Papillae and Taste Buds of the Tongue. The lingual papillae appear toward the end of the eighth week. The vallate and foliate papillae appear first, close to terminal branches of the glossopharyngeal nerve (CN IX). The fungiform papillae appear later near terminations of the chorda tympani branch of the facial nerve (CN VII). The most common lingual papillae, known as *filiform papillae* because of their threadlike shape (L. *filum*, thread), develop during the early fetal period (10 to 11 weeks). They contain afferent nerve endings that are *sensitive to touch*. For histological and anatomical details of the lingual papillae and taste buds, see Cormack (1987) and Moore (1992).

Taste buds develop during weeks 11 to 13 by inductive interaction between the epithelial cells of the tongue and invading gustatory nerve cells from the chorda tympani, glossopharyngeal, and vagus nerves (Sperber, 1989). Most taste buds form on the dorsal surface of the tongue, and some develop on the palatoglossal arches, palate, posterior surface of the epiglottis, and the posterior wall of the oropharynx. The injection of saccharine into the amniotic cavity results in increased swallowing by the fetus (Sperber, 1989). Fetal responses in the face can be induced by bitter-tasting substances at 26 to 28 weeks, indicating that reflex pathways between taste buds and facial muscles are established by this stage.

The Nerve Supply of the Tongue (Fig. 10–21). The development of the tongue explains its nerve supply. The sensory nerve supply to the mucosa of almost the entire *anterior two thirds of the tongue* (oral part) is

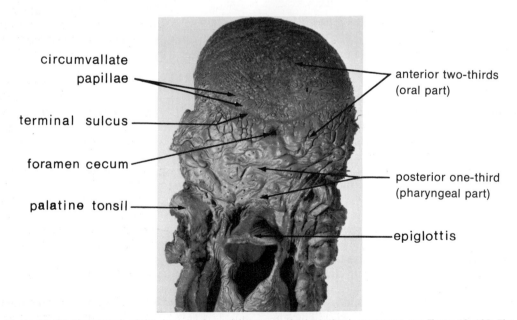

circumvallate papillae

terminal sulcus

foramen cecum

palatine tonsil

anterior two-thirds (oral part)

posterior one-third (pharyngeal part)

epiglottis

Figure 10–22. Photograph of the dorsum of an adult tongue. If orientation is necessary, see Figure 10–16*D*. The foramen cecum indicates the site of origin of the thyroid diverticulum and thyroglossal duct in the embryo. The terminal sulcus demarcates the developmentally different pharyngeal and oral parts of the tongue (see Fig. 10–21).

from the lingual branch of the mandibular division of the *trigeminal nerve* (CNV), the nerve of the first branchial or pharyngeal arch, which forms the median and distal tongue buds. Although the facial nerve is the nerve of the second branchial arch, its chorda tympani branch supplies the taste buds in the anterior two thirds of the tongue, except for the vallate papillae. Because the second arch component, the copula, is overgrown by the third arch, the facial nerve (CN VII) does not supply any of the mucosa of the tongue, except for the taste buds in the oral part of the tongue (Fig. 10–21*B* and *C*).

The *vallate papillae* in the oral part of the tongue are innervated by the *glossopharyngeal nerve* (CN IX) of the third branchial or pharyngeal arch (Fig. 10–21*C*). The reason usually given for this is that the mucosa of the posterior third of the tongue is pulled slightly anteriorly as the tongue develops. The *posterior third of the tongue* (pharyngeal part) is innervated mainly by the *glossopharyngeal nerve* of the third arch. The superior laryngeal branch of the vagus nerve (CN X) of the fourth arch supplies a small area of the tongue anterior to the epiglottis (Fig. 10–21*C*).

All **muscles of the tongue** are supplied by the *hypoglossal nerve* (CN XII), except for the palatoglossus muscle, which is supplied from the pharyngeal plexus by fibers from the *vagus nerve* (CN X).

Congenital Anomalies of the Tongue

Abnormalities of the tongue are uncommon except for fissuring of the tongue and hypertrophy of the lingual papillae, which are features of infants with Down syndrome (p. 146).

Congenital Lingual Cysts and Fistulas (Fig. 10–18). Cysts in the tongue may be derived from remnants of the thyroglossal duct. They may enlarge and produce symptoms of pharyngeal discomfort and/or *dysphagia* (difficulty in swallowing). Fistulas are derived from persistence of the thyroglossal duct; they open through the *foramen cecum* into the oral cavity (Fig. 10–22).

Ankyloglossia (Tongue-Tie). The lingual frenulum normally connects the inferior surface of the tongue to the floor of the mouth (Moore, 1992). Sometimes the frenulum is short and extends to the tip of the tongue. This interferes with its free protrusion. Tongue-tie occurs in about one in 300 North American infants but is of no functional significance (Behrman, 1992). Usually the frenulum stretches with time so that surgical correction of the anomaly is not necessary. Ankyloglossia is often found in combination with other craniofacial anomalies (van der Meulen et al., 1990).

Macroglossia. An excessively large tongue is not common. It results from generalized hypertrophy of the tongue which usually results from lymphangioma (a lymph tumor) or muscular hypertrophy. For a list of syndromes featuring macrostomia, see Jones (1988).

Microglossia. An abnormally small tongue is extremely rare and is usually associated with *micrognathia* (underdeveloped mandible and recession of the chin) and limb defects (*Hanhart's syndrome*). For a list of syndromes featuring microstomia, see Jones (1988).

Bifid or Cleft Tongue (Glossoschisis). Incomplete fusion of the distal tongue buds results in a deep median sulcus or groove in the tongue; usually the cleft does not extend to the tip of the tongue. This is a very uncommon anomaly.

DEVELOPMENT OF SALIVARY GLANDS

During the sixth and seventh weeks, these glands begin as solid epithelial proliferations or buds from the primitive oral cavity. (Fig. 10–7*C*). The club-shaped ends of these epithelial buds grow into the underlying mesenchyme. The connective tissue in the glands is derived from neural crest cells (Slavkin, 1990). All parenchymal (secretory) tissue arises by proliferation of the oral epithelium.

The *parotid glands* are the first to appear (early in the sixth week). They develop from buds that arise from the oral ectodermal lining near the angles of the stomodeum (primitive mouth). These buds grow toward the ears and branch to form solid cords with rounded ends. Later these cords are canalized (i.e., develop lumina) and become ducts by about ten weeks. The rounded ends of the cords differentiate into acini. Secretions commence at 18 weeks (Sperber, 1989). The capsule and connective tissue develop from the surrounding mesenchyme.

The *submandibular glands* appear late in the sixth week. They develop from endodermal buds from the oral epithelium in the floor of the stomodeum. Solid cellular processes grow posteriorly, lateral to the developing tongue. Later they branch and differentiate. Acini begin to form at 12 weeks and secretory activity begins at 16 weeks (Sperber, 1989). Growth of the submandibular glands continues after birth with the formation of mucous acini. Lateral to the tongue, a linear groove forms that closes over to form the *submandibular duct*.

The *sublingual glands* appear in the eighth week, two weeks later than the other salivary glands. They develop from multiple endodermal epithelial buds in the paralingual sulcus (Fig. 10–7*C*). These buds branch and canalize to form 10 to 12 ducts that open independently into the floor of the mouth.

DEVELOPMENT OF THE FACE

The facial primordia begin to appear early in the fourth week around the rather large *stomodeum*, which constitutes the primitive mouth (Figs. 10–1*E*, 10–2, 10–23*A*, and 10–24). Facial development

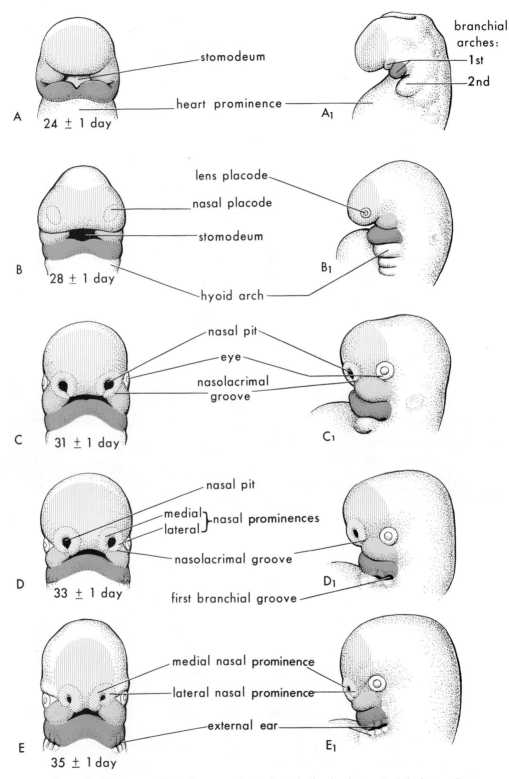

□ frontonasal prominence   ▨ maxillary prominence   ▨ mandibular prominence

Figure 10–23. Diagrams illustrating progressive stages in the development of the human face.

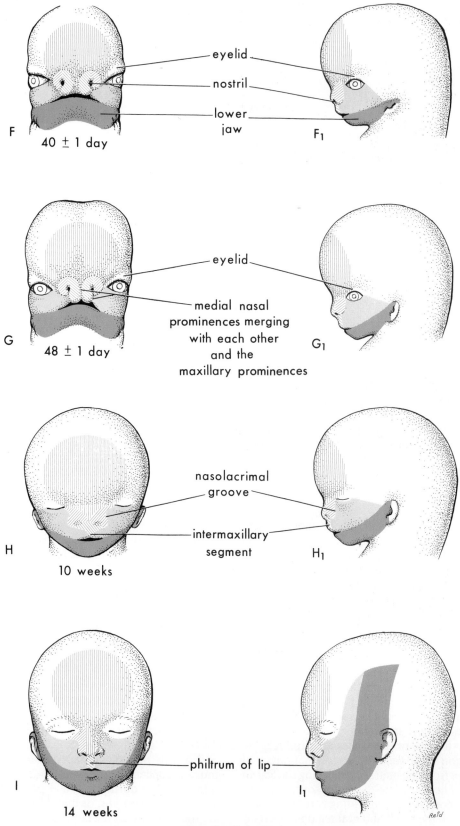

F   F₁

eyelid

nostril

lower jaw

40 ± 1 day

G   G₁

eyelid

medial nasal prominences merging with each other and the maxillary prominences

48 ± 1 day

H   H₁

nasolacrimal groove

intermaxillary segment

10 weeks

I   I₁

philtrum of lip

14 weeks

Reid

Figure 10–23 Continued

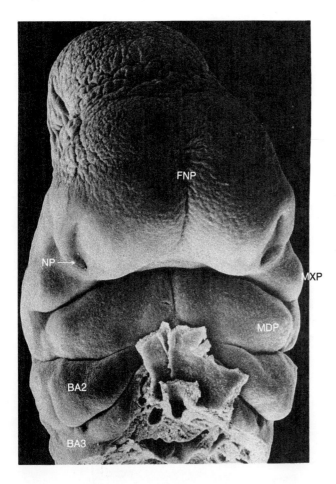

Figure 10–24. Scanning electron micrograph of a ventral view of a human embryo of about 33 days (stage 15, 8.00 mm). Observe the prominent frontonasal process (FNP) surrounding the telencephalon (forebrain). Also observe the nasal pits (NP) located in the ventrolateral regions of the frontonasal prominence (see also Fig. 10–23C). Medial and lateral nasal prominences surround these pits. The cuneiform, wedge-shaped, maxillary prominences (MXP) form the lateral boundaries of the primitive oral cavity or stomodeum. The fusing mandibular prominences (MDP) are located just caudal to the stomodeum. The second (hyoid) branchial or pharyngeal arch (BA2) is clearly visible and shows overhanging margins (opercula). The third branchial or pharyngeal arch (BA3) is also clearly visible (see also Fig. 10–23B₁). (From Hinrichsen K: *The early development of morphology and patterns of the face in the human embryo. In Advances in Anatomy, Embryology and Cell Biology.* Vol. 98. New York, Springer-Verlag, 1985).

depends upon the inductive influence of the prosencephalic and rhombencephalic **organizing centers** (Sperber, 1989). The *prosencephalic organizing center*, derived from prochordal mesoderm that migrates from the primitive streak (p. 53), is located rostral to the notochord and ventral to the prosencephalon or forebrain (Chapter 18). The *rhombencephalic organizing center* is ventral to the rhombencephalon (hindbrain).

The *five facial primordia* appear as prominences around the stomodeum (Figs. 10–1E, 10–24, and 10–25). The facial prominences are the single median frontonasal prominence and the paired maxillary and mandibular prominences. The paired prominences are derivatives of the first pair of branchial or pharyngeal arches. All these prominences are produced by the proliferation of the *neural crest cells* that migrated into the arches from the neural crest during the fourth week (p. 71). These cells are the major source of connective tissue components including cartilage, bone, and ligaments in the facial and oral regions (Sperber, 1989).

The single *frontonasal prominence* (FNP) surrounds the ventrolateral part of the forebrain which gives rise to the *optic vesicles* (p. 423) that form the eyes (Fig. 10–23C). The frontal portion of the FNP forms the forehead; the nasal part constitutes the rostral boundary of the stomodeum and forms the nose.

The paired *maxillary prominences* form the lateral boundaries of the stomodeum, and the paired *mandibular prominences* constitute the caudal boundary of the primitive mouth. The five facial prominences are active **centers of growth** in the underlying mesenchyme. This mesenchyme is continuous from one prominence to the other.

Facial development occurs mainly between the fourth and eighth weeks (Fig. 10–23A to G). By the end of this period, the face has an unquestionably human appearance (see Fig. 5–21). Facial proportions develop during the fetal period (Fig. 10–23H and I). The *lower jaw*, or mandible, and the lower lip are the first parts of the face to form. They result from merging of the medial ends of the two mandibular

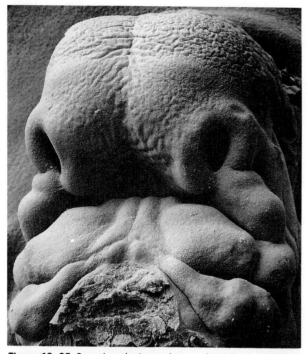

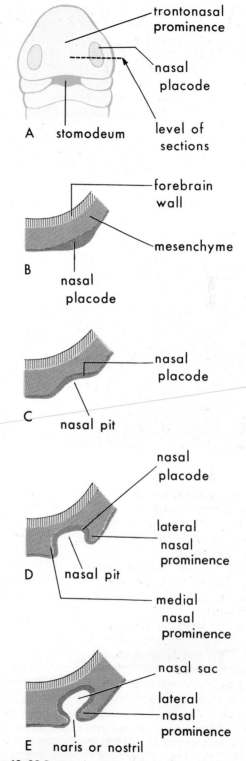

Figure 10–25. Scanning electron micrograph of the craniofacial region of a human embryo of about 37 days (stage 16, 10.5 mm). The wide stomodeum is limited caudally by the fused mandibular prominences. The nasal pits are surrounded by the medial and lateral nasal prominences and the maxillary prominences. At this stage the medial nasal prominences have not merged, but the mandibular prominences have fused. (From Hinrichsen K: *The early development of morphology and patterns of the face in the human embryo. In Advances in Anatomy, Embryology and Cell Biology.* Vol. 98. New York, Springer-Verlag, 1985.)

prominences in the median plane during the fourth week (Figs. 10–23*A* and *B*, 10–24, and 10–25).

By the end of the fourth week, bilateral oval thickenings of the surface ectoderm, called *nasal placodes* (primordia of the nose and nasal cavities), have developed on the ventrolateral parts of the frontonasal prominence (Figs. 10–1*G*, 10–23*B*, and 10–26*A*). Initially these placodes are convex, but later they are stretched to produce flat depressions in the placodes (Hinrichsen, 1985). Mesenchyme in the margins of these placodes proliferates, producing horseshoe-shaped elevations called *medial and lateral nasal prominences.* As a result, the nasal placodes now lie in depressions called *nasal pits* (Figs. 10–23*C* and 10–26*C* and *D*). These pits are the primordia of the anterior nares (nostrils) and the nasal cavities.

Proliferation of mesenchyme in the maxillary prominences causes them to enlarge and grow medially toward each other and the nasal prominences (Figs. 10–23*D* and *E*, 10–24, and 10–25). The medial migration of the maxillary prominences moves

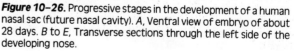

Figure 10–26. Progressive stages in the development of a human nasal sac (future nasal cavity). *A,* Ventral view of embryo of about 28 days. *B* to *E,* Transverse sections through the left side of the developing nose.

the medial nasal prominences toward the median plane and each other. Each lateral nasal prominence is separated from the maxillary prominence by a cleft called the *nasolacrimal groove* (Figs. 10–23*C* and *D*, 10–27, 10–28, and 10–29*A*).

By the end of the fifth week, the primordia of the *auricles* of the external ears have begun to develop (Figs. 10–23*E*₁ and 10–27). *Six auricular hillocks* (small elevations) form around the first branchial or pharyngeal groove (Fig. 10–27), the primordium of the external acoustic meatus (canal). *By the end of the sixth week*, each maxillary prominence has begun to merge with the lateral nasal prominence along the line of the *nasolacrimal groove* (Figs. 10–28 and 10–29). This establishes continuity between the side of the nose, formed by the lateral nasal prominence, and the cheek region formed by the maxillary prominence.

The *nasolacrimal duct* develops from a rodlike thickening of the ectoderm in the floor of the naso-

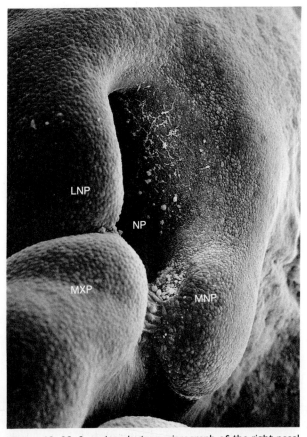

Figure 10–28. Scanning electron micrograph of the right nasal region of a human embryo of about 41 days (stage 17, 10.8 mm) showing the maxillary prominence (MXP) fusing with the medial nasal prominence (MNP). Epithelial bridges can be seen between these prominences. Observe the furrow representing the naso-lacrimal groove between the MXP and the lateral nasal promi-nence (LNP). (From Hinrichsen K: *The early development of mor-phology and patterns of the face in the human embryo. In Advances in Anatomy, Embryology and Cell Biology.* Vol. 98. New York, Springer-Verlag, 1985). Observe the large nasal pit (NP).

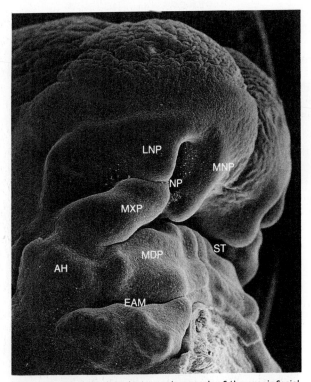

Figure 10–27. Scanning electron micrograph of the craniofacial region of a human embryo of about 41 days (stage 16, 10.8 mm), viewed obliquely. The maxillary prominence (MXP) appears puffed up laterally and is wedged between the lateral (LNP) and medial (MNP) nasal prominences surrounding the nasal pit (NP). The auric-ular hillocks can be seen on both sides of the groove between the mandibular and hyoid arches, which will form the external acous-tic meatus (EAM). (From Hinrichsen K: *The early development of morphology and patterns of the face in the human embryo. In Advances in Anatomy, Embryology and Cell Biology.* Vol. 98. New York, Springer-Verlag, 1985).

lacrimal groove. This thickening gives rise to a solid epithelial cord that separates from the ectoderm and sinks into the mesenchyme. Later, as a result of cell degeneration, this epithelial cord canalizes to form the nasolacrimal duct; its cranial end expands to form the *lacrimal sac* of the eye. By the late fetal period, the nasolacrimal duct drains into the inferior meatus in the lateral wall of the nasal cavity (Moore, 1992). The duct becomes completely patent only after birth. Part of this duct occasionally fails to canalize, resulting in a congenital defect known as *atresia of the nasolacri-mal duct.*

During the seventh week, there is a shift in the blood supply of the face from the internal to the exter-nal carotid artery (Sperber, 1989). This change is re-lated to transformation of the primitive aortic arch pattern into the postnatal arterial arrangement (p. 335). Between the seventh and tenth weeks, the medial nasal prominences merge with each other and the maxillary and lateral nasal prominences (Figs. 10–23H and G and 10–29). Merging of these prominences requires disintegration of their contacting surface epithelia. This results in intermingling of the underlying mesenchymal cells.

Merging of the medial nasal and maxillary prominences results in continuity of the upper jaw and lip and separation of the nasal pits from the stomodeum (Figs. 10–23H and 10–29). As the medial nasal prominences merge, they form an *intermaxillary segment* (Figs. 10–23H and 10–29E). This segment gives rise to: (1) the vertical groove or *philtrum* of the lip, (2) the premaxillary part of the maxilla and its

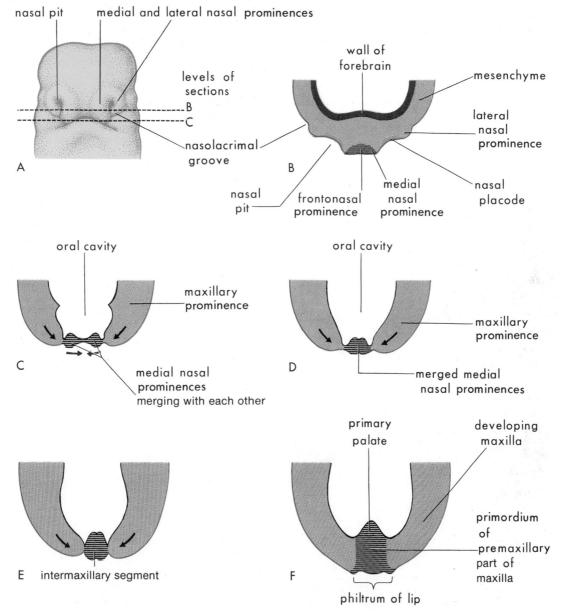

Figure 10–29. Diagrams illustrating early development of the maxilla, palate, and upper lip. *A,* Facial view of a five-week embryo. *B* and *C,* Sketches of horizontal sections at the levels shown in *A.* The arrows in *C* indicate subsequent growth of the maxillary and medial nasal prominences toward the median plane and merging of the prominences with each other (see also Fig. 10–28). *D* to *F,* Similar sections of older embryos illustrating merging of the medial nasal prominences with each other and the maxillary prominences to form the upper lip. (Modified from Patten, 1961.)

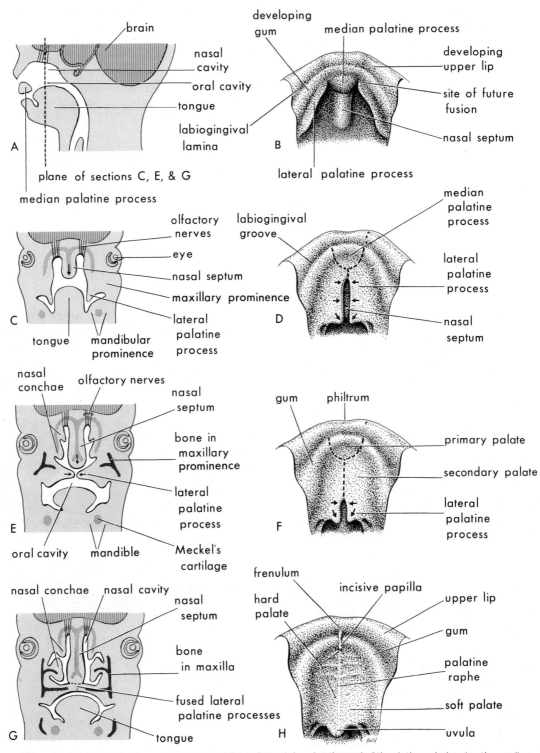

Figure 10–30. *A*, Sketch of a sagittal section of the embryonic head at the end of the sixth week showing the median palatine process or primary palate. *B, D, F,* and *H,* Drawings of the roof of the mouth from the sixth to twelfth weeks illustrating development of the palate. The broken lines in *D* and *F* indicate sites of fusion of the palatine processes. The arrows indicate medial and posterior growth of the lateral palatine processes or palatal shelves. *C, E,* and *G,* Drawings of frontal sections of the head illustrating fusion of the lateral palatine processes or palatal shelves with each other and the nasal septum, and separation of the nasal and oral cavities.

associated gingiva (gum), and (3) the *primary palate* (Figs. 10–29*F*, 10–30, and 10–31*B*).

Lateral parts of the upper lip, most of the maxilla, and the secondary palate form from the maxillary prominences (Figs. 10–23*H* and 10–30). These prominences merge laterally with the mandibular prominences. The primitive lips and cheeks are invaded by mesenchyme from the second pair of branchial or pharyngeal arches, which differentiates into the facial muscles (Fig. 10–6; Table 10–1). These *muscles of facial expression* are supplied by the facial nerve (CN VII), the nerve of the second arch. The mesenchyme in the first pair of arches differentiates into the *muscles of mastication* and a few others, all of which are innervated by the trigeminal nerves (CN V), which supply the first pair of arches (Fig. 10–6; Table 10–1).

In summary, the *frontonasal prominence* forms the forehead and the dorsum and apex of the nose. The sides (alae) of the nose are derived from the *lateral nasal prominences* (Fig. 10–23*H* and *I*), and the *nasal septum* is formed from the medial nasal prominences (Fig. 10–30*C*, *D*, and *E*). The *maxillary prominences* form the upper cheek regions and most of the upper lip (Fig. 10–23*I*). The *mandibular prominences* give rise to the chin, lower lip, and lower cheek regions. In addition to these fleshy derivatives, various bones are formed from the mesenchyme in the facial prominences (Fig. 10–5).

Until the end of the sixth week, the primitive jaws are composed of masses of mesenchymal tissue (embryonic connective tissue). The lips and *gingivae* (gums) begin to develop when a linear thickening of ectoderm, the *labiogingival lamina*, grows into the underlying mesenchyme (Fig. 10–30*B*). Gradually, most of the lamina degenerates, leaving a *labiogingi-val groove* (*lip sulcus*) between the lips and the gingivae (Fig. 10–30*H*). A small area of the labiogingival lamina persists in the median plane to form the *lingual frenulum*, which attaches the lip to the gingiva.

Final development of the face occurs slowly and results mainly from changes in the proportion and relative positions of the facial components. During the early fetal period, the nose is flat and the mandible is underdeveloped (Fig. 10–23*H*); they obtain their characteristic form as facial development is completed (Fig. 10–23*I*). As the brain enlarges it creates a prominent forehead, the eyes move medially, and the external ears rise. *The smallness of the face prenatally results* from: (1) the rudimentary upper and lower jaws, (2) the unerupted primary teeth, and (3) the small size of the nasal cavities and maxillary sinuses (Sandham and Nelson, 1985; Vermeij-Keers, 1990).

DEVELOPMENT OF NASAL CAVITIES

As the face develops, the *nasal placodes* become depressed, forming *nasal pits* (Figs. 10–23*C* to 10–26 and 10–28). Proliferation of the surrounding mesenchyme forms the medial and lateral *nasal prominences*, which results in deepening of the nasal pits and formation of primitive *nasal sacs* (Figs. 10–25 and 10–26*E*). Each nasal sac grows dorsally, ventral to the developing forebrain (Fig. 10–32*A*). At first the nasal sacs are separated from the oral cavity by the *oronasal membrane* (Fig. 10–32*A* and *B*). This membrane soon ruptures, bringing the nasal and oral cavities into communication (Fig. 10–32*C*). The regions of continuity are the *primitive choanae* (openings between the nasal cavity and the nasopharynx), which lie posterior to the primary palate (Fig. 10–32*C*).

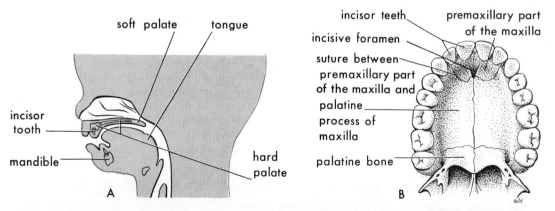

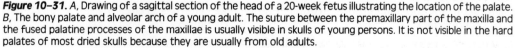

Figure 10–31. *A*, Drawing of a sagittal section of the head of a 20-week fetus illustrating the location of the palate. *B*, The bony palate and alveolar arch of a young adult. The suture between the premaxillary part of the maxilla and the fused palatine processes of the maxillae is usually visible in skulls of young persons. It is not visible in the hard palates of most dried skulls because they are usually from old adults.

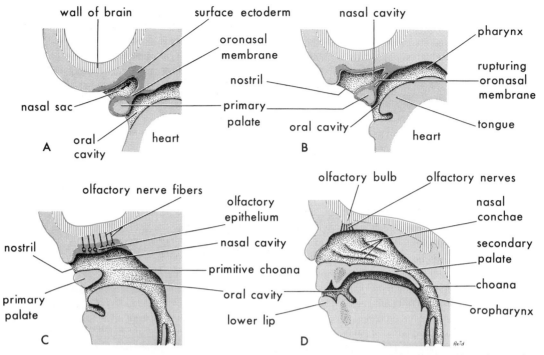

Figure 10–32. Drawings of sagittal sections of the head showing development of the nasal cavities. The nasal septum has been removed. *A*, Five weeks. *B*, Six weeks, showing breakdown of the oronasal membrane. *C*, Seven weeks, showing the nasal cavity communicating with the oral cavity and development of the olfactory epithelium. *D*, Twelve weeks, showing the palate and the lateral wall of the nasal cavity.

After the *secondary palate* develops, the choanae are located at the junction of the nasal cavity and the nasopharynx (Fig. 10–32*D*). This occurs when the lateral palatine processes fuse with each other and the nasal septum (Fig. 10–30*G*).

While these changes are occurring, the *superior, middle, and inferior conchae* develop as elevations on the lateral walls of the nasal cavities (Figs. 10–30*E* and 10–32*D*). Concurrently, the ectodermal epithelium in the roof of each nasal cavity becomes specialized to form the *olfactory epithelium* (Fig. 10–33). Some epithelial cells differentiate into *olfactory receptor cells* (neurons). The axons of these cells constitute the *olfactory nerves*, which grow into the *olfactory bulbs* of the brain (Figs. 10–30*G* and 10–32*D*).

The Paranasal Sinuses

Some paranasal (air) sinuses develop during late fetal life; the remainder develop after birth. They form as outgrowths or diverticula of the walls of the nasal cavities and become pneumatic (air-filled) extensions of the nasal cavities in the adjacent bones, e.g., the maxillary sinuses in the maxillae and the frontal sinuses in the frontal bones. The original openings of the outgrowths persist as the orifices of the adult sinuses (Moore, 1992).

Most of the paranasal sinuses are rudimentary or absent in newborn infants. The *maxillary sinuses* are small at birth (about 3 to 4 mm in diameter), and there are only a few small anterior and posterior ethmoidal cells. The maxillary sinuses grow slowly until puberty and are not fully developed until all the permanent teeth have erupted in early adulthood. No frontal or sphenoidal sinuses are present at birth. The ethmoidal cells (sinuses) are small before the age of two years, and they do not begin to grow rapidly until six to eight years of age.

Around the age of 2 years, the two most anterior ethmoidal cells grow into the frontal bone, forming a frontal sinus on each side. Usually the *frontal sinuses* are visible in radiographs by the seventh year. The septum between the right and left frontal sinuses is rarely in the median plane. The two most posterior ethmoidal cells grow into the sphenoid bone at about the age of 2 years, forming two *sphenoidal sinuses*. In adults the sphenoidal sinuses vary greatly in size (Moore, 1992). Growth of the paranasal sinuses is important in altering the size and shape of the face during infancy and childhood, and in adding resonance to the voice during adolescence.

The Vomeronasal Organs (Fig. 10–33). From the sixth to the eighth week, the nasal epithelium invaginates the nasal septum just superior to the primitive palate to form bilateral diverticula known as the *vomeronasal organs* (of Jacobson). These vestigial *chemosensory structures* form blind pouches which reach their greatest development by the twenty-fifth week. A *vomeronasal cartilage* develops ventral to each of these organs. The vomeronasal organs are lined by neurosensory epithelium similar to the olfactory epithelium. A vomeronasal nerve projects to a small accessory olfactory bulb. During late fetal life the vomeronasal organs begin to regress and usually disappear completely along with their nerves and accessory bulbs.

The *vomeronasal cartilages* are usually the only adult remnants of these vestigial organs. These narrow strips of cartilage are located between the inferior edge of the

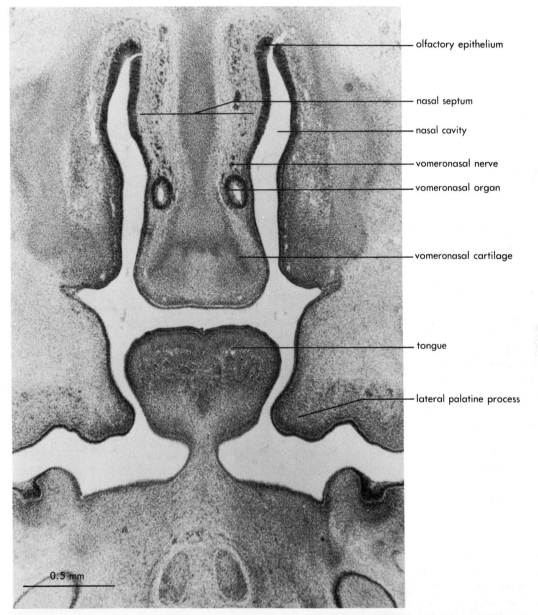

Figure 10–33. Photomicrograph of a frontal section through the developing mouth and nasal regions of a 22-mm human embryo of about 54 days (× c. 50). (Courtesy of Dr. Kunwar Bhatnagar, Professor of Anatomy, School of Medicine, University of Louisville, Louisville, Kentucky.)

cartilage of the nasal septum and the vomer (Moore, 1992).

Remnants of one or both vomeronasal organs may give rise to cysts that present wide orifices opening into the nasal vestibule on each side of the nasal septum. The remnants of these organs usually remain undetected and asymptomatic; but, in some cases, they have been linked with various pathological conditions (Gabriele, 1967). Although *atavistic remnants* in humans, the vomeronasal organs are well developed in other mammals and are olfactory chemoreceptor organs that aid the sense of smell (Bhatnagar, 1991).

DEVELOPMENT OF THE PALATE

The palate develops from two palatal primordia: the *primary palate* and the *secondary palate*. Although palatogenesis begins at the end of the fifth week, development of the palate is not complete until the twelfth week. Its *critical period of development* is from the end of the sixth week until the beginning of the ninth week (see Fig. 8–13).

The Primary Palate

Early in the sixth week the primary palate (median palatine process) begins to develop from the deep part of the *intermaxillary segment of the maxilla* (Fig. 10–29F). Initially this segment, formed by internal merging of the medial nasal prominences, is a wedge-shaped mass of mesenchyme between the internal surfaces of the maxillary prominences of the developing maxillae. The primary palate forms the *premaxillary part of the maxilla* (Figs. 10–29 and 10–31B). It represents only a small part of the adult hard palate (i.e., the part anterior to the incisive foramen that lodges the incisor teeth).

The Secondary Palate

The secondary palate is the primordium of the hard and soft parts of the palate that extend posteriorly from the incisive foramen (Figs. 10–30 to 10–32). The secondary palate begins to develop early in the sixth week from two mesenchymal projections that extend from the internal aspects of the maxillary prominences. Initially these shelflike structures, called *lateral palatine processes* (also known as *palatal shelves*), project inferomedially on each side of the tongue (Figs. 10–30C and 10–33). As the jaws develop, the tongue becomes relatively smaller and moves inferiorly.

As *palatogenesis* proceeds during the seventh and eighth weeks, the lateral palatine processes or palatal shelves elongate and ascend to a horizontal position superior to the tongue (Sandham, 1985a and c).

Gradually the processes or shelves approach each other and fuse in the median plane (Fig. 10–30 E to H and 10–34C). They also fuse with the nasal septum and the posterior part of the primary palate. Elevation of the palatal shelves to the horizontal position is believed to be caused by an intrinsic *shelf elevating force* that is generated by the hydration of hyaluronic acid in the mesenchymal cells within the palatal shelves (Ferguson, 1988).

The *nasal septum* develops as a downgrowth from internal parts of the merged medial nasal prominences (Fig. 10–30). The fusion between the nasal septum and the palatine processes begins anteriorly during the ninth week and is completed posteriorly by the twelfth week, superior to the primordium of the hard palate.

Bone gradually develops in the primary palate, forming the premaxillary part of the maxilla, which lodges the incisor teeth (Fig. 10–31B). Concurrently, bone extends from the maxillae and palatine bones into the lateral palatine processes (palatal shelves) to form the *hard palate* (Figs. 10–30C and 10–31B). The posterior parts of these processes do not become ossified. They extend posteriorly beyond the nasal septum and fuse to form the *soft palate* and its soft conical projection called the *uvula* (Fig. 10–30D, F, and H). The *palatine raphe* permanently indicates the line of fusion of the lateral palatine processes or palatal shelves during the sixth to twelfth weeks (Fig. 10–30H).

A small *nasopalatine canal* persists in the median plane of the palate between the premaxillary part of the maxilla and the palatine processes of the maxillae. This canal is represented in the adult hard palate by the *incisive fossa* (Fig. 10–31B), which is the common opening for the right and left *incisive canals* (Moore, 1992). An irregular suture runs from the incisive fossa to the alveolar process of the maxilla, between the lateral incisor and canine teeth on each side. It is visible in the anterior region of the palates of young persons (Fig. 10–31B). This suture indicates where the embryonic primary and secondary palates fused and where clefts of the anterior palate occur (Fig. 10–37G).

Cleft Lip and Palate

Clefts of the upper lip and palate are common (Sandham, 1985b; Thompson et al., 1991), and they are usually classified according to developmental criteria, with the incisive foramen as a reference landmark. These defects are especially conspicuous because they result in an abnormal facial appearance and defective speech. There are *two major groups of cleft lip and palate*: (1) clefts involving the upper lip and anterior part of the maxilla, with or without involvement of parts of the remaining hard and soft regions of the

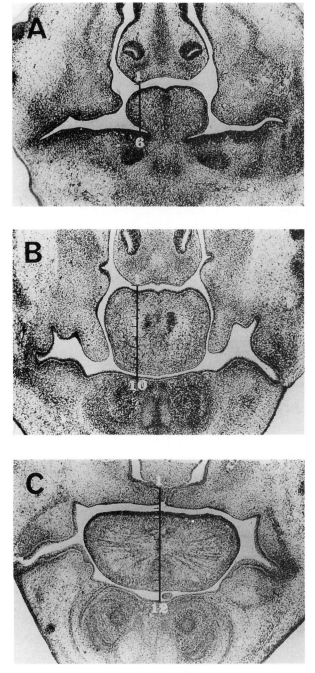

Figure 10–34. Frontal or coronal sections of human embryonic heads showing palatal shelf development during the eighth week. *A*, Embryo with a CRL of 24 mm. This section shows early development of the lateral palatine processes (palatal shelves). The scale shows 6 units from the lowest point of the nasal septum to the floor of the oral cavity. *B*, Embryo with a CRL of 27 mm. This section shows the palate just prior to palatal process or shelf elevation. The scale shows 10 units from the lowest point of the nasal septum to the floor of the oral cavity. *C*, Embryo with a CRL of 29 mm (near the end of the eighth week). The palatine processes or palatal shelves are elevated and fused. The scale shows

palate, and (2) clefts involving the hard and soft regions of the palate (see Pfeifer [1991] for a comprehensive review of craniofacial abnormalities including palatal clefting).

A complete cleft palate indicates the maximum degree of clefting of any particular type; for example, a *complete cleft of the posterior palate* (Fig. 10–37*C* and *D*) is an anomaly in which the cleft extends through the soft palate and anteriorly to the incisive foramen. The landmark for distinguishing anterior from posterior cleft anomalies is the *incisive foramen* (Fig. 10–31*B*). Anterior and posterior cleft anomalies are embryologically distinct.

Anterior cleft anomalies include cleft lip, with or without a cleft of the alveolar part of the maxilla. A complete anterior cleft anomaly is one in which the cleft extends through the lip and the alveolar part of the maxilla to the incisive foramen, separating the anterior and posterior parts of the palate. Anterior cleft anomalies result from a deficiency of mesenchyme in the maxillary prominence(s) and the intermaxillary segment (Fig. 10–29*E*).

Posterior cleft anomalies include clefts of the secondary or posterior palate that extend through the soft palate and the hard palate to the incisive foramen, separating the anterior and posterior parts of the palate. Posterior cleft anomalies are caused by defective development of the secondary palate and result from growth distortions of the lateral palatine processes (palatal shelves), which prevent their medial migration and fusion.

Cleft Lip (Figs. 10–35 and 10–36). Clefts involving the upper lip, with or without cleft palate, occur about once in 1000 births, but their frequency varies widely among ethnic groups (Thompson et al., 1991); 60 to 80 per cent of affected infants are males. The clefts vary from small notches of the vermilion border of the lip (Fig. 10–35*B*) to larger ones that extend into the floor of the nostril and through the alveolar part of the maxilla (Fig. 10–35*A*, *C*, and *D*). Cleft lip may be either unilateral or bilateral.

Unilateral cleft lip (Fig 10–35*A* and *B*) results from failure of the maxillary prominence on the affected side to unite with the merged medial nasal prominences (Fig. 10–36*C* to *H*). This is the consequence of failure of the mesenchymal masses to merge and the mesenchyme to proliferate and smooth out the overlying epithelium (Fig. 10–36*D*, *F*, and *H*). This results in a *persistent labial groove*. In addition, the epithelium in the labial groove becomes stretched, and the tissues in the floor of the persistent groove break down. As a result, the lip is divided into medial and lateral parts (Figs. 10–35*A* and 10–36 *G* and *H*). Sometimes a bridge of tissue called a *Simonart's band* joins the parts of the incomplete cleft lip (Fig. 10–35*B*).

Bilateral cleft lip (Fig. 10–35*C* and *D*) results from failure of the mesenchymal masses in the maxillary prominences to meet and unite with the merged medial nasal prominences. The epithelium in both labial grooves becomes stretched and breaks down. In bilateral clefts the

---

12 units from the lowest point of the nasal septum to the floor of the oral cavity. (From Sandham A: *Early Human Develop 12*:241, 1985c).

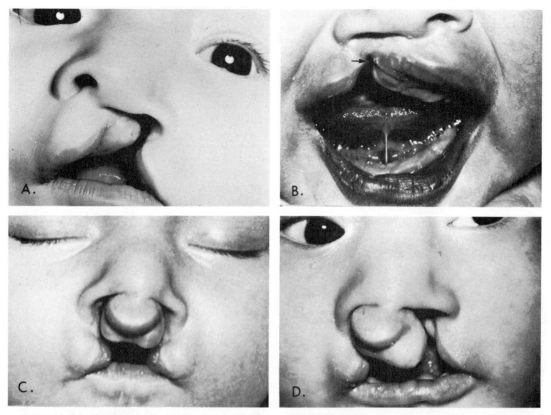

Figure 10–35. Photographs illustrating various types of cleft lip. *A* and *B*, Unilateral cleft lip. The cleft in *B* is incomplete; the *arrow* indicates a band of tissue (Simonart's band) connecting the cleft parts of the lip. *C* and *D*, Bilateral cleft lip. (Courtesy of Dr. D. A. Kernahan, The Children's Memorial Hospital, Chicago.)

defects may be dissimilar, with varying degrees of defect on each side. When there is a complete bilateral cleft of the lip and alveolar part of the maxilla, the intermaxillary segment hangs free and projects anteriorly (Figs. 10–35*C* and 10–38*B*). These defects are especially deforming because of the loss of continuity of the *orbicularis oris muscle*, which closes the mouth and purses the lips, as occurs in whistling (Moore, 1992).

Median Cleft Lip (Fig. 10–39 A) Median cleft of the upper lip, an extremely rare defect, results from a mesenchymal deficiency that causes partial or complete failure of the medial nasal prominences to merge and form the intermaxillary segment. A median cleft of the lip is a characteristic feature of the *Mohr syndrome*, which is transmitted as an autosomal recessive trait (Gorlin et al., 1990). Median cleft of the lower lip (Fig. 10–39*B*) is also very rare and is caused by failure of the mesenchymal masses in the mandibular prominences to merge completely and smooth out the embryonic cleft between them (Fig. 10–23*A*).

Cleft Palate (Figs. 10–37 and 10–38). Cleft palate, with or without cleft lip, occurs about once in 2500 births and is more common in females than in males. The cleft may involve only the uvula, giving it a fishtail appearance (Fig. 10–37*B*), or it may extend through the soft and hard regions of the palate (Figs. 10–37*C* and *D* and 10–38*C* and *D*). In severe cases associated with cleft lip, the cleft palate

Figure 10–36. Drawings illustrating the embryological basis of complete unilateral cleft lip. *A*, Five-week embryo. *B*, Horizontal section through the head illustrating the grooves between the maxillary prominences and the merging medial nasal prominences. *C*, Six-week embryo showing a persistent labial groove on the left side. *D*, Horizontal section through the head showing the groove gradually filling in on the right side following proliferation of mesenchyme (arrows). *E*, Seven-week embryo. *F*, Horizontal section through the head showing that the epithelium on the right has almost been pushed out of the groove between the maxillary prominence and medial nasal prominence. *G*, Ten-week fetus with a complete unilateral cleft lip. *H*, Horizontal section through the head after stretching of the epithelium and breakdown of the tissues in the floor of the persistent labial groove on the left side, forming a complete unilateral cleft lip.

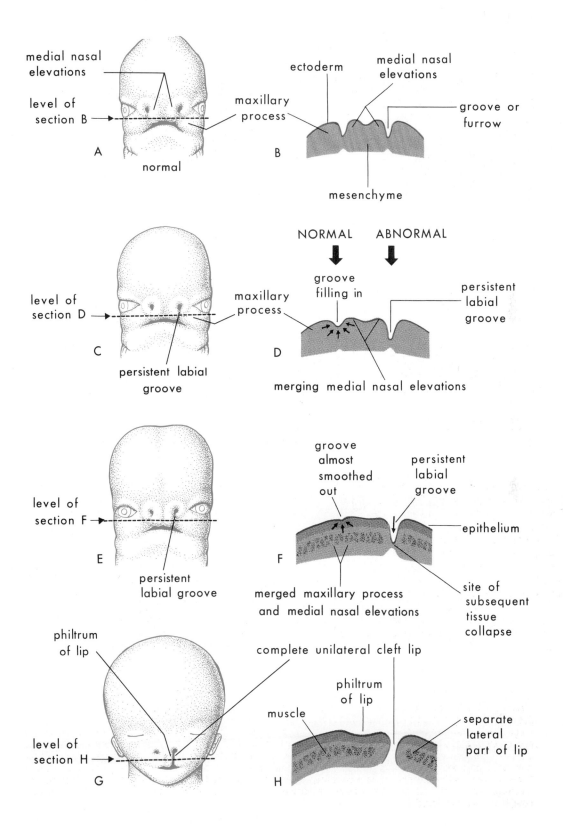

medial nasal elevations

level of section B →

maxillary process

A   normal

ectoderm

medial nasal elevations

groove or furrow

B

mesenchyme

level of section D →

maxillary process

C

persistent labial groove

NORMAL   ABNORMAL

groove filling in

persistent labial groove

D

merging medial nasal elevations

level of section F →

E

persistent labial groove

groove almost smoothed out

persistent labial groove

epithelium

F

merged maxillary process and medial nasal elevations

site of subsequent tissue collapse

philtrum of lip

complete unilateral cleft lip

philtrum of lip

muscle

level of section H →

G

separate lateral part of lip

H

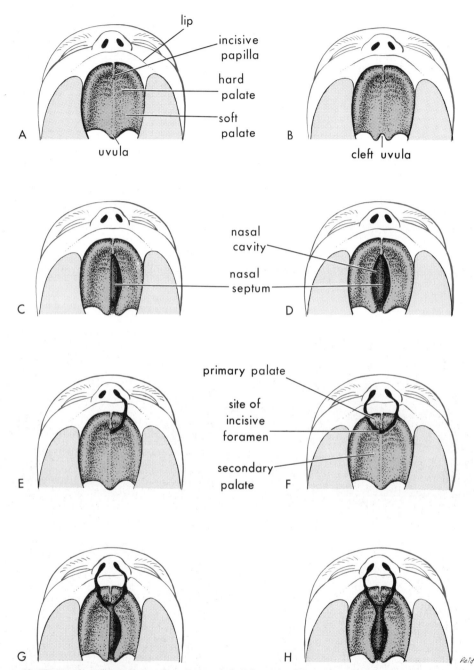

Figure 10-37. Drawings illustrating various types of cleft lip and palate. *A*, Normal lip and palate. *B*, Cleft uvula. *C*, Unilateral cleft of the posterior or secondary palate. *D*, Bilateral cleft of the posterior palate. *E*, Complete unilateral cleft of the lip and alveolar process of the maxilla with a unilateral cleft of the anterior or primary palate. *F*, Complete bilateral cleft of the lip and alveolar processes of the maxillae with bilateral cleft of the anterior palate. *G*, Complete bilateral cleft of the lip and alveolar processes of the maxillae with bilateral cleft of the anterior palate and unilateral cleft of the posterior palate. *H*, Complete bilateral cleft of the lip and alveolar processes of the maxillae with complete bilateral cleft of the anterior and posterior palate.

extends through the alveolar part of the maxilla and the lips on both sides (Figs. 10–37*G* and *H* and 10–38*B*).

The embryological basis of cleft palate is failure of the mesenchymal masses in the lateral palatine processes (palatal shelves) to meet and fuse with each other, with the nasal septum, and/or with the posterior margin of the median palatine process (Figs. 10–30*D* and 10–37). Unilateral and bilateral clefts are classified into three groups:

Clefts of the anterior (primary) palate (i.e., clefts anterior to the incisive fossa) result from failure of mesenchymal masses in the lateral palatine processes (palatal shelves) to meet and fuse with the mesenchyme in the primary palate (Fig. 10–37*E* and *F*).

Clefts of the posterior (secondary) palate (i.e., clefts posterior to the incisive fossa) result from failure of mesenchymal masses in the lateral palatine processes (palatal shelves) to meet and fuse with each other and with the nasal septum (Fig. 10–37*B*, *C*, and *D*).

Clefts of the anterior and posterior parts of the palate (i.e., clefts involving both the primary and secondary palates) result from failure of the mesenchymal masses in the lateral palatine processes (palatal shelves) to meet and fuse with mesenchyme in the primary palate, with each other, and with the nasal septum (Fig. 10–37*G* and *H*).

Causes of Cleft Lip and Palate. Most cases of cleft lip and palate are the result of multiple factors, genetic and nongenetic, each causing a minor developmental disturbance (Vanderas, 1987; Niermeyer et al., 1990; Thompson et al., 1991). This is called *multifactorial inheritance* (p. 168). How teratogenic factors induce cleft lip and palate is still unknown. Experimental studies have given us some insight into the cellular and molecular basis of these defects (Hall, 1988; Ferguson, 1988; Greene, 1989; Schubert et al., 1990).

Some clefts of the lip and/or palate appear as part of syndromes determined by single mutant genes (Fraser, 1980; Thompson et al., 1991). Other clefts are parts of chromosomal syndromes, especially trisomy 13 (see Fig. 8–5). A few cases of cleft lip and/or palate appear to have been caused by teratogenic agents (e.g., anticonvulsant drugs [Hanson, 1980]). Based on experimental findings and limited clinical experience, it has been suggested that vitamin B complex, given prophylactically to pregnant women who are at risk for cleft lip and palate, might decrease the occurrence of facial clefting in the offspring (Schubert, 1990).

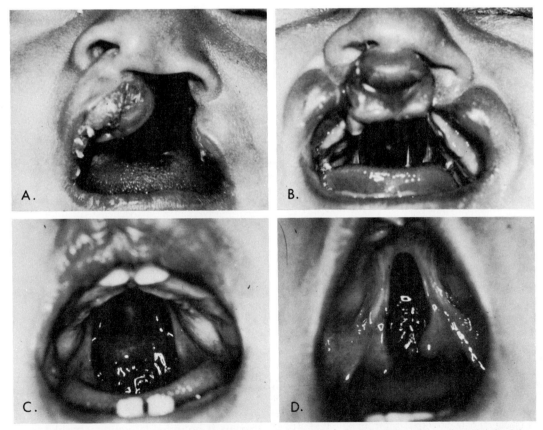

Figure 10–38. Photographs illustrating congenital anomalies of the lip and palate. *A*, Complete unilateral cleft of the lip and alveolar process. *B*, Complete bilateral cleft of the lip and alveolar process with bilateral cleft of the anterior palate. *C* and *D*, Bilateral cleft of the posterior or secondary palate; the lip is normal.

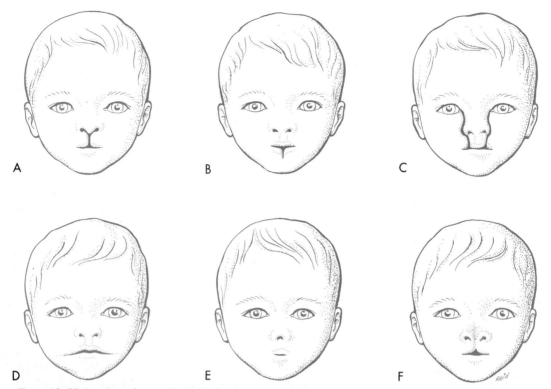

Figure 10–39. Drawings of unusual congenital anomalies of the face. *A,* Median cleft of the upper lip. *B,* Median cleft of the lower lip. *C,* Bilateral oblique facial clefts with complete bilateral cleft lip. *D,* Macrostomia. *E,* Single nostril and microstomia; these anomalies are not usually associated. *F,* Bifid nose and incomplete median cleft lip.

Studies of twins indicate that genetic factors are of more importance in cleft lip, with or without cleft palate, than in cleft palate alone. A sibling of a child with a cleft palate has an elevated risk of having a cleft palate but no increased risk of having a cleft lip. Clefts of the lip and alveolar process of the maxilla that continue through the palate are usually transmitted through a male, sex-linked gene. When neither parent is affected, the *recurrence risk* in subsequent siblings (brother or sister) is about four per cent. For further discussion of recurrence risks, see Connor and Ferguson-Smith (1987) and Thompson et al., (1991).

The fact that the palatine processes or palatal shelves fuse about a week later in females (Burdi, 1969) may explain why isolated cleft palate is more common in females than in males (e.g., among Japanese they occur in 0.63 per 1000 live births, and, of those, 34 per cent are in males and 66 per cent in females [Witkop et al., 1967]).

Facial Clefts. Various types of facial cleft may occur but they are all extremely rare. Severe clefts are usually associated with gross malformations of the head. *Oblique facial clefts* (orbitofacial fissures) are often bilateral and extend from the upper lip to the medial margin of the orbit (Fig. 10–39*C*). When this occurs the nasolacrimal ducts are open grooves (persistent nasolacrimal grooves). Oblique facial clefts associated with cleft lip result from failure of the mesenchymal masses in the maxillary prominences to merge with the lateral and medial nasal prominences. Lateral or transverse facial clefts run from the mouth toward the ear. Bilateral clefts result in a very large mouth, a condition called *macrostomia* (Fig. 10–39*D*). In severe cases the cheeks are cleft almost to the ears.

Other Facial Malformations. Congenital *microstomia* (small mouth) results from excessive merging of the mesenchymal masses in the maxillary and mandibular prominences of the first arch (Fig. 10–39*E*). In severe cases the abnormality may be associated with underdevelopment (hypoplasia) of the mandible. *Absence of the nose* occurs when no nasal placodes form. A *single nostril* results when only one nasal placode forms (Fig. 10–39*E*). *Bifid nose* results when the medial nasal prominences do not merge completely; the nostrils are widely separated and the nasal bridge is bifid (Fig. 10–39*F*). In mild forms of bifid nose, there is a groove in the tip of the nose.

SUMMARY

During the fourth and fifth weeks the primitive pharynx is bounded laterally by barlike *branchial or pharyngeal arches*. Each arch consists of a core of mesenchyme covered externally by ectoderm and internally by endoderm. The original mesenchyme of each arch is derived from the intraembryonic mesoderm. Later, *neural crest cells* migrate into the arches and are the major source of connective tissue components, including cartilage, bone, and ligaments, in the oral and facial regions. Each arch also contains an artery, a cartilage rod, a nerve, and a muscular component.

Externally the arches are separated by *branchial or pharyngeal grooves*. Internally the arches are separated by evaginations of the pharynx called *pharyngeal pouches*. Where the ectoderm of a groove contacts the endoderm of a pouch, *branchial or pharyngeal membranes* are formed. The pouches and arches, grooves, and membranes make up the branchial or pharyngeal apparatus.

Development of the tongue, face, lips, jaws, palate, pharynx, and neck largely involves transformation of the branchial apparatus into adult structures. The adult derivatives of the various arch components are summarized in Table 10–1, and the derivatives of the pouches are illustrated in Figure 10–8.

The branchial or pharyngeal grooves disappear except for the first pair, which persists as the *external acoustic meatus*. The branchial or pharyngeal membranes also disappear except for the first pair, which becomes the *tympanic membranes*. The first pharyngeal pouch gives rise to the *tympanic cavity*, mastoid antrum, and auditory tube. The second pharyngeal pouch is associated with the development of the palatine tonsil. The *thymus* is derived from the third pair of pharyngeal pouches, and the *parathyroid glands* are formed from the third and fourth pairs of pharyngeal pouches.

The *thyroid gland* develops from a downgrowth from the floor of the primitive pharynx in the region where the tongue develops. The parafollicular (C) cells in the thyroid gland are derived from the *ultimobranchial bodies*, which are derived mainly from the fourth pair of pharyngeal pouches.

Most congenital anomalies of the head and neck originate during transformation of the branchial ap-

paratus into adult structures. Branchial cysts, sinuses, and fistulas may develop from parts of the second branchial groove, the cervical sinus, or the second pharyngeal pouch that fail to obliterate.

An *ectopic thyroid gland* results when the thyroid gland fails to descend completely from its site of origin in the tongue. The thyroglossal duct may persist or remnants of it may give rise to *thyroglossal duct cysts*. Infected cysts may perforate through the skin and form *thyroglossal duct sinuses* that open anteriorly in the median plane of the neck.

Due to the complicated development of the face and palate, congenital anomalies of the face and palate are common. Anomalies result from *maldevelopment of neural crest tissue* that gives rise to the skeletal and connective tissue primordia of the face. Neural crest cells may be deficient in number, may not complete their migration to the face, or they may fail in their inductive capacity (Sperber, 1989). Anomalies of the face and palate result from an arrest of development and/or a failure of fusion of the prominences and processes involved.

Cleft lip is a common congenital anomaly. Although it is frequently associated with cleft palate, cleft lip and palate are etiologically distinct anomalies that involve different developmental processes occurring at different times. Cleft lip results from failure of mesenchymal masses in the medial nasal and the maxillary prominences to merge; whereas, *cleft palate* results from failure of mesenchymal masses in the palatine processes (palatal shelves) to meet and fuse.

Most cases of cleft lip, with or without cleft palate, are caused by a combination of genetic and environmental factors (*multifactorial inheritance*). These factors interfere with the migration of *neural crest cells* into the maxillary prominences of the first branchial or pharyngeal arch. If the number of cells is insufficient, clefting of the lip and/or palate may occur. Other cellular and molecular mechanisms may be involved (Hall, 1988; Ferguson, 1988; Greene, 1989; Sperber, 1989).

CLINICALLY ORIENTED QUESTIONS FOR PROBLEM-BASED LEARNING SESSIONS

1. A two-year-old boy had had an intermittent discharge of mucoid material from a small opening in the side of his neck, but the discharge had stopped a week ago. There was extensive redness and swelling in the inferior third of the neck, just anterior to the sternocleidomastoid muscle. What is the probable embryological basis of the intermittent discharge? Discuss the etiology of these congenital anomalies.

2. During a subtotal thyroidectomy a surgeon could locate only one inferior parathyroid gland. Where might the other one be located? What is the embryological basis for this ectopic condition?

3. A young woman consulted her physician about a swelling in the median plane of her neck, just inferior to her hyoid bone. What kind of a cyst might be present? Are they always in the median plane? Discuss its embryological basis. With what might such a swelling be confused?

4. A male infant was born with a unilateral cleft lip extending into the floor of his nose and through the alveolar process of his maxilla. What is the embryological basis of these anomalies? Neither parent had cleft lip or cleft palate. Are genetic factors likely involved? Is this anomaly more common in males? What is the chance that the next child will have a cleft lip?

5. An epileptic mother who was treated with an anticonvulsant drug during pregnancy gave birth to a child with cleft lip and palate. Is there any evidence indicating that these drugs increase the incidence of these anomalies? Discuss the respective etiologies of these two anomalies.

The answers to these questions are given on page 462.

References and Suggested Reading

Aurbach GD, Marx SJ, Spiegel AM: Parathyroid hormone, calcitonin and the calciferols. *In* Wilson JD, Foster DW (eds): *Williams Textbook of Endocrinology.* 7th ed. Philadelphia, WB Saunders, 1985.

Behrman RE (ed): *Nelson Textbook of Pediatrics.* 14th ed. Philadelphia, WB Saunders, 1992.

Bhatnager K: Personal communication, School of Medicine, University of Louisville, Louisville, Kentucky, 1991.

Bockman DE, Kirby ML: Dependence of thymus development on derivatives of the neural crest. *Science* 223:498, 1984.

Burdi AR: Sexual differences in closure of the human palatal shelves. *Cleft Palate J* 6:1, 1969.

Chetty R, Forder MD: Parathyroiditis associated with hyperthyroidism and branchial cysts. *Am J Clin Pathol* 96:348, 1991.

Connor JM, Ferguson-Smith MA: *Essential Medical Genetics.* 2nd ed. Oxford, Blackwell Scientific Publications, 1987.

Cormack DH: *Ham's Histology.* 9th ed. Philadelphia, JB Lippincott, 1987.

Cormack DH: *Introduction to Histology.* Philadelphia, JB Lippincott, 1984.

Crelin ES: Development of the upper respiratory system. *Clin Symp* 28(3), 1976.

Diewert VM: The role of craniofacial growth in palatal shelf elevation. *In* Pratt RM, Christiansen RL (eds): *Current Research Trends in Prenatal Craniofacial Development.* New York, Elsevier North–Holland, 1980.

Ferguson MWJ: Palate development. *Development* 103(Suppl):41, 1988.

Fisher DA, Polk DH: Development of the thyroid. *Bailliere's Clin Endocrin Metabol* 3:627, 1989.

Fraser FC: The genetics of cleft lip and palate: yet another look. *In* Pratt RM, Christiansen RL (eds): *Current Research Trends in Prenatal Craniofacial Development.* New York, Elsevier North–Holland, 1980.

Gabriele OF: Persistent vomeronasal organ. *Am J Roentgenol* 99:697, 1967.

Gorlin RJ, Cohen Jr, MM, Levin LS: *Syndromes of the Head and Neck.* 3rd ed. New York, Oxford Univ Press, 1990.

Goss AN: Human palatal development in vitro. *Cleft Palate J* 12:210, 1975.

Greene RM: Signal transduction during craniofacial development. *Critical Rev in Toxicology* 20:153, 1989.

Hall BK: How is mandibular growth controlled during development and evolution. *J Craniofacial Genetics and Develop Biol* 2:45, 1982.

Hall BK: Mechanisms of craniofacial development. *In* Vig KWL, Burdi AR (eds): *Craniofacial Morphogenesis and Dysmorphogenesis.* Ann Arbor, The University of Michigan, 1988.

Hanson JW: Patterns of abnormal human craniofacial development. *In* Pratt RM, Christiansen RL (eds): *Current Research Trends in Prenatal Craniofacial Development.* New York, Elsevier North-Holland, 1980.

Hayden GD, Arnold GG: The ear. *In* Kendig Jr, EL, Chernick V (eds): *Disorders of the Respiratory Tract in Children.* 4th ed. Philadelphia, WB Saunders, 1983.

Hinrichsen K: *The Early Development of Morphology and Patterns of the Face in the Human Embryo. Advances in Anatomy, Embryology and Cell Biology 98.* New York, Springer-Verlag, 1985.

Jaffee BF: The branchial arches. *In* Ferguson CF, Kendig Jr, EL (eds): *Disorders of the Respiratory Tract in Children, Vol. II: Pediatric Otolaryngology.* 2nd ed. Philadelphia, WB Saunders, 1972.

Jones KL: *Smith's Recognizable Patterns of Human Malformation.* 4th ed. Philadelphia, WB Saunders, 1988.

Karmody CS: Autosomal dominant first and second arch syndrome. *In* Bergsma D (ed): *Malformation Syndromes.* New York, International Medical Book Corp., Vol. 10, 1974.

Kendall MD: Functional anatomy of the thymic microenvironment. *J Anat* 177:1, 1991.

Kirby MF, Bockman DE: Neural crest and normal development: a new perspective. *Anat Rec* 209:1, 1984.

Martins AG: Lateral cervical sinus and pre-auricular sinuses. *Br Med J* 5:255, 1961.

McKenzie J: The first arch syndrome. *Dev Med Child Neuro.* 8:55, 1966.

Meller SM: Morphological alterations in the prefusion human palatal epithelium. *In* Pratt RM, Christiansen RL (eds): *Current Research Trends in Prenatal Craniofacial Development.* New York, Elsevier North-Holland, 1980.

Melsen B: Palatal growth studies on human autopsy material. *Am J Orthod* 68:42, 1975.

Miyauchi A, Matsuzuka F, Kima K, Katayama S: Piraform sinus

fistula and the ultimobrachial body. *Histopathology 20*:227, 1992.

Moore KL: *Clinically Oriented Anatomy.* 3rd ed. Baltimore, Williams & Wilkins, 1992.

Moore MAS, Owen JJT: Experimental studies on the development of the thymus. *J Exp Med 126*:715, 1967.

Morris HL, Bardach J: Cleft lip and palate and related disorders: issues for future research of high priority. *Cleft Palate J 26*:141, 1989.

Moseley JM, Mathews EW, Breed RH et al.: The ultimobranchial origin of calcitonin. *Lancet 1*:108, 1968.

Niermeyer MF, Van der Meulen JC: Genetics of craniofacial malformations. *In* Stricker M, Van der Meulen JC, Raphael B, Mazzola R (eds): *Craniofacial Malformations.* Edinburgh, Churchill Livingstone, 1990.

Noden DM: Interactions and fates of avian craniofacial mesenchyme. *Development 103*(Suppl):121, 1988.

Noden DM: New views on old problems. *Anat Rec 208*:1, 1984.

Pfeifer G (ed): *Craniofacial Abnormalities and Clefts of the Lip, Alveolus and Palate.* New York, Georg Thieme Verlag, 1991.

Poswillo D: The aetiology and pathogenesis of craniofacial deformity. *Development 103*(Suppl):213, 1988.

Raffensperger JG (ed): *Swenson's Pediatric Surgery.* 5th ed. Norwalk Connecticut, Appleton & Lange, 1990.

Ross RB, Johnston MC: *Cleft Lip and Palate.* Baltimore, Williams & Wilkins, 1972.

Sandham A: Classification of clefting deformity. *Early Human Development 12*:81, 1985b.

Sandham A: Embryonic facial vertical dimension and its relationship to palatal shelf elevation. *Early Human Development 12*:241, 1985c.

Sandham A: Embryonic head posture and palatal shelf elevation. *Early Human Development 11*:69, 1985a.

Sandham A, Nelson R: Embryology of the middle third of the face. *Early Human Development 10*:313, 1985.

Schubert J, Schmidt R, Raupach H-W: New findings explaining the mode of action in prevention of facial clefting and first clinical experience. *J Cranio-Max Fac Surg 18*:343, 1990.

Shepard TH: Development of the thyroid gland. *In* Gardner LI (ed): *Endocrine and Genetic Diseases of Childhood and Adolescence.* 2nd ed. Philadelphia, WB Saunders, 1975.

Slavkin HC: Cellular and molecular determinants during craniofacial development. *In* Stricker M, Van der Meulen JC, Raphael B, Mazzola R (eds): *Craniofacial Malformations.* Edinburgh, Churchill Livingstone, 1990.

Sperber GH: *Craniofacial Embryology.* 4th ed. London, Butterworth, 1989.

Steinman GG: Changes of the human thymus during ageing. *In* Müller-Hermelink HK (ed): *The Human Thymus. Histophysiology and Pathology. Current Topics in Pathology, 75.* Berlin, Springer-Verlag, 1986.

Stricker M, Raphael B, Van der Meulen J, Mazzola R: Craniofacial growth and development. *In* Stricker M, Van der Meulen JC, Raphael B, Mazzola R (eds): *Craniofacial Malformations.* Edinburgh, Churchill Livingstone, 1990.

Sulik KK, Cook CS, Webster WS: Teratogens and craniofacial malformations: relationships to cell death. *Development 103*(suppl):213, 1988.

Taeusch HW, Ballard RB, Avery ME (eds): *Schaffer & Avery's Diseases of the Newborn.* 6th ed. Philadelphia, WB Saunders, 1991.

Thompson MW, McInnes RR, Willard HF: *Thompson & Thompson Genetics in Medicine.* 5th ed. Philadelphia, WB Saunders Co, 1991.

Vanderas AP: Incidence of cleft lip, cleft palate, and cleft lip and palate among races: a review. *Cleft Palate J 24*:216, 1987.

Van der Meulen J, Mozzola B, Stricker M, Raphael B: Classification of craniofacial malformations. *In* Stricker M, Van der Meulen JC, Raphael B, Mazzola R (eds): *Craniofacial Malformations.* Edinburgh, Churchill Livingstone, 1990.

Vermeij-Keers C: Craniofacial embryology and morphogenesis: normal and abnormal. *In* Stricker M, Van der Meulen JC, Raphael B, Mazzola R (eds): *Craniofacial Malformations.* Edinburgh, Churchill Livingstone, 1990.

Warwick R: *Nomina Embryologica.* 3rd ed. Edinburgh, Churchill Livingstone, 1989.

Wedden SE, Ralphs JR, Tickle C: Pattern formation in the facial primordia. *Development 103*(Suppl):31, 1988.

Witkop CJ, MacCollum DW, Rubin A: Cleft lip and cleft palate. *In* Rubin A (ed): *Handbook of Congenital Malformations.* Philadelphia, WB Saunders, 1967.

11

The Respiratory System

The development of the *upper respiratory system* (nose, nasal cavities, paranasal sinuses, nasopharynx, and oropharynx) is described in Chapter 10. The *lower respiratory system* (larynx, trachea, bronchi, and lungs) begins to form during the fourth week (26 to 27 days). The respiratory primordium is first indicated by a median outgrowth (the **laryngotracheal groove**) from the caudal end of the ventral wall of the primitive pharynx (Fig. 11–1), caudal to the fourth pair of pharyngeal pouches.

The endoderm lining the laryngotracheal groove gives rise to the epithelium and glands of the larynx, trachea, bronchi, and the pulmonary epithelium. The connective tissue, cartilage, and smooth muscle in these structures develop from the splanchnic mesenchyme surrounding the foregut (Fig. 11–4). By the end of the fourth week, the laryngotracheal groove has evaginated to form a pouchlike *laryngotracheal diverticulum*, which is located ventral to the caudal part of the foregut (Fig. 11–2A). As this diverticulum enlongates, it is invested with splanchnic mesenchyme, and its distal end enlarges to form a globular *lung bud* (Fig. 11–2B).

The laryngotracheal diverticulum soon becomes separated from the *primitive pharynx*. Longitudinal *tracheoesophageal folds* (ridges) develop, approach each other, and fuse to form a partition known as the *tracheoesophageal septum* (Fig. 11–2D and E). This septum divides the cranial part of the foregut into a ventral portion, the *laryngotracheal tube* (primordium of the larynx, trachea, bronchi, and lungs), and a dorsal portion (primordium of the oropharynx and esophagus [Fig. 11–2F])[1] The opening of the laryngotracheal tube into the pharynx becomes the laryngeal aditus (orifice) or *inlet of the larynx* (Figs. 11–2C and 11–3C).

DEVELOPMENT OF THE LARYNX

The epithelium of the internal lining of the larynx develops from the endoderm of the cranial end of the laryngotracheal tube. The cartilages of the larynx are derived from the cartilages in the fourth and sixth pairs of branchial or pharyngeal arches (see Figs. 10–4 and 11–3A; Table 10–1). The laryngeal cartilages develop from mesenchyme which is derived from *neural crest cells* that surround the original mesoderm in these arches (p. 188).

The mesenchyme at the cranial end of the laryngotracheal tube proliferates rapidly, producing paired *arytenoid swellings* (Fig. 11–3B). These swellings grow toward the tongue, converting the slitlike aperture called the *primitive glottis* into a T-shaped *laryngeal aditus* (inlet) and reducing the developing laryngeal lumen to a narrow slit. The laryngeal epithelium proliferates rapidly, resulting in a *temporary occlusion of the laryngeal lumen* during the eighth week. Recanalization of the larynx usually occurs by the tenth week. The *laryngeal ventricles* form during this process. These lateral recesses are bounded by folds of mucous membrane that become the *vocal folds* (cords) and *vestibular folds*[2].

The epiglottis develops from the caudal part of the *hypobranchial eminence*, a prominence produced by proliferation of mesenchyme in the ventral ends of the third and fourth branchial or pharyngeal arches (Fig. 11–3B to D). The rostral part of this eminence forms the pharyngeal part of the tongue (p. 204). Because the *laryngeal muscles* develop from myoblasts in the fourth and sixth pairs of branchial or pharyngeal arches they are innervated by the laryngeal branches of the vagus nerves (CNX) that supply these arches (see Table 10–1). Growth of the larynx and epiglottis is rapid during the first three years after birth. By this time the epiglottis has reached its adult form (De Vries and De Vries, 1991).

> **Laryngeal Web.** This uncommon anomaly results from incomplete recanalization of the larynx during the tenth week. A membranous web forms at the level of the vocal folds (cords), partially obstructing the airway.

---

[1] For another interpretation of laryngotracheal tube development, see Zaw-Tun (1982) and De Vries and De Vries (1991).

---

[2] Persons desiring detailed and critical descriptions of the development of the larynx should consult Crelin (1976), Hast (1976), and Sañudo and Domenech-Mateu (1990). For a description of the adult structure of the larynx, see Moore (1992).

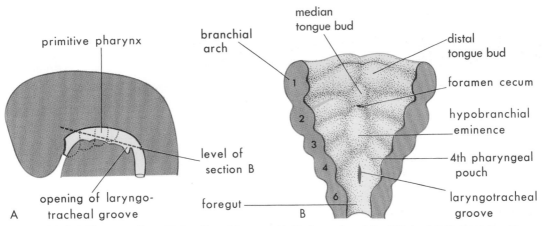

Figure 11–1. *A*, Diagrammatic sagittal section of the cranial half of an embryo (about 26 days). *B*, Horizontal section at the level shown in *A*, illustrating the floor of the primitive pharynx and the location of the laryngotracheal groove. The opening into the laryngotracheal groove represents the future inlet of the larynx or laryngeal aditus (Fig 11–3*D*).

DEVELOPMENT OF THE TRACHEA

The endodermal lining of the laryngotracheal tube distal to the larynx differentiates into the epithelium and glands of the trachea and to the pulmonary epithelium. The cartilage, connective tissue, and muscles of the trachea are derived from the splanchnic mesenchyme surrounding the laryngotracheal tube (Fig. 11–4).

Tracheoesophageal Fistula (Fig. 11–5). An abnormal communication or fistula between the trachea and esopha-

gus occurs about once in every 2500 births; most affected infants are males. In more than 85 per cent of cases, a fistula is associated with *esophageal atresia* (Herbst, 1992). Tracheoesophageal fistula is the *most common anomaly of the lower respiratory tract*. It results from incomplete division of the cranial part of the foregut into respiratory and digestive portions during the fourth week. Incomplete fusion of the tracheoesophageal folds produces a *defective tracheoesophageal septum* and an abnormal communication between the trachea and esophagus.

Four *varieties of tracheoesophageal fistula* may develop. The most common abnormality is for the superior portion

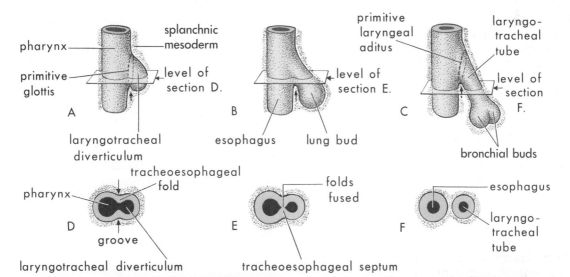

Figure 11–2. Drawings illustrating successive stages in the development of the tracheoesophageal septum during the fourth and fifth weeks. *A, B,* and *C,* Lateral views of the caudal part of the primitive pharynx, illustrating partitioning of the foregut into the esophagus and laryngotracheal tube. *D, E,* and *F,* Transverse sections illustrating formation of the tracheoesophageal septum and separation of the foregut into the laryngotracheal tube and esophagus.

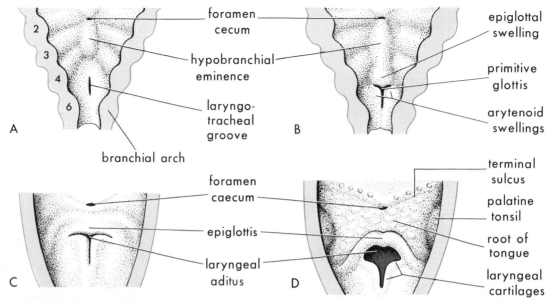

Figure 11–3. Drawings illustrating successive stages in the development of the larynx. *A*, Four weeks. *B*, Five weeks. *C*, Six weeks. *D*, Ten weeks. The epithelium of the internal lining of the larynx is of endodermal origin. The cartilages and muscles of the larynx arise from mesenchyme in the fourth and sixth pairs of branchial or pharyngeal arches. Note that the laryngeal inlet or aditus changes in shape from a slitlike opening to a T-shaped inlet as the mesenchyme proliferates.

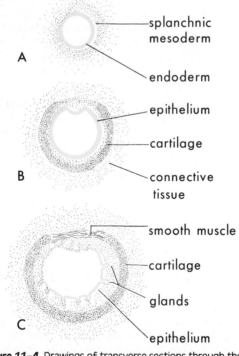

Figure 11–4. Drawings of transverse sections through the laryngotracheal tube illustrating progressive stages in the development of the trachea. *A*, Four weeks. *B*, Ten weeks. *C*, 11 weeks. Note that endoderm of the tube gives rise to the epithelium and glands of the trachea.

of the esophagus to end blindly (*esophageal atresia*) and for the inferior portion to join the trachea near its bifurcation (Fig. 11–5*A*). Other varieties of this anomaly are illustrated in Figure 11–5*B* to *D*. Infants with the common type of esophageal atresia and tracheoesophageal fistula cough and choke on swallowing due to the accumulation of excessive amounts of saliva in the mouth and upper respiratory tract. When the infant swallows milk, it rapidly fills the esophageal pouch and is regurgitated. Gastric contents may also reflux from the stomach through the fistula into the trachea and lungs. This causes chocking and may result in pneumonia or *pneumonitis* (inflammation of the lungs).

An excess of amniotic fluid, a condition known as *polyhydramnios* (p. 131), is often associated with esophageal atresia and tracheoesophageal fistula (Fig. 11–5*A*). This condition develops because amniotic fluid cannot pass to the stomach and intestines for absorption and subsequent transfer via the placenta to the mother's blood for disposal (p. 131).

Tracheal Stenosis and Atresia. Narrowing (stenosis) and obstruction (atresia) of the trachea are uncommon anomalies that are usually associated with one of the varieties of tracheoesophageal fistula (Fig. 11–5). Stenoses and atresias probably result from unequal partitioning of the foregut into the esophagus and the trachea (Fig. 11–2*D* to *F*). Sometimes there is a web of tissue obstructing airflow (*incomplete tracheal atresia*).

Tracheal Diverticulum. This extremely rare anomaly consists of a blind, bronchus-like projection from the trachea. The outgrowth or diverticulum may terminate in normal-appearing lung tissue, forming a so-called *tracheal lobe* of the lung.

DEVELOPMENT OF BRONCHI AND LUNGS

The bulb-shaped *lung bud* that develops at the caudal end of the laryngotracheal tube during the fourth week (Figs. 11–2*B* and 11–6*A*) soon divides into two knoblike *bronchial buds* (Figs. 11–2*C* and 11–6*B*). These endodermal buds grow laterally into the pericardioperitoneal canals, the primordia of the *pleural cavities* (see Figs. 9–5*A* and 11–7*A*). Together with the surrounding splanchnic mesenchyme, the bronchial buds differentiate into the bronchi and their ramifications in the lungs.

Early in the fifth week each bronchial bud enlarges to form the primordium of a main or *primary bronchus* (Fig. 11–6*E*). The embryonic right bronchus is slightly larger than the left one and is oriented more vertically; this embryonic relationship persists after birth. Consequently, a foreign body is more liable to enter the right main bronchus than the left one (Moore, 1992).

The main or primary bronchi subdivide into *secondary bronchi* (Fig. 11–6*F*). On the right, the superior secondary bronchus will supply the superior lobe of the lung; whereas, the inferior secondary bronchus subdivides into two bronchi, one to the middle lobe of the right lung and the other to the inferior lobe (Fig. 11–6*G*). On the left, the two secondary bronchi supply the superior and inferior lobes of the lung.

Each secondary bronchus subsequently undergoes progressive branching. Tertiary or *segmental bronchi*, ten in the right lung and eight or nine in the left lung, begin to form by the seventh week (Crelin, 1975). As this occurs, the surrounding mesenchymal tissue also divides (Fig. 11–6*G*). Each segmental bronchus with its surrounding mass of mesenchyme is the primordium of a *bronchopulmonary segment*[3]. By 24 weeks, about 17 orders of branches have formed and the *respiratory bronchioles* have developed (Fig. 11–8*A*). An additional seven orders of airways develop after birth.

As the bronchi develop, cartilaginous plates develop from the surrounding splanchnic mesenchyme. The bronchial smooth musculature and connective tissue and the pulmonary connective tissue and capillaries are also derived from this mesenchyme. As the lungs develop they acquire a layer of *visceral pleura*

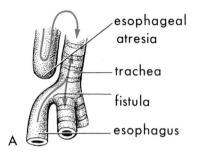

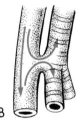

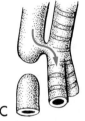

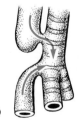

Figure 11–5. Sketches illustrating the four main varieties of tracheoesophageal fistula. Possible directions of the flow of the contents is indicated by arrows. Esophageal atresia, as illustrated in *A*, is associated with tracheoesophageal fistula in more than 85 per cent of cases. The abdomen rapidly becomes distended as the intestines fill with air. In *C*, air cannot enter the lower esophagus and stomach.

esophageal atresia
trachea
fistula
esophagus

---

[3] For a description of the adult anatomy of these clinically important segments, see Moore (1992).

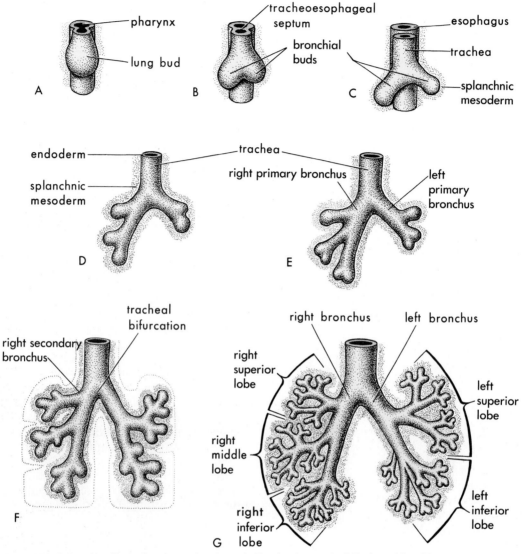

Figure 11–6. Drawings illustrating successive stages in the development of the bronchi and lungs. *A* to *C*, Four weeks. *D* and *E*, Five weeks. *F*, Six weeks. *G*, Eight weeks.

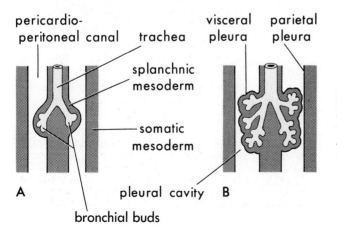

Figure 11–7. Diagrams illustrating growth of the developing lungs into the adjacent splanchnic mesenchyme of the medial walls of the pericardioperitoneal canals (primitive pleural cavities). Development of the layers of the pleura is also shown. *A*, Five weeks. *B*, Six weeks.

from the splanchnic mesenchyme (Fig. 11–7*B*). With expansion, the lungs and the pleural cavities grow caudally into the mesenchyme of the body wall and soon lie close to the heart (see Fig. 9–5). The thoracic body wall becomes lined by a layer of *parietal pleura* derived from the somatic mesoderm (Fig. 11–7*B*).

Maturation of the Lungs

Lung development can be divided into four stages: the pseudoglandular period, the canalicular period, the terminal sac period, and the alveolar period. For information on the regulation of normal lung growth and the hormonal control of lung maturation, see Ballard (1989), Scarpelli (1990), and Thurlbeck (1991).

The Pseudoglandular Period (5 to 17 weeks). The developing lung somewhat resembles an exocrine gland during this period (Fig. 11–9*A*). By 17 weeks all major elements of the lung have formed *except* those involved with gas exchange. Respiration is not possible; hence, *fetuses born during this period cannot survive.*

The Canalicular Period (16 to 25 weeks). This period overlaps the pseudoglandular period because cranial segments of the lungs mature faster than caudal ones. During the canalicular period, the lumina of the bronchi and terminal bronchioles become larger and the lung tissue becomes highly vascular (Figs. 11–8*A* and 11–9*B*). By 24 weeks, each terminal bronchiole has divided to form two or more *respiratory bronchioles.* Each of these then divides into three to six tubular passages called *alveolar ducts.*

Respiration is possible toward the end of the canalicular period because some thin-walled *terminal sacs* (primitive alveoli) have developed at the ends of the respiratory bronchioles, and these regions are *well vascularized* (Fig. 11–8*A*). Although a fetus born toward the end of this period may survive if given intensive care (see Fig. 6–10), it often dies because its respiratory and other systems are still relatively immature.

The Terminal Sac Period (24 weeks to birth). During this period many more terminal sacs develop (Figs. 11–8*C* and 11–9*C*), and their *epithelium becomes very thin.* Capillaries begin to bulge into these primitive alveoli (Fig. 11–8*B* and *C*). By 24 weeks, the terminal sacs are lined mainly by squamous epithelial cells of endodermal origin, known as *Type I alveolar cells* or pneumocytes. The capillary network proliferates rapidly in the mesenchyme around the developing alveoli, and there is concurrent active development of lymphatic capillaries (Fig. 11–8*A* and *B*).

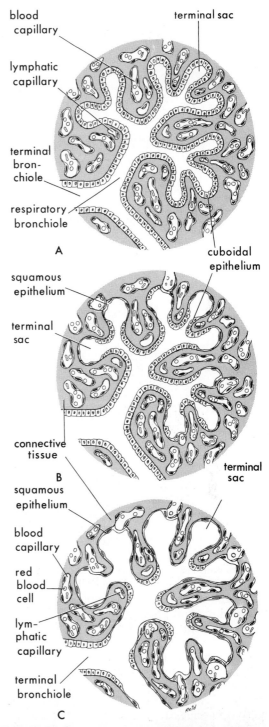

Figure 11–8. Diagrammatic sketches of histological sections, illustrating progressive stages of lung development. *A*, Late canalicular period (about 24 weeks). *B*, Early terminal sac period (about 26 weeks). *C*, Newborn infant (early alveolar period). Note that the alveolocapillary membrane is thin and that some of the capillaries have begun to bulge into the terminal sacs (future alveoli).

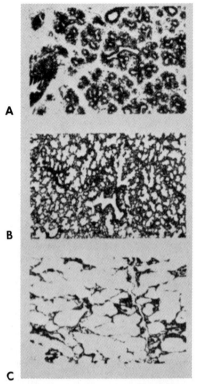

Figure 11–9. Histological sections of lungs at various stages of development, showing the changing appearance of the lung tissue. *A,* Pseudoglandular period: five to 17 weeks. *B,* Canalicular period: 16 to 25 weeks. *C,* Terminal sac period: 24 weeks to birth. (From Reid, L.: *The Pathology of Emphysema,* 1967. Courtesy of Lloyd-Luke [Medical Books] Ltd.)

Scattered among the squamous epithelial cells are rounded, secretory, epithelial cells called *Type II alveolar cells* or pneumocytes. These cells secrete **pulmonary surfactant**, a complex mixture of phospholipids, which forms as a monomolecular film over the internal walls of the terminal sacs (Whitsett, 1991). It is recognized that the maturation of alveolar type II cells and surfactant production varies widely in fetuses of different gestational ages (Chernick and Kryger, 1990). The production of surfactant increases during the terminal stages of pregnancy, particularly during the last two weeks before a full-term birth.

Surfactant counteracts surface tension forces and facilitates expansion of the terminal sacs (primitive alveoli). Consequently, fetuses born prematurely at 24 to 26 weeks after fertilization may survive if given intensive care, but they suffer from respiratory distress due to *surfactant deficiency.* Surfactant production begins by 20 weeks, but it is present in very small amounts in premature infants; it does not reach adequate levels until the late fetal period (Ballard, 1989).

By 26 to 28 weeks after fertilization the fetus usually weighs about 1000 gm, and sufficient terminal sacs and surfactant are present to permit survival of a prematurely born infant. Before this, the lungs are usually incapable of providing adequate gas exchange, partly because the alveolar surface area is insufficient and the vascularity underdeveloped. It is not the presence of thin terminal sacs or primitive alveolar epithelium so much as the development of an adequate pulmonary vasculature and sufficient surfactant that are critical to the survival of premature infants.

The Alveolar Period (late fetal period to childhood). The epithelial lining of the terminal sacs attenuates to an extremely thin, squamous epithelial layer. The type I alveolar cells become so thin that the adjacent capillaries bulge into the terminal sacs (Fig. 11–8*C*). By the late fetal period, the lungs are capable of respiration because the *alveolocapillary membrane* (respiratory membrane) is sufficiently thin to allow gas exchange. Although the lungs do not begin to perform this vital function until birth, they must be well-developed so that they are capable of functioning as soon as the baby is born.

At the beginning of the alveolar period, each respiratory bronchiole terminates in a cluster of thin-walled terminal sacs, separated from one another by loose connective tissue (Fig. 11–8*B* and *C*). These terminal sacs represent future alveolar ducts. *Characteristic mature alveoli do not form until after birth.* Before birth the immature alveoli appear as small bulges on the walls of respiratory bronchioles and terminal sacs (future alveolar ducts).

After birth the primitive alveoli enlarge as the lungs expand, but most increase in the size of the lungs results from an increase in the number of respiratory bronchioles and primitive alveoli rather than from an increase in the size of the alveoli (Crelin, 1975). From the third to the eighth year or so, the number of immature alveoli continues to increase (Thurlbeck, 1991). Unlike mature alveoli, immature alveoli have the potential for forming additional primitive alveoli. As primitive alveoli increase in size, they become mature alveoli.

Lung development during the first few months after birth is characterized by an exponential increase in the surface of the air-blood barrier (Behrman, 1992). This increase is accomplished by the multiplication of pulmonary alveoli and capillaries. About 50 million alveoli, one sixth of the adult number, are present in the lungs of a full-term newborn infant. On chest radiographs, therefore, the lungs of newborn infants are denser than adult lungs. By about the eighth year the adult complement of 300 million alveoli is present (Ballard, 1989). About 95 per cent of the alveoli develop after birth (Cormack, 1987).

Breathing movements occur before birth, exerting sufficient force to cause aspiration of amniotic fluid into the lungs. These prenatal breathing movements, which can be detected by real-time ultrasonography, are not continuous but they are essential for normal fetal lung development. The pattern of fetal breathing movements is widely used in the diagnosis of labor (p. 124) and as a predictor of fetal outcome in preterm delivery. By birth, the fetus has had the advantage of several months of breathing "exercise" (Behrman, 1992). *Fetal breathing movements*, which increase as the time of delivery approaches, probably condition the respiratory muscles. In addition, these movements stimulate lung development, possibly by creating a pressure gradient between the lungs and the amniotic fluid (Behrman, 1992).

At birth the lungs are about half filled with fluid derived from the amniotic cavity, lungs, and tracheal glands. Aeration of the lungs at birth is not so much the inflation of empty collapsed organs but rather the rapid replacement of intra-alveolar fluid by air. The fluid in the lungs is cleared at birth by three routes: (1) through the mouth and nose by pressure on the thorax during delivery, (2) into the pulmonary capillaries, and (3) into the lymphatics and pulmonary arteries and veins. In the fetus near term, the pulmonary lymphatic vessels are relatively larger and more numerous than in the adult (Crelin, 1975). Lymph flow is rapid during the first few hours after birth and then diminishes.

Of medicolegal significance is the fact that the lungs of a stillborn infant are firm and sink when placed in water because they contain fluid, not air.

Respiratory Distress Syndrome (RDS). Infants born prematurely are most susceptible to RDS (Chernick and Kryger, 1990). These infants develop rapid, labored breathing shortly after birth. **Hyaline membrane disease (HMD)** is a major cause of RDS in newborn infants (Behrman, 1992).

Surfactant deficiency is a major cause of HMD, which causes about 50 per cent of deaths in the perinatal period (Behrman, 1992). The lungs are underinflated, and the alveoli contain a fluid of high protein content that resembles a glassy or *hyaline membrane*. This membrane is believed to be derived from a combination of substances in the circulation and from the injured pulmonary epithelium. Page et al. (1981) suggested that prolonged *intrauterine asphyxia* may produce irreversible changes in the type II alveolar cells, making them incapable of producing surfactant. There appear to be, however, several causes for absence or deficiency of surfactant in premature and full-term infants.

All the growth factors and hormones controlling surfactant production have not been identified (Ballard, 1989), but *thyroxine* is known to be a potent stimulator of surfactant production (Crelin, 1975). *Glucocorticoid treatment* during pregnancy accelerates fetal lung development and surfactant production. This finding has led to the routine clinical use of corticosteroids (betamethasome) for the *prevention of RDS*.

Congenital Anomalies of the Lungs

Structural abnormalities of the lungs are uncommon. Abnormal fissures or lobes are occasionally observed, but they are usually unimportant clinically.

Lobe of the Azygos Vein. This lobe appears in the right lung in about one per cent of people. It develops when the apical bronchus grows superiorly, medial to the arch of the azygos vein, instead of lateral to it. As a result, the vein comes to lie at the bottom of a fissure in the superior lobe (Moore, 1992). It produces a linear marking on a radiograph.

Congenital Lung Cysts. These cysts (filled with fluid or air) are thought to be formed by the dilation of terminal bronchi (Salzberg, 1983). They probably result from a disturbance in bronchial development during late fetal life. If several cysts are present, the lungs have a honeycomb appearance on radiographs. The cysts are usually located at the periphery of the lung.

Agenesis of the Lungs. Absence of a lung results from failure of a bronchial bud to develop. Agenesis of one lung is more common than bilateral agenesis, yet both conditions are rare. *Unilateral pulmonary agenesis* is compatible with life. The heart and other mediastinal structures are shifted to the affected side and the existing lung is hyperexpanded.

Lung Hypoplasia. In infants with CDH (*congenital diaphragmatic hernia*), the lungs are unable to develop normally because they are compressed by the abnormally positioned abdominal viscera (p. 184). Lung hypoplasia is characterized by a markedly reduced lung weight. Most infants with CDH die of pulmonary insufficiency despite optimal postnatal care because their lungs are too hypoplastic to support extrauterine life (Harrison, 1991).

Accessory Lung. This small lung is a very uncommon congenital anomaly. It is almost always located at the base of the left lung. It does not communicate with the tracheobronchial tree, and its blood supply is usually systemic rather than pulmonary in origin.

SUMMARY

The lower respiratory system begins to develop around the middle of the fourth week from a median *laryngotracheal groove* in the floor of the primitive pharynx. The groove deepens to produce a *laryngotracheal diverticulum*, which soon becomes separated from the foregut as the tracheoesophageal folds form and fuse to form the *tracheoesophageal septum*. This results in the formation of the esophagus and the *laryngotracheal tube*. The endoderm of this tube gives rise to the epithelium of the lower respiratory organs and to the tracheobronchial glands. The splanchnic mesenchyme surrounding the laryngotracheal tube forms the connective tissue, cartilage, muscle, and blood and lymphatic vessels of these organs.

Branchial or pharyngeal arch mesenchyme contributes to formation of the epiglottis and the connective tissue of the larynx. The laryngeal muscles and the skeleton of the larynx are derived from mesenchyme in the caudal branchial or pharyngeal arches. The cartilages develop from *neural crest cells*. The laryngeal cartilages are derived from the cartilaginous bars in the fourth and sixth pairs of branchial or pharyngeal arches (see Table 10–1).

During the fourth week the laryngotracheal tube develops a *lung bud* at its distal end, which divides into two *bronchial buds* during the early part of the fifth week. Each bud soon enlarges to form a *primary bronchus*, and then each of these gives rise to two new bronchial buds, which develop into *secondary bronchi*. The right inferior secondary bronchus soon divides into two bronchi. The secondary bronchi supply the lobes of the developing lungs. Each secondary bronchus undergoes progressive branching to form *segmental bronchi*. Each segmental bronchus with its surrounding mesenchyme is the primordium of a *bronchopulmonary segment*. Branching continues until about 17 orders of branches have formed. Additional airways are formed after birth until about 24 orders of branches are present.

Lung development is divided into four stages. During the *pseudoglandular period* (5 to 17 weeks), the bronchi and terminal bronchioles form. During the *canalicular period* (16 to 25 weeks), the lumina of the bronchi and terminal bronchioles enlarge, the respiratory bronchioles and alveolar ducts develop, and the lung tissue becomes highly vascular. During the *terminal sac period* (24 weeks to birth), the alveolar ducts give rise to terminal sacs (primitive alveoli). The terminal sacs are initially lined with cuboidal epithelium that begins to attenuate to squamous epithelium at about 26 weeks. By this time, capillary networks have proliferated close to the alveolar epithelium, and the lungs are usually sufficiently well-developed to permit survival of the fetus if it is born prematurely. The *alveolar period*, the final stage of lung development, occurs from the late fetal period to about eight years of age as the lungs mature. The number of respiratory bronchioles and primitive alveoli increases.

The respiratory system develops so that it is capable of immediate function at birth. To be capable of respiration, the lungs must acquire an alveolocapillary membrane that is sufficiently thin, and an adequate amount of *surfactant* must be present. A deficiency of surfactant appears to be responsible for the failure of primitive alveoli to remain open, resulting in *hyaline membrane disease* (HMD), a major cause of the *respiratory distress syndrome* (RDS). Growth of the lungs after birth results mainly from an increase in the number of respiratory bronchioles and alveoli. New alveoli form for at least eight years after birth.

Major congenital anomalies of the lower respiratory system are uncommon except for *tracheoesophageal fistula*, which is usually associated with esophageal atresia. These anomalies result from faulty partitioning of the foregut into the esophagus and trachea during the fourth and fifth weeks.

CLINICALLY ORIENTED QUESTIONS FOR PROBLEM-BASED LEARNING SESSIONS

1. Choking and continuous coughing were observed in a newborn infant. There was an excessive amount of mucous secretion and saliva in the infant's mouth, who experienced considerable difficulty in breathing. The pediatrician was unable to pass a catheter through the esophagus into the stomach. What congenital anomalies would be suspected? Discuss the embryological basis of these defects. What kind of an examination do you think would be used to confirm the diagnosis?

2. A premature infant developed rapid, shallow respirations shortly after birth. A diagnosis of *respiratory distress syndrome* (RDS) was made. How do you think the infant might attempt to overcome his or her inadequate exchange of oxygen and carbon dioxide? What disease commonly causes RDS? What treatment is currently used clinically to prevent RDS? A deficiency of what substance is associated with RDS?

3. What is the most common type of tracheoesophageal fistula? What is its embryological basis? What anomaly of the digestive tract is frequently associated with this abnormality?

4. A newborn infant with esophageal atresia experienced respiratory distress with cyanosis shortly after birth. Radiographs demonstrated air in the infant's stomach. How did it get there? What other problem might result in an infant with this fairly common type of congenital anomaly?

The answers to these questions are given on page 463.

References and Suggested Reading

Ballard PL: Hormonal control of lung maturation. *Bailliere's Clin Endocrin Metabol 3:*723, 1989.

Beck F, Moffat DB, Davies DP: *Human Embryology.* 2nd ed. Oxford, Blackwell Scientific Publications, 1985.

Behrman RE (ed): *Nelson Textbook of Pediatrics.* 14th ed. Philadelphia, WB Saunders, 1992.

Bertalanffy FD: Respiratory tissue: Structure, histophysiology, cytodynamics. Part I. Review and basic cytomorphology. *Int Rev Cytol 16:*233, 1964.

Boyden EA: Development and growth of the airways. *In* Hodson WA (ed): *Development of the Lung.* New York, Marcel Dekker, 1977.

Boyden EA: The pattern of the terminal airspaces in a premature infant of 30–32 weeks that lived nineteen and a quarter hours. *Am J Anat 126:*31, 1969.

Broers JL, de Leij L, ter Haar A, Lane EB, Leigh IM, Wagenaar SS, Vooijs GP, Ramaekers FC: Expression of intermediate filament proteins in fetal and adult human lung tissues. *Differentiation 40:*119, 1989.

Bucher U, Reid L: Development of the intrasegmental bronchial tree: The pattern of branching and development of cartilage at various stages of intrauterine life. *Thorax 16:*207, 1961.

Chernick V, Kryger MH: Pediatric lung disease. *In* Kryger MH (ed): *Introduction to Respiratory Medicine.* 2nd ed. New York, Churchill Livingstone, 1990.

Chernick V, Mellins RB (eds): *Basic Mechanisms of Pediatric Respiratory Disease: Cellular and Integrative.* Philadelphia, BC Decker, 1991.

Conen PE, Balis JU: Electron microscopy in study of lung development. *In* Emery J (ed): *The Anatomy of the Developing Lung.* London, William Heinemann, 1969.

Cooke IR, Berger PJ: Precursor of respiratory pattern in the early gestation mammalian fetus. *Brain Res 522:*333, 1990.

Cormack DH: *Ham's Histology.* 9th ed. Philadelphia, JB Lippincott, 1987.

Crelin ES: Development of the lower respiratory system. *Clin Symp 27(4),* 1975.

Crelin ES: Development of the upper respiratory system. *Clin Symp 28(3),* 1976.

Davis JA: The first breath and development of lung tissue. *In* Philipp EE, Barnes J, Newton M (eds): *Scientific Foundations of Obstetrics and Gynecology.* London, William Heinemann, 1970.

De Vries PA, De Vries CR: Embryology and development. *In* Othersen Jr, HB (ed): *The Pediatric Airway.* Philadelphia, WB Saunders, 1991.

Emery J: *The Anatomy of the Developing Lung.* London, William Heinemann, 1969.

Endo H, Oka T: An immunohistochemical study of bronchial cells producing surfactant protein A in the developing human fetal lung. *Early Human Develop 25:*149, 1991.

Fowler CL, Pokorny WJ, Wagner ML, Kessler MS: Review of bronchopulmonary foregut malformations. *J Pediatr Surg 23:*793, 1988.

Godfrey S: Growth and development of the respiratory system–functional development. *In* Davis JA, Dobbing J (eds): *Scientific Foundations of Paediatrics.* Philadelphia, WB Saunders, 1974.

Harrison MR: The fetus with a diaphragmatic hernia: pathology, natural history, and surgical management. *In* Harrison MR, Golbus MS, Filly RA: *The Unborn Patient: Prenatal Diagnosis and Treatment.* 2nd ed. Philadelphia, WB Saunders, 1991.

Hast HM: Developmental anatomy of the larynx. *In* Hinchcliffe R, Harrison D (eds): *Scientific Foundations of Otolaryngology.* London, W Heinemann, 1976.

Herbst JL: Esophagus. *In* Behrman RE (ed): *Nelson Textbook of Pediatrics.* 14th ed. Philadelphia, WB Saunders, 1992.

Hislop A, Reid L: Growth and development of the respiratory system–anatomical development. *In* Davis JA, Dobbing J (eds): *Scientific Foundations of Paediatrics.* Philadelphia, WB Saunders, 1974.

Hodson WA (ed): *Development of the Lung.* New York, Marcel Dekker, 1977.

Hollinger PH, Johnson KC, Schiller F: Congenital anomalies of the larynx. *Ann Otol 63:*581, 1954.

Kanaan CM, O'Grady JP, Veille JC: Effect of maternal carbon dioxide inhalation on human fetal breathing movements in term and preterm labor. *Obstet Gynecol 78:*9, 1991.

Kozuma S, Nemoto A, Okai T, Mizuno M: Maturational sequence of fetal breathing movements. *Biol Neonate 60 (suppl 1):*36, 1991.

Landing BH: Pathogenetic considerations of respiratory tract malformations in humans. *In* Persaud TVN (ed): *Advances in the Study of Birth Defects. Cardiovascular, Respiratory, Gastrointestinal and Genitourinary Malformations.* Vol 6. New York, Alan R. Liss, 1982.

Lind J, Tahti E, Hirvensalo M: Roentgenologic studies of the size of the lungs of the newborn baby before and after aeration. *Ann Paediatr Fenn 12:*20, 1966.

Low FN, Sampaio MM: The pulmonary alveolar epithelium as an endodermal derivative. *Anat Rec 127:*51, 1957.

Moore KL: *Clinically Oriented Anatomy.* 3rd ed. Baltimore, Williams & Wilkins, 1992.

Oliver RE: Fetal lung liquids. *Fed Proc 36:*2669, 1977.

O'Rahilly R, Boyden E: The timing and sequence of events in the development of the human respiratory system during the embryonic period proper. *Z Anat Entwicklungsgesch 141:*237, 1973.

O'Rahilly R, Tucker JA: The early development of the larynx in staged human embryos. Part 1. Embryos of the first five weeks (to stage 15). *Ann Otol Rhinol Laryngol 82 (suppl 7):*1, 1973.

Page EW, Villee CA, Villee DB: *Human Reproduction: Essentials of Reproductive and Perinatal Medicine.* 3rd ed. Philadelphia, WB Saunders, 1981.

Patrick J, Gagnon R: Fetal breathing and body movement. *In* Creasy RK, Resnik R (eds): *Maternal-Fetal Medicine. Principles and Practice.* 2nd ed. Philadelphia, WB Saunders, 1989.

Ramenofsky ML: Bronchogenic cyst. *In* Creasy RK, Resnik R (eds): *Maternal-Fetal Medicine. Principles and Practice.* 2nd ed. Philadelphia, WB Saunders, 1989.

Salzberg AM: Congenital malformations of the lower respiratory tract. *In* Kendig EL, Jr, Chernick V (eds): *Disorders of the Respiratory Tract in Children.* 4th ed. Philadelphia, WB Saunders, 1983.

Sañudo JR, Domenech-Mateu JM: The laryngeal primordium and epithelial lamina. A new interpretation. *J Anat 171*:207, 1990.

Scarpelli EM (ed): *Pulmonary Physiology: Fetus, Newborn, Child and Adolescent.* 2nd ed. Philadelphia, Lea and Febiger, 1990.

Smith EI: The early development of the trachea and oesophagus in relation to atresia of the oesophagus and tracheo-oesophageal fistula. *Contr Embryol Carneg Instn 245*:36, 1957.

Thurlbeck WM: Pre- and postnatal organ development. *In* Chernick V, Mellins RB (eds): *Basic Mechanisms of Pediatric Respiratory Disease: Cellular and Integrative.* Philadelphia, BC Decker, 1991.

Tooley WH: Lung disease and lung development. *In* Hodson WA (ed): *Development of the Lung.* New York, Marcel Dekker, 1977.

Villee CA, Villee DB, Zuckerman J: *Respiratory Distress Syndrome.* New York, Academic Press, 1973.

Wells LJ, Boyden EA: The development of the bronchopulmonary segments in human embryos of horizons XVII and XIX. *Am J Anat 95*:163, 1954.

Whitsett JA: Molecular aspects of the pulmonary surfactant system in the newborn. *In* Chernick V, Mellins RB (eds): *Basic Mechanisms of Pediatric Respiratory Disease: Cellular and Integrative.* Philadelphia, BC Decker, 1991.

Wiseman NE, Macpherson RI: Pulmonary sequestration. *In* Persaud TVN (ed): *Advances in the Study of Birth Defects. Cardiovascular, Respiratory, Gastrointestinal and Genitourinary Malformations.* Vol 6. New York, Alan R. Liss, 1982.

Wolfson VP, Laitman JT: Ultrasound investigation of fetal human upper respiratory anatomy. *Anat Rec 227*:363, 1990.

Zaw-Tun HA: The tracheo-esophageal septum–fact or fantasy? *Acta Anat 114*:1, 1982.

The Digestive System

The **primitive gut** forms during the fourth week as the head, tail, and lateral folds incorporate the dorsal part of the yolk sac into the embryo (see Figs 5–1 and 5–2). The endoderm of the primitive gut gives rise to most of the epithelium and glands of the digestive tract. The epithelium at the cranial and caudal extremities of the tract is derived from ectoderm of the *stomodeum* (primitive mouth) and *proctodeum* (anal pit), respectively (Figs. 12–1 and 12–21). The muscular, connective tissue, and other layers comprising the wall of the digestive tract are derived from the splanchnic mesenchyme surrounding the endoderm of the primitive gut. For descriptive purposes the primitive gut is divided into three parts: foregut, midgut, and hindgut (Fig. 12–1).

THE FOREGUT

The adult derivatives of the foregut are:

1. The *primitive pharynx* and its derivatives (oral cavity, pharynx, tongue, tonsils, salivary gland, and upper respiratory system) which are discussed in Chapter 10.

2. The *lower respiratory system* (described in Chapter 11).

3. The *esophagus and stomach.*

4. The *duodenum*, proximal to the opening of the (common) bile duct.

5. The *liver, biliary apparatus* (gallbladder and bile duct system), *and pancreas.*

All these foregut derivatives, *except* the pharynx, respiratory tract, and most of the esophagus, are supplied by the *celiac artery*, the artery of the foregut (Fig. 12–1).

Development of the Esophagus

The esophagus develops from the foregut immediately caudal to the primitive pharynx (Fig. 12–1). The partitioning of the trachea from the esophagus by the *tracheoesophageal septum* is described in Chapter 11 (p. 226) and illustrated in Figure 11–2. Initially, the esophagus is short (Fig. 12–1), but it elongates rapidly, mainly due to growth and descent of the heart and lungs. The esophagus reaches its final relative length by the seventh week. Its epithelium and glands are derived from endoderm. The epithelium proliferates and partly or completely obliterates the lumen, but recanalization of the esophagus normally occurs by the end of the embryonic period.

The striated muscle constituting the muscularis externa of the superior third of the esophagus is derived from mesenchyme in the caudal branchial or pharyngeal arches. The smooth muscle, mainly in the inferior third of the esophagus, develops from the surrounding splanchnic mesenchyme (Gemonov and Kolesnikov, 1990). Both types of muscle are innervated by branches of the vagus nerves (CN X), which supply the caudal branchial or pharyngeal arches (see Table 10–1).

Esophageal Atresia. Blockage of the esophagus occurs with an incidence of 1 in 3000 to 4500 live births (Herbst, 1992). About one third of affected infants are born prematurely. Esophageal atresia is associated with *tracheoesophageal fistula* in more than 85 per cent of cases. It may occur as a separate anomaly but this is less common. Esophageal atresia results from deviation of the *tracheoesophageal septum* in a posterior direction (see Fig. 11–2); as a result, there is incomplete separation of the esophagus from the laryngotracheal tube. Isolated esophageal atresia may be associated with other congenital anomalies, e.g., *anorectal atresia* and anomalies of the urogenital system. In these cases the atresia results from *failure of recanalization of the esophagus* during the eighth week of development. The cause of this arrest of development is thought to result from defective growth of endodermal cells (Herbst, 1992).

A fetus with esophageal atresia is unable to swallow amniotic fluid; consequently, this fluid cannot pass to the intestines for absorption and transfer via the placenta to the maternal blood for disposal. This results in *polyhydramnios*, the accumulation of an excessive amount of amniotic fluid (p. 129). Newborn infants with esophageal atresia usually appear healthy, and their first swallows are normal. Suddenly, fluid returns through the nose and mouth and *respiratory distress* occurs. Inability to pass a catheter through the esophagus into the stomach strongly suggests esophageal atresia. A radiographic examination would demonstrate the anomaly by imaging the nasogastric tube

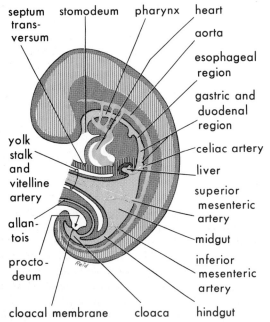

septum trans-versum
stomodeum
pharynx
heart
aorta
esophageal region
gastric and duodenal region
celiac artery
yolk stalk and vitelline artery
liver
superior mesenteric artery
allan-tois
midgut
inferior mesenteric artery
procto-deum
cloacal membrane
cloaca
hindgut

Figure 12–1. Drawing of a median section of a four-week-old embryo showing the early digestive system and its blood supply. The primitive gut is a long tube extending the length of the embryo. Its blood vessels are derived from the vessels that supplied the yolk sac.

arrested in the proximal esophageal pouch. *Surgical repair of esophageal atresia* now results in survival rates of more than 85 per cent in contrast to the less encouraging outcome of a decade ago.

Esophageal Stenosis. Narrowing of the lumen of the esophagus can exist anywhere, but it usually occurs in its distal third, either as a web or a long segment of esophagus with a threadlike lumen. Esophageal stenosis usually results from incomplete recanalization of the esophagus during the eighth week of development, but it could result from a failure of esophageal blood vessels to develop in the affected area. As a result, *atrophy* of a segment of its wall occurs.

Short Esophagus. Initially the esophagus is very short; and, if it fails to elongate sufficiently as the neck and thorax develop, a portion of the stomach may be displaced superiorly through the esophageal hiatus into the thorax. This is called a *congenital hiatal hernia*. Most hiatal hernias occur long after birth, usually in middle-aged people, and result from weakening and widening of the esophageal hiatus in the diaphragm (Moore, 1992).

Development of the Stomach

The distal part of the foregut is initially a simple tubular structure (Fig. 12–1). Around the middle of the fourth week, a slight dilation indicates the site of the future stomach. It first appears as a fusiform enlargement of the caudal part of the foregut and is initially oriented in the median plane (Figs. 12–1 and

12–2A). This primordium soon enlarges and broadens ventrodorsally. During the next two weeks the dorsal border of the primitive stomach grows faster than its ventral border; this demarcates the *greater curvature of the stomach* (Fig. 12–2B and C). (For an account of the kinetics of cell proliferation during morphogenesis of the stomach, see Menard and Arsenault, 1990).

Rotation of the Stomach (Figs. 12–2 and 12–3). As the stomach enlarges and acquires its adult shape, it slowly rotates 90 degrees in a clockwise direction around its longitudinal axis. The effects of this rotation on the stomach are as follows:

1. The ventral border (lesser curvature) moves to the right and the dorsal border (greater curvature) moves to the left.

2. The original left side becomes the ventral surface and the original right side becomes the dorsal surface.

3. Before rotation, the cranial and caudal ends of the stomach are in the median plane (Fig. 12–2A). During rotation and growth of the stomach, its cranial region (future *fundus*) moves to the left and slightly inferiorly, and its caudal region (future *pyloric antrum*[1]) moves to the right and superiorly. After rotation, the stomach assumes its final position with its long axis almost transverse to the long axis of the body (Fig. 12–2D). The rotation and growth of the stomach explain why the left vagus nerve supplies the anterior wall of the adult stomach and the right vagus nerve innervates its posterior wall.

Mesenteries of the Stomach (Figs. 12–2 and 12–3). The stomach is suspended from the dorsal wall of the abdominal cavity by a dorsal mesentery called the *dorsal mesogastrium* (Fig. 12–3A). This mesentery is originally in the median plane, but it is carried to the left during rotation of the stomach and formation of the *omental bursa* or lesser sac of peritoneum (Fig. 12–2A to C). A ventral mesentery or *ventral mesogastrium* (Fig. 12–2B) attaches the stomach and duodenum to the liver and the ventral abdominal wall (Fig. 12–2D).

The Omental Bursa (Lesser Sac of Peritoneum)

Isolated clefts (cavities) develop in the mesenchyme in the thick dorsal mesogastrium (Fig. 12–3A and B). These clefts soon coalesce to form a single cavity, which is the primordium of the *omental bursa* (Fig. 12–3C and D). Rotation of the stomach is thought to pull the dorsal mesogastrium to the left, thereby en-

---

[1] A bulging of the pyloric end of the stomach wall along the greater curvature when the organ is distended (Moore, 1992).

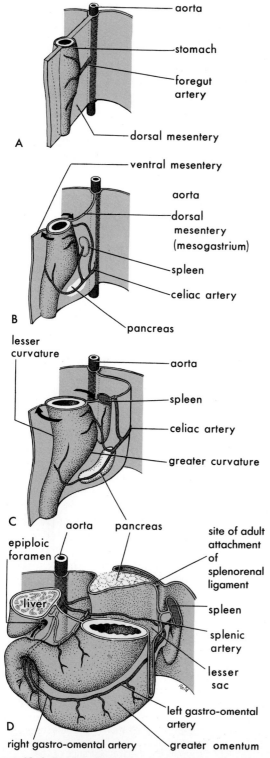

larging this recess of the peritoneal cavity. The omental bursa expands transversely and cranially and comes to lie between the stomach and the posterior abdominal wall. It is called a *bursa* (L. purse) to emphasize its importance in facilitating movement of the stomach.

The superior part of the cranial extension of the omental bursa is cut off as the diaphragm develops, forming a closed space known as the *infracardiac bursa*. If it persists, it usually lies medial to the basal part of the right lung. The inferior portion of the superior part of the cranial extension of the omental bursa persists as the *superior recess of the omental bursa* (Moore, 1992). As the stomach enlarges, the omental bursa expands and acquires an *inferior recess of the omental bursa* between the layers of the elongated dorsal mesogastrium, called the *greater omentum* (L. "fat skin"). This four-layered membrane overhangs the developing intestines (Figs. 12–3*J* and 12–13*C*). Later, the inferior recess disappears as the layers of the greater omentum fuse (Fig. 12–13*F*). The omental bursa communicates with the main part of the peritoneal cavity through a small opening called the *omental (epiploic) foramen* (Figs. 12–2*D* and 12–3*H*). In the adult, this foramen is located posterior to the free edge of the lesser omentum (Moore, 1992).

Congenital Hypertrophic Pyloric Stenosis. Anomalies of the stomach are uncommon except for hypertrophic pyloric stenosis. It affects one in every 150 males and one in every 750 females (Shandling, 1992). In infants with this abnormality, there is a marked *thickening of the pylorus*, the distal sphincteric region of the stomach. The circular and, to a lesser degree, the longitudinal muscles in the pyloric region are hypertrophied. This results in severe narrowing (stenosis) of the pyloric canal and obstruction to the passage of food. As a result, the stomach becomes markedly distended, and the infant expels the stomach's contents with considerable force (*projectile vomiting*). Surgical relief of the pyloric obstruction is the usual treatment.

The cause of congenital pyloric stenosis is unknown, but the high incidence of the condition in both infants of monozygotic twins suggests the involvement of genetic factors. Multifactorial inheritance of this disorder is likely (Shandling, 1992). For a discussion of the inheritance of congenital pyloric stenosis, see Thompson et al. (1991).

Development of the Duodenum

Early in the fourth week the duodenum begins to develop from the caudal part of the foregut, the cranial part of the midgut, and the splanchnic mesenchyme associated with these endodermal parts of the primitive gut (Fig. 12–4). The junction of the two parts of the duodenum is just distal to the origin of the bile duct (common bile duct). These parts of the

Figure 12–2. Drawings illustrating development and rotation of the stomach and formation of the omental bursa (lesser sac) and greater omentum. *A,* About 28 days. *B,* About 35 days. *C,* About 40 days. *D,* About 48 days.

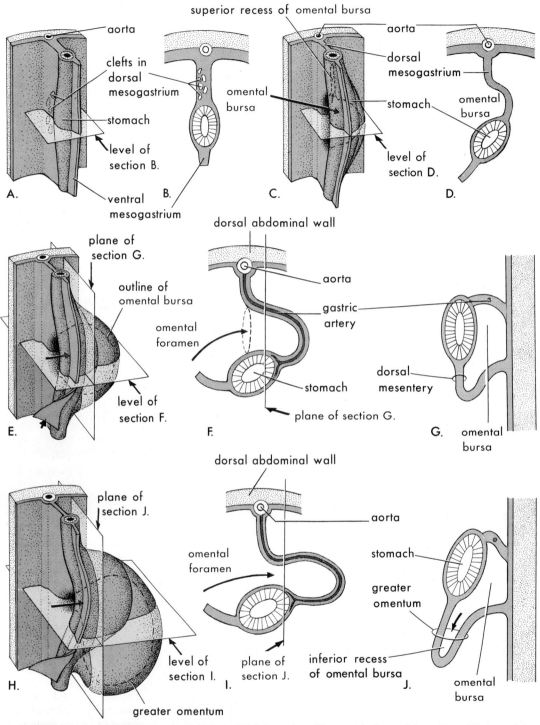

Figure 12-3. Diagrams illustrating development of the stomach and its mesenteries, and formation of the omental bursa (lesser sac). *A*, Five weeks. *B*, Transverse section showing clefts in the dorsal mesogastrium. *C*, Later stage after coalescence of the clefts to form the omental bursa. *D*, Transverse section showing the initial appearance of the omental bursa. *E*, The dorsal mesentery has elongated and the omental bursa has enlarged. *F* and *G*, Transverse and longitudinal sections, respectively, showing elongation of the dorsal mesogastrium and expansion of the omental bursa. *H*, Six weeks, showing the greater omentum and expansion of the omental bursa. *I* and *J*, Transverse and longitudinal sections, respectively, showing the inferior recess of the omental bursa and the omental (epiploic) foramen.

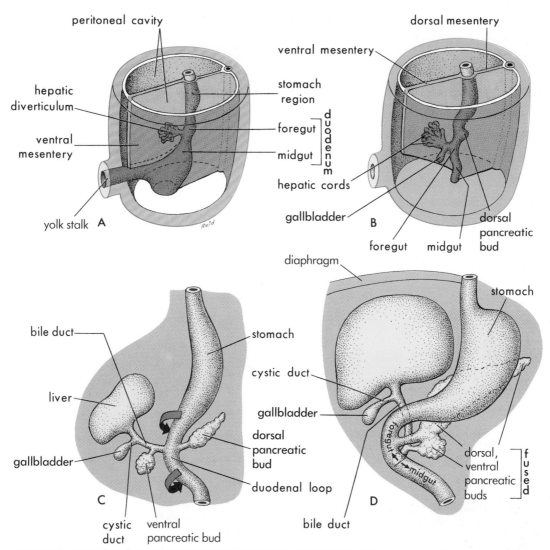

Figure 12–4. Drawings illustrating progressive stages in the development of the duodenum, liver, pancreas, and extrahepatic biliary apparatus. *A,* Four weeks. *B* and *C,* Five weeks. *D,* Six weeks. The pancreas develops from dorsal and ventral buds that fuse to form the pancreas. Note that the entrance of the bile duct into the duodenum gradually shifts from its initial position to a posterior one. This explains why the bile duct in the adult passes posterior to the duodenum and the head of the pancreas.

foregut and midgut grow rapidly and form a C-shaped loop that projects ventrally (Fig. 12–4*B* to *D*). The junction of the foregut and midgut and the attachment of the bile duct is now at the apex of this embryonic duodenal loop (Fig. 12–4*D*). As the stomach rotates, the developing duodenal loop rotates to the right where it comes to lie retroperitoneally (i.e., external to the peritoneum [Fig. 12–13*F*]). Because of its derivation from the foregut and midgut, the duodenum is supplied by branches of the celiac and supe-

rior mesenteric arteries that supply these parts of the primitive gut (Figs. 12–1 and 12–6).

During the fifth and sixth weeks, the lumen of the duodenum becomes progressively smaller and is temporarily obliterated due to the proliferation of its epithelial cells. Normally, because of vacuolation due to degeneration of the epithelial cells, the duodenum becomes recanalized by the end of the embryonic period. By this time most of the ventral mesentery of the duodenum has disappeared (Fig. 12–13).

Duodenal Stenosis (Fig. 12–5A). Partial occlusion of the duodenal lumen usually results from incomplete recanalization of the duodenum due to defective vacuolization (Fig. 12–5E_3). Duodenal stenosis may also be caused by pressure from an *anular pancreas* (Fig. 12–9). Most stenoses involve the horizontal (third) and/or ascending (fourth) parts of the duodenum. Due to the occlusion, the stomach's contents are often expelled and the vomitus usually contains bile.

Duodenal Atresia (Fig. 12–5B). Complete occlusion of the lumen of the duodenum is not common. Twenty to thirty per cent of affected infants have Down syndrome (p. 146), and an additional 20 per cent are premature (Shandling, 1992). In about 20 per cent of cases, the bile duct enters the duodenum just distal to the opening of the hepatopancreatic ampulla (Moore, 1992). During duodenal development, the lumen is completely occluded by epithelial cells. If reformation of the lumen fails to occur (Fig. 12–5D), a short segment of the duodenum is occluded. Investigation of families with *familial duodenal atresia* suggests an autosomal recessive inheritance (Best et al., 1989).

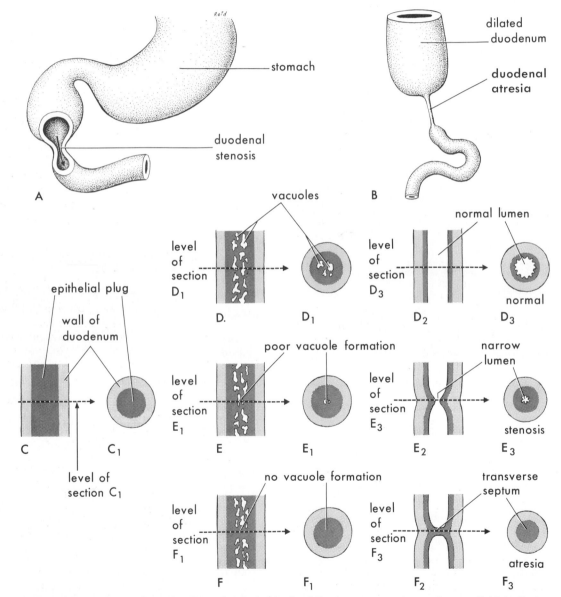

Figure 12–5. Diagrams illustrating the embryological basis of the two common types of congenital intestinal obstruction. *A,* Duodenal stenosis. *B,* Duodenal atresia. *C* to *F,* Diagrammatic longitudinal and transverse sections of the duodenum showing: (1) normal recanalization (*D* to D_3), (2) stenosis (*E* to E_3), and (3) atresia (*F* to F_3). Most duodenal atresias occur in the descending (second) and horizontal (third) parts of the duodenum.

Most atresias involve the descending (second) and horizontal (third) parts of the duodenum and are located distal to the opening of the bile duct.

In infants with duodenal atresia, vomiting begins within a few hours of birth. The vomitus almost always contains bile. Often, there is distention of the epigastrium resulting from an overfilled stomach and superior part of the duodenum. Duodenal atresia may occur as an isolated anomaly, but other severe congenital anomalies are often associated with it; e.g., Down syndrome (see Fig. 8–4), anular pancreas (Fig. 12–9), cardiovascular abnormalities, and anorectal malformations. *Polyhydramnios* (p. 129) also occurs because the duodenal atresia prevents normal absorption of amniotic fluid by the intestines.

Development of the Liver and Biliary Apparatus

The liver, gallbladder, and biliary duct system arise as a ventral outgrowth from the caudal part of the foregut early in the fourth week (Fig. 12–4A). The liver bud or *hepatic diverticulum* extends into the septum transversum, a mass of splanchnic mesoderm between the developing heart and midgut (Fig. 12–6A and B). The septum transversum forms part of the diaphragm (see Fig. 9–7) and, in this region, the ventral mesentery (Fig. 12–4A). The hepatic diverticulum enlarges rapidly and divides into two parts as it grows between the layers of the *ventral mesentery* (Fig. 12–4B).

The larger cranial part of the diverticulum is the **liver primordium**. The proliferating endodermal cells give rise to interlacing cords of hepatic cells and to the epithelial lining of the intrahepatic portion of the biliary apparatus (Fig. 12–4B). The *hepatic cords* anastomose around endothelium-lined spaces, which are the primordia of the *hepatic sinusoids*. The fibrous and *hemopoietic tissue* and the *Kupffer cells* of the liver are derived from mesenchyme in the septum transversum.

The liver grows rapidly and, from the fifth to tenth weeks, fills a large part of the abdominal cavity. The quantity of oxygenated blood flowing from the umbilical vein into the liver determines the development and functional segmentation of the liver (Champetier et al., 1989b). Initially, the right and left lobes are about the same size, but the right lobe soon becomes larger.

Hemopoiesis begins during the sixth week, giving the liver a bright reddish appearance. This hemopoietic activity is mainly responsible for the relatively large size of the liver between the seventh and ninth weeks of development (Fig. 12–12). By the ninth week, the liver accounts for about 10 per cent of the total weight of the fetus. *Bile formation* by the hepatic cells begins during the twelfth week.

The small caudal part of the hepatic diverticulum becomes the *gallbladder*, and its stalk forms the *cystic duct* (Fig. 12–4C). Initially, the extrahepatic biliary apparatus is occluded with epithelial cells, but it is later recanalized due to vacuolation resulting from degeneration of these cells. The stalk connecting the hepatic and cystic ducts to the duodenum becomes the *bile duct*. Initially, this duct attaches to the ventral aspect of the duodenal loop; but, as the duodenum grows and rotates, the entrance of the bile duct is carried to the dorsal aspect of the duodenum (Fig. 12–4C and D). The bile entering the duodenum via the bile duct after the thirteenth week gives the intestinal contents (*meconium*) a dark green color.

The Ventral Mesentery (Figs. 12–6 and 12–7). This thin, double-layered membrane gives rise to: (1) the *lesser omentum*, which passes from the liver to the lesser curvature of the stomach (*hepatogastric ligament*) and from the liver to the duodenum (*hepatoduodenal ligament*), and (2) the *falciform ligament*, which extends from the liver to the ventral abdominal wall. The *umbilical vein* passes in the free border of the falciform ligament on its way from the umbilical cord to the liver. The ventral mesentery also forms the *visceral peritoneum of the liver*. The liver is covered by peritoneum except for an area that is in direct contact with the diaphragm; this is called the *bare area of the liver*.

Anomalies of the Liver. Minor variations of liver lobulation are common and clinically insignificant, but congenital anomalies of the liver are rare. Variations of the hepatic ducts, bile duct, and cystic duct are common and clinically significant (Moore, 1992). *Accessory hepatic ducts* may be present, and awareness of their possible presence is of surgical importance. These accessory ducts are narrow channels running from the right lobe of the liver into the anterior surface of the body of the gallbladder. In some cases, the cystic duct opens into an accessory hepatic duct rather than into the common hepatic duct.

Extrahepatic Biliary Atresia. This is the most serious anomaly of the extrahepatic biliary system and occurs in 1:10,000 to 15,000 live births (Balistreri, 1992). The most common form of extrahepatic biliary atresia (85 per cent of cases) is obstruction of the ducts at or superior to the *porta hepatis*[2]. Failure of the bile ducts to canalize often results from persistence of the solid stage of duct development. It also could result from liver infection during late fetal development. Jaundice occurs soon after birth. When biliary atresia cannot be corrected surgically, the child may die if a liver transplant is not performed (Karrer and Raffensperger, 1990).

---

[2] The porta hepatis is a deep transverse fissure on the visceral surface of the liver, about 5 cm long in adults (Moore, 1992).

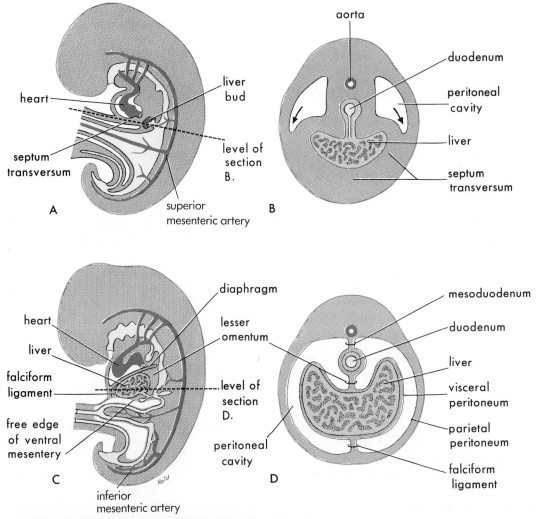

Figure 12-6. Drawings illustrating how the caudal part of the septum transversum becomes stretched and membranous as it forms the ventral mesentery. *A,* Median section of a four-week embryo. *B,* Transverse section of the embryo showing expansion of the peritoneal cavity (arrows). *C,* Sagittal section of a five-week embryo. *D,* Transverse section of the embryo after formation of the dorsal and ventral mesenteries. Note that the liver is joined to the ventral abdominal wall and to the stomach and the duodenum by the falciform ligament and the lesser omentum, respectively.

Development of the Pancreas

The pancreas develops between the layers of the ventral mesentery from dorsal and ventral *pancreatic buds* of endodermal cells that arise from the caudal part of the foregut that is developing into the proximal part of the duodenum (Figs. 12–4, 12–6, and 12–8). The larger *dorsal pancreatic bud* appears first and develops a slight distance cranial to the ventral bud. It grows rapidly between the layers of the dorsal mesentery (Figs. 12–7 and 12–10). The *ventral pancreatic bud* develops near the entry of the bile duct into the duodenum and grows between the layers of the ventral mesentery (Figs. 12–8 and 12–10).

As the duodenum rotates to the right and becomes C-shaped, the ventral pancreatic bud is carried dorsally with the bile duct (Fig. 12–8C to G). It soon lies posterior to the dorsal pancreatic bud (Fig. 12–8C) and later fuses with it (Fig. 12–8D and G). The ventral pancreatic bud forms the *uncinate process* and part of the head of the pancreas. As the stomach, duodenum, and ventral mesentery rotate, the pancreas comes to lie along the dorsal abdominal wall (Fig. 12–13C). Most of the pancreas is derived from the dorsal pancreatic bud.

As the pancreatic buds fuse, their ducts anastomose. The *main pancreatic duct* forms from the duct of the ventral bud and the distal part of the duct of the dorsal bud. The proximal part of the duct of the dorsal bud often persists as an *accessory pancreatic duct* that opens into the *minor duodenal papilla* located about 2 cm cranial to the main duct (Fig. 12–8*G*). The two ducts often communicate with each other. In about nine per cent of people, the pancreatic duct systems fail to fuse and the original two ducts persist (Moore, 1992).

Histogenesis of the Pancreas. The pancreatic parenchyma is derived from the endoderm of the pancreatic buds, which forms a network of tubules. Early in the fetal period, acini begin to develop from cell clusters around the ends of these tubules (primitive ducts). The *pancreatic islets* develop from groups of cells that separate from the tubules and soon come to lie between the acini. *Insulin* secretion begins during the early fetal period (ten weeks [von Dorsche, 1990]).

The *glucagon-* and somatostatin-containing cells develop before differentiation of the insulin secreting cells. Glucagon has been detected in fetal plasma at 15 weeks (von Dorsche, 1990). With increasing fetal age, the total pancreatic insulin and glucagon content also increases. The connective tissue sheath and the interlobular septa of the pancreas develop from the surrounding splanchnic mesenchyme. When there is *maternal diabetes mellitus,* the insulin-secreting beta cells in the fetal pancreas are chronically exposed to high levels of glucose. As a result, these cells undergo hypertrophy in order to increase the rate of insulin secretion (Carr, 1988).

> **Anomalies of the Pancreas.** Accessory pancreatic tissue is most often located in the wall of the stomach or duodenum or in an ileal (Meckel) diverticulum (Figs. 12–17 and 12–18).
>
> *Anular Pancreas.* This rare anomaly warrants description because it may cause duodenal obstruction (Fig. 12–9*C*). The ringlike or anular portion of the pancreas consists of a thin, flat band of pancreatic tissue surrounding the descending or second part of the duodenum. An anular pancreas may cause obstruction of the duodenum shortly after birth or in the adult. Blockage of the duodenum develops later in life if inflammation or malignant disease develops in an anular pancreas. An increased incidence of pancreatitis and peptic ulcer have been detected in patients with this abnormal pancreas. Males are affected much more frequently than females. Anular pancreas probably results from the growth of a bifid ventral pancreatic bud around the duodenum (Fig. 12–9). The portions of the bifid ventral bud then fuse with the dorsal bud, forming a pancreatic ring (Fig. 12–9*C*).

Development of the Spleen

Development of the spleen is described here because this *lymphatic organ* is derived from a mass of

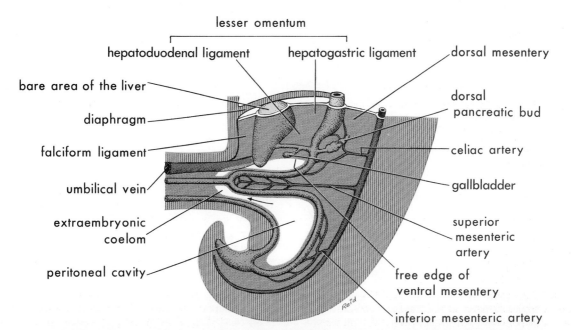

lesser omentum

hepatoduodenal ligament — hepatogastric ligament — dorsal mesentery

bare area of the liver — dorsal pancreatic bud

diaphragm — celiac artery

falciform ligament — gallbladder

umbilical vein — superior mesenteric artery

extraembryonic coelom — free edge of ventral mesentery

peritoneal cavity — inferior mesenteric artery

Figure 12–7. Diagrammatic sketch of a median section of the caudal half of an embryo at the end of the fifth week showing the liver and its associated ligaments, as viewed from the left. The *arrow* indicates the communication of the peritoneal cavity with the extraembryonic coelom. Due to the rapid growth of the liver and the midgut loop, the abdominal cavity temporarily becomes too small to contain the developing intestines; consequently, they enter the extraembryonic coelom in the umbilical cord (see also Fig. 12–12).

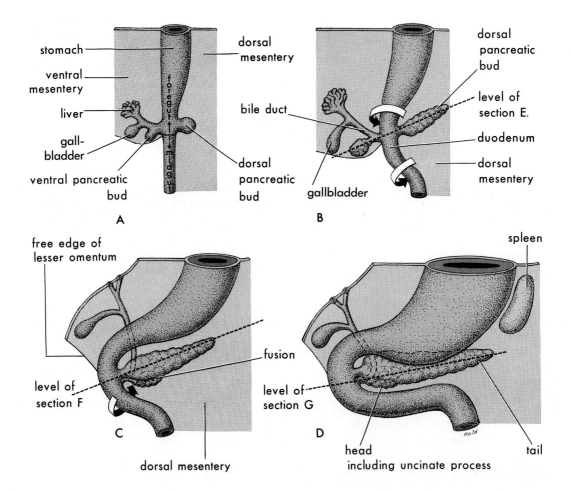

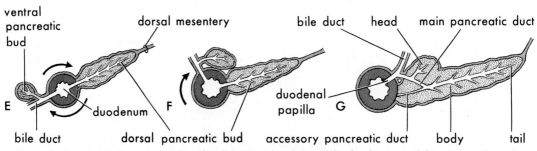

Figure 12–8. *A* to *D,* Schematic drawings showing successive stages in the development of the pancreas from the fifth to the eighth week. *E* to *G,* Diagrammatic transverse sections through the duodenum and developing pancreas. Growth and rotation (*arrows*) of the duodenum bring the ventral pancreatic bud toward the dorsal bud; they subsequently fuse. Note that the bile duct initially attaches to the ventral aspect of the duodenum and is carried around to the dorsal aspect as the duodenum rotates. The main pancreatic duct is formed by the union of the distal part of the dorsal pancreatic duct and the entire ventral pancreatic duct. The proximal part of the dorsal pancreatic duct usually obliterates, but it may persist as an accessory pancreatic duct.

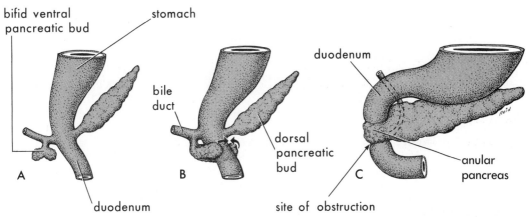

Figure 12–9. *A* and *B*, Drawings illustrating the probable embryological basis of an anular (annular) pancreas. *C*, An anular pancreas encircling the duodenum. This anomaly of the pancreas sometimes may produce complete obstruction (atresia) or partial obstruction (stenosis) of the duodenum. In most cases the anular pancreas encircles the second part of the duodenum, distal to the hepatopancreatic ampulla (see Moore [1992] for an illustration of this structure).

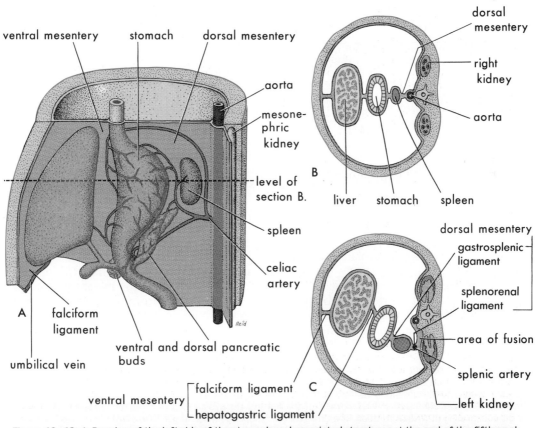

Figure 12–10. *A*, Drawing of the left side of the stomach and associated structures at the end of the fifth week. Note that the pancreas, spleen, and celiac artery are between the layers of the dorsal mesogastrium. *B*, Transverse section of the liver, stomach, and spleen at the level shown in *A*, illustrating their relationship to the dorsal and ventral mesenteries. *C*, Transverse section of a fetus showing fusion of the dorsal mesogastrium with the peritoneum on the posterior abdominal wall.

mesenchymal cells located between the layers of the dorsal mesogastrium (Figs. 12–2B and 12–10). The spleen, a large vascular lymphatic organ, begins to develop during the fifth week but does not acquire its characteristic shape until early in the fetal period (Figs. 12–8, 12–10, and 12–11E). The spleen is lobulated in the fetus, but the lobules normally disappear before birth. The notches in the superior border of the adult spleen are remnants of the grooves that separated the fetal lobules (Moore, 1992).

As the stomach rotates, the left surface of the mesogastrium fuses with the peritoneum over the left kidney. This fusion explains the dorsal attachment of the *splenorenal ligament* (lienorenal ligament) and why the adult splenic artery, the largest branch of the celiac trunk, follows a tortuous course posterior to the omental bursa and anterior to the left kidney (Fig. 12–10C).

Histogenesis of the Spleen. The mesenchymal cells in the splenic primordium differentiate to form the capsule, connective tissue framework, and parenchyma of the spleen. The spleen functions as a hematopoietic center until late fetal life, but it retains its potential for blood cell formation even in adult life.

Accessory Spleens. One or more small splenic masses may develop. They most commonly appear near the hilum of the spleen or adjacent to the tail of the pancreas. Accessory spleens occur in about 10 per cent of people; they are usually about 1 cm in diameter. An accessory spleen may be embedded partly or wholly in the tail of the pancreas or within the gastrosplenic ligament (Fig. 12–10C).

THE MIDGUT

The derivatives of the midgut are:

1. The small intestines, including most of the duodenum.

2. The cecum, vermiform appendix, ascending colon, and the right half to two thirds of the transverse colon.

All these midgut derivatives are supplied by the *superior mesenteric artery*, the artery of the midgut (Fig. 12–1). The midgut loop is suspended from the dorsal abdominal wall by an elongated mesentery (Fig. 12–11A). As the midgut elongates, it forms a ventral, U-shaped loop of gut called the *midgut loop*, which projects into the remains of the extraembryonic coelom in the proximal part of the umbilical cord (see Figs. 9–2E and 12–11A). This process is referred to as a *physiological umbilical herniation*. It occurs at the beginning of the sixth week and is a normal migration of the midgut into the umbilical cord (Figs. 12–11 and 12–12). The midgut loop communicates with the yolk sac via the narrow *yolk stalk* until the tenth week (Fig. 12–11A and C).

At this stage, the intraembryonic coelom communicates with extraembryonic coelom at the umbilicus (Fig. 12–7). Umbilical herniation occurs because there is not enough room in the abdomen for the rapidly growing midgut (Fig. 12–12). The shortage of space is caused mainly by the relatively massive liver and the two sets of kidneys that exist during this period of development (p. 265). The midgut loop has a cranial limb and a caudal limb. The *yolk stalk* is attached to the apex of the midgut loop where the two limbs join (Fig. 12–11A). The cranial limb grows rapidly and forms small intestinal loops, but the caudal limb undergoes very little change except for development of the *cecal diverticulum* (Fig. 12–11B).

Rotation of the Midgut Loop

While it is in the umbilical cord, the midgut loop rotates 90 degrees counterclockwise around the axis of the *superior mesenteric artery* (Fig. 12–11B). This brings the cranial limb of the midgut loop to the right and the caudal limb to the left (Fig. 12–11B). During rotation the midgut elongates and forms loops of small bowel (jejunum and ileum [Fig. 12–12]).

Return of the Midgut to the Abdomen (Fig. 12–11C). During the tenth week the intestines return to the abdomen. It is not known what causes the intestine to return, but the decrease in the size of the liver and kidneys and the enlargement of the abdominal cavity are important factors. This process has been called "reduction of the midgut hernia." The small intestine (formed from the cranial limb) returns first, passing posterior to the superior mesenteric artery, and occupy the central part of the abdomen. As the

---

Figure 12–11. Schematic drawings illustrating the rotation of the midgut, as seen from the left. *A*, Around the beginning of the sixth week, showing the midgut loop partially within the umbilical cord. Note the elongated, double-layered dorsal mesentery containing the superior mesenteric artery. *A₁*, Transverse section through the midgut loop, illustrating the initial relationship of the limbs of the midgut loop to the artery. *B*, Later stage showing the beginning of midgut rotation. The umbilical vein should be much larger than shown here (see Fig. 12–7). *B₁*, Illustrates the 90-degree counterclockwise rotation that carries the cranial limb of the midgut to the right. *C*, About ten weeks, showing the intestines returning to the abdomen. *C₁*, Illustrates a further rotation of 90 degrees. *D*, About 11 weeks, after return of intestines to the abdomen. *D₁*, Shows a further 90-degree rotation of the gut, for a total of 270 degrees. *E*, Later fetal period, showing the cecum rotating to its normal position in the lower right quadrant of the abdomen.

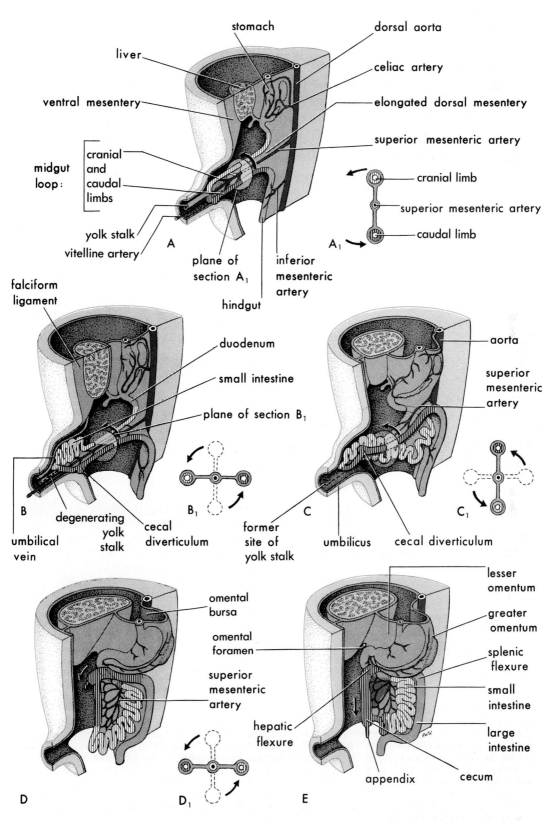

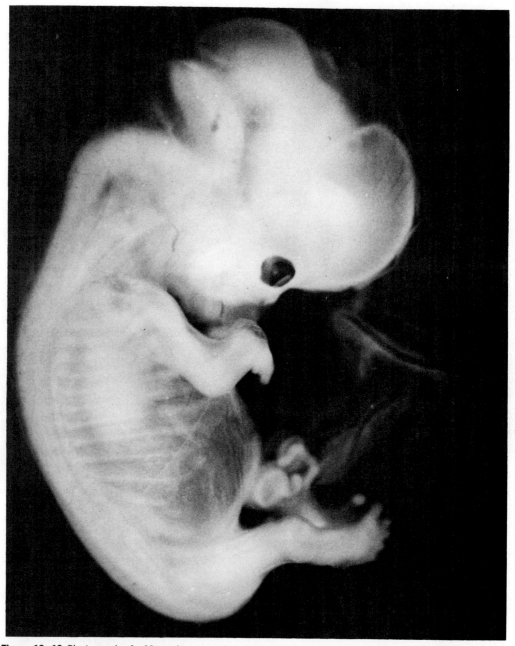

Figure 12–12. Photograph of a 28-mm human embryo (about 56 days). Note the herniated intestine derived from the midgut loop in the proximal part of the umbilical cord. Also note the umbilical blood vessels. Observe also the cartilaginous ribs, the prominent eye, the large liver, and the relatively well-developed brain. (Courtesy of Dr. Bruce Fraser, Associate Professor of Anatomy, Faculty of Medicine, Memorial University, St. John's, Newfoundland.)

large intestines return, they undergo a further 180-degree counterclockwise rotation (Fig. 12–11C_1 and D_1), making a total rotation of 270 degrees. The *cecum*, the widest part of the intestine, returns last and is located just caudal to the right lobe of the liver (Fig. 12–11D). Later it comes to occupy the right side of the abdomen (Fig. 12–11D). The ascending colon becomes recognizable as the posterior abdominal wall progressively elongates (Fig. 12–11E).

Fixation of the Intestines (Fig. 12–13). Rotation of the stomach and duodenum causes the duodenum and pancreas to fall to the right, where they are pressed against the posterior abdominal wall by the colon. The adjacent layers of peritoneum fuse and subsequently disappear (Fig. 12–13C and F); consequently, most of the duodenum and the head of the pancreas become retroperitoneal (posterior to the peritoneum).

The attachment of the dorsal mesentery to the posterior abdominal wall is greatly modified after the intestines return to the abdominal cavity. At first the dorsal mesentery is in the median plane (Fig. 12–2A). As the intestines enlarge, lengthen, and assume their final positions, their mesenteries are pressed against the posterior abdominal wall. The mesentery of the ascending colon fuses with the parietal peritoneum on this wall and disappears; consequently, the ascending colon also becomes retroperitoneal.

The colon presses the duodenum against the posterior abdominal wall. As a result, most of the duodenal mesentery is absorbed (Fig. 12–13$C, D,$ and F). Consequently, the duodenum, except for about the first 2.5 cm (derived from the foregut), has no mesentery and lies retroperitoneally (Moore, 1992). Other derivatives of the midgut loop (e.g., jejunum and ileum) retain their mesenteries (Fig. 12–13). The mesentery is at first attached to the median plane of the posterior abdominal wall (Fig. 12–11A). During rotation of the midgut, the mesentery rotates around the origin of the superior mesenteric artery (Fig. 12–11B and C). After the mesentery of the ascending colon disappears, the fan-shaped mesentery of the small intestines acquires a new line of attachment that passes from the duodenojejunal junction inferolaterally to the ileocecal junction (Fig. 12–13D).

The Cecum and Vermiform Appendix

The primordium of the cecum and appendix, called the *cecal diverticulum*, appears in the sixth week as a swelling on the antimesenteric border of the caudal limb of the midgut loop (Fig. 12–11A). The apex of the cecal diverticulum does not grow as rapidly as the rest of it; thus, the appendix is initially a small diverticulum of the cecum (Fig. 12–14B). The appendix increases rapidly in length (Fig. 12–14C) so that, by birth, it is a relatively long, worm-shaped tube arising from the distal end of the cecum (Fig. 12–14D).

After birth the wall of the cecum grows unequally, with the result that the appendix comes to enter its medial side (Fig. 12–14E). The appendix is subject to considerable variation in position. As the ascending colon elongates, the appendix may pass posterior to the cecum (*retrocecal appendix*) or colon (*retrocolic appendix*). It may also descend over the brim of the pelvis (*pelvic appendix*). *In about 64 per cent of people, the appendix is located retrocecally* (Moore, 1992).

Anomalies of the Midgut

Congenital abnormalities of the intestine are common; most of them are *anomalies of rotation* that result from incomplete rotation and/or fixation of the intestines.

Congenital Omphalocele (Fig. 12–15). This is a persistence of the herniation of abdominal contents into the proximal part of the umbilical cord (Fig. 12–12). Herniation of intestines occurs in about 1 of 5000 births and herniation of liver and intestines in 1 of about 10,000 births (Kleigman and Behrman, 1992). Omphalocele results from failure of the intestines to return to the abdominal cavity during the tenth week. The covering of the hernial sac is the epithelium of the umbilical cord, a derivative of the amnion (p. 128).

Umbilical Hernia. When the intestines return to the abdominal cavity during the tenth week and then herniate through an imperfectly closed umbilicus, an umbilical hernia forms. An umbilical hernia is different from an omphalocele. In umbilical hernia, the protruding mass (usually the greater omentum and part of the small intestine) is covered by subcutaneous tissue and skin. The hernia usually does not reach its maximum size until the end of the first month after birth. It usually ranges from 1 to 5 cm. The defect through which the hernia occurs is in the linea alba (Moore, 1992). The hernia protrudes during crying, straining, or coughing and can be easily reduced through the fibrous ring at the umbilicus. Surgery is not usually performed unless the hernia persists to the age of 3 to 5 years (Kleigman and Behrman, 1992).

Gastroschisis. This uncommon condition results from a defect in or near the median plane of the ventral abdominal wall. The linear defect permits extrusion of the abdominal viscera without involving the umbilical cord. The viscera protrude into the amniotic cavity and are bathed by amniotic fluid. The term *gastroschisis*, which literally means a "split or open stomach," is a misnomer because it is the anterior abdominal wall that is split, not the stomach. The defect usually occurs on the right side near the median plane and is more common in males than in females. The anomaly results from incomplete closure of the lateral folds during the fourth week (see Fig. 5–1).

Nonrotation of the Midgut (Fig. 12–16A). This relatively common condition, sometimes called *left-sided colon*, is generally asymptomatic, but twisting of the intestines

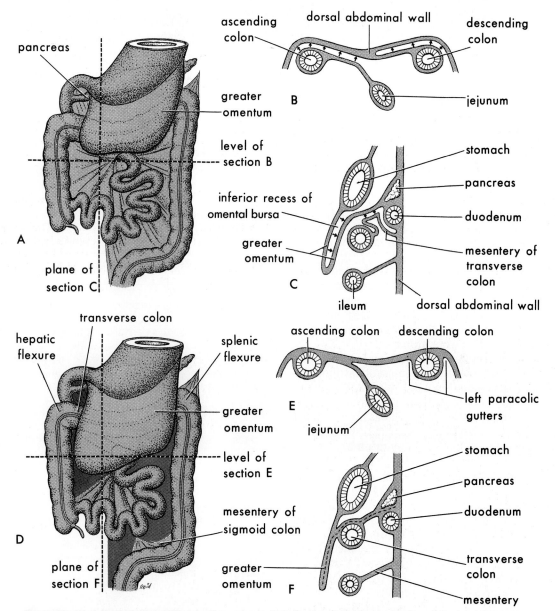

Figure 12–13. *A,* Ventral view of the intestines prior to their fixation. *B,* Transverse section at the level shown in *A.* The arrows indicate areas of subsequent fusion. *C,* Sagittal section at the plane shown in *A,* illustrating the greater omentum overhanging the transverse colon. The arrows indicate areas of subsequent fusion. *D,* Ventral view of the intestines after their fixation. *E,* Transverse section at the level shown in *D* after disappearance of the mesentery of the ascending and descending colon. *F,* Sagittal section at the plane shown in *D,* illustrating fusion of the greater omentum with the mesentery of the transverse colon and fusion of the layers of the greater omentum.

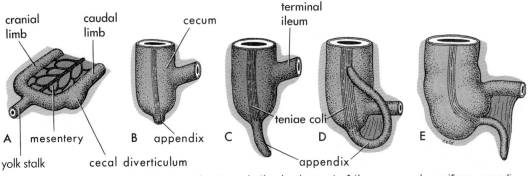

Figure 12–14. Drawings showing successive stages in the development of the cecum and vermiform appendix. *A*, Six weeks. *B*, Eight weeks. *C*, Twelve weeks. *D*, At birth. Note that the appendix is relatively long and is continuous with the apex of the cecum. *E*, Adult. Note that the appendix is relatively short and lies on the medial side of the cecum. In about 64 per cent of people, the appendix is located posterior to the cecum (retrocecal). In about 32 per cent of people, it appears as illustrated in *E*. The teniae coli are thickened bands of longitudinal muscle.

(*volvulus*) may occur (Fig. 12–16*B*). Nonrotation occurs when the midgut loop does not rotate as it enters the abdomen. As a result, the caudal limb of the loop returns to the abdomen first, and the small intestine lies on the right side of the abdomen and the entire large intestine on the left. When volvulus occurs, the superior mesenteric artery may be obstructed, resulting in infarction and gangrene of the bowel supplied by it.

Mixed Rotation and Volvulus (Fig. 12–16*B*). In this condition, the cecum lies just inferior to the pylorus of the stomach and is fixed to the posterior abdominal wall by peritoneal bands that pass over the duodenum. These bands

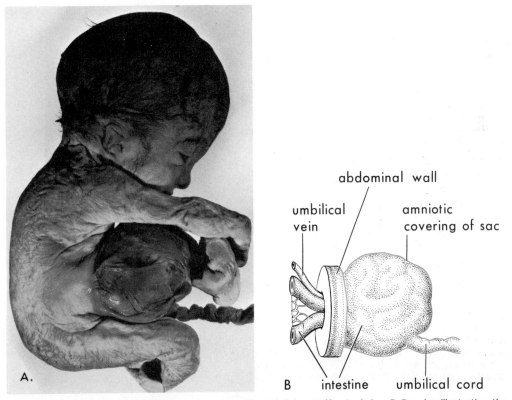

Figure 12–15. *A*, Large omphalocele in an immature 28-week fetus. Half actual size. *B*, Drawing illustrating the structure and contents of the hernial sac. The protruding mass of intestine is covered by a transparent, bilaminar membrane composed of peritoneum and amnion. Occasionally, these membranes rupture prior to or during birth. In this case, the eviscerated intestine lies freely around the gaping defect in the abdominal wall.

and the volvulus of the intestines usually cause *duodenal obstruction*. This type of malrotation results from failure of the midgut loop to complete the final 90 degrees of rotation (Fig. 12–11*D*); consequently, the terminal part of the ileum returns to the abdomen first.

Reversed Rotation (Fig. 12–16*C*). In very unusual cases, the midgut loop rotates in a clockwise rather than a counterclockwise direction. As a result, the duodenum lies anterior to the superior mesenteric artery (SMA) rather than posterior to it, and the transverse colon lies posterior to the SMA instead of anterior to it. In these cases, the transverse colon may be obstructed by pressure from the SMA. In very rare cases, the small intestine lies on the left side of the abdomen and the large intestine lies on the right side, with the cecum in the center. This unusual situation results from malrotation of the midgut followed by failure of fixation of the intestines.

Subhepatic Cecum and Appendix (Fig. 12–16*D*). If the cecum adheres to the inferior surface of the liver when it returns to the abdomen (Fig. 12–11*D*), it will be drawn superiorly as the liver diminishes in size; as a result, the cecum remains in its fetal position. Subhepatic cecum and appendix are more common in males and occur in about six per cent of fetuses. Subhepatic cecum is not common in adults; however, when it occurs, it may create a problem in the diagnosis of appendicitis and during the surgical removal of the appendix (*appendectomy*).

Mobile Cecum. In about 10 per cent of people the cecum has an unusual amount of freedom. In very unusual cases it may even herniate into the right inguinal canal. A mobile cecum results from incomplete fixation of the ascending colon. This condition is clinically significant because of the possible variations in position of the appendix (Moore, 1992) and because twisting or volvulus of the cecum may occur.

Internal Hernia (Fig. 12–16*E*). In this condition; the small intestine passes into the mesentery of the midgut loop during the return of the intestines to the abdomen. As a

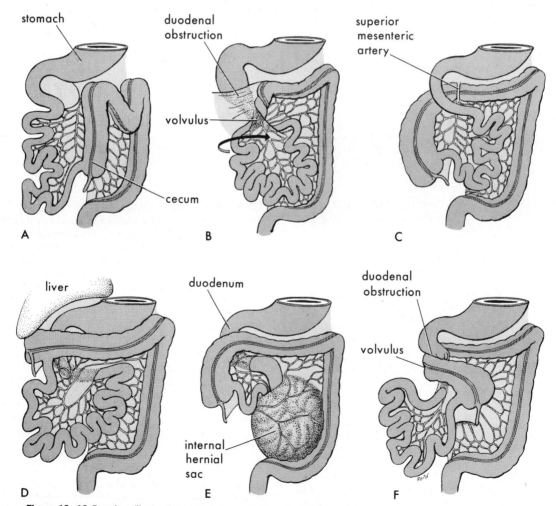

Figure 12–16. Drawings illustrating various abnormalities of midgut rotation. *A*, Nonrotation. *B*, Mixed rotation and volvulus. *C*, Reversed rotation. *D*, Subhepatic cecum and appendix. *E*, Internal hernia. *F*, Midgut volvulus.

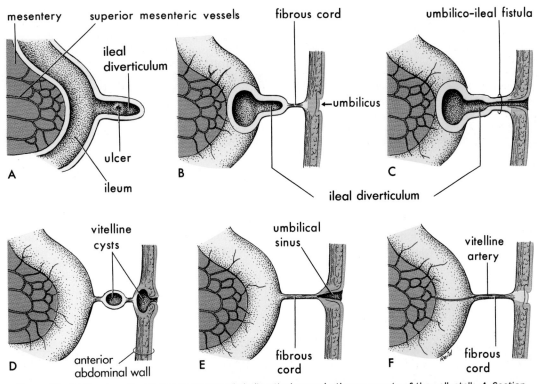

Figure 12–17. Drawings illustrating an ileal (Meckel) diverticulum and other remnants of the yolk stalk. *A*, Section of the ileum and a diverticulum with an ulcer. *B*, A diverticulum connected to the umbilicus by a fibrous cord. *C*, Umbilico-ileal fistula resulting from persistence of the entire intra-abdominal portion of the yolk stalk (see also Fig. 12–19). *D*, Vitelline cysts at the umbilicus and in a fibrous remnant of the yolk stalk. *E*, Umbilical sinus resulting from the persistence of the yolk stalk near the umbilicus. *F*, The yolk stalk has persisted as a fibrous cord connecting the ileum with the umbilicus. A persistent vitelline artery extends along the fibrous cord to the umbilicus.

result, a hernialike sac forms. This very uncommon condition usually does not produce symptoms and is often detected at autopsy or during an anatomical dissection.

Midgut Volvulus (Fig. 12–16*F*). In this condition, the small intestine fails to enter the abdominal cavity normally, and the mesenteries fail to undergo normal fixation; as a result, twisting of the intestines occurs. Only two parts of intestine are attached to the posterior abdominal wall, the duodenum and proximal colon. The small intestine hangs by a narrow stalk that contains the superior mesenteric artery and vein. These vessels are usually twisted in this stalk and become obstructed at or near the duodenojejunal junction. The circulation to the twisted segment is often restricted; and, if the vessels are completely obstructed, gangrene will develop.

Stenosis and Atresia of the Intestine (Fig. 12–5). Partial occlusion (stenosis) and complete occlusion (atresia) of the intestinal lumen account for about one third of cases of intestinal obstruction (Shandling, 1992). The obstructive lesion occurs most often in the duodenum (25 per cent) and ileum (50 per cent). The length of the area affected varies. These anomalies result from failure of an adequate number of vacuoles to form during recanalization of the intestine (Fig. 12–5). In some cases a transverse diaphragm forms,

producing a so-called *diaphragmatic atresia* (Fig. 12–5*F₂*). Another possible cause of stenoses and atresias is interruption of the blood supply to a loop of the fetal intestine due to a *fetal vascular accident*; for example, an excessively mobile loop of intestine may become twisted, thereby interrupting its blood supply and leading to necrosis of the section of bowel involved. This necrotic segment later becomes a fibrous cord connecting the proximal and distal ends of normal intestine.

Most atresias of the ileum are probably caused by infarction of the fetal bowel as the result of impairment of its blood supply due to volvulus. This impairment most likely occurs during the tenth week as the intestines return to the abdomen. Malfixation of the gut predisposes it to volvulus, strangulation, and impairment of its blood supply.

Ileal (Meckel[3]) Diverticulum (Figs. 12–17*A* to *C* and 12–18). This outpouching is one of the most common anomalies of the digestive tract. It occurs in two to four per

---

[3] Johann F. Meckel (1781–1833) was a German comparative anatomist and embryologist. He described this common ileal diverticulum which is often referred to clinically as Meckel's diverticulum.

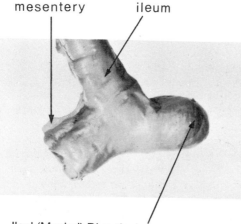

Figure 12–18. Photograph of a typical ileal (Meckel) diverticulum. Half actual size.

cent of people (Moore, 1992) and is three to five times more prevalent in males than in females. *An ileal diverticulum is of clinical significance* because it sometimes becomes inflamed and causes symptoms that mimic appendicitis. The wall of the diverticulum contains all layers of the ileum and may contain small pieces of gastric and pancreatic tissues. The gastric mucosa often secretes acid, producing ulceration and bleeding (Fig. 12–17A).

An ileal diverticulum represents the remnant of the proximal portion of the yolk stalk. It typically appears as a fingerlike pouch about 3 to 6 cm long that *arises from the antimesenteric border of the ileum* (Fig. 12–18) 40 to 50 cm from the ileocecal junction. An ileal diverticulum may be connected to the umbilicus by a fibrous cord or a fistula (Figs. 12–17B and 12–19); other possible remnants of the yolk stalk are illustrated in Figure 12–17D to F.

In rare instances there is abnormal reconstruction of the endodermal roof of the yolk sac during notochord formation (p. 57). This results in the endoderm being attached to the notochord. When the dorsal part of the yolk sac is incorporated into the embryo as the primitive gut (p. 70), a cord

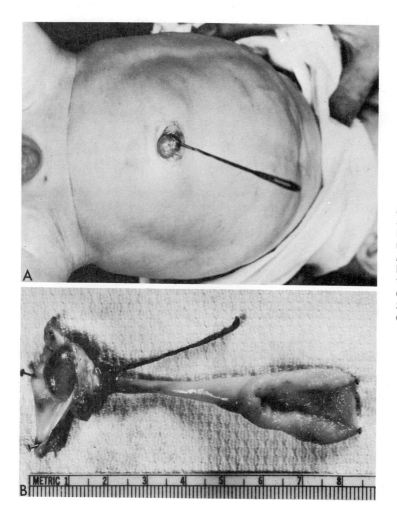

Figure 12–19. A, Photograph of the abdomen of an infant with an umbilico-ileal fistula. A probe has been inserted into the fistula. It extends from the umbilicus to the ileum (a distance of about 5 cm). B, The excised fistula with a granulomatous-looking bulge at the umbilical end and a cone-shaped diverticulum at the ileal end. See Figure 12–17C for orientation. (From Taeusch HW, Ballard RB, Avery ME: *Schaffer and Avery's Diseases of the Newborn.* 6th ed. Philadelphia, WB Saunders, 1991.)

of endodermal cells passes from the gut to the vertebral column, which develops around the notochord. This endodermal cord may give rise to a giant diverticulum on the mesenteric side of the gastrointestinal tract.

Duplication of the Intestine (Fig. 12–20). Most intestinal duplications are cystic duplications or tubular duplications. *Cystic duplications* are more common (Fig. 12–20*B*). These duplicated parts of the intestine communicate with the intestinal lumen (Fig. 12–20*C*). Almost all the duplications are caused by failure of normal recanalization; as a result, two lumina form (Fig. 12–20*H* and *I*). The duplicated segment of bowel lies on the mesenteric side of the intestine.

THE HINDGUT

The derivatives of the hindgut are:

1. The left one third to one half or distal part of the transverse colon; the descending colon and sigmoid colon; the rectum and the superior portion of the anal canal.

2. The epithelium of the urinary bladder and most of the urethra (see Chapter 13).

All these hindgut derivatives are supplied by the *inferior mesenteric artery*, the artery of the hindgut (see Fig. 12–1). The junction between the segment of transverse colon derived from the midgut and that originating from the hindgut is indicated by the change in blood supply from a branch of the superior

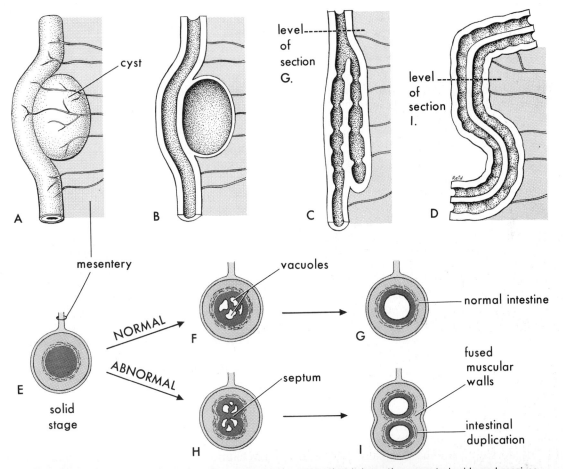

Figure 12–20. *A*, Cystic duplication of the small intestine. Note that it is on the mesenteric side and receives branches from the arteries supplying the intestine. *B*, Longitudinal section of the duplication shown in *A*. It does not communicate with the intestine, but its musculature is continuous with the gut wall. *C*, A short tubular duplication of the small intestine. *D*, A long duplication of the small intestine showing a partition consisting of the fused muscular walls. *E*, Transverse section of the intestine during the solid stage. *F*, Normal vacuole formation. *G*, Coalescence of the vacuoles and reformation of the lumen. *H*, Two groups of vacuoles have formed. *I*, Coalescence of the vacuoles illustrated in *H* results in intestinal duplication.

mesenteric artery (midgut artery) to a branch of the inferior mesenteric artery (hindgut artery).

Fixation of the Hindgut (Fig. 12–13). The descending colon becomes retroperitoneal as its mesentery fuses with the peritoneum on the left posterior abdominal wall and then disappears. The mesentery of the sigmoid colon is retained, but it is shorter than in the embryo.

The Cloaca

This terminal portion of the hindgut is an endoderm-lined cavity that is in contact with the surface ectoderm at the *cloacal membrane* (Fig. 12–21*A* and *B*). This membrane is composed of endoderm of the cloaca and ectoderm of the *proctodeum* or anal pit (Fig. 12–21*D*). The cloaca, the expanded terminal part of the hindgut, receives the *allantois* ventrally (Fig. 12–21*A*), which is a fingerlike diverticulum of the yolk sac (see Fig. 4–5*E*). For a description of this rudimentary structure, see page 61.

Partitioning of the Cloaca (Fig. 12–21). The cloaca is divided into dorsal and ventral parts by a coronal wedge of mesenchyme called the *urorectal septum*. This septum develops in the angle between the allantois and hindgut. As the septum grows toward the cloacal membrane, it develops forklike extensions that produce infoldings of the lateral walls of the cloaca (Fig. 12–21*B₁*). These folds grow toward each other and fuse, forming a partition that divides the cloaca into two parts: (1) the *rectum* and cranial part of the *anal canal* dorsally, and (2) the *urogenital sinus* ventrally (Fig. 12–21 *D* and *F*).

By the seventh week, the urorectal septum has fused with the cloacal membrane, dividing it into a dorsal *anal membrane* and a larger ventral *urogenital membrane* (Fig. 12–21*E* and *F*). The area of fusion of the urorectal septum with the cloacal membrane is represented in the adult by the *perineal body*, the tendinous center of the perineum (Moore, 1992). This fibromuscular node is the *landmark of the perineum* where several muscles converge and insert.

The urorectal septum also divides the *cloacal sphincter* into anterior and posterior parts. The posterior part becomes the *external anal sphincter*, and the anterior part develops into the superficial transverse perineal, bulbospongiosus, and ischiocavernosus muscles, and the *urogenital diaphragm* (Moore, 1992). This developmental fact explains why one nerve, the *pudendal nerve*, supplies all these muscles.

Mesenchymal proliferations produce elevations of the surface ectoderm around the *anal membrane*. As a result, this membrane is located at the bottom of an ectodermal depression called the *proctodeum* or anal pit (Fig. 12–21*E*). The *anal membrane* usually rup-

tures at the end of the eighth week, bringing the distal part of the digestive tract (anal canal) into communication with the amniotic cavity.

The Anal Canal (Fig. 12–22). The superior two thirds (about 25 mm) of the adult anal canal are derived from the *hindgut*; the inferior one third (about 13 mm) develops from the *proctodeum*. The junction of the epithelium derived from the ectoderm of the proctodeum and the endoderm of the hindgut is roughly indicated by the irregular *pectinate line*, located at the inferior limit of the anal valves (Moore, 1992). This line indicates the approximate former site of the anal membrane.

About 2 cm superior to the anus is an *anocutaneous line* ("white line"). This is approximately where the composition of the anal epithelium changes from columnar to stratified squamous cells. At the anus, the epithelium is keratinized and continuous with the skin of the anal region. The other layers of the wall of the anal canal are derived from splanchnic mesenchyme. There is scanty information on the morphological differentiation of the anal sphincter muscles (Bourdelat et al., 1990).

Due to its hindgut origin, the superior two thirds of the anal canal are mainly supplied by the *superior rectal artery*, the continuation of the inferior mesenteric artery (hindgut artery). The venous drainage of this superior part is mainly via the *superior rectal vein*, a tributary of the inferior mesenteric vein. The lymphatic drainage of this part is eventually to the *inferior mesenteric lymph nodes*. Its nerves are from the autonomic system.

Due to its origin from the proctodeum, the inferior one third of the canal is supplied mainly by the *inferior rectal arteries*, branches of the internal pudendal artery. The venous drainage is via the *inferior rectal vein*, a tributary of the internal pudendal vein that drains into the internal iliac vein. The lymphatic drainage of the inferior part of the anal canal is to the *superficial inguinal lymph nodes*. Its nerve supply is from the *inferior rectal nerve*; hence, it is sensitive to pain, temperature, touch, and pressure.

The differences in blood supply, nerve supply, and venous and lymphatic drainage of the anal canal are important clinically (Moore, 1992), e.g., when considering the metastasis of tumors. The characteristics of carcinomas in the two parts also differ. Tumors in the superior part are painless and arise from columnar epithelium, whereas those in the inferior part are painful and arise from squamous epithelium.

Anomalies of the Hindgut

Most abnormalities of the hindgut are located in the anorectal region and result from abnormal development of the

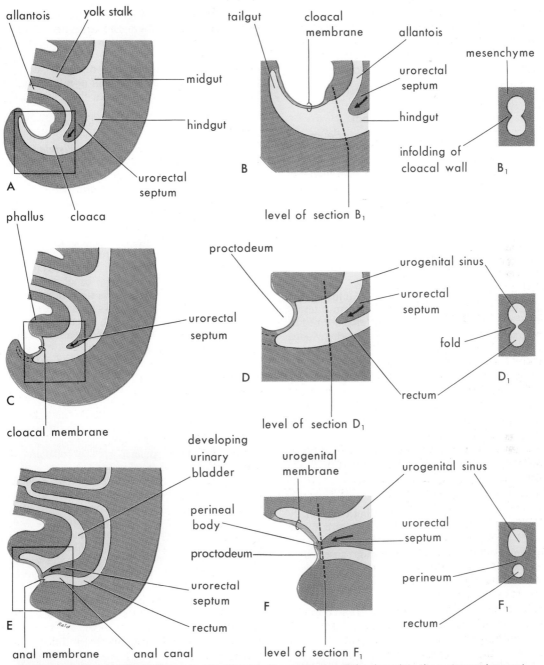

Figure 12–21. Drawings illustrating successive stages in the partitioning of the cloaca into the rectum and urogenital sinus by the urorectal septum. *A, C,* and *E,* Views from the left side at four, six, and seven weeks, respectively. *B, D,* and *F,* Enlargements of the cloacal region. $B_1, D_1,$ and $F_1,$ Transverse sections of the cloaca at the levels shown in *B, D,* and *F,* respectively. Note that the tailgut (shown in *B*) degenerates and disappears as the rectum forms from the dorsal part of the cloaca (shown in *C*).

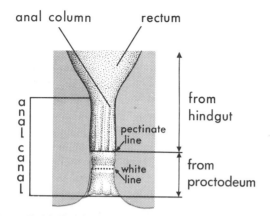

Figure 12–22. Sketch of the rectum and anal canal showing their developmental origins. Note that the superior two thirds of the anal canal are derived from the hindgut and are endodermal in origin, whereas the inferior one third of the anal canal is derived from the proctodeum and is ectodermal in origin. Because of their different embryological origins, the superior and inferior parts of the anal canal are supplied by different arteries and nerves and have different venous and lymphatic drainages.

urorectal septum. Clinically, they are divided into high and low anomalies depending on whether the rectum terminates superior or inferior to the *puborectal sling* formed by the puborectalis, a part of the levator ani muscle (Moore, 1992).

Congenital Megacolon

In infants with this condition (also referred to as Hirschsprung disease), a portion of the colon is dilated due to the *absence of autonomic ganglion cells* in the myenteric plexus distal to the dilated segment of colon. The enlarged colon, called **megacolon** (Gr. *megas*, big), has the normal number of ganglion cells. The dilation results from failure of peristalsis in the aganglionic segment, which causes failure of movement of the intestinal contents. In most cases only the rectum and sigmoid colon are involved, but occasionally ganglia are also absent from more proximal parts of the colon.

Congenital megacolon is the most common cause of neonatal obstruction of the colon and accounts for 33 per cent of all neonatal obstructions (Shandling, 1992). Males are affected more often than females (4:1). Congenital megacolon results from failure of neural crest cells to migrate into the wall of the colon during the fifth to seventh weeks. This results in failure of parasympathetic ganglion cells to develop in the *Auerbach and Meissner plexuses*. The cause of failure of some neural crest cells to complete their migration is unknown.

Imperforate Anus and Related Anorectal Anomalies

Imperforate anus occurs about once in every 5000 newborn infants; it is more common in males. *Most anorectal anomalies result from abnormal development of the urorectal septum*, resulting in incomplete separation of the cloaca into urogenital and anorectal portions (Figs. 12–21 and 12–23). There is normally a communication between the rectum and anal canal dorsally from the bladder and urethra ventrally (Fig. 12–21*C*), but it closes when the urorectal septum fuses with the cloacal membrane (Fig. 12–21*D*). Lesions are classified as "low" or "high" depending on whether the rectum ends superior or inferior to the puborectalis muscle, a major part of the levator ani muscle (Moore, 1992).

Low Anorectal Anomalies. The following are low anomalies of the anorectal region.

Anal Agenesis, With or Without a Fistula (Fig. 12–23*D* and *E*). The anal canal may end blindly or there may be an ectopic opening (*ectopic anus*) or a fistula that commonly opens into the perineum. The abnormal canal may, however, open into the vulva in females or the urethra in males. More than 90 per cent of low anorectal anomalies are associated with an external fistula (Shandling, 1992). *Anal agenesis with a fistula* results from incomplete separation of the cloaca by the urorectal septum.

Anal Stenosis (Fig. 12–23*B*). The anus is in the normal position but the anus and anal canal are narrow. This anomaly is probably caused by a slight dorsal deviation of the urorectal septum as it grows caudally to fuse with the cloacal membrane. As a result, the anal canal and anal membrane are small. Sometimes only a small probe can be inserted into the anal canal.

Membranous Atresia or Imperforate Anus (Fig. 12–23*C*). The anus is in the normal position, but a thin layer of tissue separates the anal canal from the exterior. The membrane is thin enough to bulge on straining and appears blue from the presence of meconium superior to it. This anomaly results from failure of the anal membrane to perforate at the end of the eighth week.

High Anorectal Anomalies. The following are high anomalies of the anorectal region.

Anorectal Agenesis, With or Without a Fistula (Fig. 12–23*F* and *G*). The rectum ends superior to the puborectalis muscle. This is the most common type of anorectal anomaly, which accounts for about two thirds of anorectal defects. Although the rectum ends blindly, there is usually a fistula to the bladder (*rectovesical fistula*) or the urethra (*rectourethral fistula*) in males, or to the vagina (*rectovaginal fistula*) or the vestibule of the vagina (*rectovestibular fistula*) in females. Passage of meconium or flatus (gas) in the urine is diagnostic of a rectourinary fistula.

Anorectal agenesis with a fistula is the result of incomplete separation of the cloaca by the urorectal septum. In newborn males with this condition, *meconium* (feces) may be observed in the urine; whereas fistulas in females result in the presence of meconium in the vestibule of the vagina.

Rectal Atresia (Fig. 12–23*H* and *I*). The anal canal and rectum are present but they are separated. Sometimes the two segments of bowel are connected by a fibrous cord, the remnant of the atretic portion of the rectum. The cause of rectal atresia may be abnormal recanalization of the colon or defective blood supply, as discussed, with atresia of the small intestine (p. 255).

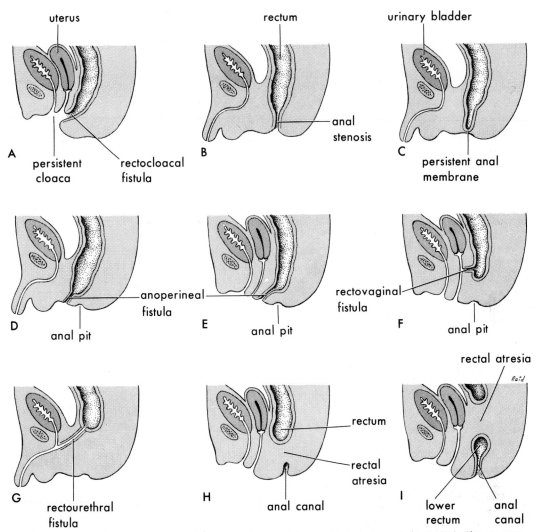

Figure 12–23. Drawings illustrating various types of anorectal anomaly. *A,* Persistent cloaca. Note the common outlet for the intestinal, urinary, and reproductive tracts. *B,* Anal stenosis. *C,* Membranous atresia (covered anus). *D* and *E,* Anal agenesis with a perineal fistula. *F,* Anorectal agenesis with a rectovaginal fistula. *G,* Anorectal agenesis with a rectourethral fistula. *H* and *I,* Rectal atresia.

SUMMARY

The **primitive gut** (foregut, midgut, and hindgut) forms during the fourth week from the part of the yolk sac that is incorporated into the embryo (p. 70). The endoderm of the primitive gut gives rise to the epithelial lining of most of the digestive tract and biliary passages together with the parenchyma of its glands including the liver and pancreas. The epithelium at the cranial and caudal extremities of the digestive tract is derived from the ectoderm of the stomodeum and proctodeum, respectively. The muscular and connective tissue components of the digestive tract are derived from the splanchnic mesenchyme surrounding the primitive gut.

The **foregut** gives rise to the pharynx, lower respiratory system, esophagus, stomach, duodenum (proximal to the opening of the bile duct), liver, pancreas, and biliary apparatus. Because the trachea and esophagus have a common origin from the foregut, incomplete partitioning by the tracheoesophageal septum results in stenoses or atresias, with or without fistulas between them.

The *hepatic diverticulum,* the primordium of the liver, gallbladder, and biliary duct system, is an outgrowth of the endodermal epithelial lining of the foregut. The epithelial liver cords and primordia of the *biliary system*, which develop from the hepatic diverticulum, grow into the septum transversum. Between the layers of the *ventral mesentery* derived from the septum transversum, these primordial cells differentiate into the *parenchyma of the liver* and the lining of the ducts of the biliary system.

Congenital duodenal atresia results from failure of the vacuolization and recanalization process to occur following the normal solid stage of the duodenum. Usually these epithelial cells degenerate and the lumen of the duodenum is restored (Fig. 12–5). Obstruction of the duodenum can also be caused by an *anular pancreas*.

The **pancreas** is formed by dorsal and ventral *pancreatic buds* that originate from the endodermal lining of the foregut. When the duodenum rotates to the right, the ventral pancreatic bud moves dorsally and fuses with the dorsal pancreatic bud. The *ventral pancreatic bud* forms most of the head of the pancreas, including the uncinate process. The *dorsal pancreatic bud* forms the remainder of the pancreas. In some fetuses the duct systems of the two buds fail to fuse, and an *accessory pancreatic duct* forms.

The **midgut** gives rise to the duodenum (distal to the bile duct), jejunum, ileum, cecum, vermiform appendix, ascending colon, and the right half to two thirds of the transverse colon. The midgut forms a U-shaped intestinal loop that herniates into the umbilical cord during the sixth week because there is no room for it in the abdomen. While in the umbilical cord, the *midgut loop* rotates counterclockwise through 90 degrees. During the tenth week, the intestines rapidly return to the abdomen, rotating a further 180 degrees during this process.

Omphaloceles, malrotations, and abnormalities of fixation result from failure of return or abnormal rotation of the intestine in the abdomen. Because the gut is normally occluded during the fifth and sixth weeks due to rapid mitotic activity of its epithelium, *stenosis* (partial obstruction), *atresia* (complete obstruction), and *duplications* result if recanalization fails to occur or occurs abnormally. Various remnants of the yolk stalk may persist. *Ileal (Meckel) diverticula* are common, but only a few of them become inflamed and produce pain.

The **hindgut** gives rise to the left one third to one half of the transverse colon, the descending and sigmoid colon, the rectum, and the superior part of the anal canal. The inferior part of the anal canal develops from the proctodeum. The caudal part of the hindgut, known as the *cloaca*, is divided by the *urorectal septum* into the urogenital sinus and rectum. The urogenital sinus mainly gives rise to the urinary bladder and urethra (see Chapter 13). At first the rectum and the superior part of the anal canal are separated from the exterior by the *anal membrane*, but this membrane normally breaks down by the end of the eighth week.

Most anorectal anomalies result from abnormal partitioning of the cloaca by the urorectal septum into the rectum and anal canal posteriorly and the urinary bladder and urethra anteriorly. Arrested growth and/or deviation of the urorectal septum in a dorsal direction causes most of the anorectal abnormalities, such as rectal atresia and abnormal connections (fistulas) between the rectum and the urethra, urinary bladder, or vagina.

CLINICALLY ORIENTED QUESTIONS FOR PROBLEM-BASED LEARNING SESSIONS

1. A female infant was born prematurely at 32 weeks' gestation to a 39-year-old woman whose pregnancy was complicated by *polyhydramnios*. Amniocentesis at 16 weeks showed that the infant had trisomy 21. The baby began to vomit within a few hours after birth, and marked dilation of the epigastrium was noted. Radiographs of the abdomen showed gas in the stomach and the superior part of the duodenum, but no other intestinal gas was observed. *A diagnosis of duodenal atresia was made.* Where does obstruction of the duodenum usually occur? What is the embryological basis of this congenital anomaly? What caused distention of the infant's epigastrium? Is duodenal atresia commonly associated with malformations such as the Down syndrome? What is the embryological basis of the *polyhydramnios* in this case?

2. The umbilicus of a newborn infant failed to heal normally. It was swollen and there was a persistent discharge from the umbilical stump. After probing, a *sinus tract* was outlined with radiopaque oil during fluoroscopy. The tract was resected on the ninth day after birth, and its distal end was found to terminate in a *diverticulum of the ileum*. What is the embryological basis of the sinus tract? What is the usual clinical name given to this type of ileal diverticulum? Is this anomaly common?

3. A female infant was born with a small dimple where the anus should have been. Examination of the infant's vagina revealed meconium and an opening of a sinus tract in the posterior wall of the vagina. Radiographic examination using a contrast medium injected through a tiny catheter inserted into the opening revealed a fistulous connection with the lower bowel. With which part of the lower bowel would the fistula probably be connected? Name this anomaly. What is the embryological basis of this condition?

4. A newborn infant was born with a light gray, shiny mass measuring the size of an orange and protruding from the umbilical region. It was covered by a thin transparent membrane. What is this congenital anomaly called? What is the origin of the membrane covering the mass? What would be the composition of the mass? What is the embryological basis of this protrusion?

5. A newborn infant appeared normal at birth, but vomiting and abdominal distention developed after a few hours. The vomitus contained bile, and only a little meconium was passed. Radiographic examination showed a gas-filled stomach and dilated, gas-filled loops of small bowel, but no air was present in the large intestine. This indicated a congenital obstruction of the small bowel. What part of the small bowel was probably obstructed? What would the condition be called? Why was only a little meconium passed? What would likely be observed at operation? What was the probable embryological basis of the condition?

The answers to these questions are given on page 463.

References and Suggested Reading

Ackerman P: Congenital defects of the abdominal wall. *In* Huff-stadt AJC (ed): *Congenital Malformations*. Amsterdam, Excerpta Medica, 1980.

Balistreri WF: Extrahepatic biliary atresia. *In* Behrman RE (ed): *Nelson Textbook of Pediatrics*. 14th ed. Philadelphia, WB Saunders, 1992.

Bear JC: Infantile hypertrophic pyloric stenosis: approaches to liability. *In* Persaud, TVN (ed): *Advances in the Study of Birth Defects. Vol. 6. Cardiovascular, Respiratory, Gastrointestinal and Genitourinary Malformations*. New York, Alan R. Liss, 1982.

Beasley SW, Myers NA, Auldist AW (eds): *Oesophageal Atresia*. London, Chapman and Hall, 1991.

Best LG, Wiseman NE, Chudley AE: Familial duodenal atresia: a report of two families and review. *Am J Med Genet 34*:442, 1989.

Bisset WM: Development of intestinal motility. *Arch Dis Child 66*:3, 1991.

Bourdelat D, Barbet JP, Hidden G: The morphological differentiation of the internal sphincter muscle of the anus in the human embryo and fetus. *Surg Radiol Anat 12*:151, 1990.

Brassett C, Ellis H: Transposition of the viscera. *Clin Anat 4*:139, 1991.

Carr BR: Fertilization, implantation, and endocrinology of pregnancy. *In* Griffin JE, Ojeda SR (eds): *Textbook of Endocrine Physiology*. New York, Oxford University Press, 1988.

Champetier J, Letoublon C, Arvieux C, Gerard P, Labrosse PA: Les variations de division des voies biliaires extrahepatiques: signification et origine, consequences chirurgicales. *J Chir (Paris) 126*:147, 1989a.

Champetier J, Yver R, Tomasella T: Functional anatomy of the liver of the human fetus: applications to ultrasonography. *Surg Radiol Anat 11*:53, 1989b.

Cobb RA, Williamson RCN: Embryology and developmental abnormalities of the large intestine. *In* Phillips SF, Pember-ton JH, Shorter RG (eds): *The Large Intestine: Physiology, Pathophysiology, and Disease*. New York, Raven Press, 1991.

Cywes S, Davies MRQ, Rode H: Congenital jejuno-ileal atresia and stenosis. *In* Persaud, TVN (ed): *Advances in the Study of Birth Defects. Vol. 6. Cardiovascular, Respiratory, Gastrointestinal and Genitourinary Malformations*. New York, Alan R. Liss, 1982.

Estrada RL: *Anomalies of Intestinal Rotation and Fixation*. Springfield, Ill., Charles C Thomas, 1968.

Fallin LT: The development and cytodifferentiation of the islets of Langerhans in human embryos and foetuses. *Acta Anat 68*:147, 1967.

Filly RA: Sonographic anatomy of the normal fetus. *In* Harrison MR, Golbus MS, Filly RA (eds): *The Unborn Patient: Prenatal Diagnosis and Treatment*. 2nd ed. Philadelphia, WB Saunders, 1991.

Fitzgerald MJT, Nolan JP, O'Neill MN: The position of the human caecum in fetal life. *J Anat 109*:71, 1971.

Gemonov VV, Kolesnikov LL: Development of oesophageal tissue structures in human embryogenesis. *Anat Anz 171*:13, 1990.

Grand RJ, Watkins JB, Torti FM: Progress in gastroenterology: Development of the human gastrointestinal tract. A review. *Gastroenterology 70*:790, 1976.

Hamilton JR: Stomach and intestines. *In* Behrman RE (ed): *Nelson Textbook of Pediatrics*. 14th ed. Philadelphia, WB Saunders, 1992.

Herbst JJ: Disorders of the esophagus. *In* Behrman RE (ed): *Nelson Textbook of Pediatrics*. 14th ed. Philadelphia, WB Saunders, 1992.

Karrer FM, Raffensperger JG: Biliary atresia. *In* Raffensperger JG (ed): *Swenson's Pediatric Surgery*. 5th ed. Norwalk, Connecticut, Appleton & Lange, 1990.

Kirillova IA, Novikova IV, Bragina ZN: Pathology of developmental defects of the digestive system in human embryos (in Russian). *Arkh Patol 52*:14, 1990.

Kleigman RM, Behrman RE: The umbilicus. *In* Behrman RE (ed): *Nelson Textbook of Pediatrics*. 14th ed. Philadelphia, WB Saunders, 1992.

Lebenthal E, Leung YK: Feeding the premature and comprised infant: gastrointestinal considerations. *Pediatr Clin North Am 35*:215, 1988.

Martinez NS, Morlach CG, Dockerty B, et al.: Heterotopic pancreatic tissue involving the stomach. *Ann Surg 147*:1, 1958.

McLean JM: Embryology of the pancreas. *In* Howat HT, Sarles H (eds): *The Exocrine Pancreas.* Philadelphia, WB Saunders, 1979.

Menard D, Arsenault P: Cell proliferation in developing human stomach. *Anat Embryol (Berl) 182*:509, 1990.

Moore KL: *Clinically Oriented Anatomy.* 3rd ed. Baltimore, Williams & Wilkins, 1992.

Noordijk JA: Omphalocele and gastroschisis. *In* Persaud, TVN (ed): Advances in the Study of Birth Defects. Vol. 6. *Cardiovascular, Respiratory, Gastrointestinal and Genitourinary Malformations.* New York, Alan R. Liss, 1982.

Raffensperger JF (ed): *Swenson's Pediatric Surgery.* Norwalk, Connecticut, Appleton & Lange, 1990.

Rawdon BB, Andrew A: Comment on "Do the pancreatic primordial buds in embryogenesis have the potential to provide all pancreatic endocrine cells?" *Medical Hypotheses 35*:275, 1991.

Severn CB: A morphological study of the development of the human liver. I. Development of the hepatic diverticulum. *Am J Anat 131*:133, 1971.

Severn CB: A morphological study of the development of the human liver. II. Establishment of liver parenchyma, extrahepatic ducts, and associated venous channels. *Am J Anat 133*:85, 1972.

Shandling B: Congenital and perinatal anomalies of the gastrointestinal tract and intestinal rotation. *In* Behrman RE (ed): *Nelson Textbook of Pediatrics.* 14th ed. Philadelphia, WB Saunders, 1992.

Taeusch HW, Ballard RB, Avery ME (eds): *Schaffer and Avery's Diseases of the Newborn.* 6th ed. Philadelphia, WB Saunders, 1991.

Thompson JC: *Atlas of Surgery of the Stomach, Duodenum, and Small Bowel.* St. Louis, Mosby Year Book, 1992.

Thompson MW, McInnes RR, Willard HF: Thompson and Thompson Genetics in Medicine. 5th ed. Philadelphia, WB Saunders, 1991.

Vaos GC: Quantitative assessment of the stage of neuronal maturation in the human fetal gut – a new dimension in the pathogenesis of developmental anomalies of the myenteric plexus. *J Pediatr Surg 24*:920, 1989.

von Dorsche HH: Inselorgan. *In* Hinrichsen KV (ed): *Humanembryologie.* Berlin, Springer-Verlag, 1990.

Wolf-Coote SA, Louw J, Poerstamper HM, Du Toit DF: Do the pancreatic primordial buds in embryogenesis have the potential to provide all pancreatic endocrine cells? *Medical Hypotheses 31*:313, 1990.

Zona JZ: Umbilical anomalies. *In* Raffensperger JG (ed): *Swenson's Pediatric Surgery.* 5th ed. Norwalk, Connecticut, Appleton & Lange, 1990.

13

The Urogenital System

The urogenital system can be divided functionally into the *urinary (excretory) system* and the *genital (reproductive) system*. Embryologically and anatomically, these systems are closely associated. They are also very closely associated in the adult male, e.g., the urethra conveys both urine and semen. Although these systems are separate in normal adult females, the urethra and vagina open into a common space between the labia minora called the vestibule of the vagina (Moore, 1992).

The *suprarenal (adrenal) glands* are described in this chapter for two reasons: (1) They are closely related to the superior poles of the kidneys, and (2) congenital, virilizing, *adrenal hyperplasia* causes virilization (masculinization) of female external genitalia (e.g., enlargement of the clitoris); this accounts for most cases of *female pseudohermaphroditism* (p. 292).

Both the urinary and genital systems develop from intermediate mesoderm, which extends along the dorsal body wall of the embryo (Fig. 13–1*B*). During folding of the embryo in the horizontal plane, this mesoderm is carried ventrally and loses its connection with the somites (see Fig. 5–1). A longitudinal elevation of mesoderm called the *urogenital ridge* forms on each side of the primitive aorta (Fig. 13–1*D*). It gives rise to parts of the urinary and genital systems. The part of the ridge giving rise to the urinary system is known as the *nephrogenic cord or ridge* (Fig. 13–1*D*), and the part that gives rise to the genital system is known as the *gonadal or genital ridge* (see Fig. 13–20).

THE URINARY SYSTEM

The urinary system consists of the following structures: (1) the *kidneys*, which excrete *urine*, (2) the *ureters*, which convey urine to (3) the *urinary bladder* where it is stored temporarily, and (4) the *urethra* through which urine is discharged to the exterior.

Development of Kidneys

Three sets of excretory organs or kidneys develop in human embryos: the *pronephros, mesonephros,* and *metanephros* (the permanent kidney). The first set of "kidneys" or *pronephroi* (plural term) are rudimentary and nonfunctional. They are analogous to the kidneys in primitive fishes. The second set of kidneys or *mesonephroi* are analogous to the kidneys of fishes and amphibians. They function for a short time during the early fetal period and are replaced by a third set of kidneys or *metanephroi*, which become the permanent kidneys. They begin to produce urine at the end of the first trimester.

The Pronephroi ("Forekidneys"). These transitory, nonfunctional structures appear in human embryos early in the fourth week as a few cell clusters and tubular structures in the cervical region (Fig. 13–2*A*). The pronephric ducts run caudally and open into the cloaca (Fig. 13–2*B*). The rudimentary pronephroi soon degenerate, but most of the pronephric ducts are utilized by the next set of kidneys.

The Mesonephroi ("Midkidneys"). These large, elongated organs appear late in the fourth week caudal to the rudimentary pronephroi (Fig. 13–2). They function as *interim kidneys* until the permanent kidneys develop and are able to function. The mesonephric kidneys consist of glomeruli and tubules (Figs. 13–2 to 13–4). The tubules open into the *mesonephric duct*, which was originally the pronephric duct. This duct opens into the *urogenital sinus*, the ventral derivative of the cloaca (see Fig. 12–21). The mesonephroi degenerate during the first trimester, but their tubules become the efferent ductules of the testes, and the mesonephric ducts have several adult derivatives (p. 288).

The Metanephroi ("Hindkidneys"). The metanephroi or *permanent kidneys* have a double origin. They begin to develop early in the fifth week and start to function about four weeks later (Behrman, 1992). *Urine formation* continues throughout fetal life. Urine is excreted into the amniotic cavity and forms a major part of the amniotic fluid. The urine mixes with

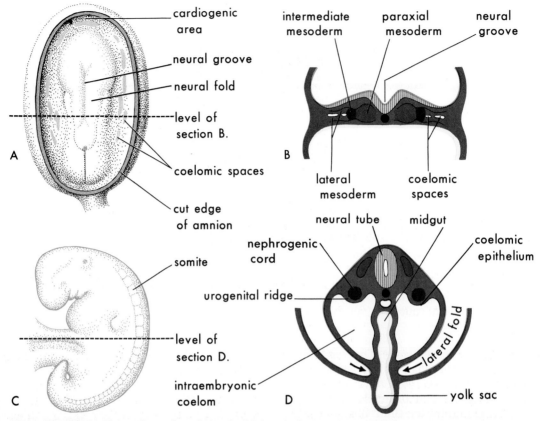

Figure 13-1. *A*, Dorsal view of an embryo during the third week (about 18 days). *B*, Transverse section of the embryo showing the position of the intermediate mesoderm before folding of the embryo. *C*, Lateral view of an embryo during the fourth week (about 26 days). *D*, Transverse section of the embryo after lateral folding showing the urogenital ridges produced by the nephrogenic cords of mesoderm.

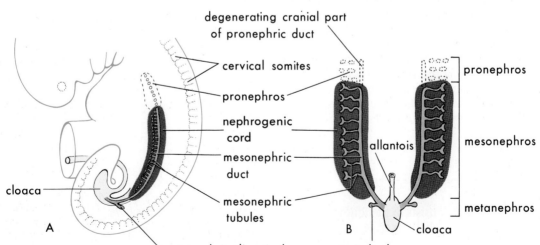

Figure 13-2. Diagrammatic sketches illustrating the three sets of excretory organs in an embryo during the fifth week. *A*, Lateral view. *B*, Ventral view. For simplicity the mesonephric tubules have been pulled to the sides of the mesonephric ducts.

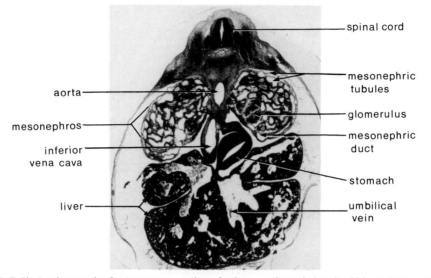

Figure 13-3. Photomicrograph of a transverse section of a 6-mm embryo during the fifth week (about 32 days), showing the mesonephroi (mesonephric kidneys) and liver. The mesonephric tubules exhibit various outlines because they are convoluted and thus are cut simultaneously at several points along their lengths (×12). (Courtesy of Professor Jean Hay, Department of Anatomy, University of Manitoba, Winnipeg, Canada.)

the amniotic fluid, which the fetus drinks. A mature fetus swallows several hundred milliliters of amniotic fluid each day. This fluid is absorbed by the intestine, and waste products are transferred through the placental membrane into the maternal blood for elimination (p. 120).

Development of the Permanent Kidneys. The permanent kidneys (*metanephroi*) develop from two sources: the *metanephric diverticulum* or ureteric bud and the *metanephric mesoderm* or metanephrogenic blastema. The metanephric diverticulum is an outgrowth from the mesonephric duct, and the metanephric mesoderm is derived from the caudal part of the nephrogenic cord (Fig. 13-5). Both primordia of the metanephros are of mesodermal origin.

The metanephric diverticulum (ureteric bud) begins as a dorsal outgrowth from the mesonephric duct near its entry into the cloaca (Fig. 13-5*A* and *B*). This diverticulum is the primordium of the *ureter, renal pelvis, calices,* and *collecting tubules* (Fig. 13-5*C* to *E*). As it elongates the metanephric diverticulum penetrates the *metanephric mesoderm,* inducing the formation of a *metanephric mass* or cap over its expanded end (Fig. 13-5*B*). Cell surface N-linked oligosaccharides appear to be important for this inductive interaction between the ureteric bud and the metanephric mesoderm (Fleming, 1990). The stalk of the metanephric diverticulum becomes the *ureter,* and its expanded cranial end forms the *renal pelvis.* Each collecting tubule undergoes repeated branching, forming successive generations of collecting tubules.

The first four generations of tubules enlarge and become confluent to form the *major calices* (Fig. 13-5*C* to *E*), and the second four generations coalesce to form the *minor calices.* The remaining generations of tubules form the collecting tubules. The end of each arched collecting tubule induces clusters of mesenchymal cells in the metanephric mesoderm to form small *metanephric vesicles* (Fig. 13-6*A*). These vesicles soon elongate and become *metanephric tubules* (Fig. 13-6*C*). As these renal tubules develop, their proximal ends are invaginated by *glomeruli.*

The renal corpuscle (glomerulus and Bowman capsule) and its proximal convoluted tubule, loop of Henle, and distal convoluted tubule constitute a **nephron** (Fig. 13-6*D*). Each distal convoluted tubule contacts an arched collecting tubule, and the two tubules become confluent.

A *uriniferous tubule* consists of two embryologically different parts: a *nephron* derived from the metanephric mesoderm and a *collecting tubule* derived from the metanephric diverticulum (Figs. 13-5 and 13-6). Tissue culture studies have shown that branching of the metanephric diverticulum is dependent upon induction by the metanephric mesoderm (cap), and that differentiation of the nephrons depends upon induction by the collecting tubules. Expression of nerve growth factor receptor in the developing nephrogenic tissue is required for the formation of the kidney tubules (Sariola et al., 1991).

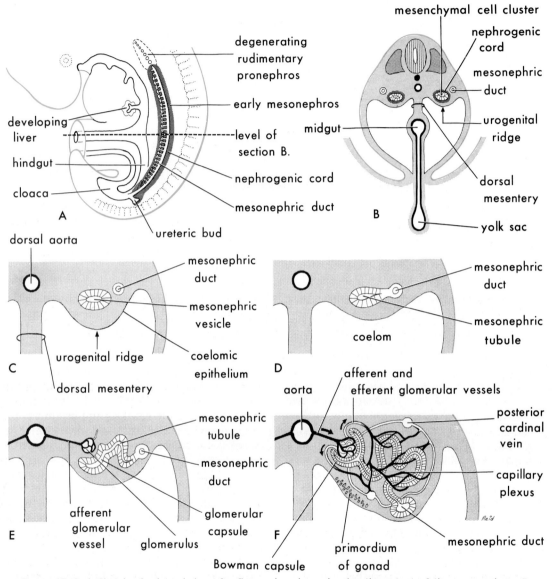

Figure 13–4. *A*, Sketch of a lateral view of a five-week embryo showing the extent of the mesonephros. *B*, Transverse section of the embryo showing the nephrogenic cords from which the mesonephric tubules develop. *C* to *F*, Sketches of transverse sections showing successive stages in the development of a mesonephric tubule between the fifth and eleventh weeks. Note that the mesenchymal cell cluster in the nephrogenic cord develops a lumen, thereby forming a mesonephric vesicle. The vesicle soon becomes an S-shaped mesonephric tubule and extends laterally to join the pronephric duct, now renamed the mesonephric duct. The expanded medial end of the mesonephric tubule is invaginated by blood vessels to form a glomerular capsule (Bowman capsule). The cluster of capillaries projecting into this capsule is known as a glomerulus.

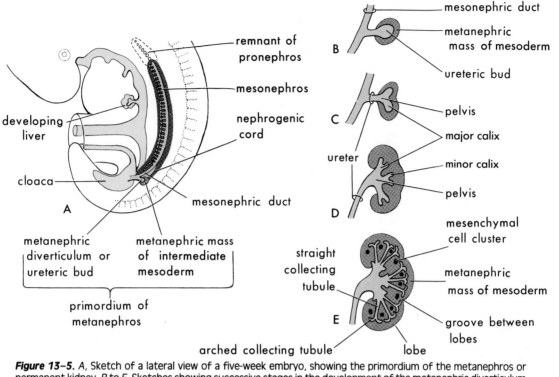

Figure 13-5. *A*, Sketch of a lateral view of a five-week embryo, showing the primordium of the metanephros or permanent kidney. *B* to *E*, Sketches showing successive stages in the development of the metanephric diverticulum or ureteric bud (fifth to eighth weeks). Observe the development of the ureter, renal pelvis, calices, and collecting tubules. The renal lobes, illustrated in *E*, are still visible in the kidneys of a 28-week fetus (Fig. 13-7).

The *fetal kidneys* are subdivided into lobes that are visible externally (Fig. 13-7). This lobation diminishes toward the end of the fetal period, but the lobes are still indicated in the kidneys of a newborn infant. The lobation usually disappears during infancy as the nephrons grow. The lobated character of the kidneys is obscured in adults; however, in very rare cases the lobes are recognizable externally, as they are in certain animals (e.g., cattle).

At term, each kidney contains 800,000 to 1,000,000 nephrons, and the increase in kidney size after birth mainly results from elongation of the proximal convoluted tubules and loops of Henle, as well as an increase of interstitial tissue. It is now believed that nephron formation is complete at birth (Behrman, 1992) except in premature infants. Functional maturation of the kidneys occurs after birth. Glomerular filtration begins around the ninth week, but the rate of filtration increases after birth (Arant, 1987; Behrman, 1992).

Prenatal Positional Changes of the Kidneys (Figs. 13-8 and 13-9). Initially the permanent (metanephric) kidneys lie close to each other in the pelvis, ventral to the sacrum. As the abdomen and pelvis grow, the kidneys gradually come to lie in the abdomen and move farther apart. They attain their adult position by the ninth week (Fig. 13-8*D*). This "migration" (relative ascent) mainly results from the growth of the embryo's body caudal to the kidneys. In effect, the caudal part of the embryo grows away from the kidneys so that they progressively occupy more cranial levels. Eventually they are retroperitoneal; that is, external or posterior to the peritoneum on the posterior abdominal wall. Initially, the hilum of the kidney faces ventrally; but, as the kidney "ascends," it rotates medially almost 90 degrees. By the ninth week its hilum is directed anteromedially (Fig. 13-8*C* and *D*).

Changes in the Blood Supply of the Developing Kidneys (Fig. 13-8). As the kidneys "ascend" from the pelvis, they receive their blood supply from vessels that are closely related to them. Initially the renal arteries are branches of the common iliac arteries (Fig. 13-8*A* and *B*). As they "ascend" further, the kidneys receive their blood supply from the distal end of the aorta. When they reach a higher level, they receive new branches from the aorta, and the inferior branches normally undergo involution and disappear. The kidneys come into contact with the *suprarenal glands* (adrenal glands) in the ninth week and the "ascent" stops. The kidneys receive their most

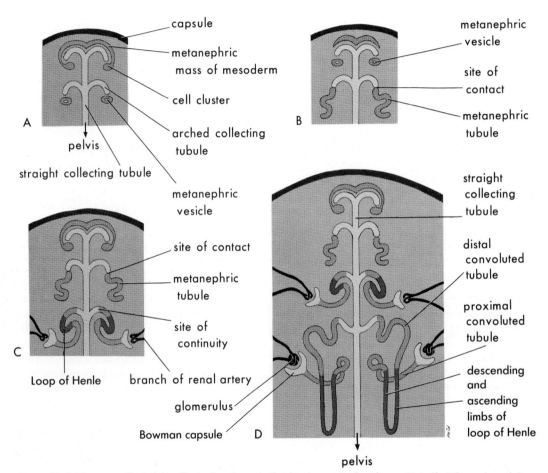

Figure 13–6. Diagrammatic sketches illustrating stages in the development of nephrons. Note that the metanephric tubules, the primordia of the nephrons, become continuous with the collecting tubules to form uriniferous tubules. This process commences around the beginning of the eighth week. The number of nephrons more than doubles from 20 weeks to 38 weeks. Observe that the nephrons are derived from the metanephric mesoderm and that the collecting system is derived from the metanephric diverticulum.

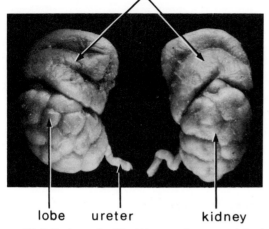

suprarenal or adrenal glands

lobe   ureter   kidney

Figure 13–7. Photograph of the kidneys and suprarenal glands of a 28-week fetus (×2). The external evidence of the lobes of the kidney normally disappears by the end of the first postnatal year. Note the large suprarenal (adrenal) glands. During the first two weeks after birth, these glands reduce to about half this size (see Fig. 13–19).

cranial branches laterally from the abdominal aorta; these branches become the permanent renal arteries. The right renal artery is longer and often more superior.

The relatively *common variations* in the blood supply to the kidneys reflect the manner in which the blood supply continually changes during fetal life (Fig. 13–8). A single

renal artery to each kidney is present in about 70 per cent of people. About 25 per cent of adult kidneys have two to four renal arteries (Moore, 1992).

Accessory renal arteries usually arise from the aorta, superior or inferior to the main renal artery, and follow it to the renal hilum. Accessory renal arteries may enter the kidneys directly, usually into the superior or inferior poles (Fig. 13–12). An accessory artery to the inferior pole may cross anterior to the ureter and obstruct it, causing *hydronephrosis.* If the artery enters the inferior pole of the right kidney, it usually crosses anterior to the inferior vena cava and ureter. It is important to be aware that accessory renal arteries are end arteries; consequently, if such an aberrant artery is damaged and/or ligated, the part of the kidney supplied by it is likely to become ischemic. Supernumerary arteries are about twice as common as supernumerary veins.

Congenital Anomalies of the Kidneys and Ureters

Some abnormality of the kidneys and ureters occurs in 3 to 4 per cent of newborn infants. Anomalies in shape and position are most common.

Renal Agenesis (Fig. 13–10 *A*). *Unilateral renal agenesis is* relatively common, occurring about once in every 1000 newborn infants. Males are affected more than females, and the left kidney is usually the absent one. Unilateral absence of a kidney often causes no symptoms and is usually not discovered during infancy because the other kidney usually undergoes compensatory hypertrophy and is able to perform the function of the missing kidney. Unilateral renal agenesis should be suspected in infants with a *single umbilical artery* (p. 128). If discovered during infancy, agenesis is usually detected during the course of evaluation for other

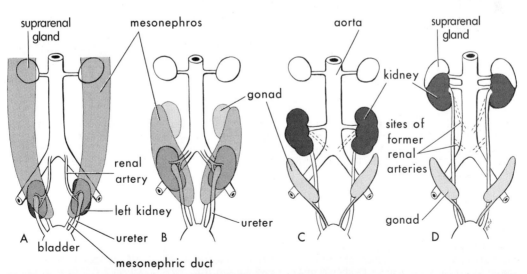

Figure 13–8. Diagrams of ventral views of the abdominopelvic region of embryos and fetuses (sixth to ninth weeks) showing medial rotation and "ascent" of the kidneys from the pelvis to the abdomen. Note that as the kidneys "ascend," they are supplied by arteries at successively higher levels and that the hilum of the kidney (where the vessels and ureter enter) is eventually directed anteromedially.

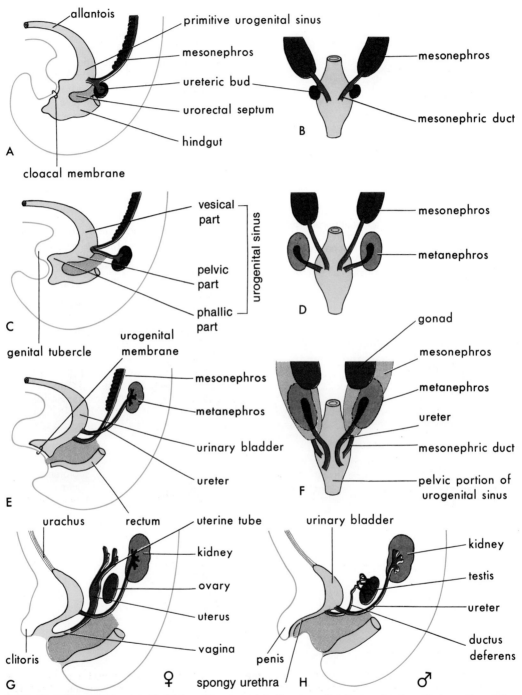

Figure 13–9. Diagrams showing: (1) division of the cloaca into the urogenital sinus and rectum, (2) absorption of the mesonephric ducts, (3) development of the urinary bladder, urethra, and urachus, and (4) changes in the location of the ureters. *A,* Lateral view of the caudal half of a five-week embryo. *B, D,* and *F,* Dorsal views. *C, E, G,* and *H,* Lateral views. The stages shown in *G* and *H* are reached by the twelfth week.

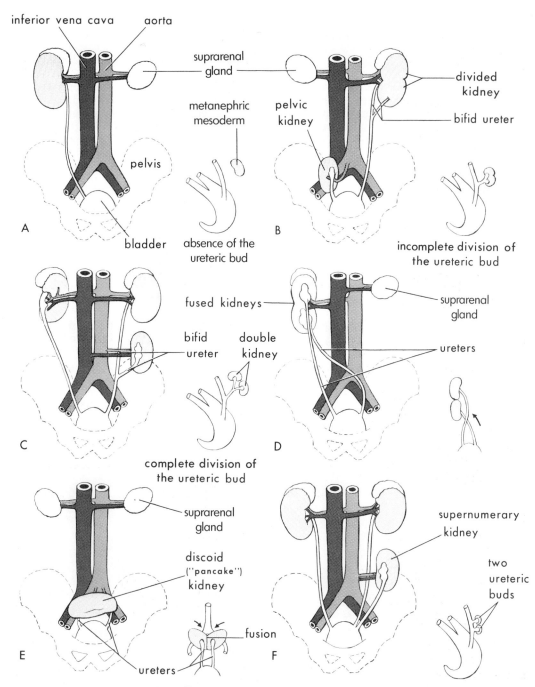

Figure 13–10. Drawings illustrating various anomalies of the urinary system. The small sketch at the lower right of each drawing illustrates the probable embryological basis of the anomaly. *A*, Unilateral renal agenesis. *B*, Right side, pelvic kidney; left side, divided kidney with a bifid ureter. *C*, Right side, malrotation of the kidney; left side, bifid ureter and double kidney. *D*, Crossed renal ectopia. The left kidney crossed to the right side and fused with the right kidney. *E*, "Pancake" or discoid kidney resulting from fusion of the kidneys while they were in the pelvis. *F*, Supernumerary left kidney resulting from the development of two ureteric buds.

congenital anomalies or for urinary tract symptoms (Behrman, 1992).

Bilateral renal agenesis is associated with oligohydramnios (p. 129) because no urine is excreted into the amniotic cavity (Peipert and Donnenfeld, 1991). Bilateral absence of the kidneys occurs about once in 3000 births and is incompatible with postnatal life. These infants have a characteristic facial appearance: the eyes are widely separated and have epicanthic folds; the ears are low set; the nose is broad and flat; the chin is receding, and there are limb defects. Fetal electrolyte stability is not impaired because it is controlled by placental exchange (Chapter 7). Most infants with bilateral renal agenesis die shortly after birth or during the first months of life. *Kidney transplants* may be performed if suitable donor sources are available.

Cause of Renal Agenesis. Absence of a kidney(s) occurs when the metanephric diverticulum fails to develop or with early degeneration of this ureteric primordium. Failure of the metanephric diverticulum to penetrate the metanephric mesoderm results in absence of kidney development because no nephrons are induced by the early collecting tubules to develop from the metanephric mesoderm.

Nonrotation and Abnormal Rotation of the Kidneys (Fig. 13–10*C*). If the kidney(s) fail to rotate, the hilum faces anteriorly; i.e., the fetal kidney retains its embryonic position (Fig. 13–8). If the hilum faces posteriorly, rotation of the kidney proceeded too far; if it faces laterally, lateral instead of medial rotation occurred. Abnormal rotation of the kidneys is often associated with ectopic kidneys.

Ectopic Kidneys (Fig. 13–10 *B, E,* and *F*). One or both kidneys may be in an abnormal position. Usually they are more inferior than usual and have not rotated, i.e., the hilum faces anteriorly. Most ectopic kidneys are located in the pelvis, but some lie in the inferior part of the abdomen. *Pelvic kidneys* and other forms of ectopia result from failure of the kidneys to "ascend." Pelvic kidneys are close to each other and are often fused to form a round mass known as a discoid or *pancake kidney* (Fig. 13–10*E*).

Ectopic kidneys receive their blood supply from blood vessels near them (internal or external iliac arteries and/or the aorta). They are often supplied by multiple vessels. Sometimes a kidney crosses to the other side resulting in *crossed renal ectopia* with or without fusion. An unusual type of abnormal kidney is *unilateral fused kidney* (Fig. 13–10*D*). The developing kidneys fuse while they are in the pelvis, and one kidney "ascends" to its normal position, carrying the other one with it. Often there are variations of the renal vessels (Fig. 13–12).

Horseshoe Kidney (Fig. 13–11). In one in about 500 persons, the poles of the kidneys are fused; usually it is the inferior poles that are fused. About seven per cent of persons with Turner syndrome (p. 146) have horseshoe kidneys (Behrman, 1992). The large, U-shaped kidney usually lies in the hypogastrium, anterior to the inferior lumbar

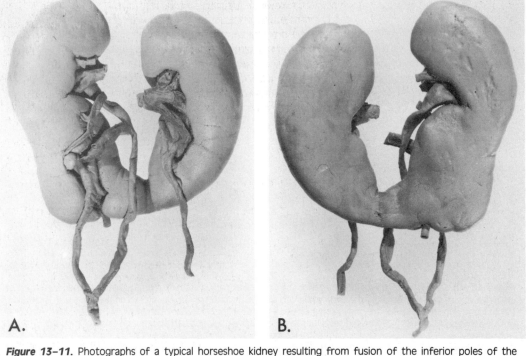

A.   **B.**

Figure 13–11. Photographs of a typical horseshoe kidney resulting from fusion of the inferior poles of the embryonic kidneys while they were in the pelvis. *A,* Anterior view. *B,* Posterior view. Half actual size. The larger right kidney has a bifid ureter.

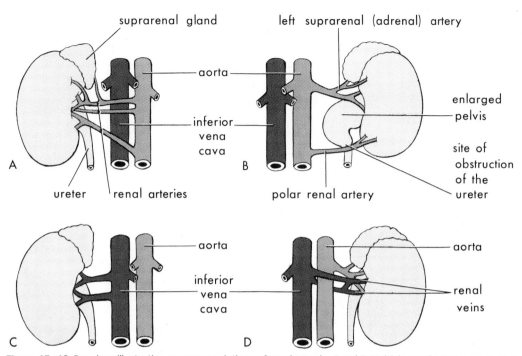

Figure 13–12. Drawings illustrating common variations of renal vessels. *A* and *B*, Multiple renal arteries. Note that some accessory vessels enter the poles of the kidney. They may arise superior or inferior to the main artery. The polar renal artery illustrated in *B* has obstructed the ureter and produced an enlarged renal pelvis. *C* and *D*, Multiple renal veins are less common than supernumerary arteries.

vertebrae. Normal ascent of the fused kidneys was prevented because it was caught by the root of the inferior mesenteric artery (Moore, 1992).

A horseshoe kidney usually produces no symptoms because its collecting system usually develops normally, and the ureters usually enter the bladder. If urinary flow is impeded, signs and symptoms of obstruction and/or infection may appear. *Wilms' tumors* are 2 to 8 times more frequent in children with horseshoe kidney than in the general population (Behrman, 1992).

Duplications of the Urinary Tract (Figs. 13–10 and 13–13). Duplications of the abdominal part of the ureter and the renal pelvis are common, but a *supernumerary kidney* is rare. These anomalies result from division of the metanephric diverticulum (ureteric bud). The extent of the duplication depends on completeness of the division of the diverticulum. Incomplete division of the ureteric primordium results in a divided kidney with a bifid ureter (Fig. 13–10*B*). Complete division results in a double kidney with a bifid ureter (Fig. 13–10*C*) or separate ureters (Fig. 13–13). A supernumerary kidney with its own ureter probably results from the formation of two ureteric primordia or buds (Fig. 13–10*F*).

Ectopic Ureteric Orifices. A ureter that opens anywhere except into the urinary bladder has an ectopic orifice. In males, an ectopic ureter usually opens into the neck of the bladder or into the prostatic portion of the urethra (Moore, 1992), but it may enter the ductus deferens, prostatic utri-

cle, or a seminal vesicle. In females, ectopic ureteric orifices may be in the bladder neck, urethra, vagina, or vestibule of the vagina (Behrman, 1992). *Incontinence* is the common complaint resulting from an ectopic ureteric orifice because the urine flowing from the ectopic orifice does not enter the bladder; instead, it continually dribbles from the urethra in males and the urethra and/or vagina in females.

Ureteric ectopia occurs when the ureter is not incorporated into the posterior part of the urinary bladder (Fig. 13–9); instead, it is carried caudally with the mesonephric duct and is incorporated into the caudal portion of the vesical part of the urogenital sinus. Because this part of the sinus becomes the prostatic urethra in males and the urethra in females, the common location of ectopic ureteric orifices is understandable. When two ureters form on one side (Fig. 13–13), they usually open into the urinary bladder (Fig. 13–10*F*). In some males the extra ureter is carried caudally and drains into the neck of the bladder or into the prostatic part of the urethra.

Congenital Polycystic Disease of the Kidney. The congenital form of this disease is relatively common. Death usually occurs shortly after birth, but an increasing number of these infants are surviving as the result of hemodialysis and kidney transplants. The kidneys contain multiple small to large cysts, which cause severe renal insufficiency. Several hypotheses have been proposed for the congenital form of the disease. For many years it was thought that the cysts were the result of failure of the ureteric bud derivatives to

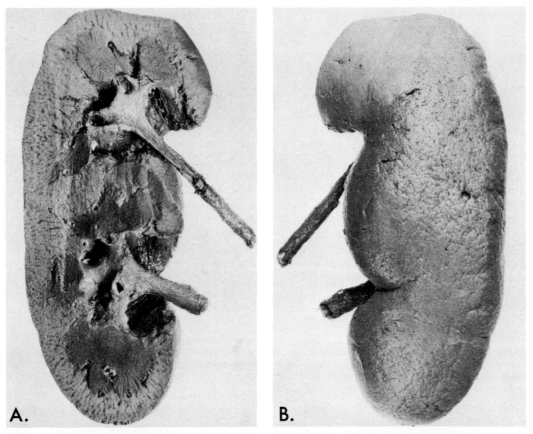

Figure 13–13. Photographs of a kidney with two ureters and renal pelves. This anomaly results from incomplete division of the metanephric diverticulum (Fig. 13–10B). A, Longitudinal section of the kidney showing the two renal pelves. B, Anterior surface. Both ureters opened into the urinary bladder as shown in Figure 13–10F.

join the tubules derived from the metanephric mesoderm. It is now widely believed that the cystlike formations are wide dilations of parts of otherwise continuous nephrons, particularly of the loops of Henle (Moffatt, 1982).

Development of the Urinary Bladder

Division of the cloaca by the *urorectal septum* into a dorsal rectum and a ventral urogenital sinus was described in Chapter 12 (p. 258; see also Fig. 12–21). For descriptive purposes, the *urogenital sinus* is divided into three parts: a cranial *vesical part* that is continuous with the allantois, a middle *pelvic part*, and a caudal *phallic part* that is closed externally by the *urogenital membrane* (Fig. 13–9E). The bladder mainly develops from the vesical part of the urogenital sinus, but its trigone region is derived from the caudal ends of the mesonephric ducts.

The epithelium of the bladder is derived from the endoderm of the vesical part of the urogenital sinus. The other layers of its wall develop from adjacent splanchnic mesenchyme. Initially the bladder is continuous with the *allantois*, a vestigial structure (p. 61). The allantois soon constricts and becomes a thick, fibrous cord called the *urachus*. It extends from the apex of the bladder to the umbilicus (Figs. 13–9 and 13–14). In the adult, the urachus is called the *median umbilical ligament* (see Fig. 7–20D).

As the bladder enlarges, distal portions of the mesonephric ducts are incorporated into its dorsal wall (Fig. 13–9B and F). These ducts contribute to the formation of the connective tissue in the *trigone of the bladder*, but the epithelium of the entire bladder is derived from the endoderm of the urogenital sinus. As the mesonephric ducts are absorbed, the ureters come to open separately into the urinary bladder (Fig. 13–9C to F). Partly because of traction exerted by the kidneys during their "ascent," the orifices of the ureters move superolaterally, and the ureters enter obliquely through the base of the bladder. The orifices of the mesonephric ducts move close together and enter the prostatic part of the urethra as the caudal

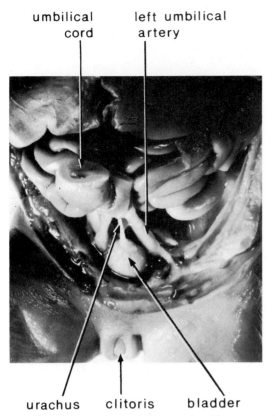

umbilical cord   left umbilical artery

urachus   clitoris   bladder

Figure 13–14. Photograph of a dissection of an 18-week female fetus showing the relation of the urachus to the urinary bladder and umbilical arteries. Note that the clitoris is relatively large at this stage.

ends of these ducts become the *ejaculatory ducts* (Fig. 13–24*A*). The distal ends of the mesonephric ducts in females degenerate (Fig. 13–23*B*).

In infants and children the urinary bladder, even when empty, is in the abdomen. It begins to enter the pelvis major at about six years of age but does not enter the pelvis minor and become a pelvic organ until after puberty (Moore, 1992).

The apex of the urinary bladder in adults is continuous with the *median umbilical ligament*, which extends posteriorly along the posterior surface of the anterior abdominal wall (Moore, 1992). This ligament is the fibrous remnant of the urachus, the tubular structure that connects the fetal bladder with the allantois (Fig. 13–14; see also Fig. 7–19). The *median umbilical ligament*, its remnant in adults, lies between the *medial umbilical ligaments*, which are the fibrous remnants of the umbilical arteries (see Fig. 14–44).

Urachal Anomalies (Fig. 13–15). A remnant of the lumen usually persists in the inferior part of the urachus in

infants and in about 50 per cent of cases, the lumen is continuous with the cavity of the bladder. The patent inferior end of the urachus may dilate to form a *urachal sinus* that opens into the bladder. The lumen in the superior part of the urachus may also remain patent and form a urachal sinus that opens at the umbilicus (Fig. 13–15*B*). Very rarely the entire urachus remains patent and forms a *urachal fistula* that allows urine to escape from its umbilical orifice (Fig. 13–15*C*). Remnants of the epithelial lining of the urachus may give rise to *urachal cysts* (Fig. 13–15*A*). Small cysts can be observed in about one third of cadavers, but urachal cysts are not detected in living persons unless they become infected and enlarge.

Exstrophy of the Bladder (Figs. 13–16 and 13–17). This severe anomaly occurs about once in every 10,000 to

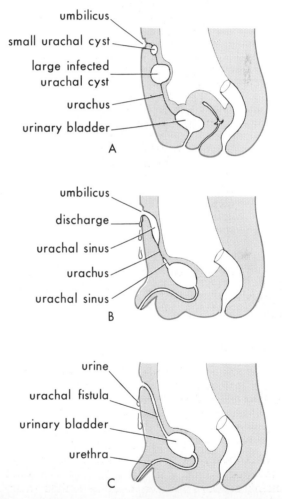

A
umbilicus
small urachal cyst
large infected urachal cyst
urachus
urinary bladder

B
umbilicus
discharge
urachal sinus
urachus
urachal sinus

C
urine
urachal fistula
urinary bladder
urethra

Figure 13–15. Diagrams illustrating malformations of the urachus. *A*, Urachal cysts. The most common site is in the superior end of the urachus just inferior to the umbilicus. *B*, Two types of urachal sinus are illustrated: one is continuous with the bladder; the other opens at the umbilicus. *C*, Patent urachus or urachal fistula connecting the bladder and umbilicus.

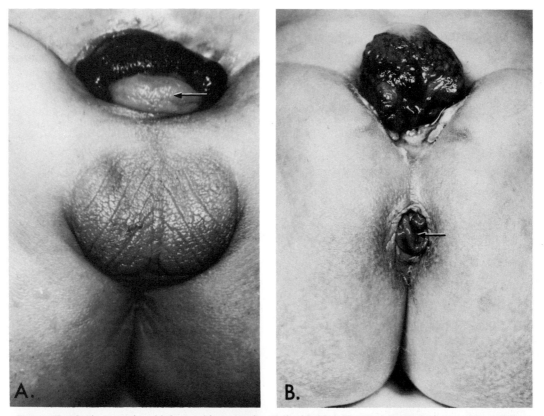

Figure 13-16. Photographs of infants with exstrophy of the bladder. Due to defective closure of the inferior portion of the anterior abdominal wall and the anterior wall of the bladder, the urinary bladder appears as an everted bulging mass inferior to the umbilicus. *A*, Male. Epispadias is also present and the penis (*arrow*) is small and flattened. (Courtesy of Dr. C. C. Ferguson, Children's Centre, Winnipeg, Canada.) *B*, Female with bladder exstrophy and a slight prolapse of the rectum, as indicated by the arrow. (Courtesy of Mr. Innes Williams, Genitourinary Surgeon, The Hospital for Sick Children, Great Ormond Street, London, England.)

40,000 births (Behrman, 1992). Exstrophy chiefly occurs in males. Exposure and *protrusion of the posterior wall of the bladder* characterize this severe congenital anomaly. The trigone of the bladder and the ureteric orifices are exposed, and urine dribbles intermittently from the everted bladder. *Epispadias* and wide separation of the pubic bones are associated with complete exstrophy of the bladder (Figs. 13-16*A* and 13-17*F*). In some cases the penis or clitoris is divided, and the halves of the scrotum or labia majora are widely separated.

Exstrophy of the bladder is caused by incomplete median closure of the inferior part of the anterior abdominal wall (Fig. 13-17*B*). The defect involves the anterior abdominal wall and the anterior wall of the urinary bladder. The anomaly is the result of failure of mesenchymal cells to migrate between the ectoderm of the abdomen and cloaca during the fourth week (Fig. 13-17*B* and *C*); as a result, no muscle and little connective tissue form in the anterior abdominal wall over the urinary bladder. Later, the thin epidermis and anterior wall of the bladder rupture, causing wide communication between the exterior and the mucous membrane of the bladder.

Development of The Urethra

The epithelium of most of the male urethra and the entire female urethra is derived from endoderm of the urogenital sinus (Figs. 13-9 and 13-18). The distal part of the urethra in the male is derived from the *glandular plate* (Fig. 13-18*A*). This ectodermal plate grows from the tip of the glans penis to meet the part of the spongy urethra derived from the phallic part of the urogenital sinus. The glandular plate becomes canalized and joins the rest of the urethra; consequently, the epithelium of the terminal part of the urethra is derived from surface ectoderm (Fig. 13-18). The connective tissue and smooth muscle of the urethra in both sexes are derived from the adjacent splanchnic mesenchyme.

THE SUPRARENAL GLANDS

The cortex and medulla of the suprarenal (adrenal) glands have different origins (Fig. 13–19). The *cortex* develops from mesoderm, and the *medulla* differentiates from *neural crest cells* (p. 62). The cortex is first indicated during the sixth week by an aggregation of mesenchymal cells on each side, between the root of the dorsal mesentery and the developing gonad (Fig. 13–20C). The cells that form the *fetal cortex* are derived from the *mesothelium* lining the posterior abdominal wall. The cells that form the medulla are

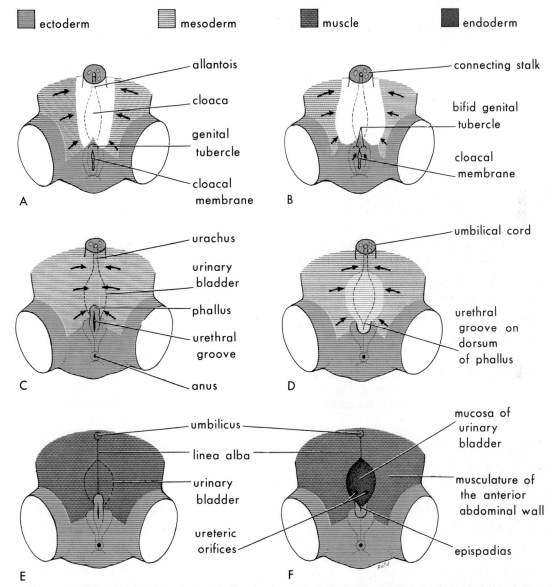

| ▨ ectoderm | ▨ mesoderm | ▨ muscle | ■ endoderm |

Figure 13–17. *A, C,* and *E,* Normal stages in the development of the infraumbilical abdominal wall and the penis during the fourth to eighth weeks. Note that mesoderm and later muscle reinforce the ectoderm of the developing anterior abdominal wall. *B, D,* and *F,* Probable stages in the development of exstrophy of the bladder and epispadias. In *B* and *D,* note that the mesenchyme (embryonic connective tissue) derived from mesoderm fails to extend into the anterior abdominal wall anterior to the urinary bladder. Also note that the genital tubercle is located in a more caudal position than usual and that the urethral groove has formed on the dorsal surface of the penis. In *F,* the surface ectoderm and endodermal anterior wall of the bladder have ruptured, resulting in exposure of the bladder mucosa. Note that the musculature of the anterior abdominal wall is present on each side of the defect. (Based on Patten BM and Barry A: *Am J Anat* 90:35, copyright © 1952. Reprinted by permission of Wiley-Liss, a division of John Wiley and Sons, Inc.)

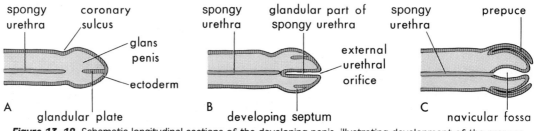

Figure 13–18. Schematic longitudinal sections of the developing penis, illustrating development of the prepuce (foreskin) and the glandular portion of the spongy urethra. *A*, 11 weeks. *B*, 12 weeks. *C*, 14 weeks. The epithelium of the spongy urethra has a dual origin; most of it is derived from the endoderm of the phallic part of the urogenital sinus. The distal portion of the urethra lining the navicular fossa is derived from surface ectoderm.

derived from an adjacent *sympathetic ganglion* (Fig. 13–20*C*), which is derived from the neural crest. Initially, the neural crest cells form a mass on the medial side of the fetal cortex (Fig. 13–19*B*). As they are surrounded by the fetal cortex, these cells differentiate into the *secretory cells* of the suprarenal medulla.

Later, more mesenchymal cells arise from the mesothelium and enclose the fetal cortex. These cells give rise to the permanent cortex (Fig. 13–19*C*). Differentiation of the characteristic suprarenal cortical zones begins during the late fetal period. The zona glomerulosa and zona fasciculata are present at birth, but the zona reticularis is not recognizable until about the end of the third year (Fig. 13–19*H*).

The suprarenal glands of the human fetus are 10 to 20 times larger than the adult glands relative to body weight and are large compared with the kidneys (Fig. 13–7). These large glands result from the extensive size of the fetal cortex. The suprarenal medulla remains relatively small until after birth. The suprarenal glands rapidly become smaller as the fetal cortex regresses during the first year. The glands lose about one third of their weight during the first two or three weeks after birth and do not regain their original weight until the end of the second year. For a review of the regulation of fetal suprarenal growth, differentiation, maturation, and subcellular mechanisms controlling fetal suprarenal function, see Pepe and Albrecht, 1990.

Congenital Adrenal Hyperplasia (CAH). An abnormal increase in the cells of the suprarenal cortex results in excessive androgen production during the fetal period. In females, this usually causes *female pseudohermaphroditism* (Fig. 13–28). Affected male infants have normal external genitalia and may go undetected in early infancy. Later in childhood in both sexes, androgen excess leads to rapid growth and accelerated skeletal maturation (Thompson et al., 1991). The adrenogenital syndrome associated with congenital *virilizing adrenal hyperplasia* manifests itself in various clinical forms that can be correlated with enzymatic deficiencies of cortisol biosynthesis (Zurbrügg, 1975). CAH is a group of *autosomal recessive disorders* that result in

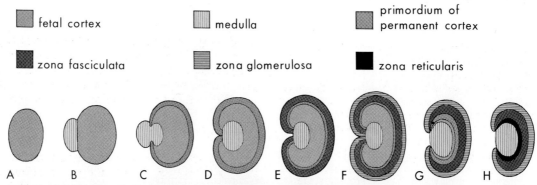

Figure 13–19. Schematic drawings illustrating development of the suprarenal glands (adrenal glands). *A*, Six weeks, showing the mesodermal primordium of the fetal cortex. *B*, Seven weeks, showing the addition of the neural crest cells to the suprarenal medulla. *C*, Eight weeks, showing the fetal cortex and the early permanent cortex beginning to encapsulate the medulla. *D* and *E*, Later stages of encapsulation of the medulla by the cortex. *F*, Newborn, showing the fetal cortex and two zones of the permanent cortex. *G*, One year; the fetal cortex has almost disappeared. *H*, Four years, showing the adult pattern of cortical zones. Note that the fetal cortex has disappeared and that the gland is smaller than it was at birth.

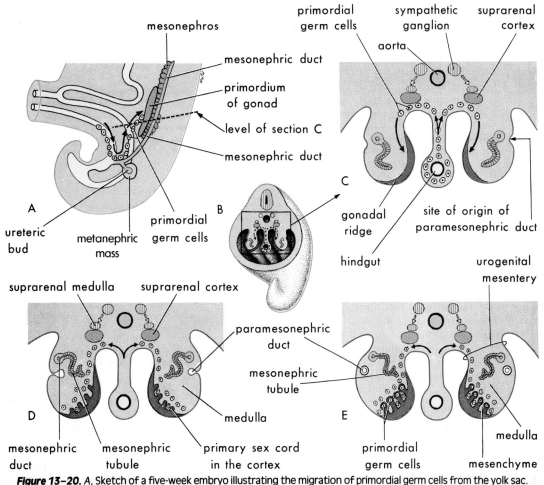

Figure 13–20. *A*, Sketch of a five-week embryo illustrating the migration of primordial germ cells from the yolk sac. *B*, Three-dimensional sketch of the caudal region of a five-week embryo, showing the location and extent of the gonadal ridges. *C*, Transverse section showing the primordium of the suprarenal (adrenal) glands, the gonadal ridges, and the migration of primordial germ cells into the developing gonads. *D*, Transverse section of a six-week embryo showing the primary sex cords and developing paramesonephric ducts. *E*, Similar section at later stage showing the indifferent gonads and mesonephric and paramesonephric ducts.

virilization of female fetuses. For details about the adrenal hyperplasias and their genetic basis, see New et al. (1989) and Thompson et al. (1991).

CAH is caused by a genetically determined deficiency of adrenal cortical enzymes necessary for the synthesis of various steroid hormones. The reduced hormone output results in an increased release of adrenocorticotropic hormone (ACTH), which causes adrenal hyperplasia and overproduction of androgens by the hyperplastic suprarenal glands.

THE GENITAL SYSTEM

Although the chromosomal and genetic sex of an embryo is determined at fertilization by the kind of sperm that fertilizes the ovum (p. 32), male and fe-

male morphological characteristics do not begin to develop until the seventh week. The early genital systems in the two sexes are similar; therefore, the initial period of early genital development is often referred to as the indifferent stage of sexual development.

Development of Gonads

The gonads (testes and ovaries) are derived from three sources (Fig. 13–20): the *mesothelium* (mesodermal epithelium) lining the posterior abdominal wall, the underlying *mesenchyme*, and the *primordial germ cells*.

The Indifferent or Undifferentiated Gonads (Figs. 13–20 and 13–21). The initial stages of gonadal development occur during the fifth week when a

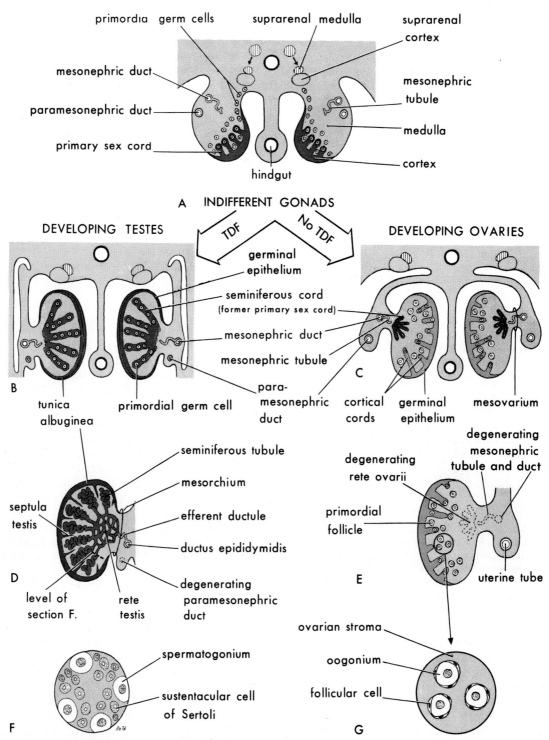

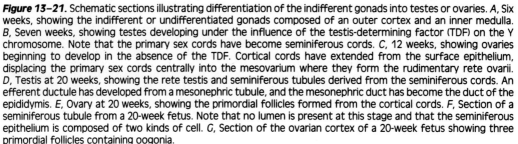

Figure 13-21. Schematic sections illustrating differentiation of the indifferent gonads into testes or ovaries. *A*, Six weeks, showing the indifferent or undifferentiated gonads composed of an outer cortex and an inner medulla. *B*, Seven weeks, showing testes developing under the influence of the testis-determining factor (TDF) on the Y chromosome. Note that the primary sex cords have become seminiferous cords. *C*, 12 weeks, showing ovaries beginning to develop in the absence of the TDF. Cortical cords have extended from the surface epithelium, displacing the primary sex cords centrally into the mesovarium where they form the rudimentary rete ovarii. *D*, Testis at 20 weeks, showing the rete testis and seminiferous tubules derived from the seminiferous cords. An efferent ductule has developed from a mesonephric tubule, and the mesonephric duct has become the duct of the epididymis. *E*, Ovary at 20 weeks, showing the primordial follicles formed from the cortical cords. *F*, Section of a seminiferous tubule from a 20-week fetus. Note that no lumen is present at this stage and that the seminiferous epithelium is composed of two kinds of cell. *G*, Section of the ovarian cortex of a 20-week fetus showing three primordial follicles containing oogonia.

thickened area of mesodermal epithelium develops on the medial side of the *mesonephros* (Figs. 13-4*F* and 13-20). Proliferation of this epithelium and of the underlying mesenchyme produces a bulge on the medial side of the mesonephros known as the *gonadal ridge* (Fig. 13-20*C*). Fingerlike epithelial cords called *primary sex cords* soon grow into the underlying mesenchyme (Fig. 13-20*D*). The "indifferent gonad" now consists of an external *cortex* and an internal *medulla.*

In embryos with an XX sex chromosome complex, the cortex of the indifferent gonad normally differentiates into an ovary and the medulla regresses. In embryos with an XY sex chromosome complex, the medulla normally differentiates into a testis, and the cortex regresses except for vestigial remnants (Table 13-1).

Primordial Germ Cells (Fig. 13-20). These large, spherical, primitive sex cells are visible early in the fourth week among the endodermal cells of the yolk sac near the origin of the allantois. During folding of the embryo (p. 70; see also Fig. 5-1), the dorsal part of the yolk sac is incorporated into the embryo. As this occurs, the primordial germ cells migrate along the dorsal mesentery of the hindgut to the gonadal ridges. During the sixth week the primordial germ cells enter the underlying mesenchyme and are incorporated in the *primary sex cords* (Fig. 13-20*E*).

Sex Determination. Chromosomal and genetic sex is established at fertilization and depends upon whether an X-bearing sperm or a Y-bearing sperm fertilizes the X-bearing ovum (p. 32). The type of gonads that develop is determined by the sex chromosome complex (XX or XY). Before the seventh week the gonads of the two sexes are identical in appearance and are referred to as "indifferent" or undifferentiated gonads (Fig. 13-21*A*). Development of the male phenotype requires a Y chromosome, but only the short arm of this chromosome is critical for sex determination. The gene for a *testis-determining factor* (TDF) has been localized in the "sex-determining region of the Y" (SRY) chromosome (Berta et al., 1990; Thompson et al., 1991). Two X chromosomes are required for the development of the female phenotype. A number of genes and regions of the X chromosome have special roles in sex determination.

The Y chromosome has a strong, testis-determining effect on the medulla of the indifferent gonad. It is the TDF (testis-determining factor) regulated by the Y chromosome that determines testicular differentiation. Under the influence of this organizing factor, the primary sex cords differentiate into seminiferous tubules (Fig. 13-21*B* and *D*). The absence of a Y chromosome (i.e., an XX sex chromosome complement) results in the formation of an ovary (Fig. 13-21*C* and

E); thus, the type of sex chromosome complex established at fertilization determines the type of gonad that differentiates from the indifferent gonad (Mittwoch, 1992).

The type of gonads present then determines the type of sexual differentiation that occurs in the genital ducts and external genitalia (p. 290). It is the androgen testosterone, produced by the fetal testes, that determines maleness. Primary female sexual differentiation in the fetus does not depend on hormones; it occurs even if the ovaries are absent and apparently is not under hormonal influence.

In embryos with abnormal sex chromosome complexes (e.g., XXX or XXY), the number of X chromosomes appears to be unimportant in sex determination. If a *normal* Y chromosome is present, the embryo develops as a male. If no Y chromosome is present or the testis-determining region of the Y chromosome has been lost, female development occurs. The loss of an X chromosome does not appear to interfere with the migration of primordial germ cells to the gonadal ridges because some germ cells have been observed in the fetal gonads of 45,X females with Turner syndrome (Carr et al., 1968). Two X chromosomes are needed, however, to bring about complete ovarian development.

Development of Testes (Figs. 13-21*B*, *D*, and *F*, and 13-22*A* and *C*). Embryos with a Y chromosome in their sex chromosome complement usually develop testes. A coordinated sequence of genes leads to development of testes (Thompson et al., 1991). A gene on the short arm of the Y chromosome, designated as the *testis-determining factor* (TDF), acts as the switch that directs development of the indifferent or undifferentiated gonad into a testis (Berta et al., 1990; DiGeorge, 1992). TDF induces the primary sex cords to condense and extend into the medulla of the indifferent gonad where they branch and anastomose to form the *rete testis.* The connection of the prominent sex cords, now called *seminiferous (testicular) cords,* with the surface epithelium is disrupted when a thick, fibrous capsule called the tunica albuginea develops (Fig. 13-21*B* and *D*). The development of the dense *tunica albuginea* is the characteristic and diagnostic feature of testicular development. Gradually the enlarging testis separates from the degenerating mesonephros and becomes suspended by its own mesentery, the *mesorchium.* The seminiferous cords develop into the seminiferous tubules, tubuli recti, and rete testis (Fig. 13-21*D*).

The seminiferous tubules become separated by mesenchyme that gives rise to the *interstitial cells* (of Leydig). By about the eighth week, these cells begin to produce the male sex hormone *testosterone,* which induces masculine differentiation of the mesonephric ducts and the external genitalia. Testosterone production is stimulated by hCG (p. 40), which

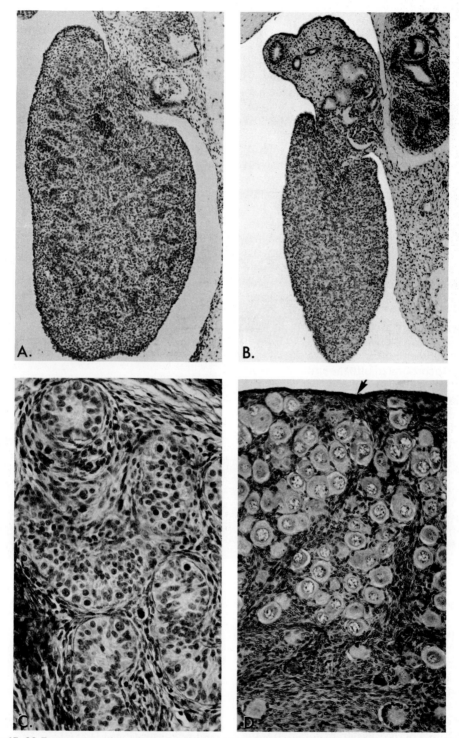

Figure 13–22. Transverse sections of gonads of human embryos and fetuses. *A*, Testis from an embryo of about 43 days, showing prominent seminiferous (testicular) cords (×175). *B*, From an embryo of about the same age, a gonad that may be assumed to be an ovary because of the absence of prominent primary sex cords (×125). *C*, Section of a testis from a male fetus born prematurely at about 21 weeks, showing seminiferous tubules composed mostly of sustentacular or Sertoli cells. A few large spermatogonia are visible (×475). *D*, Section of an ovary from a 14-day-old female infant showing numerous primordial follicles in the cortex, each of which contains a primary oocyte. The arrow indicates the relatively thin surface epithelium (×275). (From van Wagenen G, Simpson ME: *Embryology of the Ovary and Testis. Homo sapiens and Macaca mulatta.* 1965. Courtesy of Yale University Press.)

reaches peak amounts during the 8- to 12-week period (DiGeorge, 1992). In addition to testosterone, the fetal testes produce *müllerian-inhibiting factor* (MIF). It is first produced by the sustentacular cells (of Sertoli). MIF suppresses development of the paramesonephric (müllerian) ducts (p. 288).

The walls of the seminiferous tubules are composed of two kinds of cells (Fig. 13-21*F*): supporting cells or *Sertoli cells* derived from the surface epithelium, and *spermatogonia* derived from the primordial germ cells. Sertoli cells constitute most of the seminiferous epithelium in the fetal testis (Figs. 13-21*F* and 13-22*C*). During later development, the surface epithelium of the testes flattens to form the mesothelium on the external surface of the adult testis. The rete testis becomes continuous with 15 to 20 mesonephric tubules that become *efferent ductules* (ductuli efferentes). These ductules are connected with the mesonephric duct, which becomes the *ductus epididymis* (Figs. 13-21*B* and *D*, and 13-23*A*).

Development of Ovaries (Figs. 13-21*C, E,* and *G*, and 13-22*B* and *D*). In female 46,XX embryos, gonadal development occurs slowly. The X chromosomes bear genes for ovarian development, but an autosomal gene also appears to play a role in ovarian organogenesis (DiGeorge, 1992). The ovary is not identifiable histologically until about the tenth week. *Primary sex cords* do not become prominent, but they extend into the medulla and form a rudimentary *rete ovarii*. This structure and the primary sex cords normally degenerate and disappear (Fig. 13-21*E*).

During the early fetal period *secondary sex cords*, often called **cortical cords**, extend from the surface epithelium of the developing ovary into the underlying mesenchyme (Fig. 13-21*C*). This epithelium is derived from the mesothelium. As the cortical cords increase in size, primordial germ cells are incorporated into them. At about 16 weeks these cords begin to break up into isolated cell clusters composed of *primordial follicles*, each of which consists of an *oogonium* derived from a primordial germ cell surrounded by a single layer of flattened follicular cells derived from a cortical cord (Fig. 13-21*E* and *G*). Active mitosis of oogonia occurs during fetal life, producing thousands of these primitive germ cells. *No oogonia form postnatally.* Although many oogonia degenerate before birth, the two million or so that remain enlarge to become primary oocytes before birth.

After birth the surface epithelium of the ovary flattens to a single layer of cells continuous with the mesothelium of the peritoneum at the hilum of the ovary. The surface epithelium used to be called the "germinal epithelium" even though there was no convincing evidence that it was the site of germ cell formation in human embryos. The use of the term germinal epithelium is inappropriate because it is well established that the germ cells differentiate from primordial germ cells (Figs. 13-20 and 13-21). The surface epithelium becomes separated from the follicles in the cortex by a thin, fibrous capsule, the *tunica albuginea*. As the ovary separates from the regressing mesonephros, it becomes suspended by its own mesentery, the *mesovarium* (Fig. 13-21*C*).

Development of Genital Ducts

Both male and female embryos have two pairs of genital (sex) ducts. The mesonephric (wolffian) ducts play an important part in the development of the male reproductive system, and the paramesonephric (müllerian) ducts have a leading role in the development of the female reproductive system.

The Indifferent or Undifferentiated Stage (Fig. 13-24). During the fifth and sixth weeks when both pairs of genital ducts are present, the genital system is in the "indifferent" or undifferentiated stage. When the mesonephroi (p. 265) cease to function at the end of the first trimester, its ducts are taken over by the genital system.

The *mesonephric ducts*, which drained urine from the mesonephric kidneys, play an essential role in the development of the *male reproductive system* (Fig. 13-23*A*). Under the influence of testosterone produced by the fetal testes in the eighth week, the proximal part of each mesonephric duct becomes highly convoluted to form the *epididymis*. The remainder of this duct forms the *ductus (vas) deferens* and *ejaculatory duct*. In female fetuses the mesonephric ducts almost completely disappear; only a few nonfunctional remnants persist (Fig. 13-23*B* and *C*; Table 13-1).

The *paramesonephric ducts* develop lateral to the gonads and mesonephric ducts (Fig. 13-21). They play an essential role in the development of the *female reproductive system*. The paramesonephric ducts form on each side from longitudinal invaginations of the mesothelium on the lateral aspects of the mesonephroi (Fig. 13-20*C*). The edges of these invaginations approach each other and fuse to form the paramesonephric ducts (Fig. 13-20*D* and *E*). The funnel-shaped cranial ends of these ducts open into the future peritoneal cavity (Fig. 13-24*A*).

The paramesonephric ducts pass caudally, parallel to the mesonephric ducts, until they reach the future pelvic region of the embryo. Here they cross ventral to the mesonephric ducts, approach each other in the median plane, and fuse to form a Y-shaped *uterovaginal primordium* (Fig. 13-24*A*). This tubular structure projects into the dorsal wall of the urogenital

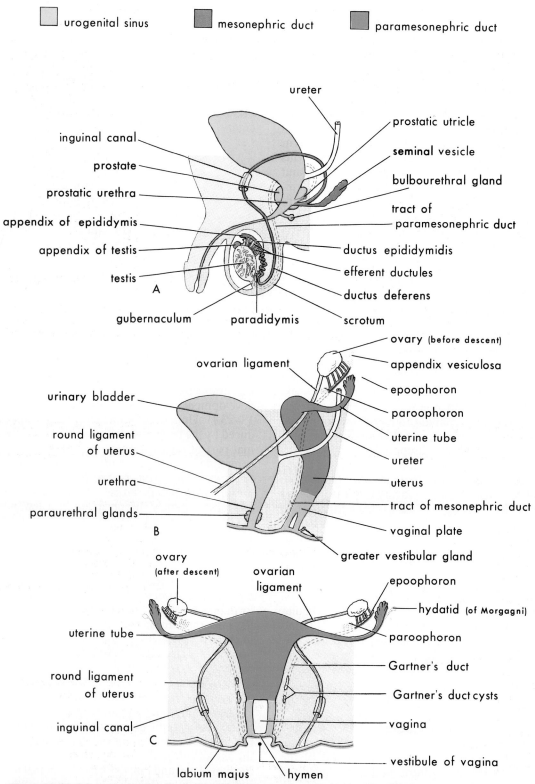

□ urogenital sinus   ■ mesonephric duct   ■ paramesonephric duct

Figure 13–23. Schematic drawings illustrating development of the male and female reproductive systems from the genital ducts and the urogenital sinus. Vestigial structures are also shown. *A,* Reproductive system in a newborn male. *B,* Female reproductive system in a 12-week fetus. *C,* Reproductive system in a newborn female.

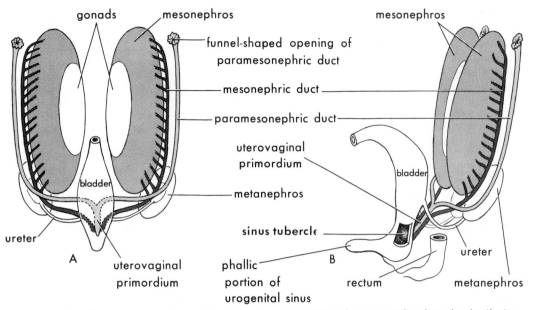

Figure 13–24. *A*, Sketch of a frontal view of the posterior abdominal wall of a seven-week embryo showing the two pairs of genital ducts present during the indifferent stage. *B*, Lateral view of a nine-week fetus showing the sinus tubercle (müllerian tubercle) on the posterior wall of the urogenital sinus. It becomes the hymen in females and the seminal colliculus in males.

Table 13–1. ADULT DERIVATIVES AND VESTIGIAL REMAINS OF EMBRYONIC UROGENITAL STRUCTURES*

Male	Embryonic Structure	Female
Testis	***Indifferent Gonad***	*Ovary*
Seminiferous tubules	***Cortex***	*Ovarian follicles*
Rete testis	***Medulla***	Rete ovarii
Gubernaculum testis	***Gubernaculum***	*Ovarian ligament*
		Round ligament of uterus
Ductuli efferentes	***Mesonephric Tubules***	Epoophoron
Paradidymis		Paroophoron
Appendix of epididymis	***Mesonephric Duct***	Appendix vesiculosa
Duct of epididymis		Duct of epoophoron
Ductus deferens		Duct of Gartner
Ureter, pelvis, calyces and collecting tubules		*Ureter, pelvis, calyces and collecting tubules*
Ejaculatory duct and seminal vesicle		
Appendix of testis	***Paramesonephric Duct***	Hydatid (of Morgagni)
		Uterine tube
		Uterus
Urinary bladder	***Urogenital Sinus***	*Urinary bladder*
Urethra (except *navicular fossa*)		*Urethra*
Prostatic utricle		*Vagina*
Prostate gland		*Urethral and paraurethral glands*
Bulbourethral glands		*Greater vestibular glands*
Seminal colliculus	***Sinus Tubercle***	Hymen
Penis	***Phallus***	*Clitoris*
Glans penis		*Glans clitoridis*
Corpora cavernosa penis		*Corpora cavernosa clitoridis*
Corpus spongiosum penis		*Bulb of the vestibule*
Ventral aspect of penis	***Urogenital Folds***	*Labia minora*
Scrotum	***Labioscrotal Swellings***	*Labia majora*

* Functional derivatives are in *italics*.

sinus and produces an elevation called the *sinus (müllerian) tubercle* (Fig. 13–24*B*).

Development of Male Genital Ducts and Auxiliary Glands (Figs. 13–23 and 13–25). The fetal testes produce a *masculinizing hormone* (testosterone) and a *müllerian-inhibiting factor* (MIF). The Sertoli cells produce MIF beginning at six to seven weeks, and the interstitial cells begin producing testosterone in the eighth week (DiGeorge, 1992). Testosterone, the production of which is stimulated by hCG (p. 40), stimulates the mesonephric ducts to form male genital ducts; whereas, MIF suppresses development of the paramesonephric ducts.

As the mesonephros (interim kidney) degenerates, some mesonephric tubules near the testis persist and are transformed into *efferent ductules* (Fig. 13–23*A*). These ductules open into the mesonephric duct, which has been transformed into the *ductus epididymis* in this region. Distal to the epididymis, the mesonephric duct acquires a thick investment of smooth muscle and becomes the *ductus deferens*. A lateral outgrowth from the caudal end of each mesonephric duct gives rise to the *seminal vesicle*. This pair of glands produces a secretion that nourishes the sperms (Cormack, 1987). The part of the mesonephric duct between the duct of this gland and the urethra becomes the *ejaculatory duct*.

The Prostate (Fig. 13–25). Multiple endodermal outgrowths arise from the prostatic portion of the urethra and grow into the surrounding mesenchyme. The glandular epithelium of the prostate differentiates from these endodermal cells, and the associated mesenchyme differentiates into the dense stroma and smooth muscle of the prostate.

The Bulbourethral Glands (Fig. 13–23*A*). These pea-sized structures develop from paired outgrowths from the spongy part of the urethra. The smooth muscle fibers and the stroma differentiate from the adjacent mesenchyme. The secretions of these glands contribute to the semen (Moore, 1992).

Development of Female Genital Ducts and Auxiliary Glands (Figs. 13–23*B* and *C* and 13–26). In embryos with ovaries, the mesonephric ducts regress due to the lack of testosterone, and the paramesonephric ducts develop due to the absence of MIF[1]. The paramesonephric ducts form most of the female genital tract.

The *uterine (fallopian) tubes* develop from the cranial, unfused portions of the paramesonephric ducts.

---

[1] Although testosterone is essential for the stimulation of male sexual development, female sexual development does not depend on the presence of ovaries or hormones.

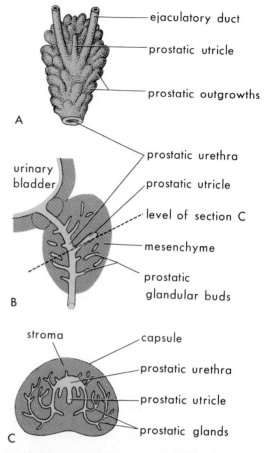

Figure 13–25. *A,* Dorsal view of the developing prostate in an 11-week fetus. *B,* Sketch of a median section of the developing urethra and prostate, showing the numerous endodermal outgrowths from the prostatic urethra. The vestigial prostatic utricle is also shown. *C,* Section of the prostate at the level shown in *B* (16 weeks).

The caudal fused portions of these ducts form the *uterovaginal primordium* (canal). As the name of this structure indicates, it gives rise to the uterus and vagina (superior part). The endometrial stroma and myometrium are derived from the adjacent splanchnic mesenchyme.

Similar development of the paramesonephric ducts occurs in males if the testes fail to develop (*agonadal males*) due to the absence of MIF. When the testes are removed in animals before the initiation of differentiation of the genital ducts, the female duct system also develops. Removal of the ovaries of female embryos, however, has no effect on fetal sexual development. This indicates that the testes impose masculinity and repress femininity and that the ovaries are not necessary for primary sexual development.

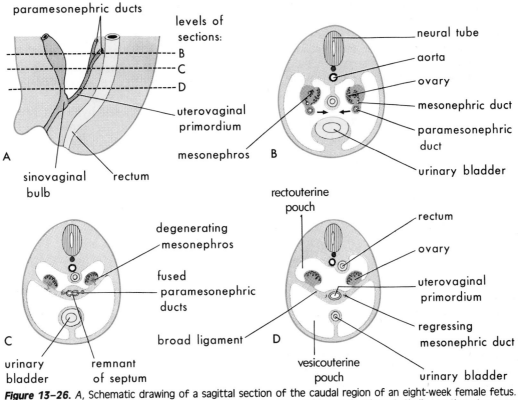

Figure 13–26. *A*, Schematic drawing of a sagittal section of the caudal region of an eight-week female fetus. *B*, Transverse section showing the paramesonephric ducts approaching each other. *C*, Similar section at a more caudal level illustrating fusion of the paramesonephric ducts. A remnant of the septum that initially separates them is shown. *D*, Similar section showing the uterovaginal primordium, broad ligament, and pouches in the pelvic cavity. Note that the mesonephric ducts have regressed.

Fusion of the paramesonephric ducts also brings together two peritoneal folds that form the right and left *broad ligaments* and forms two peritoneal compartments, the *rectouterine pouch* and the *vesicouterine pouch* (Fig. 13–26B to D). Along the sides of the uterus between the layers of the broad ligament, the mesenchyme proliferates and differentiates into the *parametrium*, which is composed of loose connective tissue and smooth muscle.

Development of the Vagina (Fig. 13–23B and C and 13–24). The vaginal epithelium is derived from the endoderm of the urogenital sinus, and the fibromuscular wall of the vagina develops from the surrounding splanchnic mesenchyme. Contact of the uterovaginal primordium with the urogenital sinus, forming the *sinus (müllerian) tubercle* (Fig. 13–24B), induces the formation of paired endodermal outgrowths called *sinovaginal bulbs*. They extend from the urogenital sinus to the caudal end of the uterovaginal primordium. The sinovaginal bulbs fuse to form a solid *vaginal plate* (Fig. 13–23B). Later, the

central cells of this plate break down, forming the lumen of the vagina. Its peripheral cells form the vaginal epithelium[2] (Fig. 13–23C).

Until late fetal life, the lumen of the vagina is separated from the cavity of the urogenital sinus by a membrane called the *hymen* (Figs. 13–23C and 13–27H). The hymen is formed by invagination of the posterior wall of the urogenital sinus, resulting from expansion of the caudal end of the vagina. The hymen usually ruptures during the perinatal period and remains as a thin fold of mucous membrane just within the entrance to the vagina (vaginal orifice).

[2] There is a difference of opinion concerning the origin of the lining of the vagina. Some authorities consider the superior third of the vaginal epithelium to be derived from the uterovaginal primordium and the inferior two thirds to arise from the urogenital sinus (Persaud, 1992). Most people believe that the lining of the entire vagina is derived from the vaginal plate (Minh et al., 1989; Persaud, 1992).

Auxiliary Genital Glands in the Female. Buds grow from the urethra into the surrounding mesenchyme and form *urethral glands* and *paraurethral glands* (of Skene). These glands correspond to the prostate in the male. Outgrowths from the urogenital sinus form the *greater vestibular glands* (of Bartholin), which are homologous to the bulbourethral glands in the male (Table 13–1).

Vestigial Structures Derived From the Embryonic Genital Ducts.

(Fig. 13–23; Table 13–1). During conversion of the mesonephric and paramesonephric ducts into adult structures, parts of them remain as vestigial structures. These vestiges are rarely seen unless pathological changes develop in them.

Mesonephric Remnants in Males (Fig. 13–23*A*). The blind cranial end of the mesonephric duct may persist as an *appendix of the epididymis*; it is usually attached to the head of the epididymis. Caudal to the efferent ductules, some mesonephric tubules may persist as a small body called the *paradidymis.*

Mesonephric Remnants in Females (Fig. 13–23*B* and *C*). The cranial end of the mesonephric duct may persist as an *appendix vesiculosa.* A few blind tubules and a duct called the *epoophoron* correspond to the efferent ductules and duct of the epididymis in the male. The epoophoron may persist in the mesovarium between the ovary and uterine tube (Moore, 1992). Closer to the uterus, some rudimentary tubules may persist as the *paroophoron.* Parts of the mesonephric duct, corresponding to the ductus deferens and ejaculatory duct, may persist as the *duct of Gartner* between the layers of the broad ligament along the lateral wall of the uterus or in the wall of the vagina. These mesonephric duct remnants may give rise to Gartner's duct cysts (Fig. 13–23*C*).

Paramesonephric Remnants in Males. The cranial end of the paramesonephric duct may persist as a vesicular *appendix of the testis.* It is attached to the superior pole of the testis (Fig. 13–23*A*). The *prostatic utricle*, a small, saclike structure that opens on the seminal colliculus in the prostatic urethra (Fig. 13–23*A*), is homologous to the vagina. The lining of the prostatic utricle is derived from the epithelium of the urogenital sinus. Within its epithelium endocrine cells containing neuron-specific enolase and serotonin have been detected (Wernert, 1990). The *seminal colliculus*, a small elevation in the posterior wall of the prostatic urethra (Moore, 1992), is the adult derivative of the sinus tubercle (Fig. 13–24*B*). It is homologous to the hymen in the female (Table 13–1).

Paramesonephric Remnants in Females. Part of the cranial end of the paramesonephric duct that does not contribute to the infundibulum of the uterine tube may persist as a vesicular appendage called a *hydatid of Morgagni* (Fig. 13–23*C*).

Development of External Genitalia

Up to the seventh week of development the external genitalia are similar in both sexes. Distinguishing sexual characteristics begin to appear during the ninth week, but the external genitalia are not fully differentiated until the twelfth week.

The Indifferent or Undifferentiated Stage

(Fig. 13–27*A* and *B*). From the fourth to the seventh week the external genitalia are sexually undifferentiated (i.e., they are in a *sexless state*). Early in the fourth week, proliferating mesenchyme produces a *genital tubercle* in both sexes at the cranial end of the cloacal membrane. *Labioscrotal swellings* (genital swellings) and *urogenital folds* (urethral folds) soon develop on each side of the cloacal membrane. The genital tubercle soon elongates to form a *phallus.*

When the urorectal septum fuses with the cloacal membrane at the end of the sixth week, it divides the cloacal membrane into a dorsal *anal membrane* and a ventral *urogenital membrane* (see Figs. 12–21 and 13–27*B*). The urogenital membrane lies in the floor of a median cleft known as the *urogenital groove*, which is bounded by the urogenital folds. These membranes rupture a week or so later, forming the *anus* and *urogenital orifice*, respectively. In the female fetus, the urethra and vagina open into a common *vestibule of the vagina.* In male fetuses, the *urethral groove* extends along the ventral surface of the phallus.

Development of Male External Genitalia

(Figs. 13–15 and 13–27*C, E,* and *G*). Masculinization of the indifferent external genitalia is caused by testosterone produced by the fetal testes (p. 283). As the phallus enlarges and elongates to become the penis, *urogenital folds* develop and form the lateral walls of the *urethral groove* on the ventral surface of the penis. This groove is lined by a proliferation of endodermal cells called the *urethral plate* (Fig. 13–27C_1), which extends from the phallic portion of the urogenital sinus.

The *urogenital folds* fuse with each other along the ventral surface of the penis to form the *spongy urethra* (Fig. 13–27E_1–E_3). The surface ectoderm fuses in the median plane of the penis, forming the *penile raphe* and enclosing the spongy urethra within the penis. At the tip of the glans penis, an ectodermal ingrowth forms a cellular cord called the *glandular plate.* It grows caudally toward the root of the penis to meet the spongy urethra (Fig. 13–18*A*). This plate canalizes and joins the previously formed spongy urethra. This completes the terminal part of the urethra and moves the external urethral orifice to the tip of the glans penis (Fig. 13–18*C*).

During the twelfth week a circular ingrowth of ectoderm occurs at the periphery of the glans penis (Fig. 13–18*B*). When this cellular ingrowth breaks down, it forms the *prepuce* and separates it from the glans penis (Fig. 13–18*C*); however, for some time the

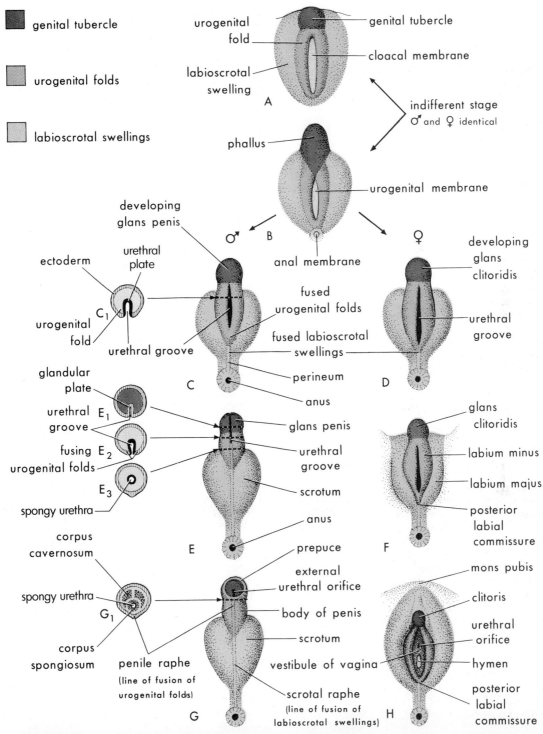

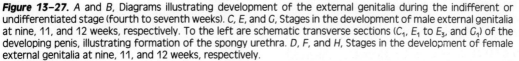

Figure 13–27. *A* and *B*, Diagrams illustrating development of the external genitalia during the indifferent or undifferentiated stage (fourth to seventh weeks). *C, E,* and *G,* Stages in the development of male external genitalia at nine, 11, and 12 weeks, respectively. To the left are schematic transverse sections (*C₁, E₁* to *E₃,* and *G₁*) of the developing penis, illustrating formation of the spongy urethra. *D, F,* and *H,* Stages in the development of female external genitalia at nine, 11, and 12 weeks, respectively.

prepuce is adherent to the glans and is usually not retractable at birth. Breakdown of the adherent surfaces normally occurs during infancy. The *corpora cavernosa penis* and *corpus spongiosum penis* develop from mesenchyme in the phallus. The *labioscrotal swellings* grow toward each other and fuse to form the scrotum (Fig. 13–27*E* and *G*). The line of fusion of these folds is clearly visible as the *scrotal raphe*.

Development of Female External Genitalia (Fig. 13–27*D, F*, and *H*). Feminization of the indifferent external genitalia occurs without the presence of a sex hormone. Growth of the phallus gradually ceases, and it becomes the *clitoris*, a very sensitive sexual organ. The clitoris, still relatively large at 18 weeks (Fig. 13–14), develops like the penis, but the urogenital folds do not fuse, except posteriorly where they join to form the *frenulum of the labia minora*. The unfused parts of the urogenital folds form the *labia minora*. The labioscrotal folds fuse posteriorly to form the *posterior labial commissure* and anteriorly to form the *anterior labial commissure* and *mons pubis* (Fig. 13–27*H*). Most parts of the labioscrotal folds remain unfused and form two large folds of skin called the *labia majora*. The labia majora (L. large lips) are two symmetrical folds of skin that are homologous to the scrotum.

Congenital Anomalies of the Genital System

When sexual differentiation is normal, the appearance of the external and internal genitalia is consistent with the sex chromosome complement (i.e., XX or XY). Because early embryos have the potential to develop as either males or females, errors in sex determination and differentiation result in various degrees of intermediate sex, a condition known as *hermaphroditism* or **intersexuality**. Hermaphroditism implies a discrepancy between the morphology of the gonads (testes/ovaries) and the appearance of the external genitalia. A person with ambiguous external genitalia is called an **intersex** or a *hermaphrodite*. Intersexual conditions are classified according to the histological appearance of the gonads.

True hermaphrodites have both ovarian and testicular tissue. *Male pseudohermaphrodites* have testes and *female pseudohermaphrodites* have ovaries (Rutgers, 1991).

True Hermaphroditism. Persons with this *extremely rare condition* usually have chromatin-positive nuclei, and 80 per cent of them have a 46,XX chromosome constitution. The causes of true hermaphroditism or intersexuality are still poorly understood (DiGeorge, 1992). Most true hermaphrodites are reared as females (Behrman, 1992) and have both testicular and ovarian tissue (e.g., an ovary and a testis or an ovotestis). These tissues are not usually functional. True hermaphroditism results from an error in sex determination. The phenotype may be male or female, but the external genitalia are ambiguous. *Ovotestes* form if both the medulla and cortex of the indifferent gonads develop (Fig. 13–21).

Female Pseudohermaphroditism (Figs. 13–28 and 13–29). Persons with this intersexual condition have *chromatin-positive nuclei* (see Fig. 8–7*B*) and a 46,XX chromosome constitution. This anomaly results from exposure of the female fetus to excessive androgens (p. 158), and the effects are principally virilization of the external genitalia (clitoral enlargement and labial fusion [see Fig. 8–15]). The most common cause of female pseudohermaphroditism is CAH (p. 280). There is no ovarian abnormality, but the excessive production of androgens by the fetal suprarenal glands causes masculinization of the external genitalia, varying from enlargement of the clitoris to almost masculine genitalia (Fig. 13–28*C* and *D*). Commonly, there is clitoral hypertrophy, partial fusion of the labia majora, and a persistent urogenital sinus (Fig. 13–29). In very unusual cases, the masculinization may be so intense that a complete *clitoral urethra* results (DiGeorge, 1992).

Female pseudohermaphrodites who do not have CAH are very rare. The administration of *androgenic agents* to women during pregnancy may cause similar anomalies of the fetal external genitalia (see Fig. 8–15; Table 8–6). Most cases have resulted from the use of certain progestational compounds for the treatment of threatened abortion (p. 158). *Masculinizing maternal tumors* can also cause virilization of female fetuses (e.g., benign adrenal adenoma and ovarian tumors, especially *arrhenoblastoma*).

Male Pseudohermaphroditism. Persons with this intersexual condition have *chromatin-negative nuclei* (see Fig. 8–7*A*) and a 46,XY chromosome constitution. The external and internal genitalia are variable due to varying degrees of development of the external genitalia and paramesonephric ducts. These abnormalities are caused by inadequate production of testosterone and MIF by the fetal testes (p. 285). Testicular development in these males ranges from rudimentary to normal. Five genetic defects have been described in the enzymatic synthesis of testosterone by the fetal testes, and a defect in Leydig cell differentiation has been described (DiGeorge, 1992). These defects produce male pseudohermaphroditism through inadequate virilization of the male fetus.

Androgen Insensitivity Syndrome (Testicular Feminization). Persons with this unusual condition (1 in 20,000 live births) are normal-appearing females despite the presence of testes and a 46,XY chromosome constitution (Fig. 13–30). The external genitalia are female, but the vagina usually ends blindly, and the uterus and uterine tubes are absent or rudimentary. At puberty there is normal development of breasts and female characteristics, but menstruation does not occur and pubic hair is scanty or absent. The psychosexual orientation of these women is entirely female and medically, legally, and socially, they are females.

The testes are usually in the abdomen or the inguinal canals, but they may descend into the labia majora. The failure of masculinization to occur in these individuals results from a resistance to the action of testosterone at the cellular level in the labioscrotal and urogenital folds. Current evidence suggests that *the defect is in the androgen receptor mechanism*. Embryologically these females repre-

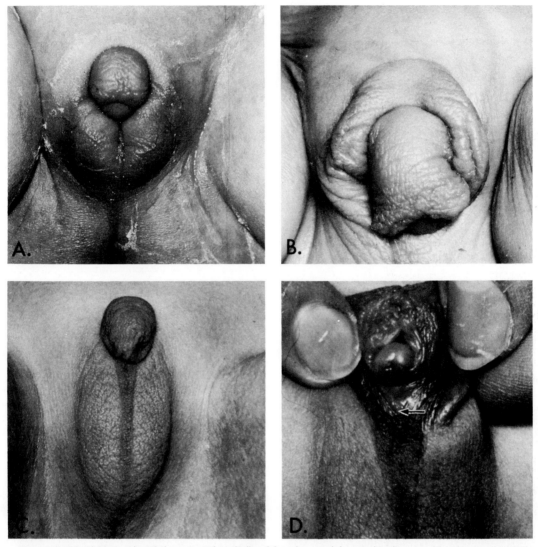

Figure 13–28. Photographs of the external genitalia of female pseudohermaphrodites resulting from congenital adrenal hyperplasia (CAH). The degree of labioscrotal fusion and clitoral hypertrophy depends upon the stage of differentiation at which the fetus is exposed to masculinizing hormones. *A,* External genitalia of a newborn female exhibiting enlargement of the clitoris and fusion of the labia majora. *B,* External genitalia of a female infant showing considerable enlargement of the clitoris. The unfused labia majora are rugose as in a scrotum. *C* and *D,* External genitalia of a six-year-old girl showing an enlarged clitoris and fused labia majora that have formed a scrotumlike structure. In *D,* note the glans clitoris and the location of the opening of the urogenital sinus (*arrow*).

sent an extreme form of male pseudohermaphroditism, but they are not intersexes because they have normal external genitalia. Usually the testes are removed as soon as they are discovered because, in about one third of these women, malignant tumors develop by 50 years of age (Behrman, 1992). The androgen insensitivity syndrome follows X-linked recessive inheritance, and the gene encoding the androgen receptor has been localized (DiGeorge, 1992). For details on the genetics of this condition, see Thompson et al., 1991.

Mixed Gonadal Dysgenesis. Persons with this very rare condition usually have chromatin-negative nuclei (see Fig. 8–7*A*), a testis on one side and an undifferentiated gonad on the other side. The internal genitalia are female, but male derivatives of the mesonephric ducts are sometimes present (Table 13–1). The external genitalia range from normal female, through intermediate states, to normal male. At puberty neither breast development nor menstruation occurs, but varying degrees of virilization are common (McDonough, 1990).

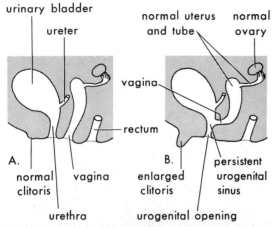

Figure 13–29. Schematic lateral views of the female urogenital system. *A*, Normal. *B*, Female pseudohermaphrodite caused by congenital virilizing adrenal hyperplasia. Note the enlarged clitoris and persistent urogenital sinus that were induced by androgens produced by the hyperplastic suprarenal glands.

Hypospadias (Fig. 13–31*A* to *C*). In about one of every 300 male infants, the external urethral orifice is on the ventral surface of the glans penis (*glandular hypospadias*) or on the ventral surface of the body (shaft) of the penis (*penile hypospadias*). Usually the penis is underdeveloped and curved ventrally, a condition known as *chordee*. Although there are four types of hypospadias (*glandular, penile, penoscrotal,* and *perineal*), the glandular and penile types constitute about 80 per cent of cases.

Hypospadias is the result of inadequate production of androgens by the fetal testes and/or inadequate receptor sites for the hormones. These defects result in failure of canalization of the glandular plate (Fig. 13–18) and/or failure of fusion of the urogenital folds (Fig. 13–27); as a consequence, there is incomplete formation of the spongy urethra. Differences in the timing and degree of hormonal failure and/or in the failure of the development of receptor sites account for the different types of hypospadias.

In *perineal hypospadias* the labioscrotal folds fail to fuse, and the external urethral orifice is located between the unfused halves of the scrotum. Because the external genitalia in this severe type of hypospadias are ambiguous, persons with perineal hypospadias and cryptorchidism (undescended testes) are sometimes diagnosed as male pseudohermaphrodites.

Epispadias (Fig. 13–31*D*). In about one of every 30,000 male infants, the urethra opens on the dorsal surface of the penis. Although epispadias may occur as a separate entity, it is *often associated with exstrophy of the bladder* (Figs. 13–16*A* and 13–17*F*). The embryological basis of epispadias is unclear, but it appears that the genital tubercle develops more dorsally than in normal embryos (Fig. 13–17*B*); consequently, when the urogenital membrane ruptures, the urogenital sinus opens on the dorsal surface of the penis. Urine is expelled at the root of the malformed penis.

Agenesis of the Penis. This extremely rare condition is the result of failure of the genital tubercle to develop. The urethra usually opens into the perineum near the anus.

Bifid Penis and Double Penis. These abnormalities are very rare. Bifid penis occurs when two genital tubercles develop. This malformation is often associated with exstrophy of the bladder (Fig. 13–16). It may also be associated with urinary tract abnormalities and imperforate anus.

Micropenis. The penis is so small that it is almost hidden by the suprapubic pad of fat. This condition results from a hormonal deficiency of the fetal testes and is commonly associated with hypopituitarism.

Anomalies of the Uterus and Vagina

Various types of uterine duplication and vaginal anomaly result from arrests of development of the uterovaginal primordium during the eighth week (Fig. 13–32): (1) incomplete fusion of the paramesonephric ducts, (2) incomplete development of a paramesonephric duct, (3) failure of parts of one or both paramesonephric ducts to develop, and (4) incomplete canalization of the vaginal plate (Fig. 13–23*B*).

Double uterus (uterus didelphys) results from failure of fusion of the inferior parts of the paramesonephric ducts. It may be associated with a double or a single vagina (Fig. 13–32*A* and *B*). In some cases the uterus appears normal externally but is divided internally by a thin septum (Fig. 13–32*F*). If the duplication involves only the superior portion of the body of the uterus, the condition is called *bicornuate uterus* (Fig. 13–32*C* and *D*). If one paramesonephric duct is retarded in its growth and does not fuse with the other one, a *bicornuate uterus with a rudimentary horn (cornu)* develops (Fig. 13–32*D*). The rudimentary horn may not communicate with the cavity of the uterus. Very rarely one paramesonephric duct fails to develop. This results in a *unicornuate uterus* with one uterine tube (Fig. 13–32*F*).

Absence of the Vagina and Uterus. Once in about every 4000 female births, absence of the vagina occurs. This results from failure of the sinovaginal bulbs to develop and form the vaginal plate (Fig. 13–23). When the vagina is absent, the uterus is usually also absent because the developing uterus (uterovaginal primordium) induces the formation of the vaginal plate.

Vaginal Atresia. Failure of canalization of the vaginal plate results in blockage of the vagina. Failure of its inferior end to perforate results in a condition known as *imperforate hymen*.

Development of the Inguinal Canals

The inguinal canals form pathways for the testes to descend from the abdomen through the anterior abdominal wall into the scrotum. *Inguinal canals develop in both sexes.* As the mesonephros (interim kidney) degenerates, a ligament called the *gubernaculum*

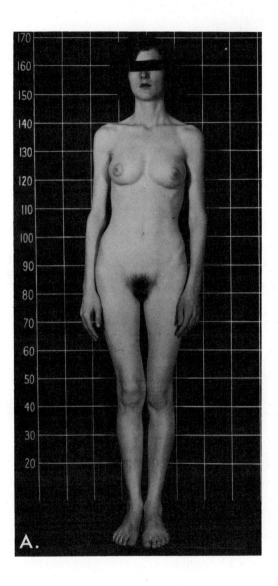

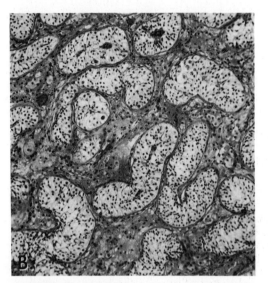

Figure 13–30. *A*, Photograph of a 17-year-old woman with the androgen insensitivity syndrome (testicular feminization syndrome). The external genitalia are female, but the patient has a 46,XY karyotype and testes. *B*, Photomicrograph of a section through a testis removed from the inguinal region of this woman, showing seminiferous tubules lined by Sertoli cells. There are no germ cells and the interstitial cells are hypoplastic. Medically, legally, and socially, these individuals are females. (From Jones HW, Scott WW: *Hermaphroditism, Genital Anomalies and Related Endocrine Disorders*. 1958. Courtesy of Williams & Wilkins, Baltimore.)

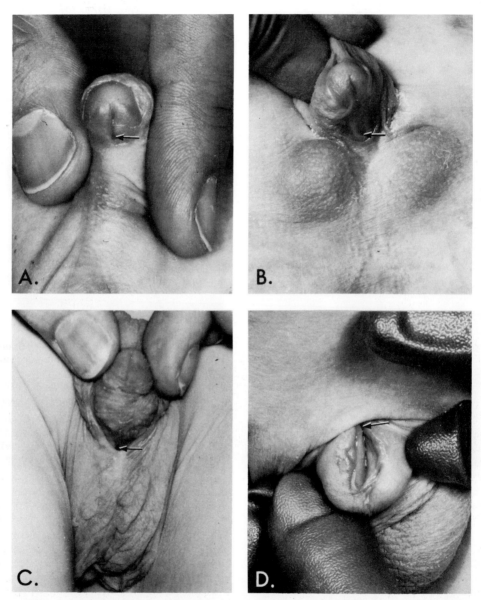

Figure 13–31. Photographs of penile malformations. *A,* Glandular hypospadias. This constitutes the simplest and most common form of hypospadias. The external urethral orifice is indicated by the arrow. There is a shallow pit in the glans penis at the usual site of the orifice. Note that the prepuce does not encircle the glans and that there is a moderate degree of chordee, causing the penis to curve ventrally. (From Jolly H: *Diseases of Children.* 2nd ed. 1968. Courtesy of Blackwell Scientific Publications.) *B,* Penile hypospadias. The penis is short and curved (chordee). The external urethral orifice (*arrow*) is near the penoscrotal junction. *C,* Penoscrotal hypospadias. The external urethral orifice (*arrow*) is located at the penoscrotal junction. *D,* Epispadias. The external urethral orifice (*arrow*) is on the dorsal surface of the penis. (Courtesy of Mr. Innes Williams, Genitourinary Surgeon, The Hospital for Sick Children. Great Ormond Street, London, England.)

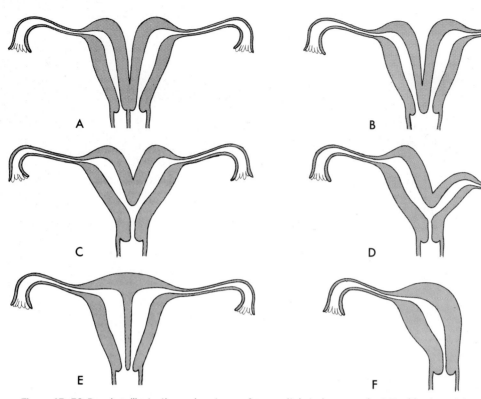

Figure 13–32. Drawings illustrating various types of congenital uterine anomaly. *A,* Double uterus (uterus didelphys) and double vagina. *B,* Double uterus with single vagina. *C,* Bicornuate uterus. *D,* Bicornuate uterus with a rudimentary left horn. *E,* Septate uterus. *F,* Unicornuate uterus.

descends on each side of the abdomen from the inferior pole of the gonad (Fig. 13–33*A*). The gubernaculum passes obliquely through the developing anterior abdominal wall at the site of the future inguinal canal. It attaches to the internal surface of the *labioscrotal swelling* (future half of the scrotum or labium majus).

An evagination of peritoneum called the *processus vaginalis* develops on each side ventral to the gubernaculum and herniates through the abdominal wall along the path formed by the gubernaculum (Fig. 13–33*B*). Each processus vaginalis carries before it extensions of the layers of the abdominal wall that form the walls of the inguinal canal. In males these layers also become the coverings of the spermatic cord and testis (Fig. 13–33*F*). The opening produced in the transversalis fascia by the processus vaginalis becomes the *deep inguinal ring,* and the opening created in the external oblique aponeurosis forms the *superficial inguinal ring* (Moore, 1992).

Descent of the Testes (Fig. 13–33). By about 28 weeks the testes have descended from the posterior abdominal wall to the deep inguinal rings. This change in position occurs as the pelvis enlarges and the trunk of the embryo elongates. This "descent" in

the abdomen is largely a relative movement that results from growth of the cranial part of the abdomen away from the caudal part (future pelvic region). Little is known about the cause of testicular descent through the inguinal canals into the scrotum, but the process is controlled by androgens produced by the fetal testes (Wensing, 1988).

The role of the gubernaculum in testicular descent is uncertain. Initially it forms a path through the anterior abdominal wall for the processus vaginalis to follow during formation of the inguinal canal. The gubernaculum also anchors the testis to the scrotum and appears to guide its descent. Passage of the testis through the inguinal canal may also be aided by the increase in intra-abdominal pressure that results from the growth of the abdominal viscera.

Descent of the testes through the inguinal canals usually begins during the twenty-eighth week and takes two or three days. The testes pass external to the peritoneum and processus vaginalis. About four weeks later (32 weeks) the testes enter the scrotum. After the testes pass into the scrotum, the inguinal canal contracts around the spermatic cord. More than 97 per cent of full-term newborn boys have both testes

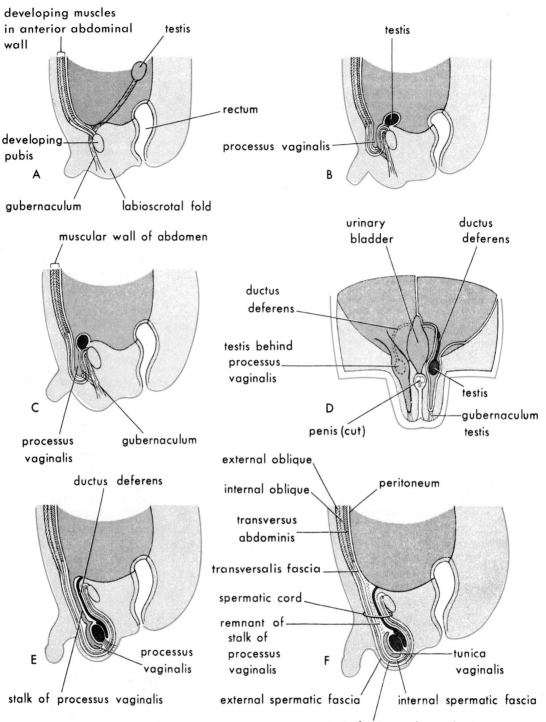

Figure 13–33. Schematic diagrams illustrating formation of the inguinal canals and descent of the testes. *A*, Sagittal section of a seven-week embryo showing the testis before its descent from the dorsal abdominal wall. *B* and *C*, Similar sections at about 28 weeks showing the processus vaginalis and the testis beginning to pass through the inguinal canal. Note that the processus vaginalis carries fascial layers of the abdominal wall before it. *D*, Frontal section of a fetus about three days later illustrating descent of the testis posterior to the processus vaginalis. The processus vaginalis has been cut away on the left side to show the testis and ductus deferens. *E*, Sagittal section of a newborn infant showing the processus vaginalis communicating with the peritoneal cavity by a narrow stalk. *F*, Similar section of a one-month-old infant after obliteration of the stalk of the processus vaginalis. Note that the extended fascial layers of the abdominal wall now form the coverings of the spermatic cord.

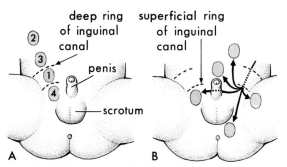

Figure 13–34. Diagrams showing the possible sites of cryptorchid and ectopic testes. *A*, Positions of cryptorchid testes, numbered in order of frequency. *B*, Positions of ectopic testes.

in the scrotum. During the first three months after birth, most testes, undescended at birth, descend into the scrotum.

The mode of descent of the testis explains why the ductus deferens crosses anterior to the ureter (Fig. 13–23*A*); it also explains the course of the testicular vessels. These vessels form when the testis is high on the posterior abdominal wall. When the testis de-

scends it carries its ductus deferens and vessels with it. As the testis and ductus deferens descend, they are ensheathed by the fascial extensions of the abdominal wall (Fig. 13–33*F*). The extension of the transversalis fascia becomes the *internal spermatic fascia*; the internal oblique muscle gives rise to the *cremasteric fascia* and muscle, and the external oblique aponeurosis forms the *external spermatic fascia* (Moore, 1992). Within the scrotum the testis projects into the distal end of the processus vaginalis. During the perinatal period, the connecting stalk of the processus vaginalis normally obliterates, isolating the *tunica vaginalis* as a peritoneal sac related to the testis (Fig. 13–33*F*).

Descent of the Ovaries. The ovaries also descend from the posterior abdominal wall to a point just inferior to the pelvic brim. The gubernaculum is attached to the uterus near the attachment of the uterine tube. The cranial part of the gubernaculum becomes the *ovarian ligament*; the caudal part forms the round ligament of the uterus (Fig. 13–23*C*). The *round ligament of the uterus* passes through the inguinal canal and terminates in the labium majus. The relatively small processus vaginalis in the female usually

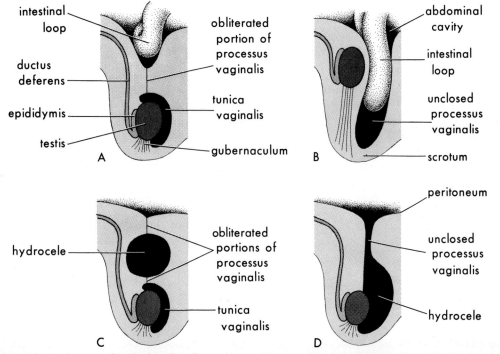

Figure 13–35. Diagrams of sagittal sections illustrating conditions resulting from failure of closure of the processus vaginalis. *A*, Incomplete congenital inguinal hernia resulting from persistence of the proximal part of the processus vaginalis. *B*, Complete congenital inguinal hernia into the scrotum resulting from persistence of the processus vaginalis. Cryptorchidism, a commonly associated malformation, is also illustrated. *C*, Large cyst that arose from an unobliterated portion of the processus vaginalis. This condition is called a hydrocele of the spermatic cord. *D*, Hydrocele of the testis and spermatic cord resulting from peritoneal fluid passing into an unclosed processus vaginalis.

obliterates and disappears long before birth; if it persists, it is called the *canal of Nuck.*

Cryptorchidism or Undescended Testes (Fig. 13–34*A*). This condition occurs in about 30 per cent of premature males and in about 3 per cent of full-term males. Cryptorchidism may be unilateral or bilateral. In most cases the testes descend into the scrotum by the end of the first year. If both testes remain within or just outside the abdominal cavity, they fail to mature and sterility is common. Undescended testes are unable to produce mature sperms, presumably because of the higher temperature in the abdominal cavity or inguinal canal. A *cryptorchid testis* may be located in the abdominal cavity or anywhere along the usual path of descent of the testis, but usually it lies in the inguinal canal. The cause of most cases of cryptorchidism is unknown, but a deficiency of androgen production by the fetal testes is an important factor.

Ectopic Testis (Fig. 13–34*B*). After traversing the inguinal canal, the testis may deviate from its usual path of descent and become lodged in various abnormal locations: interstitial (external to the aponeurosis of the external oblique muscle), in the thigh, dorsal to the penis, or on the opposite side (crossed ectopia). All types of ectopic testis are rare, but *interstitial ectopia* occurs most frequently. Ectopic testis occurs when a portion of the gubernaculum passes to an abnormal location and the testis follows it (Wensing, 1988).

Congenital Inguinal Hernia (Fig. 13–35). If the communication between the tunica vaginalis and the peritoneal cavity fails to close, a condition known as *persistent processus vaginalis* exists. A loop of intestine may herniate through it into the scrotum or labium majus (Fig. 13–35*B*). Embryonic remnants resembling the ductus deferens or epididymis are often found in inguinal hernial sacs (Popek, 1990). Congenital inguinal hernia is much more common in males and is often associated with cryptorchidism.

Hydrocele (Fig. 13–35). Occasionally the abdominal end of the processus vaginalis remains open but is too small to permit herniation of intestine. Peritoneal fluid passes into the patent processus vaginalis and forms a *hydrocele of the testis and spermatic cord* (Fig. 13–35*D*). If the middle portion of the canal of the processus vaginalis remains open, fluid may accumulate and give rise to a *hydrocele of the spermatic cord* (Fig. 13–35*C*).

SUMMARY

The urogenital system develops from the intermediate mesoderm, the mesothelium lining the peritoneal cavity, and the endoderm of the urogenital sinus. Three successive sets of kidneys develop: (1) the nonfunctional *pronephroi*, (2) the *mesonephroi*, which serve as temporary excretory organs, and (3) the functional *metanephroi* or permanent kidneys.

The metanephroi develop from two sources: (1) the *metanephric diverticulum* or *ureteric bud*, which gives rise to the ureter, renal pelvis, calices, and collecting tubules, and (2) the *metanephric mesoderm* which gives rise to the nephrons. At first the kidneys are located in the pelvis, but they gradually "ascend" to the abdomen. This apparent migration results from disproportionate growth of the lumbar and sacral regions.

The *urinary bladder* develops from the urogenital sinus and the surrounding splanchnic mesenchyme. The female urethra and almost all of the male urethra have a similar origin.

Developmental abnormalities of the kidneys and ureters are common. Incomplete division of the metanephric diverticulum results in double ureter and supernumerary kidney. Failure of the kidney to "ascend" from its embryonic position in the pelvis results in ectopic kidney that is abnormally rotated.

The genital or reproductive system develops in close association with the urinary or excretory system. Genetic sex is established at fertilization, but the gonads do not begin to attain sexual characteristics until the seventh week. The *primordial germ cells* form in the wall of the yolk sac during the fourth week and migrate into the developing gonads and differentiate into the definitive germ cells (oogonia/spermatogonia). The external genitalia do not acquire distinct masculine or feminine characteristics until the twelfth week.

The reproductive organs develop from primordia that are identical in both sexes. During this *indifferent or undifferentiated stage* an embryo has the potential to develop into either a male or a female.

Gonadal sex is determined by the *testis-determining factor* (TDF) *on the Y* chromosome. The TDF is located in the "sex-determining region of the Y" (SRY) of the short arm of the Y chromosome. The TDF directs testicular differentiation. The Leydig cells produce testosterone that stimulates development of the mesonephric ducts into male genital ducts. These androgens also stimulate development of the indifferent external genitalia into the penis and scrotum. A *müllerian inhibiting factor* (MIF) produced by the Sertoli cells of the testes inhibits development of the paramesonephric ducts.

In the absence of a Y chromosome and the presence of two X chromosomes, ovaries develop, the mesonephric ducts regress, the paramesonephric ducts develop into the uterus and uterine tubes, the vagina develops from the vaginal plate derived from the urogenital sinus, and the indifferent external genitalia develop into the clitoris and labia (majora and minora).

Persons with *true hermaphroditism*, an extremely rare intersexual condition, have both ovarian and testicular tissue and variable internal and external genitalia. Errors in sexual differentiation cause pseudohermaphroditism. *Male pseudohermaphroditism* is the result of failure of the fetal testes to produce adequate amounts of masculinizing hormones or from the tissue insensitivity of the sexual structures.

Female pseudohermaphroditism usually results from virilizing adrenal hyperplasia, a disorder of the fetal suprarenal (adrenal) glands that causes excessive production of androgens and masculinization of the external genitalia.

Most abnormalities of the female genital tract result from incomplete fusion of the paramesonephric ducts (e.g., double uterus).

Cryptorchidism and ectopic testes result from abnormalities of testicular descent. *Congenital inguinal hernia* and hydrocele result from persistence of the processus vaginalis. In males failure of the urogenital folds to fuse normally results in various types of *hypospadias*.

CLINICALLY ORIENTED QUESTIONS FOR PROBLEM-BASED LEARNING SESSIONS

1. A three-year-old girl was still in diapers because she was continually wet. The pediatrician saw urine coming from the infant's vagina. An *intravenous urogram* showed two renal pelves and two ureters on the right side. One ureter was clearly observed to enter the bladder, but the termination of the other one was not clearly seen. A pediatric urologist examined the child under general anesthesia and observed a small opening in the posterior wall of the vagina. He passed a tiny catheter into it and injected a radiopaque solution. This procedure showed that the opening in the vagina was the orifice of the second ureter. What is the embryological basis of the two renal pelves and ureters? Describe the embryological basis of the ectopic ureteric orifice. What is the anatomical basis of the continual dribbling of urine into the vagina?

2. A seriously injured young man suffered a cardiac arrest. After cardiopulmonary resuscitation (CPR), his heart began to beat again, but spontaneous respirations did not occur. Artificial respiration was instituted but there was no electroencephalographic (EEG) evidence of brain activity. After two days the man's family agreed that there was no hope of his recovery, and they asked that his kidneys be donated for transplantation. The radiologist carried out femoral artery catheterization and aortography (radiographic visualization of the aorta and its branches). This technique showed a single large renal artery on the right but two renal arteries on the left, one medium in size and the other small. Only the right kidney was used for transplantation because it is more difficult to implant small arteries than large ones. Grafting of the small accessory renal artery into the aorta would be difficult because of its size, and part of the kidney would die if one of the arteries was not successfully grafted. Are accessory renal arteries common? What is the embryological basis of the two left renal arteries? In what other circumstance might an accessory renal artery be of clinical significance?

3. A 32-year-old woman with a short history of cramping, lower abdominal pain and tenderness underwent a laparotomy because of a suspected ectopic pregnancy. The operation revealed a pregnancy in a *rudimentary right uterine horn*. The gravid uterine horn was totally removed. Is this type of uterine anomaly common? What is the embryological basis of the rudimentary uterine horn?

4. During physical examination of a newborn male infant, it was observed that the urethra opened on the ventral surface of the penis at the junction of its glans and body (shaft). The glans was curved toward the undersurface of the penis. Give the medical terms for the anomalies described. What is the embryological basis of the abnormal urethral orifice? Is this anomaly common? Discuss its etiology.

5. A 10-year-old boy suffered pain in his left groin while attempting to lift a heavy box. He later noticed a lump in his groin. When he told his mother about the lump, she arranged an appointment with the family physician. After a physical examination, a diagnosis of indirect inguinal hernia was made. Explain the embryological basis of this type of inguinal hernia. On the basis of your embryological knowledge, list the layers of the spermatic cord that would cover the hernial sac.

The answers to these questions are given on page 464.

References and Suggested Reading

Arant BS, Jr: Postnatal development of renal function during the first year of life. *Pediatr Nephrol 1*:308, 1987.

Austin CR: Sex chromatin in embryonic and fetal tissue. *In* Moore KL (ed): *The Sex Chromatin.* Philadelphia, WB Saunders, 1966.

Barr ML: Correlations between sex chromatin patterns and sex chromosome complexes in man. *In* Moore KL (ed): *The Sex Chromatin.* Philadelphia, WB Saunders, 1966.

Bartrina J: Hypospadias. *In* Rashad MN, Morton WRM (eds): *Selected Topics on Genital Anomalies and Related Subjects.* Springfield Ill, Charles C Thomas, 1969.

Behrman RE (ed): *Nelson Textbook of Pediatrics.* 14th ed. Philadelphia, WB Saunders, 1992.

Berta P, Hawkins JR, Sinclair AH, et al.: Genetic evidence equating SRY and the testis-determining factor. *Nature 348*:448, 1990.

Carr DH, Haggar RA, Hart AG: Germ cells in the ovaries of XO female infants. *Am J Clin Pathol 49*:521, 1968.

Cormack DH: *Ham's Histology.* 9th ed. Philadelphia, JB Lippincott, 1987.

Cunha GR: The dual origin of vaginal epithelium. *Am J Anat 143*:387, 1975.

Dewhurst CJ: Foetal sex and development of genitalia. *In* Philipp EE, Barnes J, Newton M (eds): *Scientific Foundations of Obstetrics and Gynecology.* London, William Heinemann, 1970.

DiGeorge AM: Hermaphroditism. *In* Behrman RE (ed): *Nelson Textbook of Pediatrics.* 14th ed. Philadelphia, WB Saunders, 1992.

Federman DD: *Abnormal Sexual Development: A Genetic and Endocrine Approach to Differential Diagnosis.* Philadelphia, WB Saunders, 1967.

Fleming S: N-linked oligosaccharides during human renal organogenesis. *J Anat 170*: 151, 1990.

Fukuda T: Ultrastructure of primordial germ cells in human embryos. *Virchows Arch B Cell Pathol 20*:85, 1975.

Gardner LI: Development of the normal fetal and neonatal adrenal. *In* Gardner LI (ed): *Endocrine and Genetic Diseases of Childhood and Adolescence.* 2nd ed. Philadelphia, WB Saunders, 1975.

Gray SW, Skandalakis JE: *Embryology for Surgeons.* 2nd ed. Baltimore, Williams & Wilkins, 1993.

Grobstein C: Some transmission characteristics of the tubule inducing influence on mouse metanephrogenic mesenchyme. *Exp Cell Res 13*:575, 1957.

Grumbach MM, Barr ML: Cytologic tests of chromosomal sex in relation to sexual anomalies in man. *Recent Prog Horm Res 14*:255, 1958.

Houston IB, Oetliker O: The growth and development of the kidneys. *In* Davis JA, Dobbing J (eds): *Scientific Foundations of Paediatrics.* Philadelphia, WB Saunders, 1974.

Jones HH, Scott WW: *Hermaphroditism, Genital Anomalies and Related Endocrine Disorders.* Baltimore, Williams & Wilkins, 1958.

Jost A: Development of sexual characteristics. *Sci J 6*:67, 1970.

Lennox B: The sex chromatin in hermaphroditism. *In* Moore KL (ed): *The Sex Chromatin.* Philadelphia, WB Saunders, 1966.

Mack WS: Testicular maldescent. *In* Rashad MN, Morton WRM (eds): *Selected Topics on Genital Anomalies and Related Subjects.* Springfield Ill, Charles C Thomas, 1969.

Mahony BS: The genitourinary system. *In* Callen PW (ed): *Ultrasonography in Obstetrics and Gynecology.* 2nd ed. Philadelphia, WB Saunders, 1988.

McCrory WW: *Developmental Nephrology.* Cambridge, Mass, Harvard University Press, 1972.

McDonough PG: Gonadal dysgenesis. *In* Quilligan EJ, Zuspan FP (eds): *Current Therapy in Obstetrics and Gynecology.* Vol. 3. Philadelphia, WB Saunders, 1990.

Minh HN, Hervé de Sigalony JP, Smadja A, Orcel L: Nouvelles acquisitions sur l'embryogénèse du vagin. *J Gynecol Obstet Biol Reprod 18*:589, 1989.

Mittwoch U: Sex determination and sex reversal: genotype, phenotype, dogma and semantics. *Hum Genet 89*:467, 1992.

Moffatt DB: Developmental abnormalities of the urogenital system. *In* Chisholm GD, Williams DI (eds): *Scientific Foundations of Urology.* 2nd ed. London, Heinemann Medical, 1982.

Moore KL: *Clinically Oriented Anatomy.* 3rd ed. Baltimore, Williams & Wilkins, 1992.

Moore KL: The development of clinical sex chromatin tests. *In* Moore KL (ed): *The Sex Chromatin.* Philadelphia, WB Saunders, 1966.

Moore KL: Sex determination, sexual differentiation and intersex development. *Can Med Assoc J 7*:292, 1967.

Morton WRM: Development of the urogenital systems. *In* Rashad MN, Morton WRM (eds): *Selected Topics on Genital Anomalies and Related Subjects.* Springfield Ill, Charles C Thomas, 1969.

Nader S: Polycystic ovary syndrome and the androgen-insulin connection. *Obstet Gynecol 165*:346, 1991.

New MI, White PC, Pang S et al.: The adrenal hyperplasias. *In* Scriver CR, Beaudet AL, Sly WS, Valle D (eds): *The Metabolic Basis of Inherited Diseases.* 6th ed. New York, McGraw-Hill, 1989.

O'Rahilly R: The development of the vagina in the human. *In* Blandau RJ, Bergsma D (eds): *Morphogenesis and Malformations of the Genital Systems.* Original Article Series. New York, Alan R Liss, 1977.

Pearson PL, Borrow M, Vosa CG: Technique for identifying Y chromosomes in human interphase nuclei. *Nature 226*:78, 1970.

Peipert JF, Donnenfeld AE: Oligohydramnios: a review. *Obstet Gynecol Surv 46*:325, 1991.

Pepe GJ, Albrecht ED: Regulation of the primate fetal adrenal cortex. *Endocr Rev 11*:151, 1990

Persaud TVN: Embryology of the female genital tract and gonads. *In* Copeland LJ, Jarrell J, McGregor J (eds): *Textbook of Gynecology.* Philadelphia, WB Saunders, 1992.

Polani P: Hormonal and clinical aspects of hermaphroditism and the testicular feminizing syndrome in man. *Philos Trans R Soc Lond [Biol Sci] 259*:187, 1970.

Popek EJ: Embryonal remnants in inguinal sac hernias. *Human Path 21*:339, 1990.

Rutgers JL: Advances in the pathology of intersex conditions. *Human Path 22*:884, 1991.

Sariola H, Saarma M, Sainio K, Arumäe U, Palgi J, Vaahtokari A, Thesleff I, Karavanov A: Dependence of kidney morphogenesis on the expression of nerve growth factor receptor. *Science 254*:571, 1991.

Saxen L: Embryonic induction. *Clin Obstet Gynecol 18*:149, 1975.

Schlegel RJ, Gardner LI: Ambiguous and abnormal genitalia in infants: differential diagnosis and clinical management. *In* Gardner LI (ed): *Endocrine and Genetic Diseases of Childhood and Adolescence.* 2nd ed. Philadelphia, WB Saunders, 1975.

Scorer CG, Farrington GH: *Congenital Deformities of the Testis and Epididymis.* London, Butterworth, 1971.

Simpson JL: *Disorders of Sexual Differentiation: Etiology and Clinical Delineation.* New York, Academic Press, 1976.

Stempfel RS, Jr.: Abnormalities of sexual differentiation. *In* Gardner LI (ed): *Endocrine and Genetic Diseases of Childhood and Adolescence.* 2nd ed. Philadelphia, WB Saunders, 1975.

Thompson MW, McInnes RR, Willard HF: *Thompson & Thompson Genetics in Medicine.* 5th ed. Philadelphia, WB Saunders, 1991.

van Wagenen G, Simpson ME: *Embryology of the Ovary and Testis–Homo sapiens and Macaca mulatta.* New York, Yale University Press, 1965.

Vaughan ED, Jr, Middleton GW: Pertinent genitourinary embryology. Review for the practicing urologist. *Urology* 6:139, 1975.

Villee DB: *Human Endocrinology: A Developmental Approach.* Philadelphia, WB Saunders, 1975.

Welling LW, Grantham JJ: Cystic and developmental diseases of the kidney. *In* Brenner BM, Rector Jr. FC (eds): *The Kidney.* 4th ed. Philadelphia, WB Saunders, 1991.

Wensing CJG: The embryology of testicular descent. *Hormone Res* 30:144, 1988.

Wernert N, Kern L, Heitz P, Bonkhoff H, Goebbels R, Seitz G, Inniger R, Remberger K, Dhom G: Morphological and immunohistochemical investigations of the utriculus prostaticus from the fetal period up to adulthood. *Prostate* 17:19, 1990.

Witschi E: Migration of the germ cells of human embryos from the yolk sac to the primitive gonadal folds. *Contr Embryol Carneg Instn* 32:67, 1948.

Zurbrügg RP: Congenital adrenal hyperplasia. *In* Gardner LI (ed): *Endocrine and Genetic Diseases in Childhood and Adolescence.* 2nd ed. Philadelphia, WB Saunders, 1975.

14

The Cardiovascular System

The cardiovascular system is the first system to function in the embryo; blood begins to circulate by the end of the third week. This precocious development is necessary because the rapidly growing embryo needs an efficient method of acquiring oxygen and nutrients and disposing of carbon dioxide and waste products.

The cardiovascular system is derived from *angioblastic tissue*, which arises from mesenchyme, an aggregation of mesenchymal cells derived from mesoderm. The process of blood vessel development called *angiogenesis* is described in Chapter 4 (see Figs. 4–9 and 4–10). Primitive blood vessels cannot be distinguished structurally as arteries or veins but are named according to their future fates and relationship to the heart.

EARLY DEVELOPMENT OF THE HEART AND PRIMITIVE CIRCULATORY SYSTEM

The earliest sign of the heart is the appearance of paired endothelial strands called *angioblastic cords* during the third week (Fig. 14–1). These cords canalize to form *endothelial heart tubes* that soon fuse to form a single heart tube (Figs. 14–2 and 14–6). Three paired veins drain into the tubular heart of four-week-old embryos (Figs. 14–2 and 14–3): (1) the *vitelline veins* return blood from the yolk sac; (2) the *umbilical veins* bring oxygenated blood from the chorion (embryonic part of the placenta); and (3) the *common cardinal veins* return blood from the body of the embryo.

The **vitelline veins** follow the yolk stalk into the embryo. After passing through the septum transversum, they enter the venous end of the heart known as the *sinus venosus* (Fig. 14–2). As the endodermal liver bud grows into the septum transversum (see Chapter 12, Fig. 12–6), the *hepatic cords* anastomose around pre-existing endothelium-lined spaces. These spaces, the primordia of the *hepatic sinusoids*, later become linked to the vitelline veins. The *hepatic veins* form from the remains of the right vitelline vein in the region of the developing liver. The *portal vein* devel-

ops from an anastomotic network formed around the duodenum by the vitelline veins (Fig. 14–4B).

The **umbilical veins** are transformed as follows: (1) the right umbilical vein and the part of the left umbilical vein between the liver and the sinus venosus degenerate (Fig. 14–4B); and (2) the persistent part of the left umbilical vein carries all the blood from the placenta to the fetus. Concurrently, a large shunt called the *ductus venosus* develops within the liver and connects the umbilical vein with the inferior vena cava (Fig. 14–4B). The ductus venosus forms a bypass through the liver, enabling some blood from the placenta to pass directly to the heart (Fig. 14–43). After birth the umbilical vein and ductus venosus become the *ligamentum teres* and *ligamentum venosum*, respectively (Fig. 14–44).

The **cardinal veins** (colored blue in Fig. 14–3A) constitute the main venous drainage system of the embryo. The anterior and posterior cardinal veins drain cranial and caudal parts of the embryo, respectively. The anterior and posterior cardinal veins empty into a common cardinal vein which enters the *sinus venosus* of the primitive heart (Figs. 14–2 to 14–4).

During the eighth week the *anterior cardinal veins* become connected by an oblique anastomosis (Fig. 14–4B). This communication shunts blood from the left to the right anterior cardinal vein. This anastomosis becomes the *left brachiocephalic vein* when the caudal part of the left anterior cardinal vein degenerates (Fig. 14–4C). The right anterior cardinal vein and the right common cardinal vein become the *superior vena cava* (Figs. 14–3 and 14–4).

The *posterior cardinal veins* develop primarily as the vessels of the mesonephric kidneys (p. 265) and largely disappear with these organs. The only adult derivatives of the posterior cardinal veins are the *root of the azygos vein* and the *common iliac veins* (Fig. 14–3D). The subcardinal and supracardinal veins gradually replace and supplement the posterior cardinal veins. The *subcardinal veins* appear first (colored red in Fig. 14–3). They are connected with each other via the subcardinal anastomosis and with the posterior cardinal veins through the mesonephric sinu-

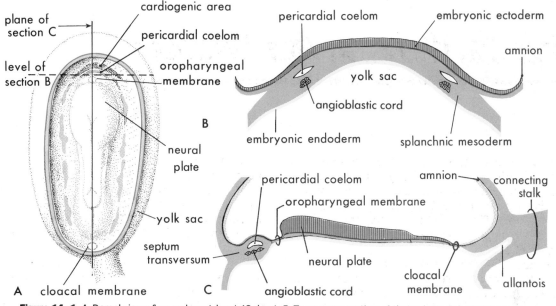

Figure 14–1. *A*, Dorsal view of an embryo (about 18 days). *B*, Transverse section of the embryo demonstrating the angiogenic cords and their relationship to the pericardial coelom. *C*, Longitudinal section through the embryo illustrating the relationship of the angioblastic cords to the oropharyngeal membrane, pericardial coelom, and septum transversum.

soids. The subcardinal veins form the stem of the left renal vein, the suprarenal veins, the gonadal veins (testicular and ovarian), and a segment of the inferior vena cava (Fig. 14–3*D*). The *supracardinal veins* (colored yellow in Fig. 14–3) are the last set of vessels to develop. They become disrupted in the region of the kidneys (Fig. 14–3*C*). Cranial to this, they become united by an anastomosis that is represented in the adult by the *azygos* and *hemiazygos veins* (Figs. 14–3 and 14–4). Caudal to the kidneys, the left supracardinal vein degenerates, but the right supracardinal vein becomes the inferior part of the inferior vena cava.

Development of the Inferior Vena Cava (IVC)

The IVC forms during a series of changes in the primitive veins of the trunk (Fig. 14–2) that occur as blood, returning from the caudal part of the embryo, is shifted from the left to the right side of the body. The inferior vena cava is composed of four main segments (Fig. 14–3*D*): (1) a *hepatic segment* (colored purple) derived from the hepatic vein (proximal part of right vitelline vein) and hepatic sinusoids, (2) a *prerenal segment* (colored red) derived from the right subcardinal vein, (3) a *renal segment* (colored green) derived from the subcardinal-supracardinal anastomosis, and

(4) a *postrenal segment* (colored yellow) derived from the right supracardinal vein.

Anomalies of the Venae Cavae

Because of the many transformations that occur during the formation of the superior and inferior venae cavae (Figs. 14–3 and 14–4), variations in their adult form may occur, but they are not common.

Double Superior Venae Cavae (Fig. 14–5). Persistence of the left anterior cardinal vein results in the presence of a left superior vena cava (SVC); hence, there are two superior venae cavae. The anastomosis that usually forms the left brachiocephalic vein (Figs. 14–3 and 14–4) is small or absent (Fig. 14–5). The abnormal left SVC, derived from the left anterior cardinal and common cardinal veins, opens into the right atrium via the coronary sinus.

Left Superior Vena Cava. The left anterior cardinal vein and the left common cardinal vein may form a left SVC, and the right anterior cardinal vein and the common cardinal vein, which usually form the SVC, degenerate. As a result, blood from the right side is carried by the brachiocephalic vein to the unusual left SVC.

Absence of Hepatic Portion of IVC. Occasionally the hepatic segment of the IVC fails to form. As a result, blood from inferior parts of the body drains into the right atrium through the azygos and hemiazygos veins and the superior vena cava (Fig. 14–3*D*). The hepatic veins open separately into the right atrium.

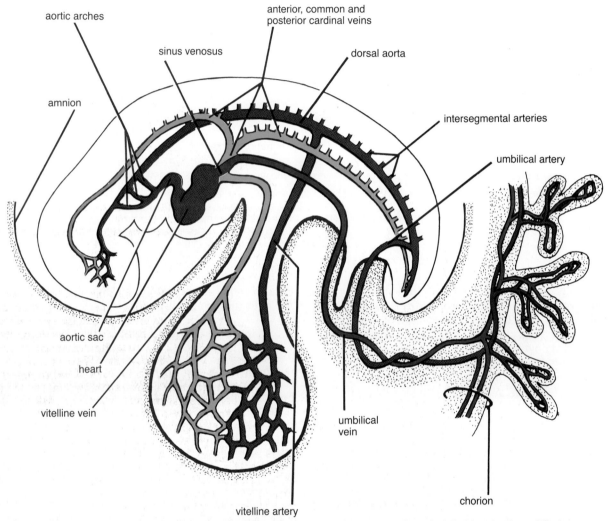

Figure 14–2. Sketch of the cardiovascular system (about 26 days) showing vessels on the left side only. The umbilical vein is shown in red because it carries well-oxygenated blood and nutrients from the chorion (embryonic part of the placenta) to the embryo. The umbilical arteries carry poorly oxygenated blood and waste products to the chorion. (See Chapter 7 for a description of the placenta at this stage).

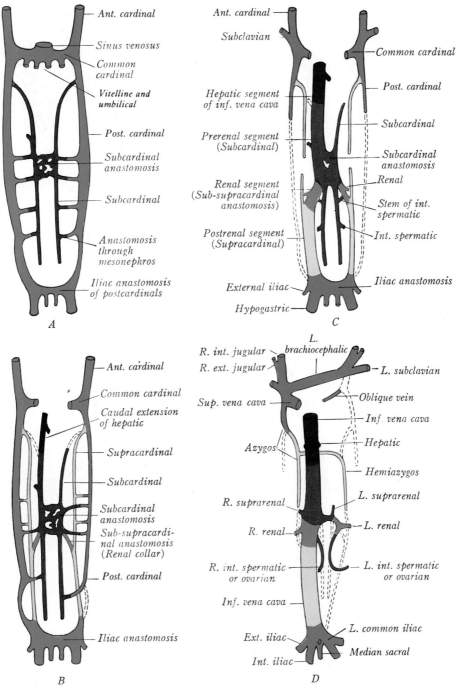

Figure 14–3. Drawings illustrating the primitive veins of the trunk in the human embryo (ventral views). Initially, three systems of veins are present (colored blue): the umbilical veins from the chorion, the vitelline veins from the yolk sac, and the cardinal veins from the body of the embryo. Next, the subcardinal veins (colored red) appear, and finally the supracardinal veins (colored yellow) develop. The transformations resulting in the adult venous pattern are shown in *D. A*, Six weeks. *B*, Seven weeks. *C*, Eight weeks. *D*, Adult. (From Arey LB: *Developmental Anatomy*. Revised 7th ed. Philadelphia, WB Saunders, 1974.)

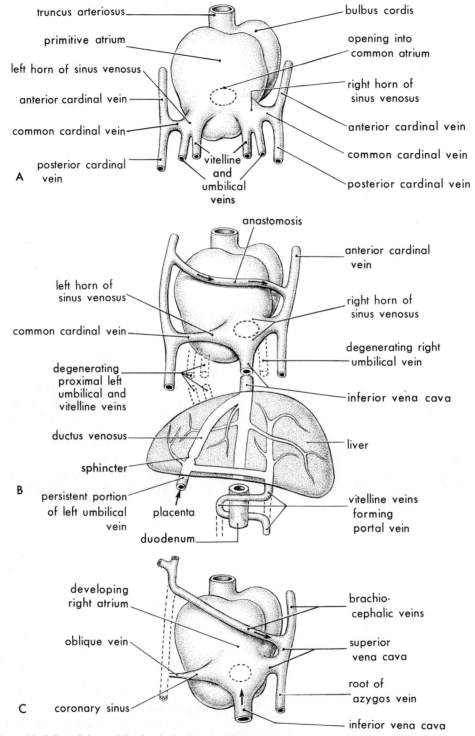

Figure 14–4. Dorsal views of the developing heart. *A*, The heart during the fourth week (about 24 days), showing the primitive atrium and sinus venosus. *B*, Seven weeks, showing the enlarged right horn of the sinus venosus and the venous circulation through the liver. The organs are not drawn to scale. *C*, Eight weeks, indicating the adult derivatives of the cardinal veins.

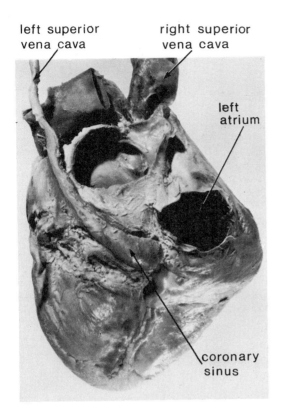

left superior
vena cava

right superior
vena cava

left
atrium

coronary
sinus

Figure 14–5. Photograph of the posterior aspect of an adult heart with double superior venae cavae. The small left superior vena cava opens into the coronary sinus. Parts of the walls of the atria have been removed.

Double Inferior Venae Cavae. In these unusual cases, the IVC inferior to the renal veins is represented by two vessels; usually, the one on the left is much smaller (Moore, 1992). This condition probably results from failure of an anastomosis to develop between the primitive veins of the trunk (Fig. 14–3*B*). As a result, the inferior part of the left supracardinal vein fails to disappear (as illustrated in Figure 14–3*D*) and persists as a second IVC.

Aortic Arches and Branches of the Dorsal Aorta

As the *branchial or pharyngeal arches* form during the fourth and fifth weeks (p. 188), they are penetrated by arteries called *aortic arches.* They arise from the *aortic sac* and terminate in a dorsal aorta (Figs. 14–2). Initially, the paired dorsal aortae run through the entire length of the embryo, but they soon fuse to form a single *dorsal aorta* just caudal to the branchial or pharyngeal arches.

The Intersegmental Arteries

Thirty or so branches of the dorsal aorta called *intersegmental arteries* (Fig. 14–2) pass between and carry blood to the somites and their derivatives. The dorsal intersegmental arteries in the neck join to form a longitudinal artery on each side called the *vertebral artery.* Most of the original connections of the intersegmental arteries to the dorsal aorta disappear. In the thorax, the dorsal intersegmental arteries persist as the *intercostal arteries.* Most of the dorsal intersegmental arteries in the abdomen become *lumbar arteries,* but the fifth pair of lumbar intersegmental arteries becomes the *common iliac arteries.* In the sacral region, the intersegmental arteries form the lateral *sacral arteries.* The caudal end of the dorsal aorta becomes the median sacral artery (Moore, 1992).

Fate of the Vitelline and Umbilical Arteries

The unpaired, ventral branches of the dorsal aorta pass to the yolk sac, allantois, and chorion (Fig. 14–2). The vitelline arteries pass to the yolk sac and later to the primitive gut, which forms from the incorporated part of the yolk sac (see Fig. 12–1). Three vitelline arteries remain as the *celiac artery* to the foregut, the *superior mesenteric artery* to the midgut, and the *inferior mesenteric artery* to the hindgut.

The paired umbilical arteries pass through the connecting stalk (later the *umbilical cord*) and become continuous with the chorionic vessels in the chorion, the embryonic part of the placenta. The umbilical arteries carry poorly oxygenated blood to the placenta (Figs. 14–2 and 14–43). Proximal parts of the umbilical arteries become the *internal iliac arteries* and *superior vesical arteries*; whereas, the distal parts obliterate after birth and become the *medial umbilical ligaments* (Fig. 14–44). The major changes leading to the definitive arterial system, especially the *transformation of the aortic arches* (Fig. 14–36), are described later (p. 335).

DEVELOPMENT OF THE PRIMITIVE HEART

As previously described, heart development is first indicated around the middle of the third week. In the *cardiogenic area*, splanchnic mesenchymal cells ventral to the pericardial coelom aggregate and arrange themselves side by side to form two longitudinal cellular strands called *angioblastic cords* (Fig. 14–1). These cords become canalized to form two, thinwalled *endothelial heart tubes* (Figs. 14–6 and 14–7*B*). As lateral embryonic folding occurs (p. 71), these tubes gradually approach each other and fuse to form a single *endothelial heart tube* (Figs. 14–6*A* and *B* and 14–7*C* and *D*). Fusion of these tubes begins at the cranial end of the developing heart and extends caudally.

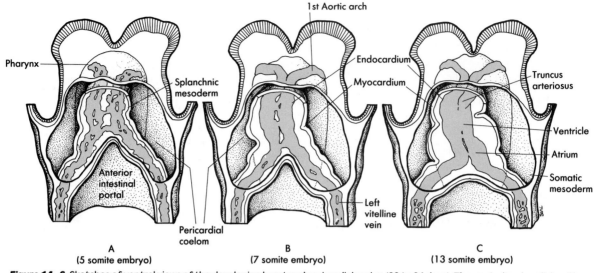

Figure 14–6. Sketches of ventral views of the developing heart and pericardial region (22 to 24 days). The ventral pericardial wall has been removed to show the developing myocardium and fusion of the endothelial tubes to form a single endothelial heart tube.

As the endothelial heart tubes fuse, an external layer of the embryonic heart is formed from splanchnic mesoderm surrounding the pericardial coelom. This layer represents the *primitive myocardium* (Fig. 14–7*D*). At this stage the developing heart is composed of an endothelial tube separated from another tube, the primitive myocardium, by gelatinous connective tissue called *cardiac jelly*. The endothelial tube becomes the internal endothelial lining of the heart called the *endocardium*, and the primitive myocardium becomes the muscular wall or *myocardium*. The visceral pericardium or *epicardium* (Fig. 14–7*F*) is derived from mesothelial cells that arise from the external surface of the sinus venosus and spread over the myocardium (Hirakow, 1992).

During folding of the head (p. 70), the heart and pericardial cavity come to lie ventral to the foregut and caudal to the oropharyngeal membrane (Fig. 14–8). Concurrently, the tubular heart elongates and develops alternate dilatations and constrictions (Fig. 14–6): truncus arteriosus, bulbus cordis, ventricle, atrium, and sinus venosus. The truncus arteriosus is continuous cranially with the *aortic sac*, from which the *aortic arches* arise (Fig. 14–9). The large sinus venosus receives the umbilical, vitelline, and common cardinal veins from the chorion, yolk sac and embryo, respectively (Figs. 14–2 and 14–6*B*).

The arterial and venous ends of the heart tube are fixed by the branchial or pharyngeal arches and the septum transversum, respectively (Fig. 14–6*A*). Because the bulbus cordis and ventricle grow faster than other regions, the heart tube bends upon itself, forming a U-shaped *bulboventricular loop* (Fig. 14–7*E*). As the primitive heart bends, the atrium and sinus venosus come to lie dorsal to the truncus arteriosus, bulbus cordis, and ventricle (Fig. 14–9). By this stage, the sinus venosus has developed lateral expansions called right and left horns (Fig. 14–9*B*).

As the heart elongates and bends, it gradually invaginates into the pericardial cavity (Figs. 14–7*C* and *D* and 14–8*C*). The heart is initially suspended from the dorsal wall of this cavity by a mesentery, the *dorsal mesocardium* (Fig. 14–7*D*), but the central part of this mesentery soon degenerates. This forms a communication, the *transverse pericardial sinus*, between the right and left sides of the pericardial cavity (Fig. 14–7*E* and *F*). The heart tube is now attached only at its cranial and caudal ends.

Circulation Through the Primitive Heart

Contractions of the heart begin on days 21 to 22. These originate in the muscle, i.e., they are of myogenic origin. The muscle layers of the atrium and ventricle are continuous, and contractions occur in

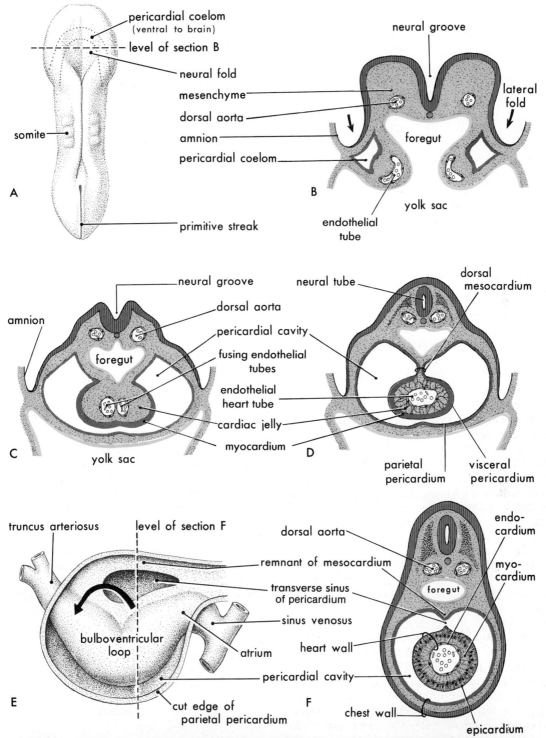

Figure 14-7. *A*, Dorsal view of an embryo (about 20 days). *B*, Schematic transverse section of the heart region of the embryo illustrated in *A*, showing the endothelial tubes and the lateral body folds (*arrows*). *C*, Transverse section of a slightly older embryo, showing the formation of the pericardial cavity and the endothelial tubes which are about to fuse. *D*, Similar section (about 22 days), showing the single heart tube suspended by the dorsal mesocardium. Note that a primitive myocardium is present. *E*, Schematic drawing of the heart (about 28 days), showing degeneration of the central part of the dorsal mesocardium and formation of the transverse sinus of the pericardium. *F*, Transverse section of this embryo, showing the layers of the heart wall.

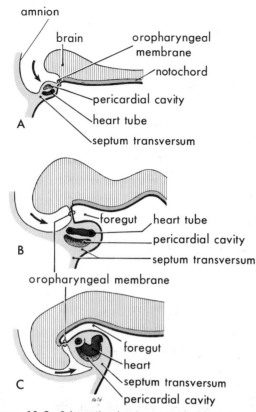

Figure 14-8. Schematic drawings of longitudinal sections through the cranial half of human embryos during the fourth week, showing the effect of the head fold (*arrow*) on the position of the heart and other structures. As the head fold develops, the heart tube and the pericardial cavity come to lie ventral to the foregut and caudal to the oropharyngeal membrane. Note that the positions of the pericardial cavity and the septum transversum have reversed with respect to each other. The septum transversum now lies posterior to the pericardial cavity where it will form the central tendon of the diaphragm (see Fig. 9-7).

peristalsis-like waves that begin in the sinus venosus. At first circulation through the primitive heart is of an ebb and flow type; but, by the end of the fourth week, coordinated contractions of the heart result in unidirectional flow.

Blood enters the *sinus venosus* from: (1) the embryo via the common cardinal veins, (2) the developing placenta via the umbilical veins, and (3) the yolk sac via the vitelline veins (Figs. 14-2, 14-4, and 14-6). Blood from the sinus venosus enters the *primitive atrium*; flow through it is controlled by *sinoatrial valves* (Figs. 14-9A and 14-10A). The blood then passes through the atrioventricular canal into the *primitive ventricle*. When the ventricle contracts, blood is pumped through the *bulbus cordis* and *truncus arteriosus* into the aortic sac from which it is distributed to the *aortic arches* in the branchial or pha-

ryngeal arches (Fig. 14-9C). The blood then passes into the dorsal aorta for distribution to the embryo, yolk sac, and placenta (Fig. 14-2).

PARTITIONING OF THE PRIMITIVE HEART

Partitioning of the atrioventricular canal and the primitive atrium and ventricle begins around the middle of the fourth week and is essentially completed by the end of the fifth week. Although described separately, these processes occur concurrently.

Partitioning of the Atrioventricular Canal

During the fourth week, swellings called *endocardial cushions* form on the dorsal and ventral walls of the atrioventricular canal. As they are invaded by mesenchymal cells during the fifth week, the atrioventricular endocardial cushions approach each other and fuse, dividing the atrioventricular canal into right and left *atrioventricular canals* (Figs. 14-10D and 14-11D).

Partitioning of the Primitive Atrium

The primitive atrium is divided into right and left atria by the formation and subsequent modification and fusion of two septa, the septum primum and the septum secundum (Figs. 14-10 to 14-12). The septum primum also unites with the fused endocardial cushions.

The **septum primum**, a thin, crescent-shaped membrane, grows toward the fusing endocardial cushions from the dorsocranial wall or roof of the primitive atrium. As this curtainlike septum grows, a large opening, the *foramen primum*, forms between its crescentic free edge and the endocardial cushions (Figs. 14-10 to 14-12). The foramen primum becomes progressively smaller and disappears when the septum primum fuses with the fused endocardial cushions (atrioventricular septum). Before the foramen primum is obliterated, perforations appear in the central part of the septum primum that coalesce to form another opening, the *foramen secundum* (Figs. 14-11 and 14-12). Concurrently, the free edge of the septum primum fuses with the left side of the fused endocardial cushions, obliterating the foramen primum (Figs. 14-11D and 14-12D).

The **septum secundum**, another crescentic membrane, grows from the ventrocranial wall of the atrium, immediately to the right of the septum primum (Fig. 14-12D). As this thick septum grows during the fifth and sixth weeks, it gradually overlaps the

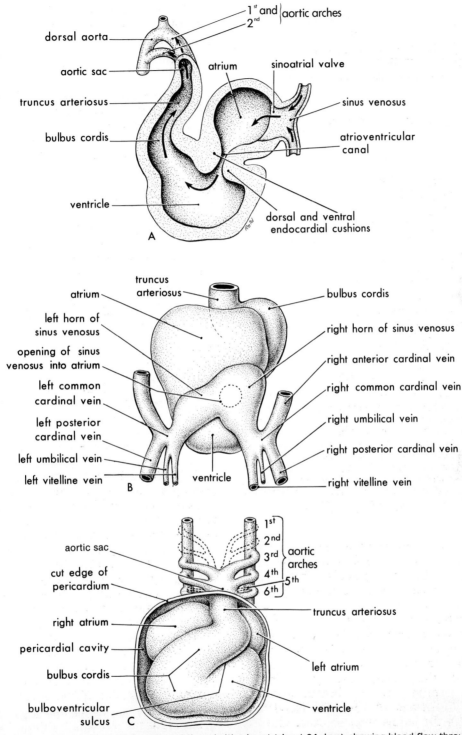

Figure 14–9. *A,* Schematic sagittal section of the primitive heart (about 24 days), showing blood flow through it. *B,* Dorsal view of the heart (about 26 days) illustrating the horns of the sinus venosus and the location of the primitive atrium. *C,* Ventral view of the heart and aortic arches (about 35 days). The ventral wall of the pericardial sac has been removed to show the heart in the pericardial cavity.

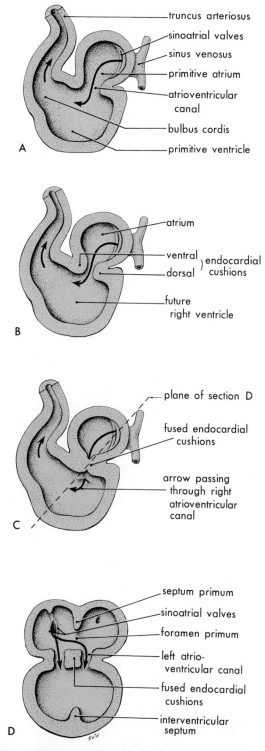

truncus arteriosus
sinoatrial valves
sinus venosus
primitive atrium
atrioventricular canal
bulbus cordis
primitive ventricle

A

atrium
ventral ⎫ endocardial
dorsal ⎭ cushions
future right ventricle

B

plane of section D
fused endocardial cushions
arrow passing through right atrioventricular canal

C

septum primum
sinoatrial valves
foramen primum
left atrio-ventricular canal
fused endocardial cushions
interventricular septum

D

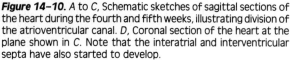

Figure 14–10. A to C, Schematic sketches of sagittal sections of the heart during the fourth and fifth weeks, illustrating division of the atrioventricular canal. D, Coronal section of the heart at the plane shown in C. Note that the interatrial and interventricular septa have also started to develop.

foramen secundum in the septum primum. The septum secundum forms an incomplete partition between the atria, forming an oval opening called the **foramen ovale** (Fig. 14–12E_1). The cranial part of the septum primum, initially attached to the roof of the left atrium, gradually disappears (Fig. 14–12 G_1). The remaining part of the septum primum, attached to the fused endocardial cushions, forms the flap-type *valve of the foramen ovale* (Fig. 14–12H_1).

Before birth the foramen ovale allows most of the blood entering the right atrium from the inferior vena cava to pass into the left atrium (Fig. 14–13); however, it prevents the passage of blood in the opposite direction because the septum primum closes against the relatively rigid septum secundum.

After birth the foramen ovale normally closes, and the interatrial septum becomes a complete partition between the atria when the septum primum fuses with the septum secundum (Figs. 14–13 and 14–16A).

Changes in the Sinus Venosus and Associated Veins (Figs. 14–1, 14–9, and 14–14). Initially the sinus venosus opens into the center of the dorsal wall of the primitive atrium, and its right and left horns are about the same size. Progressive enlargement of the right horn of the sinus venosus results from two left-to-right shunts of blood. By the end of the fourth week, the right horn is noticeably larger than the left (Figs. 14–4C and 14–9B). As this occurs, the sinoatrial orifice moves to the right and opens in the part of the primitive atrium that will become the adult right atrium (Fig. 14–21B).

The first left-to-right shunt of blood results from transformation of the vitelline and umbilical veins, discussed previously (p. 309). The second left-to-right shunt of blood occurs when the anterior cardinal veins become connected by an oblique anastomosis (Fig. 14–4B and C). This communication shunts blood from the left to the right anterior cardinal vein. The shunt eventually becomes the left *brachiocephalic vein* (Figs. 14–3D and 14–4C). The right anterior cardinal vein and the right common cardinal vein become the superior vena cava.

The results of these two left-to-right venous shunts are: (1) the left horn of the sinus venosus decreases in size and importance; and (2) the right horn enlarges and receives all the blood from the head and neck via the superior vena cava and from the placenta and caudal regions of the body via the inferior vena cava (Figs. 14–4C and 14–43).

The Sinus Venosus and the Right Atrium (Fig. 14–14). Initially the sinus venosus is a separate chamber of the primitive heart and opens into the dorsal wall of the right atrium (Figs. 14–4A and 14–9A and B). As development proceeds, the left horn of the sinus venosus forms the *coronary sinus,* and the right

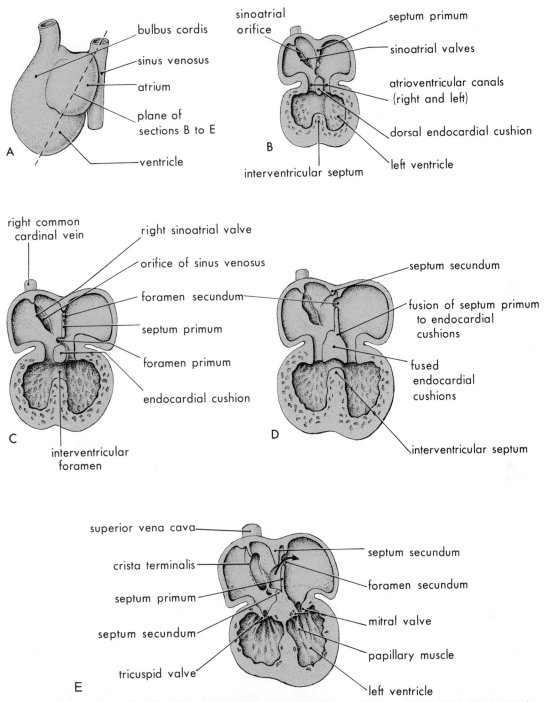

Figure 14-11. Schematic drawings of the developing heart showing partitioning of the atrioventricular canal, primitive atrium, and ventricle. *A*, Sketch showing the plane of the coronal sections. *B*, During the fourth week (about 28 days), showing the early appearance of the septum primum, interventricular septum, and dorsal endocardial cushion. *C*, Section of the heart (about 32 days), showing perforations in the dorsal part of the septum. *D*, Section of the heart (about 35 days), showing the foramen secundum. *E*, About eight weeks, showing the heart after it is partitioned into four chambers.

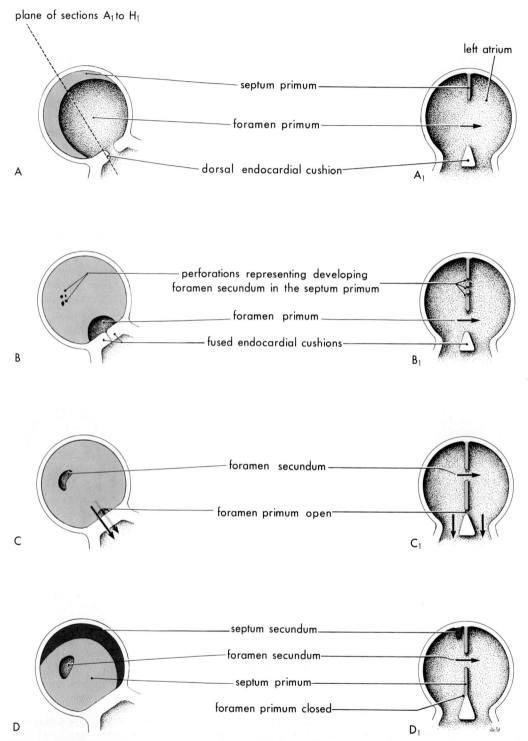

plane of sections A₁ to H₁

septum primum

foramen primum

dorsal endocardial cushion

left atrium

A

A₁

perforations representing developing
foramen secundum in the septum primum

foramen primum

fused endocardial cushions

B

B₁

foramen secundum

foramen primum open

C

C₁

septum secundum

foramen secundum

septum primum

foramen primum closed

D

D₁

Figure 14–12. Diagrammatic sketches illustrating partitioning of the primitive atrium. *A* to *H* are views of the developing interatrial septum as viewed from the right side. *A₁* to *H₁* are coronal sections of the developing interatrial septum at the plane shown in *A*.

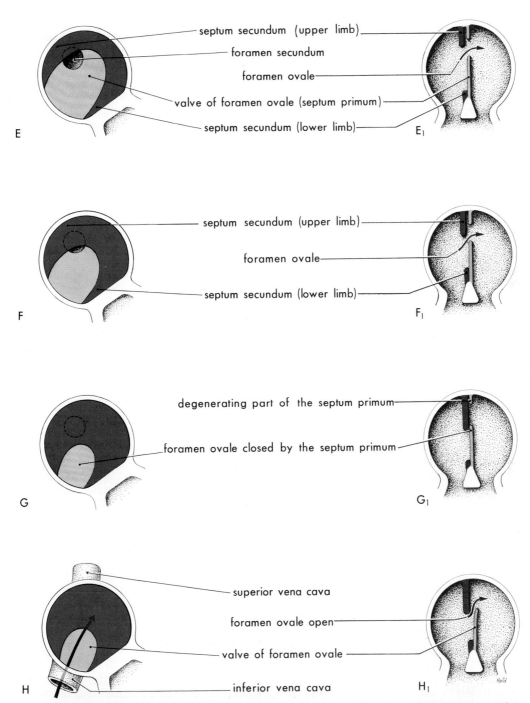

Figure 14–12 (continued). As the septum secundum grows, note that it overlaps the opening in the septum primum (foramen secundum). Observe the valvelike nature of the foramen ovale in G_1 and H_1. When pressure in the right atrium exceeds that in the left atrium, blood passes from the right to the left side of the heart. When the pressures are equal or higher in the left atrium, the septum primum closes the foramen ovale.

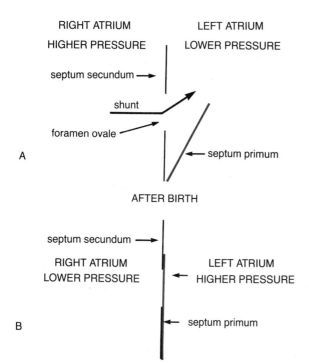

Figure 14–13. Diagrams illustrating the relationship of the septum primum to the foramen ovale and septum secundum. *A,* Before birth blood is shunted from the right atrium through the foramen ovale into the left atrium when the pressure rises. When the pressure falls in the right atrium, the flaplike valve of the foramen ovale formed by the septum primum is pressed against the relatively rigid septum secundum. This closes the foramen ovale. *B,* After birth the pressure in the left atrium rises as the blood returns from the lungs, which are now functioning. Eventually, the septum primum is pressed against the septum secundum and adheres to it. This permanently closes the foramen ovale.

horn becomes incorporated into the wall of the right atrium (Fig. 14–14*B* and *C*).

Because it is derived from the sinus venosus, the smooth part of the wall of the right atrium is called the *sinus venarum* (Fig. 14–14*B* and *C*). The remainder of the internal surface of the wall of the right atrium and the conical muscular pouch called the *auricle* (auricular appendage) have a rough, trabeculated appearance (Moore, 1992). These two parts are derived from the primitive atrium. The smooth part (sinus venarum) and the rough part (primitive atrium) are demarcated internally in the right atrium by a vertical ridge, the *crista terminalis* (Fig. 14–14*C*), and externally by a shallow inconspicuous groove, the *sulcus terminalis* (Fig. 14–14*B*). The crista terminalis represents the cranial part of the right sinoatrial valve (Fig. 14–14*C*); the caudal part of this valve forms the valves of the inferior vena cava and the coronary

sinus. The left sinoatrial valve fuses with the septum secundum and is incorporated with it into the interatrial septum.

The Primitive Pulmonary Vein and the Left Atrium (Fig. 14–15). The wall of the left atrium is smooth and is formed by incorporation of the primitive pulmonary vein. This vein develops as an outgrowth of the dorsal atrial wall, just to the left of the septum primum. As the atrium expands, the primitive pulmonary vein and its main branches are gradually incorporated into the wall of the left atrium; as a result, four pulmonary veins are formed that have separate openings (Fig. 14–15*C* and *D*). The small left auricle (auricular appendage) is derived from the primitive atrium; its internal surface has a rough, trabeculated appearance (Moore, 1992).

Anomalous Pulmonary Venous Connections. In total anomalous pulmonary venous connections, none of the pulmonary veins connects with the left atrium. They open into the right atrium or into one of the systemic veins or into both. In partial anomalous pulmonary venous connections, one or more pulmonary veins have similar anomalous connections; the others have normal connections.

Partitioning of the Primitive Ventricle

Division of the primitive ventricle into right and left ventricles is first indicated by a median muscular ridge in the floor of the ventricle near its apex (Fig. 14–11). This thick, crescentic fold has a concave free edge (Fig. 14–16*A*). Initially, most of its increase in height results from dilation of the ventricles on each side of it (Fig. 14–16*B*). Later, there is active proliferation of myoblasts as the thick muscular part of the interventricular septum forms.

Until the seventh week there is a crescentic **interventricular foramen** between the free edge of the interventricular septum and the fused endocardial cushions. This foramen permits communication between the right and left ventricles (Figs. 14–16 and 14–17). The interventricular foramen usually closes by the end of the seventh week as the bulbar ridges fuse (Fig. 14–18). *Closure of the interventricular foramen* results from the fusion of tissue from three sources: (1) the right bulbar ridge, (2) the left bulbar ridge, and (3) the endocardial cushions.

The *membranous part of the interventricular septum* is derived from an extension of tissue from the right side of the fused endocardial cushions. This tissue merges with the aorticopulmonary septum and the thick muscular part of the interventricular septum (Fig. 14–18*C*). After closure of the interventricular foramen, the pulmonary trunk is in communication with the right ventricle, and the aorta communicates with the left ventricle.

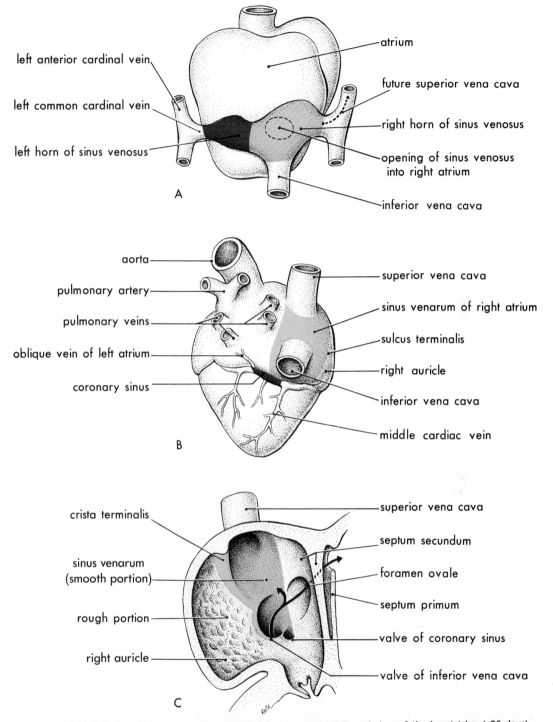

Figure 14-14. Diagrams illustrating the fate of the sinus venosus. *A,* Dorsal view of the heart (about 26 days), showing the sinus venosus. The umbilical and vitelline veins are not shown (see Fig. 14–9*B*). *B,* Dorsal view at eight weeks after incorporation of the right horn of the sinus venosus into the right atrium. The left horn of the sinus venosus has become the coronary sinus. *C,* Internal view of the fetal right atrium showing: (1) the smooth part of the wall of the right atrium (sinus venarum) derived from the right horn of the sinus venosus, and (2) the crista terminalis and the valves of the inferior vena cava and coronary sinus derived from the right sinoatrial valve. The primitive right atrium becomes the right auricle, a conical muscular pouch, which lies against the root of the aorta in the adult.

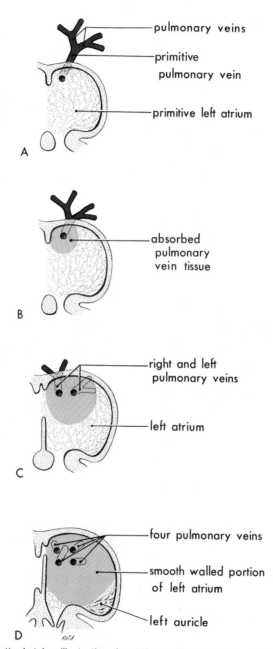

Figure 14-15. Diagrammatic sketches illustrating absorption of the pulmonary veins into the left atrium. *A*, Five weeks, showing the common pulmonary vein opening into the primitive left atrium. *B*, Later stage, showing partial absorption of the common pulmonary vein. *C*, Six weeks, showing the openings of two pulmonary veins into the left atrium resulting from absorption of the common pulmonary vein. *D*, Eight weeks, showing four pulmonary veins with separate atrial orifices. The primitive left atrium becomes the left auricle, a tubular appendage of the left atrium.

Partitioning of the Bulbus Cordis and Truncus Arteriosus

During the fifth week active proliferation of mesenchymal cells in the walls of the bulbus cordis result in the formation of *bulbar ridges* (Fig. 14–19). Similar ridges form in the truncus arteriosus that are continuous with the bulbar ridges. The spiral orientation of the bulbar and *truncal ridges*, possibly caused by the streaming of blood from the ventricles, results in the formation of a spiral *aorticopulmonary septum* when the bulbar and truncal ridges fuse (Fig. 14–19D to G). This septum divides the bulbus cordis and truncus arteriosus into two arterial channels, the aorta and pulmonary trunk. Because of the spiralling of the aorticopulmonary septum, the pulmonary trunk twists around the ascending aorta (Figs. 14–18 and 14–19H).

The results of experimental studies suggest that *neural crest cells* contribute substantially to the development of the aorticopulmonary septum as well as to other parts of the heart (Kirby et al., 1983; Clark, 1986). This is now a major area of interest in cardiac embryology.

The bulbus cordis is incorporated into the walls of the ventricles; and, in the adult right ventricle, it is represented by the *conus arteriosus* (infundibulum) that gives origin to the pulmonary trunk (Moore, 1992). In the left ventricle, the bulbus cordis forms the walls of the *aortic vestibule*, the part of the ventricular cavity just inferior to the aortic valve (Fig. 14–17B).

Development of the Ventricular Walls (Figs. 14–11 and 14–21). Cavitation of the ventricular walls forms a spongework of muscular bundles. Some of these remain as the *trabeculae carneae*, and others become the *papillary muscles* and *chordae tendineae*. These tendinous cords run from the papillary muscles to the atrioventricular valves (Fig. 14–21C and D).

Development of the Cardiac Valves (Figs. 14–20 and 14–21). The *semilunar valves* develop from three *valve swellings* of subendocardial tissue around the orifices of the aorta and pulmonary trunk. These swellings are hollowed out and reshaped to form three, thin-walled cusps. The *atrioventricular valves* (tricuspid and mitral valves) develop similarly from localized proliferations of tissue around the atrioventricular canals.

Development of the Conducting System of the Heart

Initially the muscle layers of the atrium and ventricle are continuous. The primitive atrium acts as the temporary pacemaker of the heart, but the sinus venosus soon takes over this function.

The **sinoatrial node** develops during the fifth week. It is originally in the right wall of the sinus venosus, but it is incorporated into the wall of the right atrium with the sinus venosus (Fig. 14–21D). After incorporation of the sinus venosus, cells from its left wall are found in the base of the interatrial septum just anterior to the opening of the coronary sinus. Together with cells from the atrioventricular region, they make up the **atrioventricular node** and bundle. This specialized tissue is normally the only pathway from the atria to the ventricles because, as the four chambers of the heart develop, a band of connective tissue grows in

Text continues on page 326.

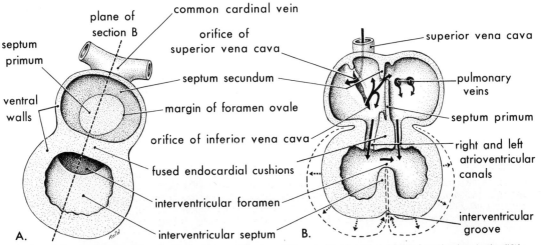

Figure 14–16. Schematic diagrams illustrating partitioning of the primitive heart. *A*, Sagittal section late in the fifth week, showing the cardiac septa and foramina. *B*, Coronal section at a slightly later stage, illustrating the directions of blood flow through the heart and the expansion of the ventricles.

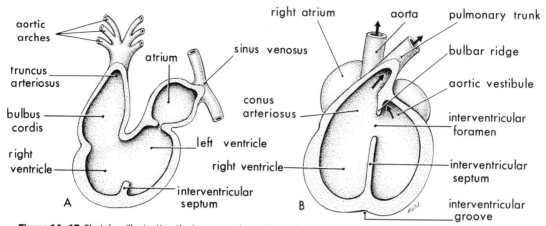

Figure 14-17. Sketches illustrating the incorporation of the bulbus cordis into the ventricles and partitioning of the bulbus cordis and truncus arteriosus into the aorta and pulmonary trunk. *A,* Sagittal section at five weeks, showing the bulbus cordis as one of the five primitive chambers of the heart. *B,* Schematic coronal section at six weeks after the bulbus cordis has been incorporated into the ventricles to become the conus arteriosus (infundibulum) of the right ventricle and the aortic vestibule of the left ventricle.

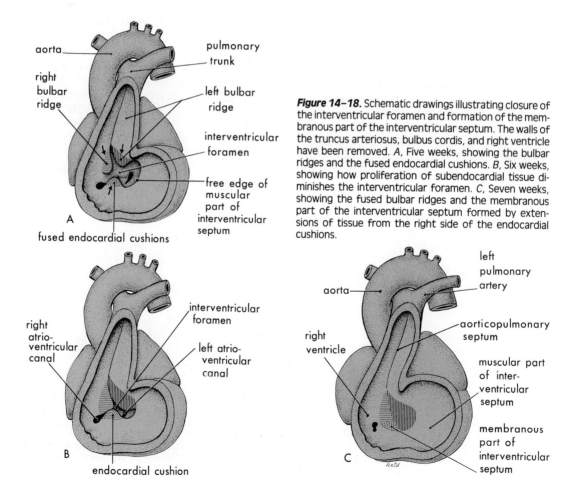

Figure 14-18. Schematic drawings illustrating closure of the interventricular foramen and formation of the membranous part of the interventricular septum. The walls of the truncus arteriosus, bulbus cordis, and right ventricle have been removed. *A,* Five weeks, showing the bulbar ridges and the fused endocardial cushions. *B,* Six weeks, showing how proliferation of subendocardial tissue diminishes the interventricular foramen. *C,* Seven weeks, showing the fused bulbar ridges and the membranous part of the interventricular septum formed by extensions of tissue from the right side of the endocardial cushions.

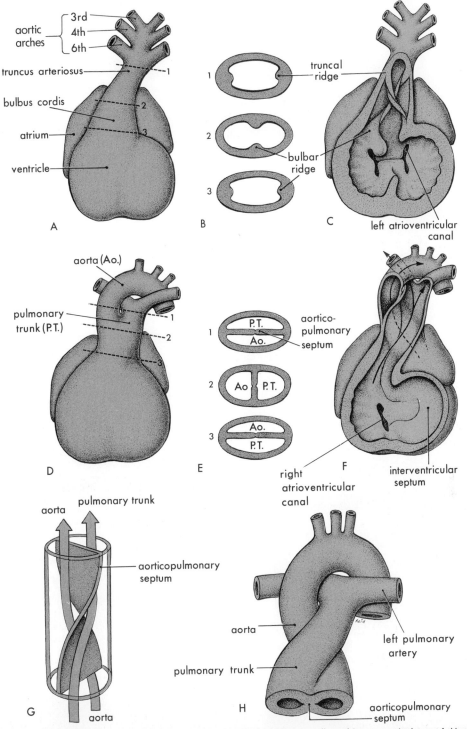

Figure 14-19. Schematic drawings illustrating partitioning of the bulbus cordis and truncus arteriosus. *A*, Ventral aspect of the heart at five weeks. *B*, Transverse sections of the truncus arteriosus and bulbus cordis, illustrating the truncal and bulbar ridges. *C*, The ventral wall of the heart and truncus arteriosus has been removed to demonstrate these ridges. *D*, Ventral aspect of the heart after partitioning of the truncus arteriosus. *E*, Sections through the newly formed aorta (Ao.) and pulmonary trunk (P.T.), showing the aorticopulmonary septum. *F*, Six weeks. The ventral wall of the heart and pulmonary trunk have been removed to show the aorticopulmonary septum. *G*, Diagram illustrating the spiral form of the aorticopulmonary septum. *H*, Drawing showing the great arteries twisting around each other as they leave the heart.

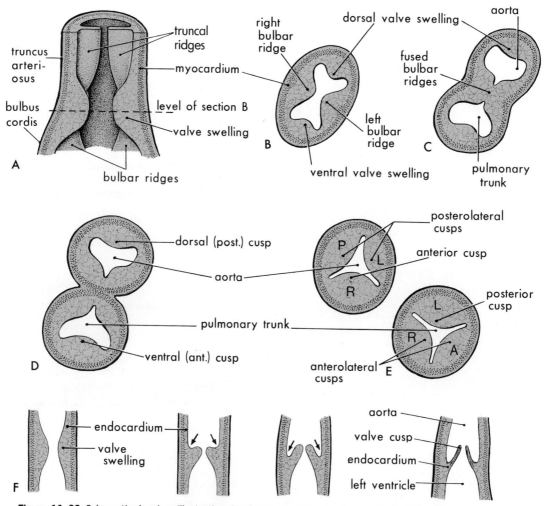

Figure 14–20. Schematic drawings illustrating development of the semilunar valves of the aorta and pulmonary trunk. *A,* Sketch of a sagittal section of the truncus arteriosus and bulbus cordis, showing the valve swellings. *B,* Transverse section of the bulbus cordis. *C,* Similar section after fusion of the bulbar ridges. *D,* Formation of the walls and valves of the aorta and pulmonary trunk. *E,* Rotation of the vessels has established the adult relations of the valves. *F,* Longitudinal sections of the aorticoventricular junction, illustrating successive stages in the hollowing (*arrows*) and thinning of the valve swellings to form the valve cusps.

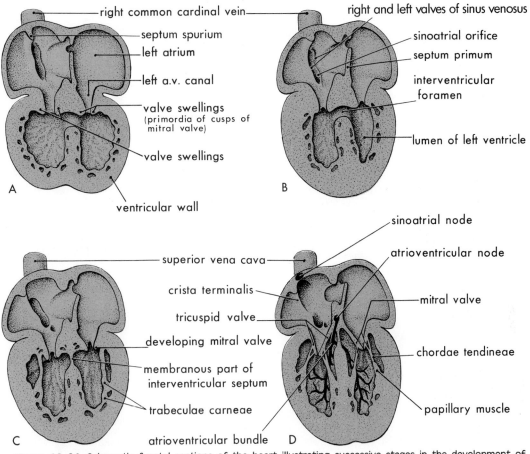

Figure 14-21. Schematic frontal sections of the heart illustrating successive stages in the development of the atrioventricular valves, chordae tendineae, and papillary muscles. *A*, Five weeks. *B*, Six weeks. *C*, Seven weeks. *D*, Twenty weeks, showing the conducting system of the heart.

from the epicardium. This tissue subsequently separates the muscle of the atria from that of the ventricles and forms part of the adult *cardiac skeleton*. The sinoatrial node, atrioventricular node, and atrioventricular bundle soon become richly supplied with nerves.

Abnormalities of the conducting tissue may cause unexpected death during infancy. Anderson and Ashley (1974) observed conducting tissue abnormalities in the hearts of several infants who died unexpectedly from a disorder classified as "crib death" or *sudden infant death syndrome* (SIDS). There remains a lack of consensus that a single mechanism is responsible for the sudden and unexpected deaths of apparently healthy infants. Some findings in infants who later died of SIDS suggest that they have an abnormality in the autonomic nervous system (Behrman, 1992).

CONGENITAL ANOMALIES OF THE HEART AND GREAT VESSELS

Congenital heart defects (CHDs) are common, with a frequency of six to eight cases per 1000 births (Thompson et al., 1991; Behrman, 1992). Some cases of CHD are caused by single-gene or chromosomal mechanisms (Chapter 8), and others are the result of exposure to teratogens, such as the *rubella virus* (p. 165), but, in most cases, the cause is unknown. Most CHDs, however, are thought to be caused by multiple factors, genetic and environmental, each of which has a minor effect, i.e., multifactorial inheritance (p. 168). Recent technology, such as real-time, two-dimensional echocardiography, permits detection of fetal CHDs as early as the seventeenth or eighteenth week of gestation (Schmidt and Silverman, 1988; Veille et al., 1989).

Most heart defects are well tolerated during fetal life. It is only after birth, when the maternal circulation is eliminated, that the impact of the CHDs becomes apparent. Some types of CHD cause very little disability, but others are incompatible with extrauterine life. Due to recent advances in cardiovascular surgery, many types of CHD can be corrected surgically, and fetal cardiac surgery may soon be possible for complex CHD (Verrier et al., 1991).

Not all CHDs are described in this text. Emphasis is placed on those that are compatible with life or are currently amenable to surgery. For a detailed description of congenital heart disease, see Behrman (1992).

Abnormal Positions of the Heart

Dextrocardia. If the heart tube bends to the left instead of to the right (Fig. 14–22), the heart is displaced to the right, and there is transposition in which the heart and its vessels are reversed left to right, as in a mirror image. Dextrocardia is the most frequent positional abnormality of the heart, but it is still relatively uncommon. In *dextrocardia with situs inversus* (transposition of the viscera, e.g., the liver being on

the left side and the heart on the right), the incidence of accompanying cardiac defects is low. If there are no other associated vascular abnormalities, these hearts function normally. In *isolated dextrocardia*, the abnormal position of the heart is not accompanied by displacement of other viscera. This anomaly is usually complicated by severe cardiac anomalies (e.g., single ventricle and arterial transposition). For a discussion of the prognosis and treatment of dextrocardia, see Behrman (1992).

Ectopia Cordis (Fig. 14–23). In this extremely rare condition, the heart is in an abnormal location. In the thoracic form of ectopia cordis, the heart is partly or completely exposed on the surface of the thorax. It is usually associated with widely separated halves of the sternum and an open pericardial sac. Death occurs in most cases during the first few days after birth, usually from infection, cardiac failure, or hypoxemia (Behrman, 1992). If there are not severe cardiac defects, surgical therapy consists of covering the heart with skin. In some cases of ectopia cordis the heart protrudes through the diaphragm into the abdomen. Occasional patients with this type of ectopia have survived to adulthood.

The most common thoracic form of ectopia cordis is the result of faulty development of the sternum and pericardium due to failure of complete fusion of the lateral folds in the thoracic region during the fourth week (p. 71).

Atrial Septal Defects (ASDs)

ASD is a common congenital heart anomaly. It occurs more frequently in females than in males. The most com-

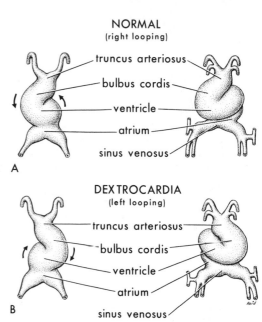

NORMAL
(right looping)

truncus arteriosus
bulbus cordis
ventricle
atrium
sinus venosus

A

DEXTROCARDIA
(left looping)

truncus arteriosus
bulbus cordis
ventricle
atrium
sinus venosus

B

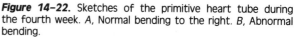

Figure 14–22. Sketches of the primitive heart tube during the fourth week. *A*, Normal bending to the right. *B*, Abnormal bending.

mon form of ASD is *patent foramen ovale* (Figs. 14–24 to 14–27). An isolated patent foramen ovale is of no hemodynamic significance; however, if there are other defects (e.g., pulmonary stenosis or atresia [p. 334]), blood is shunted through the foramen ovale into the left atrium and produces *cyanosis,* a dark, bluish or purplish coloration of the skin and mucous membranes due to deficient oxygenation of the blood.

Probe Patent Foramen Ovale (Fig. 14–24*B*). In up to 25 per cent of people, a probe can be passed from one atrium to the other through the superior part of the floor of the fossa ovalis. This defect, usually small, is not considered to be clinically significant, but a probe patent foramen ovale may be forced open as a result of other cardiac defects and contribute to the functional pathology of the heart. Probe patent foramen ovale is the result of incomplete adhesion between the original flap of the valve of the foramen ovale and the septum secundum after birth (Fig. 14–13).

Clinically Significant Types of ASD (Figs. 14–25 and 14–26). There are four main types of ASD: (1) secundum ASDs, (2) endocardial cushion defects with primum ASDs, (3) sinus venosus ASD, and (4) common atrium. The first two types are relatively common.

Secundum ASDs (Figs. 14–25*A* to *D* and 14–26). These defects are in the area of the fossa ovalis (Fig. 14–24*A)* and include both defects of the septum primum and septum secundum. The defects may be multiple; and, in symptomatic older children, defects of 2 cm or more in diameter are not unusual (Behrman, 1992). Females with these defects outnumber males three to one.

Secundum ASDs are one of the most common types of congenital heart defect. The patent foramen ovale usually results from abnormal resorption of the septum primum

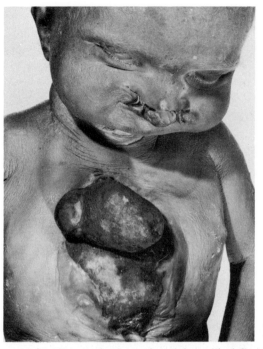

Figure 14–23. Photograph of a newborn infant with cleft sternum, ectopia cordis, and bilateral cleft lip. Death occurred in the first days of life from infection, cardiac failure, and hypoxemia.

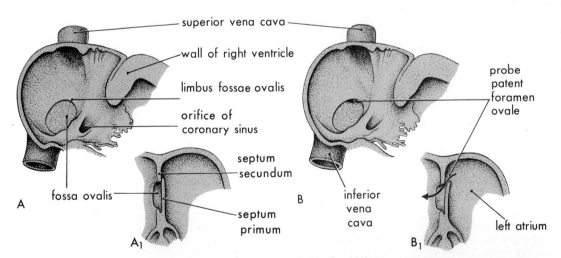

Figure 14–24. *A,* Drawing illustrating the normal appearance of the right side of the interatrial septum after adhesion of the septum primum to the septum secundum. *A₁,* Sketch of a frontal section of the interatrial septum, illustrating formation of the fossa ovalis in the right atrium. Note that the floor of this fossa is formed by the septum primum. *B* and *B₁,* Similar views of a probe patent foramen ovale resulting from incomplete adhesion of the septum primum to the septum secundum.

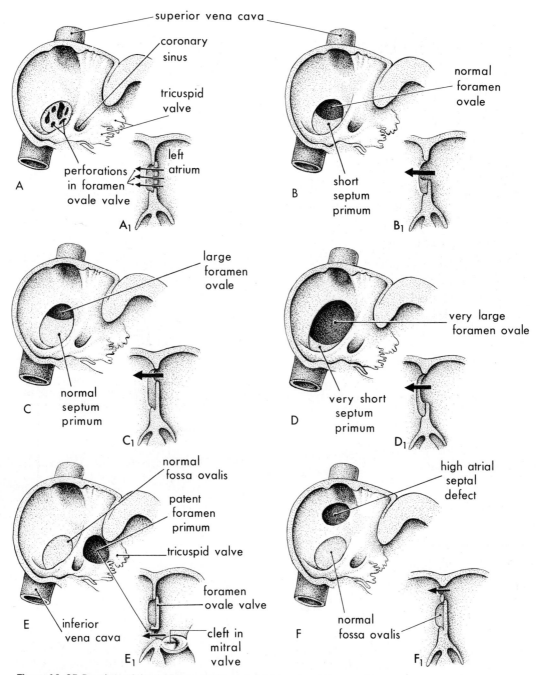

Figure 14–25. Drawings of the right aspect of the interatrial septum (*A* to *F*) and sketches of coronal sections of the septum (*A₁* to *F₁*), illustrating various types of atrial septal defect (ASD). *A*, Patent foramen ovale resulting from resorption of the septum primum in abnormal locations. *B*, Patent foramen ovale caused by excessive resorption of the septum primum, sometimes called a "short flap defect." *C*, Patent foramen ovale resulting from an abnormally large foramen ovale. *D*, Patent foramen ovale resulting from an abnormally large foramen ovale and excessive resorption of the septum primum. *E*, Endocardial cushion defect with primum-type atrial septal defect. The section *E₁* also shows the cleft in the anterior cusp of the mitral valve. *F*, Sinus venosus ASD. The high septal defect resulted from abnormal absorption of the sinus venosus into the right atrium. Note that in *E* and *F*, the fossa ovalis has formed normally.

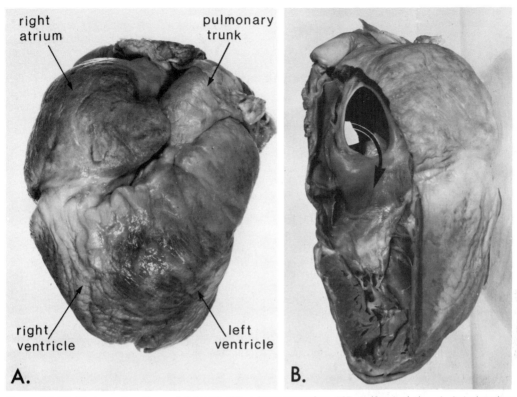

Figure 14-26. Photographs of an adult heart with a large secundum ASD. Half actual size. *A*, Anterior view (sternocostal aspect of the heart), showing the large right ventricle, right atrium, and pulmonary trunk. *B*, Right atrial aspect, showing the large ASD (*arrow*) resulting from an abnormally large foramen ovale and excessive resorption of the septum primum (see Fig. 14-25 *D*).

during the formation of the foramen secundum (Fig. 14-12*B*). If resorption occurs in abnormal locations, the septum primum is fenestrated or netlike (Fig. 14-25*A*). If excessive resorption of the septum primum occurs, the resulting short septum primum will not close the foramen ovale (Fig. 14-25*B*).

If an abnormally large foramen ovale occurs due to defective development of the septum secundum, a normal septum primum will not close the abnormal foramen ovale at birth (Fig. 14-25*C*). Large secundum ASDs may occur due to a combination of excessive resorption of the septum primum and a large foramen ovale (Figs. 14-25*D* and 14-26*B*). Secundum ASDs are well tolerated during childhood; symptoms (e.g., pulmonary hypertension) usually appear in the 30s or later. Closure of the ASD is carried out at open heart surgery, and the mortality rate is less than one per cent (Behrman, 1992).

Endocardial Cushion and AV Septal Defects with Primum ASDs (Fig. 14-25*E*). The incomplete form of endocardial cushion defect is relatively common. Several cardiac abnormalities are grouped together under this heading because they are the result of the same developmental defect, a deficiency of the endocardial cushions and the atrioventricular septum. The septum primum does not fuse with the endocardial cushions (Fig. 14-12*D*); as a result, there is a

patent foramen primum (Fig. 14-25*E*). Usually, there is also a cleft in the anterior cusp of the mitral valve.

In the less common complete form of endocardial cushion and AV septal defects, fusion of the endocardial cushions fails to occur. As a result, there is a large defect in the center of the heart known as atrioventricular (AV) canal or AV septal defect (Figs. 14-27 and 14-28). This type of ASD occurs in about 20 per cent of persons with Down syndrome; otherwise, it is a relatively uncommon cardiac defect. It consists of a continuous interatrial and interventricular defect with markedly abnormal atrioventricular valves (Behrman, 1992). This severe cardiac defect can be detected during an evaluation of the fetal heart by ultrasound (Fig. 14-28; Schmidt and Silverman, 1991).

Sinus Venosus ASD (Fig. 14-25*F*). All sinus venosus defects are located in the superior part of the interatrial septum close to the entry of the superior vena cava. Sinus venosus ASD is one of the rarest types of defect. It results from incomplete absorption of the sinus venosus into the right atrium and/or abnormal development of the septum secundum. This type of ASD is commonly associated with partial anomalous pulmonary venous connections.

Common Atrium. In this rare condition the interatrial septum is absent. This situation is the result of failure of the septum primum and septum secundum to develop.

Ventricular Septal Defects (VSDs)

VSD is the most common type of cardiac defect and accounts for about 25 per cent of congenital heart disease (Behrman, 1992). VSD occurs more frequently in males than in females (Fink, 1985). Most defects involve the membranous part of the interventricular septum. Many small VSDs (30 to 50 per cent) close spontaneously, most frequently during the first year. Isolated VSDs are detected at a rate of 10 to 12 per 10,000 between birth and five years. Most patients with a large VSD have a massive left-to-right shunt of blood. For a discussion of the complications of VSDs, see Behrman (1992).

Membranous VSD (Fig. 14–27*B*). This is the most common type of VSD. Incomplete closure of the interventricular foramen is the result of failure of the membranous part of the interventricular septum to develop. It arises from failure of extensions of subendocardial tissue to grow from the right side of the fused endocardial cushions and fuse with the aorticopulmonary septum and the muscular part of the interventricular septum (Fig. 14–18*C*).

Muscular VSD. The perforation(s) in this less common type of VSD may appear anywhere in the muscular part of the interventricular septum. Sometimes there are multiple defects, the so-called *Swiss-cheese VSD*. Muscular VSDs probably occur because of excessive cavitation of myocardial tissue during formation of the ventricular walls and the muscular part of the interventricular septum (p. 321).

Absence of the Interventricular Septum (Common Ventricle). Failure of the septum to form is extremely rare and results in a three-chambered heart, cor triloculare biatriatum. With a single ventricle, both atria empty through a common valve or two separate atrioventricular valves into a single ventricular chamber. The aorta and pulmonary trunk arise from this single ventricle. *Transposition of the great arteries* (Fig. 14-30) and an abnormal outlet chamber are present in most infants. Some patients die during infancy from congestive heart failure, but others survive until early adult life. For discussion of the treatment of this defect, see Behrman (1992).

Abnormal Division of the Truncus Arteriosus (TA)

Truncus Arteriosus (Fig. 14–29). Persistence of the TA is the result of failure of the truncal ridges and aorticopulmonary septum to develop normally and divide the truncus arteriosus into the aorta and pulmonary trunk. The most common type of TA is a single arterial vessel that gives rise to the pulmonary trunk and ascending aorta (Fig. 14–29*A* and *B*). In the next most common type, the right and left pulmonary arteries arise close together from the dorsal wall of the TA (Fig. 14–29*C*). Less common types are illustrated in Figure 14–29*D* and *E*.

Aorticopulmonary Septal Defect. In this rare condition there is an opening (*aortic window*) between the aorta and pulmonary trunk near the aortic valve. This defect is the result of a localized defect in the formation of the aorticopulmonary septum (Fig. 14–19).

Transposition of the Great Arteries (Fig. 14–30). Transposition of the great arteries (TGA) is the most common cause of *cyanotic heart disease* in newborn infants. TGA is

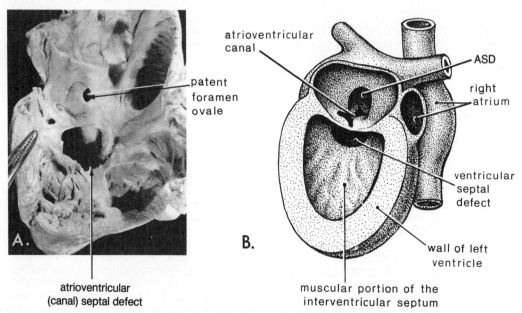

Figure 14–27. *A,* Photograph of an infant's heart, sectioned and viewed from the right side, showing a patent foramen ovale and an atrioventricular (canal) septal defect. (From Lev M: *Autopsy Diagnosis of Congenitally Malformed Hearts.* 1953. Courtesy of Charles C Thomas, Springfield, Ill.) *B,* Schematic drawing of a heart illustrating various septal defects.

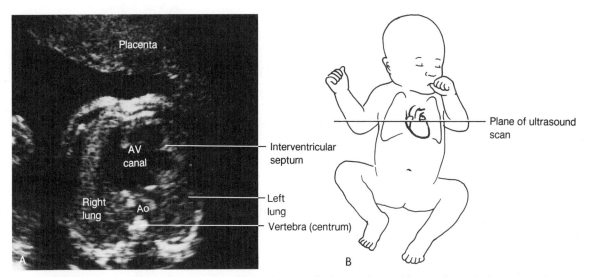

Figure 14–28. *A,* Ultrasound image of the heart of a second trimester fetus with an atrioventricular (AV) canal (atrioventricular septal) defect. An ASD and VSD are also present. (Courtesy of Dr. B. Benacerraf, Diagnostic Ultrasound Associates, P.C., Boston, MA.). *B,* Orientation drawing.

often associated with other cardiac anomalies. In typical cases the aorta lies anterior to the pulmonary trunk and arises anteriorly from the morphological right ventricle, and the pulmonary trunk arises from the morphological left ventricle. There is also an *atrial septal defect* (with or without an associated *patent ductus arteriosus* [p. 346] or VSD) that permits some interchange between the pulmonary and systemic circulations. Because of these anatomical abnormalities, deoxygenated systemic venous blood returning to the right atrium enters the right ventricle and then passes to the body via the aorta. Oxygenated pulmonary venous blood passes via the left ventricle back into the pulmonary circulation. Because of the patent foramen ovale, there is some mixing of the blood; but, without surgical correction of the transposition, the baby will die within a few months.

Many attempts have been made to explain the embryological basis of TGA, but the *conal growth hypothesis* is favored by many investigators. According to this explanation, the aorticopulmonary septum fails to pursue a spiral course during partitioning of the bulbus cordis and truncus arteriosus. This defect is thought to be the result of failure of the conus arteriosus to develop normally during incorporation of the bulbus cordis into the ventricles (p. 319).

Unequal Division of the Truncus Arteriosus (Figs. 14–31*B* and *C* and 14–32*A*). If partitioning of the truncus arteriosus superior to the valves is unequal, one great artery is large and the other small. As a result, the aorticopulmonary septum is not aligned with the interventricular septum and a ventricular septal defect results. The larger vessel (aorta or pulmonary trunk) usually straddles (overrides) the ventricular septal defect.

Pulmonary Stenosis (Figs. 14–31 and 14–32). In *pulmonary valve stenosis*, the cusps of the pulmonary valve are fused together to form a dome with a narrow central open-

ing (Fig. 14–31*D*). In *infundibular pulmonary stenosis*, the conus arteriosus (infundibulum) of the right ventricle is underdeveloped. The two types of pulmonary stenosis may occur together. Depending upon the degree of obstruction to blood flow, there is a variable degree of hypertrophy of the right ventricle.

Tetralogy of Fallot (Figs. 14–32*B* and 14–33). This classic and common group of four cardiac defects consists of: (1) pulmonary stenosis, (2) ventricular septal defect (VSD), (3) overriding aorta, and (4) hypertrophy of the right ventricle. *Cyanosis* (p. 327) is one of the obvious signs of tetralogy, but it may not be present at birth (Behrman, 1992).

Pulmonary Atresia. If the division of the truncus arteriosus is so unequal that the pulmonary trunk has no lumen or there is no orifice at the level of the pulmonary valve, the anomaly is called pulmonary atresia. There may or may not be an associated VSD.

Aortic Stenosis and Atresia (Fig. 14–31*D*). In *aortic valve stenosis*, the edges of the valve are usually fused together to form a dome with a narrow opening. This condition may be present at birth (congenital) or may develop after birth (acquired). The *valvular stenosis* causes extra work for the heart and results in hypertrophy of the left ventricle and abnormal heart sounds (heart murmurs). In *subaortic stenosis* there is often a band of fibrous tissue just inferior to the aortic valve. The narrowing of the aorta results from persistence of tissue that normally degenerates as the valve forms. When obstruction of the aorta or its valve is complete, the condition is called *aortic atresia.*

Hypoplastic Left Heart Syndrome (Fig. 14–34). The left ventricle is small and nonfunctional; the right ventricle maintains both pulmonary and systemic circulations (Behrman, 1992). The blood passes through an ASD or a dilated foramen ovale from the left to the right side of the

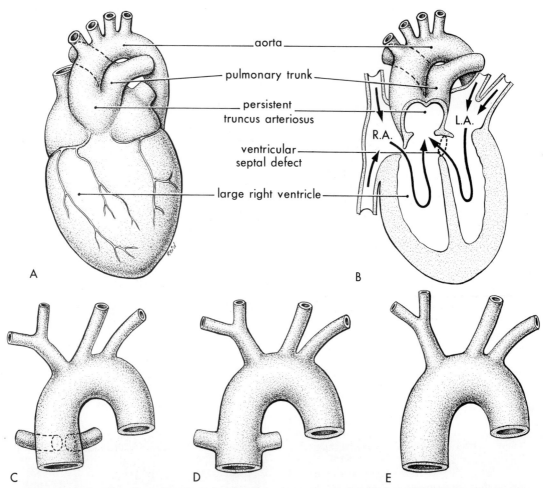

aorta

pulmonary trunk

persistent
truncus arteriosus

ventricular
septal defect

large right ventricle

A

B

R.A.

L.A.

C

D

E

Figure 14-29. Drawings illustrating the main types of persistent truncus arteriosus. *A,* The common trunk divides into an aorta and short pulmonary trunk. *B,* Coronal section of the heart shown in *A.* Observe the circulation in this heart and the VSD. *C,* The right and left pulmonary arteries arise close together from the truncus arteriosus. *D,* The pulmonary arteries arise independently from the sides of the truncus arteriosus. *E,* No pulmonary arteries are present. In such cases the lungs are supplied by the bronchial arteries.

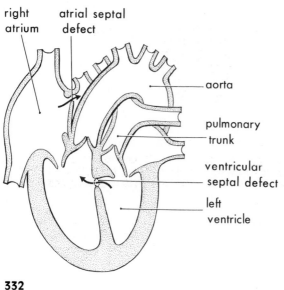

right
atrium

atrial septal
defect

aorta

pulmonary
trunk

ventricular
septal defect

left
ventricle

Figure 14-30. Diagram of a malformed heart illustrating transposition of the great arteries (TGA), also known as transposition of the great vessels. The ventricular and atrial septal defects allow mixing of the arterial and venous blood. TGA is the most common single cause of cyanotic heart disease in newborn infants. As here, it is often associated with other cardiac malformations (VSD and ASD).

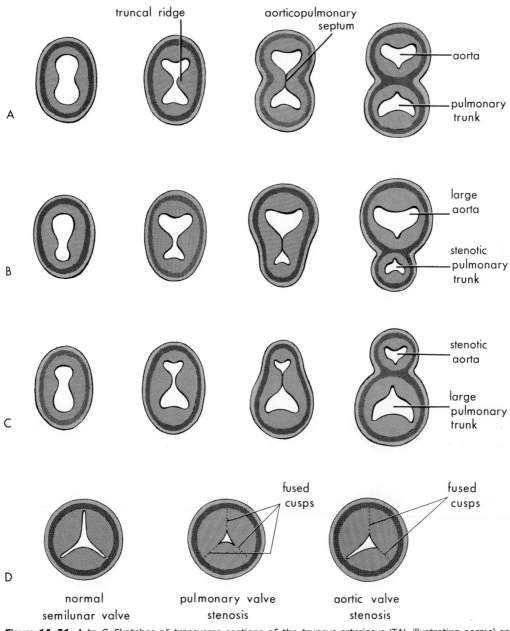

Figure 14–31. *A* to *C*, Sketches of transverse sections of the truncus arteriosus (TA), illustrating normal and abnormal partitioning of the TA. *A*, Normal. *B*, Unequal partitioning resulting in a small pulmonary trunk. *C*, Unequal partitioning resulting in a small aorta. *D*, Sketches illustrating a normal semilunar valve and stenotic pulmonary and aortic valves.

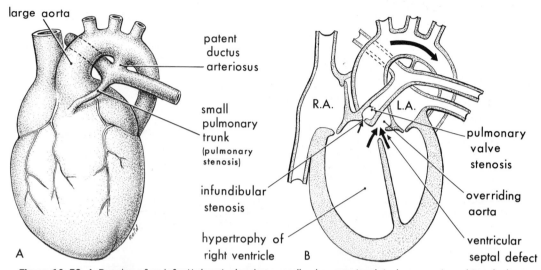

Figure 14-32. *A*, Drawing of an infant's heart, showing a small pulmonary trunk (pulmonary stenosis) and a large aorta resulting from unequal partitioning of the truncus arteriosus (see Fig. 14-32*B*). There is also hypertrophy of the right ventricle and a patent ductus arteriosus. *B*, Frontal section of a heart illustrating tetralogy of Fallot. Observe the four cardiac deformities: pulmonary valve stenosis, VSD, overriding aorta, and hypertrophy of the right ventricle. In this case, there is also infundibular stenosis, which is not considered to be part of the classical tetralogy of Fallot. Note that the large aorta overrides (straddles) the VSD.

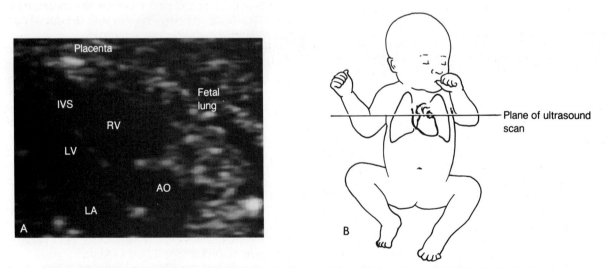

Figure 14-33. *A*, Ultrasound image of the heart of a 20-week fetus with tetralogy of Fallot. Note that the large overriding aorta (AO) straddles the interventricular septum. As a result, it receives blood from the left (LV) and right (RV) ventricles. (Courtesy of Dr. B. Benacerraf, Diagnostic Ultrasound Associates, P.C., Boston, MA.) *B*, Orientation drawing.

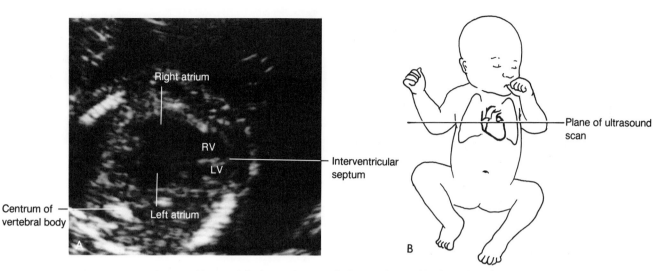

Figure 14–34. *A*, Ultrasound image of the heart of a second trimester fetus with a hypoplastic left heart. Note that the left ventricle (LV) is much smaller than the right ventricle (RV). This is an oblique scan of the fetal thorax through the long axis of the ventricles. (Courtesy of Dr. B. Benacerraf, Diagnostic Ultrasound Associates, P.C., Boston, MA.) *B*, Orientation drawing.

heart where it mixes with the systemic venous blood. In addition to the underdevelopment of the left side of the heart, there is atresia of the aortic or mitral orifice and hypoplasia of the ascending aorta. Infants with this severe anomaly usually die during the first few weeks after birth.

Disturbances in the migration of neural crest cells, in hemodynamic function, in cell death, and in the proliferation of the extracellular matrix are likely responsible for the pathogenesis of many CHDs (Clark, 1986).

DERIVATIVES OF THE AORTIC ARCHES

As the branchial or pharyngeal arches develop during the fourth week (see Figs. 10–1 and 10–2), they receive arteries from the aortic sac called *aortic arches* (Figs. 14-9, 14–35, and 14–36). The aortic arches terminate in the dorsal aorta of the corresponding side. Although six pairs of aortic arches may develop, they are not all present at the same time. By the time the sixth pair of aortic arches has formed, the first two pairs have disappeared (Fig. 14–35*C*). During the sixth to eighth weeks the primitive aortic arch pattern is transformed into the adult arterial arrangement (Fig. 14–36).

Derivatives of the First Pair of Aortic Arches. These vessels largely disappear, but the remaining parts form the maxillary arteries. These aortic arches may also contribute to the development of the external carotid arteries.

Derivatives of the Second Pair of Aortic Arches. Dorsal portions of these vessels persist and form the stems of the stapedial arteries.

Derivatives of the Third Pair of Aortic Arches. The proximal parts of these arteries form the *common carotid arteries*; distal portions join with the dorsal aortae to form the *internal carotid arteries*.

Derivatives of the Fourth Pair of Aortic Arches. The *left fourth aortic arch* forms part of the arch of the aorta. The proximal part of the arch of the aorta develops from the aortic sac, and the distal part is derived from the left dorsal aorta (Fig. 14–36*D*). The *right fourth aortic arch* becomes the proximal part of the *right subclavian artery*. The distal part of the subclavian artery forms from the right dorsal aorta and the right seventh intersegmental artery. The left subclavian artery is not derived from an aortic arch; it forms from the left seventh intersegmental artery (Fig. 14–36*A*). As development proceeds, differential growth shifts the origin of the left subclavian artery cranially so it comes to lie close to the origin of the left common carotid artery (Fig. 14–33*D*).

Derivatives of the Fifth Pair of Aortic Arches. In about 50 per cent of embryos, the fifth pair of aortic arches are rudimentary vessels that soon degenerate, leaving no derivatives. In about as many embryos, these arteries never develop.

Derivatives of the Sixth Pair of Aortic Arches. The *left sixth aortic arch* develops as follows: (1) the

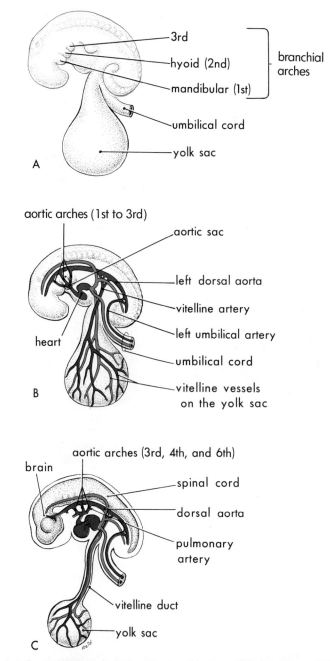

Figure 14–35. Drawings illustrating the branchial or pharyngeal arches and their arteries, called aortic arches. *A*, Left side of an embryo (about 26 days). *B*, Schematic drawing of this embryo, showing the left aortic arches arising from the aortic sac, running through the branchial arches, and terminating in the left dorsal aorta. *C*, An embryo (about 37 days), showing the single dorsal aorta and that most of the first two pairs of aortic arches have degenerated.

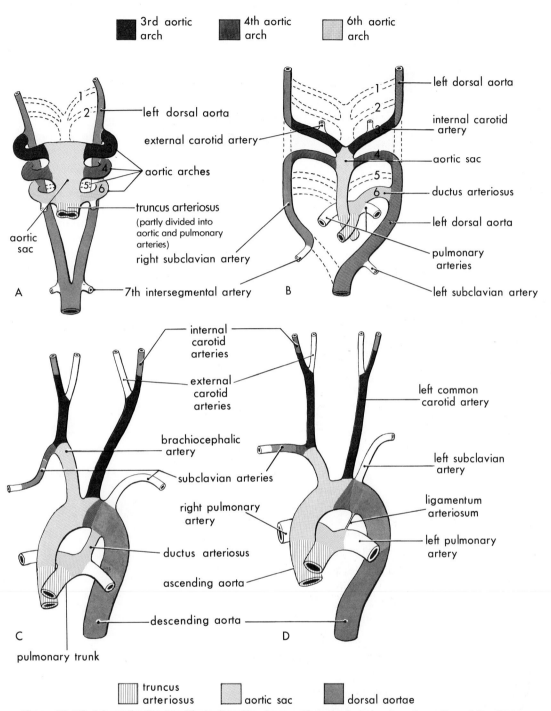

3rd aortic arch
4th aortic arch
6th aortic arch

A

left dorsal aorta

external carotid artery

aortic arches

truncus arteriosus
(partly divided into aortic and pulmonary arteries)

right subclavian artery

7th intersegmental artery

aortic sac

B

left dorsal aorta

internal carotid artery

aortic sac

ductus arteriosus

left dorsal aorta

pulmonary arteries

left subclavian artery

C

internal carotid arteries

external carotid arteries

brachiocephalic artery

subclavian arteries

right pulmonary artery

ductus arteriosus

ascending aorta

descending aorta

pulmonary trunk

D

left common carotid artery

left subclavian artery

ligamentum arteriosum

left pulmonary artery

truncus arteriosus
aortic sac
dorsal aortae

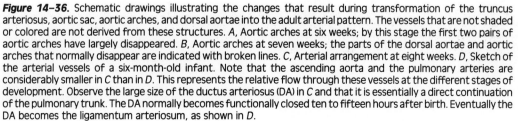

Figure 14–36. Schematic drawings illustrating the changes that result during transformation of the truncus arteriosus, aortic sac, aortic arches, and dorsal aortae into the adult arterial pattern. The vessels that are not shaded or colored are not derived from these structures. *A,* Aortic arches at six weeks; by this stage the first two pairs of aortic arches have largely disappeared. *B,* Aortic arches at seven weeks; the parts of the dorsal aortae and aortic arches that normally disappear are indicated with broken lines. *C,* Arterial arrangement at eight weeks. *D,* Sketch of the arterial vessels of a six-month-old infant. Note that the ascending aorta and the pulmonary arteries are considerably smaller in *C* than in *D.* This represents the relative flow through these vessels at the different stages of development. Observe the large size of the ductus arteriosus (DA) in *C* and that it is essentially a direct continuation of the pulmonary trunk. The DA normally becomes functionally closed ten to fifteen hours after birth. Eventually the DA becomes the ligamentum arteriosum, as shown in *D.*

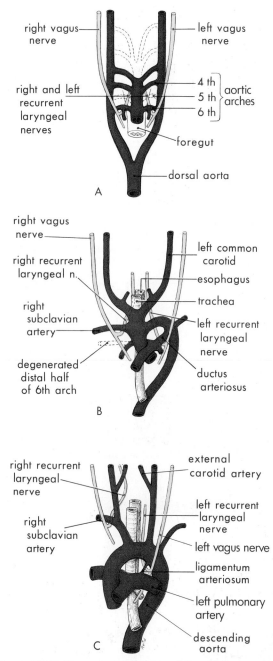

Figure 14–37. Diagrams showing the relation of the recurrent laryngeal nerves to the aortic arches and their derivatives. A, Six weeks, showing the recurrent laryngeal nerves hooked around the sixth pair of aortic arches. B, Eight weeks, showing the right recurrent laryngeal nerve hooked around the right subclavian artery and the left recurrent laryngeal nerve hooked around the ductus arteriosus and the arch of the aorta. C, Adult, showing the left recurrent laryngeal nerve hooked around the ligamentum arteriosum and the arch of the aorta.

proximal part persists as the proximal part of the left pulmonary artery, and (2) the distal part, which passes from the left pulmonary artery to the dorsal aorta, persists as a shunt called the *ductus arteriosus* (Figs. 14–36C and 14–37B). The **right sixth aortic arch** develops as follows: (1) the proximal part persists as the proximal part of the right pulmonary artery, and (2) the distal part degenerates.

The Course of the Recurrent Laryngeal Nerves (Fig. 14–37). The transformation of the sixth pair of aortic arches explains why the course of the recurrent laryngeal nerves differs on the two sides. The recurrent laryngeal nerves supply the sixth pair of branchial arches and hook around the sixth pair of aortic arches on their way to the developing larynx.

On the right, because the distal part of the right sixth aortic arch and the fifth aortic arch degenerate, the right recurrent laryngeal nerve moves superiorly and hooks around the proximal part of the right subclavian artery (the derivative of the fourth aortic arch).

On the left, the left recurrent laryngeal nerve hooks around the ductus arteriosus (the persistent distal portion of the sixth aortic arch). When this vessel obliterates after birth, the nerve hooks around its ligamentous derivative, the ligamentum arteriosum, and the arch of the aorta.

Anomalies of the Aortic Arches

Because of the many changes involved in transformation of the embryonic aortic arch system into the adult arterial pattern, it is understandable that variations may occur. Most anomalies result from the persistence of parts of aortic arches that normally disappear or from disappearance of parts that normally persist.

Coarctation of the Aorta (Fig. 14–38). This malformation is characterized by constrictions of varying lengths of the aorta. Most of them (98 per cent) occur just distal to the origin of the left subclavian artery near the insertion of the ductus arteriosus. The classification into preductal and postductal coarctations is commonly used; but, in a significant number of instances, the coarctation is directly opposite the ductus arteriosus. Coarctation of the aorta occurs twice as often in males as in females (Behrman, 1992).

Postductal Coarctation (Fig. 14–38A and B). In this common type the constriction is just inferior to the ductus arteriosus. This location allows for development of a collateral circulation during the fetal period, thus assisting with passage of blood to inferior parts of the body.

Preductal Coarctation (Fig. 14–38C and D). In this less common type the constriction is just superior to the ductus arteriosus. If the ductus arteriosus is patent, there is a communication between the pulmonary artery and the aorta and more blood flow to the lower body. The narrowed segment may be extensive (Fig. 14–38D).

Causes of Coarctation of the Aorta. The causes of coarctation are not clearly understood. This abnormality is a common finding in cases of Turner syndrome (p. 146), a

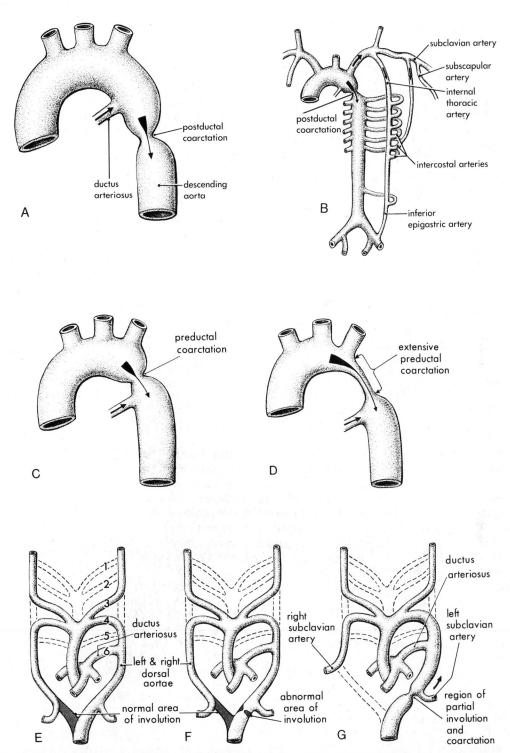

Figure 14–38. *A,* Postductal coarctation of the aorta; 98 per cent occur just distal to the origin of the left subclavian artery and ductus arteriosus. *B,* Diagrammatic representation of the common routes of collateral circulation that develop in association with postductal coarctation of the aorta. *C* and *D,* Preductal coarctation. The type (illustrated in *D*) is usually associated with major cardiac defects. *E,* Sketch of the aortic arch pattern in a seven-week embryo showing the areas that normally involute. Note that the distal segment of the right dorsal aorta normally involutes as the right subclavian artery develops. *F,* Abnormal involution of a small distal segment of the left dorsal aorta. *G,* Later stage, showing the abnormally involuted segment appearing as a coarctation of the aorta. This moves (follow arrow) to the region of the ductus arteriosus with the left subclavian artery, as illustrated in *B.* These drawings (*E to G*) illustrate one hypothesis about the embryological basis of coarctation of the aorta.

condition caused by the loss of a sex chromosome. This and other observations suggest that genetic and/or environmental factors cause coarctation. The embryological basis of coarctation of the aorta is also unclear. There are three main views:

1. During formation of the arch of the aorta, muscle tissue of the ductus arteriosus may be incorporated into the wall of the aorta; then, when the ductus arteriosus contracts at birth, the ductal muscle in the aorta also contracts, forming a coarctation.

2. There may be abnormal involution of a small segment of the left dorsal aorta (Fig. 14–38F). Later this stenotic segment (area of coarctation) moves cranially with the left subclavian artery to the region of the ductus arteriosus (Fig. 14–38G).

3. During fetal life the segment of the arch of the aorta between the left subclavian artery and the ductus arteriosus is normally narrow (Fig. 14–36C) because it carries little blood. Following normal closure of the ductus arteriosus, this region called the *isthmus* normally enlarges until it is the same diameter as the aorta (Fig. 14–33D). If the narrow region persists, a coarctation forms.

Anomalies of the Arch of the Aorta

Double Aortic Arch (Fig. 14–39). This rare abnormality is characterized by a *vascular ring* around the trachea and esophagus. Varying degrees of compression of these structures occur. The ring occurs due to failure of the distal portion of the right dorsal aorta to disappear; as a result,

right and left arches arise from the ascending aorta. Usually the right arch of the aorta is larger and passes posterior to the trachea and esophagus.

Right Arch of the Aorta (Fig. 14–40). When the entire right dorsal aorta persists and the distal segment of the left dorsal aorta involutes, a right aortic arch results. There are two main types:

Right Arch of the Aorta Without a Retroesophageal Component (Fig. 14–40 B). The ductus arteriosus (or ligamentum arteriosum) passes from the right pulmonary artery to the right arch of the aorta. Because no vascular ring is formed, this condition is usually asymptomatic.

Right Arch of the Aorta With a Retroesophageal Component (Fig. 14–40C). Originally there was probably a small left arch of the aorta (Fig. 14–39B) which then disappeared, leaving the right arch of the aorta posterior to the esophagus. The normal left ductus arteriosus (or ligamentum arteriosum) attaches to the descending aorta and forms a *vascular ring*, which may constrict the esophagus and trachea, as in Figure 14–39C. If there is tracheal compression, a surgical procedure is usually performed for release of the compression.

Abnormal Origin of the Right Subclavian Artery (Fig. 14–41). The right subclavian artery arises from the descending aorta and passes posterior to the trachea and esophagus to supply the right upper limb (*retroesophageal subclavian artery*). This abnormal origin of the right subclavian artery occurs when the right fourth aortic arch and the right dorsal aorta disappear cranial to the seventh intersegmental artery. As a result, the right subclavian artery forms from the right seventh intersegmental artery and the distal

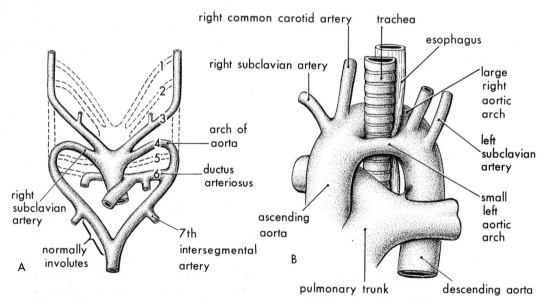

Figure 14–39. *A,* Drawing of the embryonic aortic arches illustrating the embryological basis of double aortic arch. The distal portion of the right dorsal aorta persists and forms a right aortic arch. *B,* A large right aortic arch and a small left aortic arch arise from the ascending aorta and form a vascular ring around the trachea and esophagus. Note that there is compression of the esophagus. The right common carotid and subclavian arteries arise separately from the large right arch.

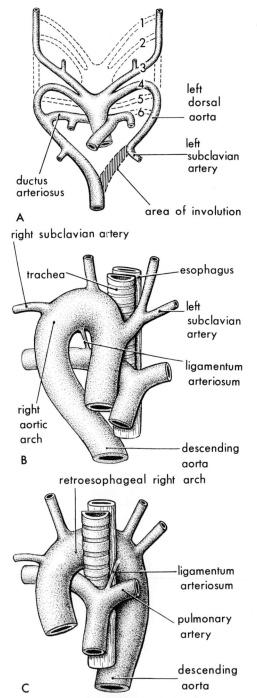

Figure 14–40. *A,* Sketch of the aortic arches, showing abnormal involution of the distal portion of the left dorsal aorta. There is also persistence of the entire right dorsal aorta and the distal portion of the right sixth aortic arch artery. *B,* Right aortic arch without a retroesophageal component. *C,* Right aortic arch with a retroesophageal component. The abnormal arch and the normal ligamentum arteriosum form a vascular ring that compresses the esophagus and trachea.

part of the right dorsal aorta. As development proceeds, differential growth shifts the origin of the right subclavian artery cranially until it comes to lie close to the origin of the left subclavian artery. Although this abnormality, often called **anomalous right subclavian artery**, is common and always forms a vascular ring, it is rarely clinically significant because the ring is usually not tight enough to constrict the esophagus and trachea.

FETAL AND NEONATAL CIRCULATION

The fetal cardiovascular system is cleverly designed to serve prenatal needs and to permit modifications at birth that establish the postnatal circulatory pattern. Good respiration in the newborn infant is dependent upon normal circulatory changes occurring at birth.

The Fetal Circulation (Figs. 14–42 and 14–43). Well-oxygenated blood returns from the placenta in the *umbilical vein.* About half the blood from the placenta passes through the hepatic sinusoids; whereas, the remainder bypasses the liver and goes through the *ductus venosus* into the inferior vena cava.

The blood flow through the ductus venosus is regulated by a *sphincter* close to the umbilical vein. When the sphincter relaxes, more blood passes through the ductus venosus. When the sphincter contracts, more blood is diverted through the *portal sinus* to the portal vein and into the hepatic sinusoids. Although the presence of an *anatomical sphincter* in the ductus venosus is not universally accepted, it is generally agreed that there is a *physiological sphincter* that prevents overloading of the heart when venous flow in the umbilical vein is high, e.g., during uterine contractions.

After a short course in the inferior vena cava, the blood enters the right atrium of the heart. Because the inferior vena cava also contains poorly oxygenated blood from the lower limbs, abdomen, and pelvis, the blood entering the right atrium is not as well oxygenated as that in the umbilical vein, but it is still well-oxygenated blood.

Most blood from the inferior vena cava is directed by the inferior border of the septum secundum called the *crista dividens* through the **foramen ovale** into the left atrium (Figs. 14–43 and 14–45). Here it mixes with the relatively small amount of deoxygenated blood returning from the lungs via the pulmonary veins. The fetal lungs extract oxygen from the blood instead of providing it. From the left atrium, the blood passes into the left ventricle and leaves via the ascending aorta. *The arteries supplying the heart, head, neck, and upper limbs receive well-oxygenated blood. The*

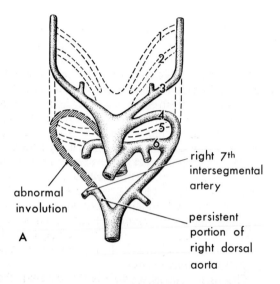

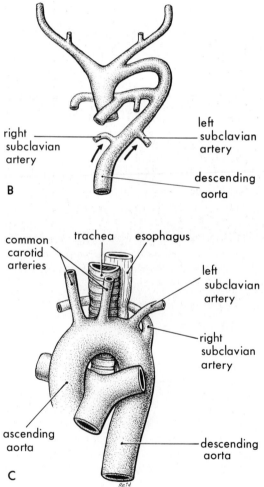

Figure 14–41. Sketches illustrating the probable embryological basis of abnormal origin of the right subclavian artery. *A,* The right fourth aortic arch and the cranial portion of the right dorsal aorta have involuted. As a result, the right subclavian artery forms from the right seventh intersegmental artery and the distal segment of the right dorsal aorta. *B,* As the arch of the aorta forms, the right subclavian artery is carried cranially (*arrows*) with the left subclavian artery. *C,* The abnormal right subclavian artery arises from the aorta and passes posterior to the trachea and esophagus.

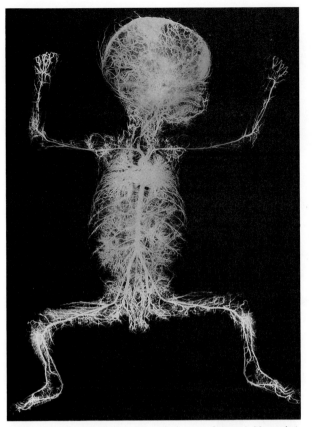

Figure 14–42. Arteriogram of male human fetus at 22 weeks' gestation, showing the entire primary arterial network. The arteries were perfused with an aqueous suspension of a radiopaque media (cinnabar or mercury sulfide) via the ascending thoracic aorta. (From Maher, WP: *Am J Anat 187*:201, 1990).

rest of the blood supplies the viscera and the inferior half of the body.

The Neonatal Circulation (Fig. 14–44). Important circulatory adjustments occur at birth when the circulation of fetal blood through the placenta ceases and the infant's lungs begin to function. The three shunts that permitted much of the blood to bypass the liver and the lungs cease to function. As soon as the baby is born, *the foramen ovale, ductus arteriosus, ductus venosus, and umbilical vessels are no longer needed.* The sphincter in the ductus venosus constricts so that all blood entering the liver passes through the hepatic sinusoids. Occlusion of the placental circulation causes an immediate fall of blood pressure in the inferior vena cava and right atrium.

Aeration of the lungs is associated with a dramatic fall in pulmonary vascular resistance, a marked increase in pulmonary blood flow, and a progressive thinning of the walls of the pulmonary arteries. The thinning of the walls of these arteries results mainly from stretching as the lungs increase in size with the first few breaths. Due to increased pulmonary blood flow, the pressure in the left atrium is raised above that in the right atrium. This increased left atrial pressure closes the foramen ovale by pressing the valve of the foramen ovale against the septum secundum (Figs. 14–13 and 14–44).

The right ventricular wall is thicker than the left ventricular wall in fetuses and in newborn infants because the right ventricle has been working harder. By the end of the first month, the left ventricular wall is thicker than the right ventricular wall because the left ventricle is now working harder than the right one; furthermore, the right ventricular wall becomes thinner because of the atrophy associated with its lighter workload.

The ductus arteriosus constricts at birth, but there is often a small shunt of blood from the aorta to the left pulmonary artery for a few days. The ductus arteriosus usually becomes functionally closed soon after birth; but, in premature infants and in those with persistent hypoxia, it may remain open much longer. Oxygen is the most important factor in controlling closure of the ductus arteriosus. Closure of the ductus appears to be mediated by *bradykinin*, a substance released from the lungs during their initial inflation (Rudolph et al., 1977). The action of this substance appears to be dependent on the high oxygen content of the aortic blood that results from ventilation of the lungs at birth. When the PO_2 of the blood passing through the ductus arteriosus reaches about 50 mmHg, the wall of the ductus constricts. The mechanisms by which oxygen causes ductal restrictions is not well understood. The effects of oxygen on

liver also receives well oxygenated blood from the umbilical vein (Fig. 14–43).

A small amount of well-oxygenated blood from the inferior vena cava remains in the right atrium (Figs. 14–43 and 14–45). This blood mixes with poorly oxygenated blood from the superior vena cava and coronary sinus and passes into the right ventricle. This blood with a medium saturation of oxygen leaves via the pulmonary trunk. Some of it goes to the lungs, but most of it passes through the *ductus arteriosus* into the aorta. Because of the high pulmonary vascular resistance in fetal life, pulmonary blood flow is low. Only five to ten per cent of the cardiac output goes to the lungs, which is adequate because they are not functioning as respiratory organs.

Forty to 50 per cent of the blood in the descending aorta passes into the umbilical arteries and is returned to the placenta for reoxygenation (Fig. 14–43). The

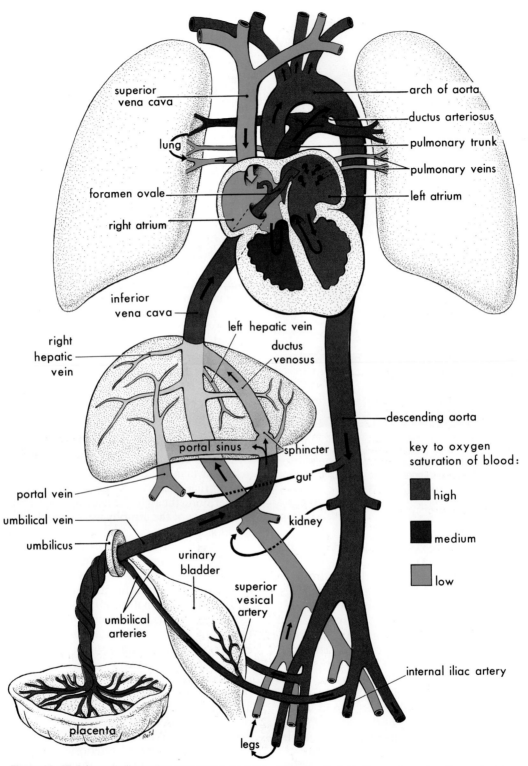

Figure 14–43. Schematic illustration of the fetal circulation. The colors indicate the oxygen saturation of the blood and the arrows show the course of the blood. The organs are not drawn to scale. Observe that three shunts permit most of the blood to bypass the liver and the lungs: (1) the ductus venosus, (2) the foramen ovale, and (3) the ductus arteriosus.

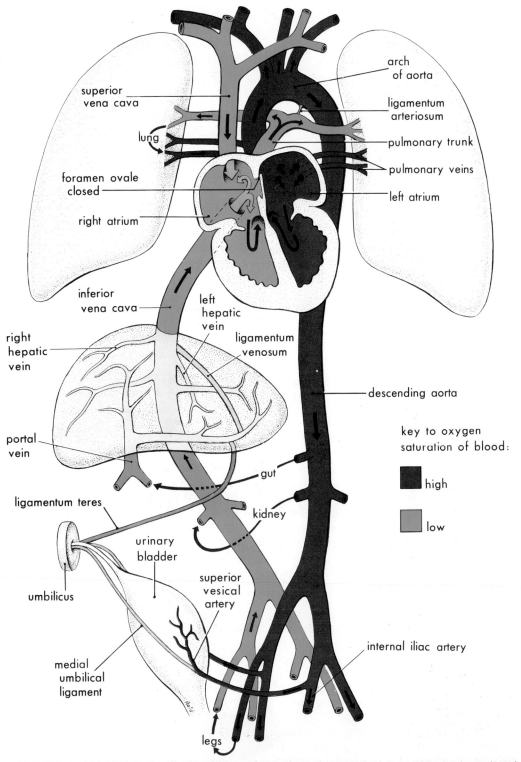

Figure 14–44. A schematic illustration of the neonatal circulation. The adult derivatives of the fetal vessels and structures that become nonfunctional at birth are also shown. The arrows indicate the course of the blood in the infant. The organs are not drawn to scale. After birth the three shunts that short circuited the blood during fetal life cease to function, and the pulmonary and systemic circulations become separated.

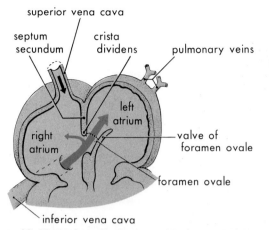

Figure 14–45. A schematic diagram of blood flow through the fetal atria, illustrating how the crista dividens (lower edge of the septum secundum) separates the blood from the inferior vena cava into two streams. The larger stream passes through the foramen ovale into the left atrium where it mixes with a small volume of deoxygenated blood from the pulmonary veins. The smaller stream of blood from the inferior vena cava remains in the right atrium and mixes with poorly oxygenated blood from the superior vena cava and coronary sinus.

the ductal smooth muscle may be direct or may be mediated by its effects on prostaglandin secretion (Behrman, 1992). The ductus of the premature infant is less responsive to oxygen.

During fetal life, the patency of the ductus arteriosus before birth is controlled by the low content of oxygen in the blood passing through it and by endogenously produced *prostaglandins* that act on the muscle cells in the wall of the ductus arteriosus, causing them to relax (Page et al., 1981). *Hypoxia* and other ill-defined influences cause the local production of prostaglandin E_1 and E_2, which keep the ductus arteriosus open. Inhibitors of prostaglandin synthesis such as *indomethacin* can cause constriction of a patent ductus arteriosus in premature infants (Behrman, 1992).

The umbilical arteries constrict at birth, preventing loss of the infant's blood. If the umbilical cord is not tied for a minute or so, blood flow through the umbilical vein continues, transferring fetal blood in the placenta to the infant.

The change from the fetal to the adult pattern of blood circulation is not a sudden occurrence. Some changes occur with the first breath, and others are effected over hours and days (Behrman, 1992). During the transitional stage, there may be a right-to-left flow through the foramen ovale. Although the ductus arteriosus constricts at birth, it usually remains patent for two to three months. The closure of the fetal vessels and the foramen ovale is initially a functional

change. Later, anatomical closure occurs due to proliferation of endothelial and fibrous tissues.

ADULT DERIVATIVES OF FETAL VESSELS AND OTHER FETAL CIRCULATORY STRUCTURES (FIGS. 14–40, 14–43, AND 14–44). Because of the changes in the cardiovascular system at birth, certain vessels and structures are no longer required.

The intra-abdominal portion of the umbilical vein eventually becomes the *ligamentum teres*, which passes from the umbilicus to the porta hepatis (Moore, 1992); here it is attached to the left branch of the portal vein (Fig. 14–46B). The umbilical vein remains patent for a long time and may be used for *exchange transfusions* during early infancy. This is done to prevent brain damage and death of anemic erythroblastotic infants. Most of the infant's blood is replaced with donor blood. The lumen of the umbilical vein usually does not disappear completely; hence, the ligamentum teres can usually, if necessary, be cannulated in adults for the injection of contrast medium or chemotherapeutic drugs. The potential patency of this vein may also be of functional significance in hepatic cirrhosis.

The ductus venosus becomes the *ligamentum venosum*. It passes through the liver from the left branch of the portal vein to the inferior vena cava, to which it is attached (Fig. 14–46B). Most of the intra-abdominal portions of the umbilical arteries become the *medial umbilical ligaments*; the proximal parts of these vessels persist as the *superior vesical arteries* (Fig. 14–43).

The **foramen ovale** normally closes at birth (Fig. 14-44). This is a functional closure for several weeks. Anatomical closure occurs by the third month and is the result of tissue proliferation and adhesion of the septum primum (the valve of the foramen ovale) to the left margin of the septum secundum (Fig. 14–13). The septum primum forms the floor of the fossa ovalis (Fig. 14–47). The inferior edge of the septum secundum forms a rounded fold, the *limbus fossae ovalis* (anulus ovalis). It marks the former boundary of the foramen ovale. There is often a lunate impression on the left side of the interatrial septum, which indicates the site of the foramen ovale in the prenatal heart.

The ductus arteriosus becomes the *ligamentum arteriosum* (Figs. 14–37C and 14–44). It passes from the left pulmonary artery to the arch of the aorta. Anatomical closure of the ductus normally occurs by the twelfth week.

Patent Ductus Arteriosus (PDA). This is a common anomaly that is two to three times more frequent in females than in males (Fig. 14–48). The reason for this preponderance is not known. Functional closure of the ductus usually

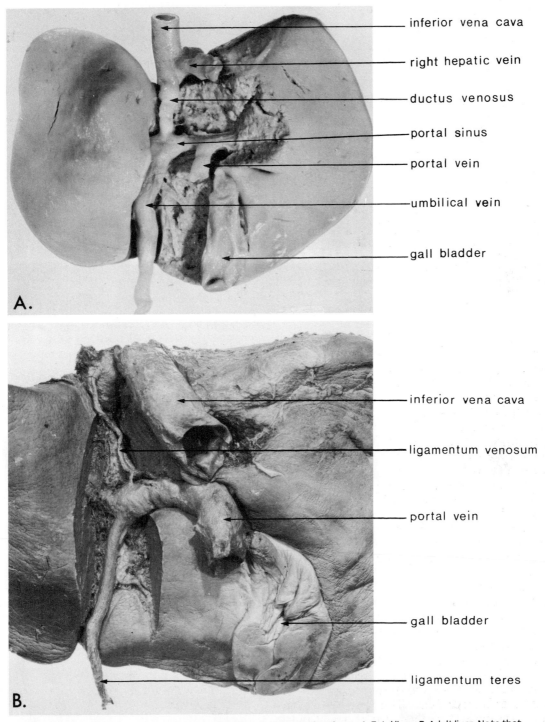

inferior vena cava

right hepatic vein

ductus venosus

portal sinus

portal vein

umbilical vein

gall bladder

A.

inferior vena cava

ligamentum venosum

portal vein

gall bladder

ligamentum teres

B.

Figure 14–46. Photographs of dissected livers showing their visceral surfaces. *A*, Fetal liver. *B*, Adult liver. Note that the umbilical vein is represented in the adult by the ligamentum teres and the ductus venosus by the ligamentum venosum.

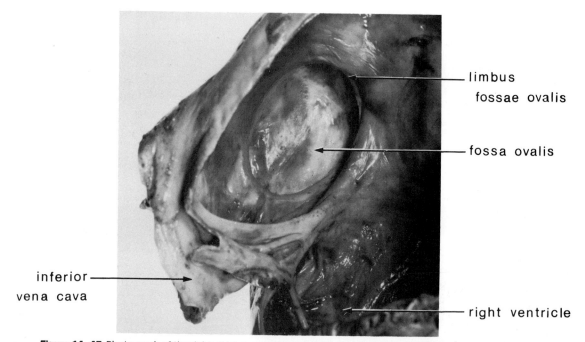

limbus
fossae ovalis

fossa ovalis

inferior
vena cava

right ventricle

Figure 14–47. Photograph of the right atrial aspect of an adult interatrial septum, showing the fossa ovalis and the limbus fossae ovalis (×1.5). The floor of the fossa ovalis is derived from the septum primum; whereas, the limbus fossae ovalis represents the free edge of the septum secundum (also see Fig. 14–24).

occurs soon after birth; however, if it remains patent, aortic blood is shunted into the pulmonary artery. PDA is the most common congenital anomaly associated with maternal rubella infection during early pregnancy (p. 165), but the mode of action of the rubella virus is unclear.

Premature infants usually have a PDA; the patency is the result of hypoxia and immaturity. Virtually all infants whose birth weight is less than 1750 gm have a PDA in the

first 24 hours of postnatal life. PDA in a full-term infant occurs as a pathologic entity (Behrman, 1992). Surgical closure of a PDA is the usual treatment. Closure is achieved by ligation and division.

The embryological basis of PDA is failure of the ductus arteriosus to involute after birth and form the ligamentum arteriosum. Failure of contraction of the muscular wall of the ductus arteriosus after birth is the primary cause of

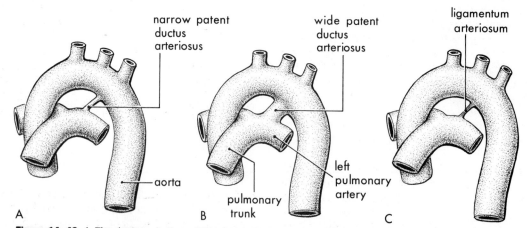

narrow patent ductus arteriosus

wide patent ductus arteriosus

ligamentum arteriosum

aorta

pulmonary trunk

left pulmonary artery

A   B   C

Figure 14–48. *A,* The ductus arteriosus (DA) of a newborn infant. The DA is normally patent for about two weeks after birth. *B,* Abnormal patent DA in a six-month-old infant. The large ductus is nearly the same size as the left pulmonary artery. *C,* The ligamentum arteriosum, the normal remnant of the ductus arteriosus, in a six-month-old infant.

patency. There is some evidence that the low oxygen content of the blood in infants with *neonatal respiratory distress* can adversely affect closure of the ductus arteriosus; for example, PDA commonly occurs in small premature infants with respiratory difficulties associated with a deficiency of surfactant. Isolated PDA is more common in infants born at high altitude.

PDA may occur as an isolated malformation or in association with cardiac defects. Large differences between aortic and pulmonary pressures can cause heavy flow of blood through the ductus arteriosus, thereby preventing normal constriction. Such pressure differences may be caused by preductal coarctation of the aorta (Fig. 14–38C), transposition of the great arteries (Fig. 14–30), or pulmonary stenosis and atresia (Fig. 14–31).

THE LYMPHATIC SYSTEM

The lymphatic system begins to develop at the end of the fifth week, about two weeks after the primordia of the cardiovascular system are recognizable. Lymphatic vessels develop in a manner similar to that previously described for blood vessels (see Fig. 4–9) and make connections with the venous system. The early lymph capillaries join each other to form a network of lymphatics (Fig. 14–49).

Development of Lymph Sacs and Ducts

There are *six primary lymph sacs* (Fig. 14–49A): (1) two *jugular lymph sacs* near the junction of the subclavian veins with the anterior cardinal veins (the future internal jugular veins), (2) two *iliac lymph sacs* near the junction of the iliac veins with the posterior cardinal veins, (3) one *retroperitoneal lymph sac* in the root of the mesentery on the posterior abdominal wall, and (4) one *cisterna chyli*, located dorsal to the retroperitoneal lymph sac.

Lymph vessels pass from the lymph sacs principally along main veins to the head, neck, and upper limbs from the jugular lymph sacs; to the lower trunk and lower limbs from the iliac lymph sacs; and to the primitive gut from the retroperitoneal lymph sac and cisterna chyli. Two large channels (right and left thoracic ducts) connect the jugular lymph sacs with the cisterna chyli. Soon a large anastomosis forms between these channels (Fig. 14–49B).

The Thoracic Duct. This duct develops from: (1) the caudal part of the right thoracic duct, (2) the anastomosis, and (3) the cranial part of the left thoracic duct. Because there initially are right and left thoracic ducts, there are many variations in the origin, course, and termination of the adult thoracic duct. The *right lymphatic duct* is derived from the cranial part of the right thoracic duct (Fig. 14–49C). The thoracic duct

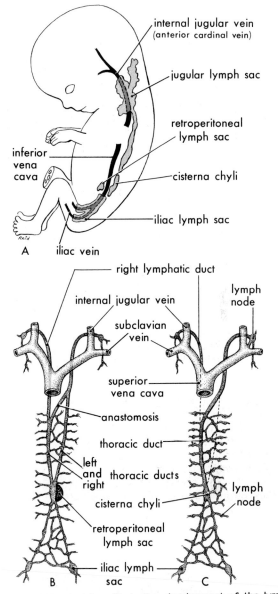

Figure 14–49. Drawings illustrating development of the lymphatic system. *A,* Left side of an eight-week embryo, showing the primary lymph sacs. *B,* Ventral view of the lymphatic system at nine weeks, showing the paired thoracic ducts. *C,* Later in the fetal period, illustrating formation of the definitive thoracic duct and right lymphatic duct.

and right lymphatic duct connect with the venous system at the angle between the internal jugular and subclavian veins (Fig. 14–49C). The superior portion of the embryonic cisterna chyli persists. In the adult the *cisterna chyli* is about 5 cm long and 6 mm wide (Moore, 1992).

Development of Lymph Nodes

Except for the superior part of the cisterna chyli, the lymph sacs are transformed into groups of lymph nodes during the early fetal period. Mesenchymal cells invade each lymph sac and break up its cavity into a network of lymphatic channels, the primordia of the *lymph sinuses*. Other mesenchymal cells give rise to the capsule and connective tissue framework of the lymph node.

Development of Lymphocytes. The lymphocytes are originally derived from primitive stem cells in the yolk sac mesenchyme and later from the liver and spleen. These lymphocytes eventually enter the bone marrow where they divide to form *lymphoblasts*. The lymphocytes that appear in lymph nodes before birth are derived from the *thymus gland*, a derivative of the third pair of pharyngeal pouches (p. 195). Small lymphocytes leave the thymus and circulate to other lymphoid organs. Later, some mesenchymal cells in the lymph nodes differentiate into lymphocytes. Lymph nodules do not appear in the lymph nodes until just before and/or after birth.

The **spleen** develops from an aggregation of mesenchymal cells in the dorsal mesentery of the stomach (p. 245). The *palatine tonsils* develop from the second pair of pharyngeal pouches (p. 193). The *tubal tonsils* develop from aggregations of lymph nodules around the pharyngeal openings of the auditory (eustachian) tubes. The *pharyngeal tonsils* ("adenoids") develop from an aggregation of lymph nodules in the wall of the nasopharynx. The *lingual tonsil* develops from an aggregation of lymph nodules in the root of the tongue. Lymph nodules also develop in the mucosa of the respiratory and digestive systems.

Abnormalities of the Lymphatic System

Congenital anomalies of the lymphatic system are uncommon. There may be diffuse swelling of a part of the body (*congenital lymphedema*). This condition may result from dilation of primitive lymphatic channels or from a congenital hypoplasia of lymphatic vessels. More rarely, diffuse cystic dilatation of lymphatic channels involves widespread portions of the body.

Cystic Lymphangioma or Hygroma. These large swellings usually appear in the inferolateral part of the neck and consist of large single or multilocular fluid-filled cavities. Hygromas may be present at birth, but they often enlarge and become evident during infancy. Most hygromas appear to be derived from abnormal transformation of the jugular lymph sacs. Hygromas are believed to arise from portions of a jugular lymph sac that are pinched off or from lymphatic spaces that fail to establish connections with the main lymphatic channels.

SUMMARY

The cardiovascular system begins to develop toward the end the third week, and the heart starts to beat at 21 to 22 days. Mesenchymal cells derived from the splanchnic mesoderm proliferate and form isolated cell clusters, which soon develop into endothelial tubes that join to form the primitive vascular system.

The heart develops from splanchnic mesenchyme in the *cardiogenic area*. Paired endothelial tubes form and fuse into a single endothelial heart tube. Splanchnic mesoderm surrounding the heart tube forms the *primitive myocardium*. The primordium of the primitive heart consists of four chambers (sinus venosus, atrium, ventricle, and bulbus cordis). The *truncus arteriosus* is continuous caudally with the *bulbus cordis* and enlarges cranially to form the *aortic sac* (Fig. 14–9).

As the heart grows, it bends to the right and soon acquires the general external appearance of the adult heart. The heart becomes partitioned into four chambers between the fourth and seventh weeks.

Three systems of paired veins drain into the primitive heart: (1) the *vitelline system*, which becomes the *portal system*, (2) the *cardinal veins*, which form the *caval system*, and (3) the *umbilical system*, which involutes after birth.

As the branchial or pharyngeal arches form during the fourth and fifth weeks, they are penetrated by arteries, referred to as *aortic arches*. They arise from the *aortic sac*. During the sixth to eighth weeks, the aortic arches are transformed into the adult arterial arrangement of the carotid, subclavian, and pulmonary arteries.

The critical period of heart development is from day 20 to day 50 after fertilization. Numerous critical events occur during cardiac development, and deviation from the normal pattern at any time may produce one or more congenital heart defects. Because partitioning of the primitive heart results from complex processes, defects of the cardiac septa are relatively common, particularly VSDs. Some congenital anomalies result from abnormal transformation of the aortic arches into the adult arterial pattern.

Because the lungs are nonfunctional during prenatal life, the fetal cardiovascular system is structurally designed so that the blood is oxygenated in the placenta and largely bypasses the lungs. The modifications that establish the postnatal circulatory pattern at birth are not abrupt but extend into infancy. Failure of these changes in the circulatory system to occur at birth results in two of the most common congenital abnormalities of the heart and great vessels: patent foramen ovale and patent ductus arteriosus.

The *lymphatic system* begins to develop during the fifth week in close association with the venous system. Six primary *lymph sacs* develop, which later become interconnected by lymph vessels. Lymph nodes develop along the network of lymphatic vessels; lymph nodules do not appear until just before and/or after birth. Sometimes a part of a jugular lymph sac becomes pinched off and may give rise to a mass of dilated lymphatic vessels called a *hygroma*.

CLINICALLY ORIENTED QUESTIONS FOR PROBLEM-BASED LEARNING SESSIONS

1. What is the most common type of congenital cardiac anomaly? What per centage of congenital heart disease results from this defect? Discuss blood flow in infants with this defect. What problems would the infant likely encounter if the defect was large?

2. A female infant was born normally after a pregnancy complicated by a *rubella infection* during the first trimester of pregnancy. She had *congenital cataracts* and *congenital heart disease*. A radiograph of the infant's chest at three weeks showed generalized *cardiac enlargement* with some increase in pulmonary vascularity. What congenital cardiovascular abnormality is commonly associated with *maternal rubella* during early pregnancy? What probably caused the cardiac enlargement?

3. In *tetralogy of Fallot* there are four cardiac abnormalities. What are they? What is one of the most obvious signs of tetralogy? What radiographic technique might be used to confirm a tentative diagnosis of this type of congenital heart disease? What do you think would be the main aim of therapy in these cases?

4. A male infant was born after a full-term normal pregnancy. Severe, generalized cyanosis was observed on the first day. A chest film revealed a *slightly enlarged heart* with a narrow base and increased pulmonary vascularity. A clinical diagnosis of TGA was made. What radiographic technique would likely be used to verify the diagnosis? What would this technique reveal in the present case? How was the infant able to survive after birth with this severe congenital anomaly of the great arteries?

5. During an autopsy on a 72-year-old man who had died following *chronic heart failure*, it was observed that his heart was very large and that the pulmonary artery and its main branches were dilated. Opening the heart revealed a very large *atrial septal defect*. What type of ASD was probably present? Where would the defect likely be located? Explain why the pulmonary artery and its main branches were dilated.

The answers to these questions are given on page 465.

References and Suggested Reading

Anderson RH, Ashley GT: Growth and development of the cardiovascular system. *In* Davis JA, Dobbing J (eds): *Scientific Foundation of Paediatrics.* Philadelphia, WB Saunders, 1974.

Anderson RH, Taylor IM: Development of atrioventricular specialized tissue in human heart. *Br Heart J* 34:1205, 1972.

Barry A: The aortic arch derivatives in the human adult. *Anat Rec* 111:221, 1951.

Beck F, Moffat DB, Davies DP: *Human Embryology.* 2nd ed. Oxford, Blackwell Scientific Publications, 1985.

Behrman RE (ed): *Nelson Textbook of Pediatrics.* 14th ed. Philadelphia, WB Saunders, 1992.

Blausen BE, Johannes RS, Hutchins GM: Computer-based reconstructions of the cardiac ventricles of human embryos. *Am J Cardiovasc Pathol* 3:37, 1989.

Bowman JM: Hemolytic disease (erythroblastosis fetalis). *In* Creasy RK, Resnik R (eds): *Maternal-Fetal Medicine: Principles and Practice.* Philadelphia, WB Saunders, 1989.

Bruyer Jr, HJ, Kargas SA, Levy JM: The causes and underlying developmental mechanisms of congenital cardiovascular malformation: A critical review. *Am J Med Genet (Suppl)* 3:411, 1987.

Butler J, Vincent RN, Reed M, Collins GF: Cardiac embryogenesis: a three-dimensional approach. *Can J Card* 3:111, 1987.

Campbell M: Natural history of atrial septal defect. *Br Heart J* 32:820, 1970.

Campbell MS, Sack DA: Anomalies of the heart and great vessels. *In* Pearson AA, Sauter RW (eds): *The Development of the Cardiovascular System*. Portland, University of Oregon Medical School Printing Department, 1968.

Chinn A, Fitzsimmons J, Shepard TH, Fantel AG: Congenital heart disease among spontaneous abortuses and stillborn fetuses: prevalence and associations. *Teratology 40*:475, 1989.

Clark EB: Cardiac embryology. Its relevance to congenital heart disease. *Am J Dis Child 140*:41, 1986.

Coffin JD, Poole TJ: Embryonic vascular development: immunohistochemical identification of the origin and subsequent morphogenesis of the major vessel primordia in quail embryos. *Development 102*:735, 1988.

Collet RW, Edwards JE: Persistent truncus arteriosus: A classification according to anatomic types. *Surg Clin North Am 29*:1245, 1949.

Conte G, Grieco M: Closure of the interventricular foramen and morphogenesis of the membranous septum and ventricular septal defects in the human heart. *Anat Anz 155*:39, 1984.

Conte G, Pellegrini A: On the development of the coronary arteries in human embryos, stages 14–19. *Anat Embryol 169*:209, 1984.

Dawes GS: Foetal blood gas homeostasis. *In* Wolstenholme GEW, O'Connor M (eds): *Foetal Autonomy*. London, J & A Churchill, 1969.

Deanfield JE: Transposition of the great arteries: To switch or not to switch? *Curr Opin Pediatr 1*:85, 1989.

Dickson AD: The development of the ductus venosus in man and the goat. *J Anat 91*:358, 1957.

Edwards JE, Dry TJ, Parker RL, et al.: *An Atlas of Congenital Anomalies of the Heart and Great Vessels*. Springfield, Ill, Charles C Thomas, 1954.

Eidemiller LR, Keane JM: Development of the heart. *In* Pearson AA, Sauter RW (eds): *The Development of the Cardiovascular System*. Portland, University of Oregon Medical School Printing Department, 1968.

Fananapazir K, Kaufman MH: Observations on the development of the aortico-pulmonary spiral septum in the mouse. *J Anat 158*:157, 1988.

Feinberg RN (ed): *The Development of the Vascular System*. Farmington, S Karger Publishers, 1990.

Feinberg RN, Sherer GK, Auerbach R (eds): *The Development of the Vascular System*. Basel, Karger, 1991.

Ferencz C: The etiology of congenital cardiovascular malformations: observations on genetic risks with implications for further birth defects research. *J Med 16*:497, 1985.

Ferencz C, Rubin JD, McCarter RB, Boughman JA, Wilson PD, Brenner J, Neil CA, Perry LW, Hepner S, Downing JW: Cardiac and noncardiac malformations; observations in a population-based study. *Teratology 35*:367, 1987.

Fink BW: *Congenital Heart Disease*. 2nd ed. Chicago, Year Book Medical Publishers, 1985.

Gootman N, Gootman PM (eds): *Perinatal Cardiovascular Function*. New York, Marcel Dekker, 1983.

Gray SW, Skandalakis JE: *Embryology for Surgeons*. 2nd ed. Baltimore, Williams & Wilkins, 1993.

Hayek H von: Der funktionelle Bau der Nabelarterien und des Ductus Botalli. *Z Anat Entwicklungs-gesch 105*:15, 1935.

Hirakow R: Development of the vertebrate heart and the extracellular matrix. *Congenital Anomalies 26*:205, 1986.

Hirakow R: Personal communication, 1992.

Keith JD, Rowe RD, Vlad P: *Heart Disease in Infancy and Childhood*. 3rd ed. New York, The Macmillan Company, 1978.

Kessler RE, Zimman DS: Umbilical vein angiography. *Radiology 87*:841, 1966.

Kirby ML, Gale TF, Stewart DE: Neural crest cells contribute to normal aorticopulmonary septation. *Science 220*:1059, 1983.

Kirklin JW, Colvin EV, McConnell ME, et al.: Complete transposition of the great arteries: Treatment in the current era. *Pediatr Clin North Am 37*:171, 1990.

Krediet P: A hypothesis of the development of coarctation in man. *Acta Morphol Neerlando Scand 6*:207, 1965.

Lind J: Normal perinatal circulation. *In* Emery J (ed): *The Anatomy of the Developing Lung*. London, William Heinemann, 1969.

Long WA: *Fetal and Neonatal Cardiology*. Philadelphia, WB Saunders, 1990.

Lucas RV, Schmidt RE: Anomalous venous connections, pulmonary and systemic. *In* Moss AJ, Adams FH (eds): *Heart Disease in Infants, Children and Adolescents*. 2nd ed. Baltimore, Williams & Wilkins, 1977.

Merrill WH, Bender HW: The surgical approach to congenital heart disease. *Current Problems in Surg 22*:4, 1985.

Moller JF, Neal WA: *Fetal, Neonatal and Infant Cardiac Disease*. Norwalk, Appleton & Lange, 1989.

Moore KL: *Clinically Oriented Anatomy*. 2nd ed. Baltimore, Williams & Wilkins, 1992.

Morris GK, Hampton J: Congenital heart lesions–an introduction. *Medicine International 18*:745, 1985.

Moscoso GV, Pexieder T: Variations in microscopic anatomy and ultrastructure of human embryonic hearts subjected to three different modes of fixation. *Path Res Pract 186*:768, 1990.

Moss AJ, Emmanouilides GC, Adams FH, Chuang K: Response of ductus arteriosus and pulmonary and systemic arterial pressure to changes in oxygen environment in newborn infants. *Pediatrics 33*:937, 1964.

Neill CA: Development of the pulmonary veins. *Pediatrics 18*:880, 1956.

O'Rahilly R: The timing and sequence of events in human cardiogenesis. *Acta Anat 79*:70, 1971.

Page EW, Villee CA, Villee DB: *Human Reproduction. Essentials of Reproductive and Perinatal Medicine*. 3rd ed. Philadelphia, WB Saunders, 1981.

Papp JG: Autonomic responses and neurohumoral control in the human early antenatal heart. *Basic Res Cardiol 83*:2, 1988.

Pearson AA, Sauter RW: Observation on the innervation of the umbilical vessels in human embryos and fetuses. *Anat Rec 160*:406, 1968.

Pearson AA, Sauter RW (eds): *The Development of the Cardiovascular System*. Portland, University of Oregon Medical School Printing Department, 1968.

Persaud TVN: Historical development of the concept of a pulmonary circulation. *Can J Cardio 5*:12, 1989.

Pexieder T: Genetic aspects of congenital heart disease. *In* Pexieder T (ed): *Perspectives in Cardiovascular Research*. Vol 5. *Mechanisms of Cardiac Morphogenesis and Teratogenesis*. New York, Raven Press, 1981.

Riva E, Hearse DK: *The Developing Myocardium*. New York, Futura Publishing, 1991.

Rosenquist GC, Bergsma D (eds): *Morphogenesis and Malformation of the Cardiovascular System*. The National Foundation–March of Dimes. Birth Defects: Original Article Series, Vol. XIV, No. 7. New York, Alan R. Liss, 1978.

Rudolph AM, Heymann MA, Lewis AB: Physiology and pharmacology of the pulmonary circulation in the fetus and newborn. *In* Hodson WA (ed): *Development of the Lung*. New York, Marcel Dekker, 1977.

Schats R, Jansen CAM, Wladimiroff JW: Embryonic heart activity: appearance and development in early pregnancy. *Brit J Obstet Gynaecol 97*:989, 1990.

Schmidt KG, Silverman WH: Evaluation of the fetal heart by ultrasound. *In* Callen PW: *Ultrasonography in Obstetrics and Gynecology*. 2nd ed. Philadelphia, WB Saunders, 1988.

Schmidt KG, Silverman NH: The fetus with a cardiac malformation. *In* Harrison MR, Golbus MS, Filly RA (eds): *The Unborn Patient: Prenatal Diagnosis and Treatment.* 2nd ed. Philadelphia, WB Saunders, 1991.

Schwartz SM, Heimark RL, Majesky MW: Developmental mechanisms underlying pathology of arteries. *Physiol Rev 70*:1177, 1990.

Skovránek J: Prenatal development of the heart and the blood circulatory system. *Physiol Res 40*:25, 1991.

Thompson MW, McInnes RR, Willard HF: *Thompson & Thompson Genetics in Medicine.* 5th ed. Philadelphia, WB Saunders, 1991.

Ueland K: Cardiac diseases. *In* Creasy RK, Resnik R (eds): *Maternal-Fetal Medicine: Principles and Practice.* Philadelphia, WB Saunders, 1989.

van Mierop LHS: Transposition of the great arteries. I. Clarification of further confusion. *Am J Cardiol 28*:735, 1971.

van Praagh R, van Praagh S, Nebasar RA, et al.: Tetralogy of Fallot: Underdevelopment of the pulmonary infundibulum and its sequelae. *Am J Cardiol 26*:25, 1970.

Veille JC, Mahowald MB, Sivakoff M: Ethical dilemmas in fetal echocardiography. *Obstet Gynecol 73*:710, 1989.

Vernall DG: The human embryonic heart in the seventh week. *Am J Anat 111*:17, 1962.

Verrier ED, Vlahakes GJ, Hanley FL, Bradley SM: Experimental Fetal Cardiac Surgery. *In* Harrison MR, Golbus MS, Filly RA (eds): *The Unborn Patient: Prenatal Diagnosis and Treatment.* 2nd ed. Philadelphia, WB Saunders, 1991.

Virmani R, Atkinson JD, Fenoglio JJ: *Cardiovascular Pathology.* Philadelphia, WB Saunders, 1991.

Yoffey JM, Courtice, FC: *Lymphatics, Lymph and Lymphomyeloid Complex.* London, Academic Press, 1970.

15

The Skeletal System

The skeletal system develops from mesoderm and neural crest cells (p. 71). As the notochord and neural tube form, the *intraembryonic mesoderm* lateral to these structures condenses to form two longitudinal columns of *paraxial mesoderm* (Fig. 15–1). Toward the end of the third week, these columns become segmented into blocks of tissue called somites (see Fig. 4–7).

Externally, the **somites** appear as pairs of beadlike elevations along the dorsolateral surface of the embryo (see Figs. 5–8 to 5–10). Each somite differentiates into two parts (Fig. 15–1*B* and *C*). The ventromedial part is known as the *sclerotome*; its cells form the vertebrae and ribs. The remainder of the somite is known as the *dermomyotome*; cells from its *myotome* region form myoblasts (primitive muscle cells), and cells from its *dermatome* region form the dermis of the skin.

Mesodermal cells give rise to *mesenchyme*, which is loosely organized embryonic connective tissue. Some mesenchyme in the head region is also derived from *neural crest cells*. These cells migrate into the branchial or pharyngeal arches (p. 187) and form the bones and connective tissue of craniofacial structures. Regardless of their source, mesenchymal cells have the ability to differentiate in many different ways (e.g., into fibroblasts, chondroblasts, or osteoblasts).

DEVELOPMENT OF BONE AND CARTILAGE

Bones first appear as condensations of mesenchymal cells that form models of the bones. Some bones develop in mesenchyme by *intramembranous bone formation*. In other cases the mesenchymal bone models are transformed into cartilage bone models that later become ossified by endochondral bone formation. There are significant differences in the kinetics of the mineralization process in endochondral and intramembranous bone formation (Dziedzic-Goclawska et al., 1988).

Histogenesis of Cartilage. Cartilage develops from mesenchyme and first appears in embryos during the fifth week. In areas where cartilage is to develop, the mesenchyme condenses and the cells proliferate and become rounded. Subsequently, collagenous and/or elastic fibers are deposited in the intercellular substance or matrix. The cartilage-forming cells, called *chondroblasts*, secrete collagenous fibrils and the ground substance of the matrix. *Three types of cartilage* (hyaline cartilage, fibrocartilage, and elastic cartilage) are distinguished according to the type of matrix that is formed. Hyaline cartilage is the most widely distributed type.

Histogenesis of Bone. Bone develops in two types of connective tissue: mesenchyme and cartilage. Like cartilage, bone consists of cells and an organic intercellular substance called matrix, which comprises collagen fibrils embedded in an amorphous component. For an account of bone cells with respect to the regulation of development, structure, matrix formation, and mineralization, see Marks Jr and Popoff (1988) and Dziedzic-Goclawska et al. (1988).

Intramembranous Ossification. This type of bone formation occurs in mesenchyme that has formed a membranous layer (Fig. 15–2). This is why ossification that occurs in mesenchyme is called intramembranous ossification. The mesenchyme condenses and becomes highly vascular; some cells differentiate into *osteoblasts* (bone-forming cells) and begin to deposit matrix or intercellular substances called *osteoid tissue* or prebone. The osteoblasts are almost completely separated from one another, contact being maintained by a few tiny processes. Calcium phosphate is then deposited in the osteoid tissue as it is organized into bone. Bone osteoblasts are trapped in the matrix and become *osteocytes*.

At first new bone has no organized pattern. Spicules of bone soon become organized and coalesce into lamellae or layers. Concentric lamellae develop around blood vessels, forming *haversian systems*. Some osteoblasts remain at the periphery of the developing bone and continue to lay down layers, forming plates of compact bone on the surfaces. Between the surface plates, the intervening bone remains spiculated or spongy. This spongy environment is somewhat accentuated by the action of cells with a different origin called *osteoclasts*, which absorb bone. In the interstices of spongy bone, the mesenchyme differentiates into bone marrow. During fetal and postnatal

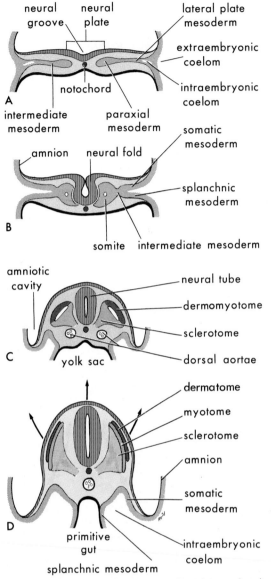

Figure 15–1. Transverse sections through embryos of various ages, illustrating the formation and early differentiation of somites. *A,* Presomite embryo (about 18 days), showing the paraxial mesoderm from which the somites are derived. *B,* Embryo of about 22 days. *C,* Embryo of about 26 days. The dermomyotome region of the somite gives rise to a myotome and a dermatome (future dermis). *D,* Embryo of about 28 days. The arrows indicate the directions of somite remnants and the neural tube in relation to the notochord.

life, there is continuous remodeling of bone by the simultaneous action of osteoclasts and osteoblasts. Studies of the cellular and molecular events during embryonic bone formation suggest that osteogenesis and chondrogenesis are programmed early in development and are independent events under the influence of vascular factors.

Intracartilaginous Ossification. This type of bone formation occurs in pre-existing cartilaginous models (Fig. 15–3). In a long bone, for example, the **primary ossification center** appears in the *diaphysis* (the portion of a long bone between its ends). This part is later called the body or shaft. Here the cartilage cells increase in size (hypertrophy), the matrix becomes calcified, and the cells die. Concurrently, a thin layer of bone is deposited under the *perichondrium* surrounding the diaphysis; thus, the perichondrium becomes the *periosteum.* Invasion of vascular connective tissue from the periosteum breaks up the cartilage. Some invading cells differentiate into the *hemopoietic cells* of the bone marrow, and others differentiate into osteoblasts that deposit bone matrix on the spicules of calcified cartilage. This process continues toward the *epiphyses* or ends of the bone. The spicules of bone are remodeled by the action of osteoclasts and osteoblasts.

Lengthening of long bones occurs at the *diaphyseal-epiphyseal junction.* Cartilage cells in this region proliferate by mitosis. Toward the diaphysis, the cartilage cells hypertrophy, and the matrix becomes calcified and broken up into spicules by vascular tissue from the marrow or medullary cavity. Bone is deposited on these spicules; absorption of this bone keeps the spongy bone masses relatively constant in length and enlarges the marrow cavity.

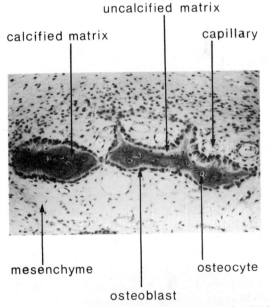

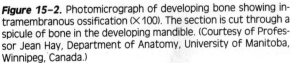

Figure 15–2. Photomicrograph of developing bone showing intramembranous ossification (×100). The section is cut through a spicule of bone in the developing mandible. (Courtesy of Professor Jean Hay, Department of Anatomy, University of Manitoba, Winnipeg, Canada.)

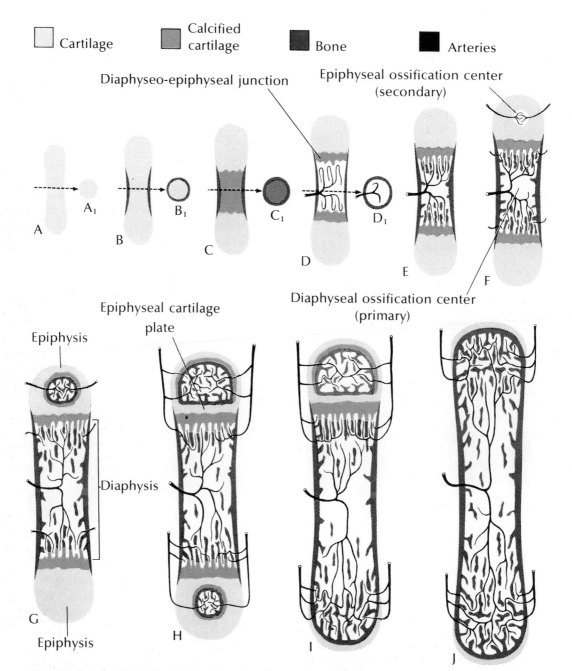

Figure 15–3. Schematic diagrams illustrating intracartilaginous or endochondral ossification and the development of a typical long bone. *A* to *J* are longitudinal sections, and A_1 to D_1 are cross sections at the levels indicated. *A*, Cartilage model of the bone. *B*, A subperiosteal ring of bone appears. *C*, Cartilage begins to calcify. *D*, Vascular mesenchyme enters the calcified cartilage. *E*, At each diaphyseal-epiphyseal junction there is a zone of ossification. *F*, Blood vessels and mesenchyme enter the superior epiphyseal cartilage. *G*, The epiphyseal ossification center grows. *H*, A similar center develops in the inferior epiphyseal cartilage plate. *I*, The inferior epiphyseal cartilage plate is ossified. *J*, The superior epiphyseal cartilage plate ossifies, forming a continuous bone marrow cavity. When the epiphyseal plates ossify, the bone can no longer grow in length. (Modified from Bloom W, Fawcett DW: *A Textbook of Histology.* 11th ed. Philadelphia, WB Saunders, 1986.)

Ossification of limb bones begins at the end of the embryonic period and thereafter makes demands on the maternal supply of calcium and phosphorus. Pregnant women are therefore advised to maintain an adequate intake of these elements in order to preserve healthy bones and teeth. The region of bone formation at the center of the body (shaft) of a long bone is called the *primary ossification center* (Fig. 15–3F). At birth, the bodies or diaphyses are largely ossified, but most of the ends or *epiphyses* are still cartilaginous.

Most *secondary ossification centers* appear in the epiphyses during the first few years after birth. The epiphyseal cartilage cells hypertrophy, and there is invasion by vascular connective tissue. As previously described, ossification spreads in all directions, and only the articular cartilage and a transverse plate of cartilage, the *epiphyseal cartilage plate*, remain cartilaginous. Upon completion of growth, this plate is replaced by spongy bone; the epiphyses and diaphyses are united, and further elongation of the bone does not occur.

In most bones the epiphyses have fused with the diaphyses by about the age of 20 years. Growth in the diameter of a bone results from deposition of bone at the periosteum and from absorption on the medullary surface. The rate of deposition and absorption is balanced to regulate the thickness of the compact bone and the size of the marrow cavity. The internal reorganization of bone continues throughout life. The development of irregular bones is similar to that of the epiphyses of long bones. Ossification begins centrally and spreads in all directions. In addition to membranous and endochondral ossification, *chondroid tissue*, which also differentiates from mesenchyme, is now recognized as an important factor for skeletal growth (Dhem et al., 1989).

DEVELOPMENT OF JOINTS

The terms articulation and joint are used synonymously to refer to the structural arrangements that join two or more bones together at their place of meeting. Joints are classified in several ways. Joints with little or no movement are classified according to the type of material holding the bones together; e.g., the bones involved in fibrous joints are joined by fibrous tissue (Fig. 15–4D). Joints begin to develop during the sixth week, and by the end of the eighth week, they resemble adult joints.

Synovial Joints

During the development of this type of joint, the mesenchyme between the developing bones, known

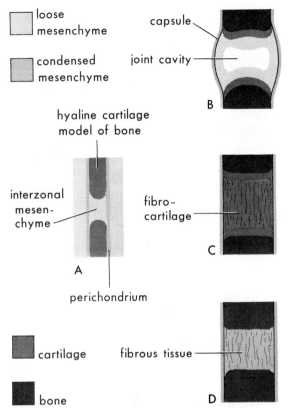

Figure 15–4. Schematic drawings illustrating the development of joints during the sixth and seventh weeks. A, Condensed mesenchyme continues across the gap, or interzone, between the developing bones, enclosing some mesenchyme (the interzonal mesenchyme) between them. This primitive joint may differentiate into B, a synovial joint, C, a cartilaginous joint, or D, a fibrous joint.

as *interzonal mesenchyme*, differentiates as follows (Fig. 15–4B): (1) peripherally, it gives rise to the capsular and other ligaments, (2) centrally, it disappears and the resulting space becomes the joint cavity, and (3) where it lines the fibrous capsule and articular surfaces, it forms the synovial membrane. Probably as a result of joint movement, the mesenchymal cells subsequently disappear from the surfaces of the articular cartilages. Examples of this type of joint are the knee and elbow joints. An abnormal intrauterine environment restricting embryonic and fetal movement may interfere with limb development and cause joint fixation (Davis and Kalousek, 1988).

Cartilaginous Joints

During the development of this type of joint, the interzonal mesenchyme between the developing bones differentiates into hyaline cartilage; e.g., the costochondral joints, or fibrocartilage (Fig. 15–4C);

e.g., the pubic symphysis between the bodies of the pubic bones (Moore, 1992).

Fibrous Joints

During the development of this type of joint, the interzonal mesenchyme between the developing bones differentiates into dense fibrous tissue (Fig. 15–4D); e.g., the sutures of the skull (Fig. 15–8).

THE AXIAL SKELETON

The axial skeleton is composed of the skull, vertebral column, ribs, and sternum. During formation of this part of the skeleton, the cells in the sclerotomes of the somites change their position (Fig. 15–1). During

the fourth week they surround the neural tube (primordium of spinal cord) and the notochord (primordium of the vertebral column). This positional change is effected by differential growth of the surrounding structures and not by active migration of sclerotome cells (Gasser, 1979).

Development of the Vertebral Column

Precartilaginous or Mesenchymal Stage. Mesenchymal cells from the sclerotomes are found in three main areas (Figs. 15–1D and 15–5A):

1. *Surrounding the notochord.* In a frontal section of a four-week embryo, the sclerotomes appear as paired condensations of mesenchymal cells around the notochord (Fig. 15–5B). Each sclerotome consists of loosely arranged cells cranially and densely packed

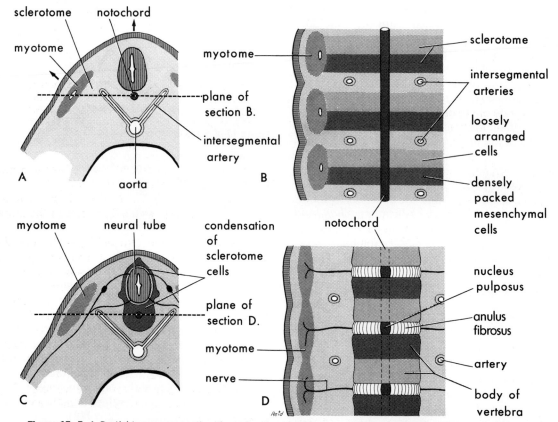

Figure 15–5. *A,* Partial transverse section through a four-week embryo. The arrows indicate the dorsal growth of the neural tube and the simultaneous dorsolateral movement of the somite remnant leaving behind a trail of sclerotomal cells. *B,* Diagrammatic frontal section of this embryo showing that the condensation of sclerotome cells around the notochord consists of a cranial area of loosely packed cells and a caudal area of densely packed cells. *C,* Partial transverse section through a five-week embryo, showing the condensation of sclerotome cells around the notochord and neural tube, which forms a mesenchymal vertebra. *D,* Diagrammatic frontal section, illustrating that the vertebral body forms from the cranial and caudal halves of two successive sclerotome masses. The intersegmental arteries now cross the bodies of the vertebrae, and the spinal nerves lie between the vertebrae. The notochord is degenerating except in the region of the intervertebral disc where it forms the nucleus pulposus.

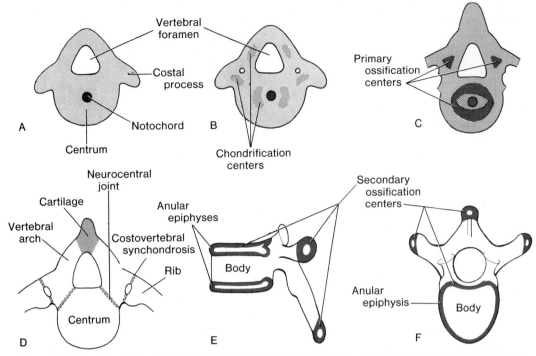

Figure 15-6. Drawings illustrating the stages of vertebral development. *A*, Mesenchymal vertebra at five weeks. *B*, Chondrification centers in a mesenchymal vertebra at six weeks. *C*, Primary ossification centers in a cartilaginous vertebra at seven weeks. *D*, A thoracic vertebra at birth consisting of three bony parts. Note the cartilage between the halves of the vertebral arch and between the arch and the centrum (the neurocentral joint). *E* and *F*, Two views of a typical thoracic vertebra at puberty showing the location of the secondary centers of ossification.

cells caudally. Some of the densely packed cells move cranially opposite the center of the myotome and form the *intervertebral disc* (Fig. 15-5D). The remaining densely packed cells fuse with the loosely arranged cells of the immediately caudal sclerotome to form the mesenchymal *centrum*, the primordium of the body of a vertebra. Thus, each centrum develops from two adjacent sclerotomes and becomes an intersegmental structure. The nerves now lie in close relationship to the intervertebral discs, and the *intersegmental arteries* lie on each side of the vertebral bodies. In the thorax, the dorsal intersegmental arteries become the *intercostal arteries*.

The **notochord** degenerates and disappears where it is surrounded by the developing vertebral bodies. Between the vertebrae the notochord expands to form the gelatinous center of the intervertebral disc called the *nucleus pulposus* (Fig. 15-5D). This nucleus is later surrounded by the circularly arranged fibers of the *anulus fibrosus*. The nucleus pulposus and anulus fibrosus together constitute the intervertebral disc. Remnants of the notochord may persist and give rise to a *chordoma*. This slow-growing neoplasm occurs most frequently in the base of the skull and in the lumbosacral region.

2. *Surrounding the neural tube.* These mesenchymal cells form the vertebral (neural) arch.

3. *In the body wall.* These mesenchymal cells form the costal processes, which form ribs in the thoracic region.

Cartilaginous Stage. During the sixth week chondrification centers appear in each mesenchymal vertebra (Fig. 15-6). The two centers in each centrum fuse at the end of the embryonic period to form a cartilaginous centrum. Concomitantly, the centers in the vertebral arches fuse with each other and with the centrum. The spinous and transverse processes develop from extensions of chondrification centers in the vertebral arch. Chondrification spreads until a *cartilaginous vertebral column* is formed.

Bony Stage. Ossification of typical vertebrae begins during the embryonic period and usually ends by the twenty-fifth year.

Prenatal Period. There are two primary ossification centers, ventral and dorsal, for the centrum (Fig. 15-6C). These **primary ossification centers** soon fuse to form one center. Three primary centers are present by the end of the embryonic period: one in the centrum and one in each half of the vertebral arch. Ossification becomes evident in the vertebral arches during the eighth week. At birth each vertebra consists of three bony parts connected by cartilage (Fig. 15–6D).

Postnatal Period. The halves of the vertebral arch usually fuse during the first three to five years. The laminae of the arches first unite in the lumbar region and union progresses cranially. The vertebral arch articulates with the centrum at cartilaginous *neurocentral joints*. These articulations permit the vertebral arches to grow as the spinal cord enlarges. These joints disappear when the vertebral arch fuses with the centrum during the third to sixth years.

Five **secondary ossification centers** appear *in the vertebrae after puberty*: one for the tip of the spinous process, one for the tip of each transverse process, and two rim or *anular epiphyses*, one on the superior and one on the inferior rim of the vertebral body (Fig. 15–6E). The *vertebral body* is a composite of the superior and inferior anular epiphyses and the mass of bone between them. It includes the centrum, parts of the vertebral arch, and the facets for the heads of the ribs. All secondary centers unite with the rest of the vertebra at about 25 years of age.

Ossification of Atypical Vertebrae. Exceptions to the typical ossification of vertebrae occur in the atlas (C1), axis (C2), C7, lumbar vertebrae, sacrum, and coccyx. For details of their ossification, consult Williams et al. (1989).

Variation in the Number of Vertebrae. About 95 per cent of people have seven cervical, 12 thoracic, five lumbar, and five sacral vertebrae. About three per cent of people have one or two more vertebrae, and about two per cent have one less. To determine the number of vertebrae, it is necessary to examine the entire vertebral column because an apparent extra (or absent) vertebra in one segment of the column may be compensated for by an absent (or extra) vertebra in an adjacent segment; e.g., 11 thoracic-type vertebrae with six lumbar-type vertebrae.

Development of Ribs

The ribs develop from the mesenchymal costal processes of the thoracic vertebrae (Fig. 15–6A). They become cartilaginous during the embryonic period and ossify during the fetal period. The original site of union of the costal processes with the vertebra is replaced by *costovertebral joints*. These are the plane type of synovial joint (Fig. 15–6D). Seven pairs of ribs (1 to 7) called *true ribs* attach via their own cartilages to the sternum. Five pairs of ribs (8 to 12) are called *false ribs* because they attach to the sternum through the cartilage of another rib or ribs. The last two pairs of ribs (11 and 12) do not attach to the sternum and, because of this, are called *floating ribs*.

Development of the Sternum

A pair of mesenchymal vertical bands called *sternal bars* develop ventrolaterally in the body wall. *Chondrification* occurs in these bars as they move medially and fuse craniocaudally in the median plane to form cartilaginous models of the manubrium, sternebrae (segments of the body), and xiphoid process. Fusion at the inferior end of the sternum is sometimes incomplete. As a result, the xiphoid process in these infants is bifid or perforated. Centers of ossification appear craniocaudally in the sternum before birth except that for the xiphoid process, which appears during childhood.

Development of the Skull

The skull develops from mesenchyme around the developing brain. It consists of the *neurocranium*, a protective case for the brain, and the *viscerocranium*, the skeleton of the face.

Cartilaginous Neurocranium (Fig. 15–7). Initially, the cartilaginous neurocranium or *chondrocranium* consists of the cartilaginous base of the developing skull, which forms by fusion of several cartilages. Later, endochondral ossification of the chondrocranium forms the bones of the base of the skull. The ossification pattern of the cranial bones has a definite sequence, beginning with the frontal bone and followed by the occipital bone, basisphenoid bone, and ethmoid bone (Kjaer, 1990).

The *parachordal cartilage*, or basal plate, forms around the cranial end of the notochord and fuses with the cartilages derived from the sclerotome regions of the occipital somites. This cartilaginous mass contributes to the base of the occipital bone; later, extensions grow around the cranial end of the spinal cord and form the boundaries of the foramen magnum.

The *hypophyseal cartilage* forms around the developing hypophysis cerebri, or pituitary gland, and fuses to form the body of the sphenoid bone. The *trabeculae cranii* fuse to form the body of the ethmoid bone. The *ala orbitalis* forms the lesser wing of the sphenoid bone.

Otic capsules appear around the developing internal ears or otic vesicles (see Chapter 19) and form the petrous and mastoid portions of the temporal bone. *Nasal capsules* develop around the nasal sacs (see Chapter 10) and contribute to the formation of the ethmoid bone.

Membranous Neurocranium (Figs. 15–7D and 15–8). Intramembranous ossification occurs in the mesenchyme at the sides and top of the brain, forming the *calvaria* (cranial vault). During fetal life and in-

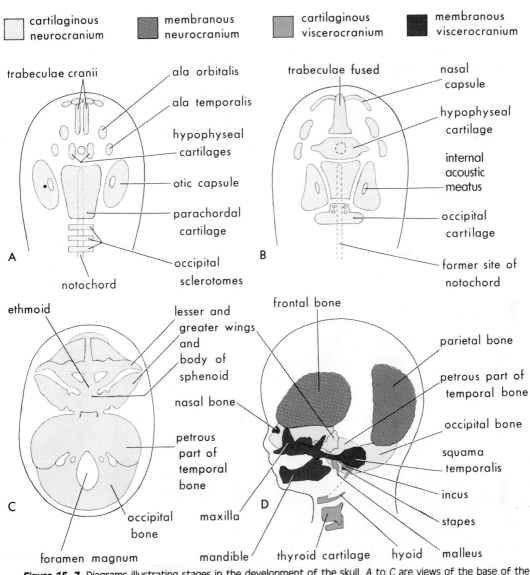

cartilaginous neurocranium

membranous neurocranium

cartilaginous viscerocranium

membranous viscerocranium

Figure 15–7. Diagrams illustrating stages in the development of the skull. *A* to *C* are views of the base of the developing skull (as viewed superiorly). *D* is a lateral view. *A*, Six weeks, showing the various cartilages that will fuse to form the chondrocranium. *B*, Seven weeks after fusion of some of the paired cartilages. *C*, 12 weeks, showing the cartilaginous base of the skull or chondrocranium formed by the fusion of various cartilages. *D*, 20 weeks, indicating the derivation of the bones of the fetal skull.

fancy, the flat bones of the calvaria are separated by dense connective tissue membranes that constitute fibrous joints called *sutures* (Fig. 15–8). Six large fibrous areas called **fontanelles** are present where several sutures meet (Sundaresan, 1990). The softness of the bones and their loose connections at the sutures enable the calvaria to undergo changes of shape during birth called molding. During **molding of the fetal skull**, the frontal bone becomes flat, the occipital bone is drawn out, and one parietal bone slightly

overrides the other one. Within a day or so after birth, the shape of the calvaria returns to normal.

Cartilaginous Viscerocranium. This part of the fetal skull is derived from the cartilaginous skeleton of the first two pairs of branchial or pharyngeal arches (see Fig. 10–4). The dorsal end of the *first arch cartilage* (Meckel cartilage) forms two middle ear bones: the malleus and the incus (see Fig. 19–16). The dorsal end of the *second arch cartilage* (Reichert cartilage) forms the stapes of the middle ear and the styloid

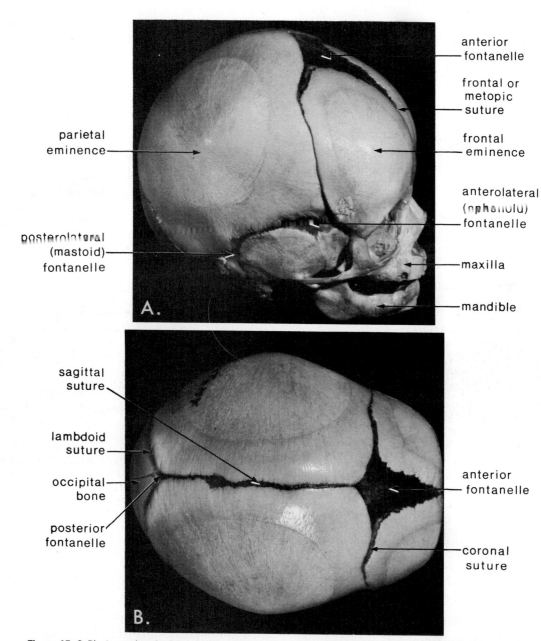

anterior
fontanelle

frontal or
metopic
suture

frontal
eminence

anterolateral
(sphenoid)
fontanelle

maxilla

mandible

parietal
eminence

posterolateral
(mastoid)
fontanelle

A.

sagittal
suture

lambdoid
suture

occipital
bone

posterior
fontanelle

anterior
fontanelle

coronal
suture

B.

Figure 15–8. Photographs of a fetal skull showing the bones, fontanelles, and connecting sutures. *A*, Lateral view. *B*, Superior view. The posterior and anterolateral fontanelles disappear, due to growth of surrounding bones, within two or three months after birth, but they remain as sutures for several years. The posterolateral fontanelles disappear in a similar manner by the end of the first year and the anterior fontanelle by the end of the second year. The two halves of the frontal bone normally begin to fuse during the second year, and the frontal or metopic suture is often obliterated by the eighth year. The other sutures begin to disappear during adult life, but the times when the sutures close are subject to wide variations.

process of the temporal bone. Its ventral end ossifies to form the lesser cornu and superior part of the body of the hyoid bone. The *third, fourth, and sixth arch cartilages* form only in the ventral portions of the arches. The third arch cartilages give rise to the greater cornua and inferior part of the body of the hyoid bone. The fourth and sixth arch cartilages fuse to form the laryngeal cartilages except for the epiglottis (see Fig. 10–4).

Membranous Viscerocranium. Intramembranous ossification occurs in the maxillary prominence of the first branchial or pharyngeal arch (see Fig. 10–1*F*) and subsequently forms the squamous temporal, maxillary, and zygomatic bones. The squamous temporal bones become part of the neurocranium. The mesenchyme in the mandibular prominence of the first arch condenses around its cartilage (Meckel cartilage) and undergoes intramembranous ossification to form the mandible. Some endochondral ossification occurs in the median plane of the chin and in the mandibular condyle.

The Newborn Skull. After recovering from molding (p. 361), the newborn skull is rather round and its bones are thin. Like the fetal skull (Fig. 15–8), it is large in proportion to the rest of the skeleton, and the face is relatively small compared with the calvaria. The small facial region is a result of the small size of the jaws, the virtual absence of paranasal air sinuses, and the general underdevelopment of the facial bones at this stage.

Postnatal Growth of the Skull. The fibrous sutures of the newborn calvaria permit the brain to enlarge during infancy and childhood. The increase in the size of the calvaria is greatest during the first two years, the period of most rapid postnatal growth of the brain. The calvaria normally increases in capacity until 15 to 16 years of age. After this, it usually increases slightly in size for three to four years due to thickening of its bones.

There is also rapid growth of the face and jaws, coinciding with the eruption of the primary or deciduous teeth. These changes are still more marked after the secondary or permanent teeth erupt (see Chapter 20). There is concurrent enlargement of the frontal and facial regions associated with the increase in the size of the paranasal sinuses. Most paranasal sinuses are rudimentary or absent at birth. Growth of these sinuses is important in altering the shape of the face and in adding resonance to the voice.

Anomalies of the Axial Skeleton

Klippel-Feil Syndrome (Brevicollis). The main features of this syndrome are short neck, low hairline, and restricted neck movements. In most cases the number of cervical vertebral bodies is less than normal. In some cases there is a lack of segmentation of several elements of the cervical region of the vertebral column. The number of cervical nerve roots may also be normal, but they are small, as are the intervertebral foramina. Patients with this syndrome are often otherwise normal, but the association of this malformation with other congenital anomalies is not uncommon.

Spina Bifida (see Fig. 18–12*A*). Defective closure of the neural tube leads to a condition known as spina bifida. Most cases (80 per cent) are "open" and covered by a thin membrane; whereas, the "closed" spina bifida or spina bifida occulta is covered by a thick membrane or skin. This defect of the vertebral arch is a consequence of failure of fusion of the halves of the vertebral arch. It is commonly observed in radiographs of the cervical, lumbar, and sacral regions. Frequently only one vertebra is affected. Spina bifida occulta is a relatively minor, insignificant abnormality of the vertebral column that usually causes no clinical symptoms. It can be diagnosed *in utero* by sonography (Filly, 1991a).

Spina bifida occulta of the first sacral vertebra occurs in about 20 per cent of vertebral columns that are examined radiographically (Behrman, 1992). The spinal cord and spinal nerves are usually normal, and neurological symptoms are commonly absent. The skin over the bifid spine is intact, and there may be no external evidence of the vertebral defect. Sometimes the anomaly is indicated by a dimple or a tuft of hair. In about three per cent of normal adults, there is spina bifida occulta of the atlas. At other cervical levels, this condition is rare; and, when present, it is sometimes accompanied by other abnormalities of the cervical region of the vertebral column.

Spina bifida cystica (see Fig. 18–14), a severe type of spina bifida involving the spinal cord and meninges, is discussed in Chapter 18 (p. 395). Neurological symptoms are usually present in these patients.

Accessory Ribs (Fig. 15–9*A*). Accessory ribs, which may be rudimentary or well developed, result from the development of the costal processes of cervical or lumbar vertebrae. These processes form ribs in the thoracic region. The most common type of accessory rib is a *lumbar rib*, but it causes no problems (Moore, 1992). *Cervical ribs* are less common (0.5 to one per cent of people), and genetic factors may play a role in their occurrence. A cervical rib is attached to the seventh cervical vertebra and may be unilateral or bilateral (McNally et al., 1990). Pressure of a cervical rib on the brachial plexus or the subclavian artery often produces symptoms (Moore, 1992).

Fused Ribs. Fusion of ribs occasionally occurs posteriorly when two or more ribs arise from a single vertebra. Fused ribs are often associated with a hemivertebra.

Hemivertebra (Fig. 15–9*B*). The developing vertebral bodies have two chondrification centers that soon unite (Fig. 15–6*B*). A hemivertebra results from failure of one of the chondrification centers to appear and subsequent failure of half of the vertebra to form. These defective vertebrae produce *scoliosis* (lateral curvature) of the vertebral column (Moore, 1992). There are other causes of scoliosis, e.g., myopathic scoliosis due to weakness of the spinal muscles.

Rachischisis (Fig. 15–10*C*). The term *rachischisis* (cleft vertebral column) refers to the vertebral abnormalities in a

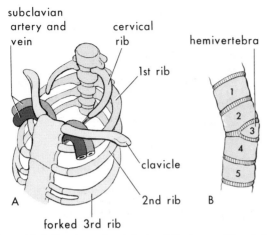

Figure 15–9. Drawings of vertebral and rib abnormalities. *A,* Cervical and forked ribs. Observe that the left cervical rib has a fibrous band that passes posterior to the subclavian vessels and attaches to the sternum. This condition very likely produced neurovascular changes in the left upper limb. *B,* Anterior view of the vertebral column showing a hemivertebra. The right half of the third thoracic vertebra is absent. Note the associated lateral curvature (scoliosis) of the vertebral column.

complex group of anomalies (*axial dysraphic disorders*) that primarily affect axial structures. In these infants the neural folds fail to fuse, either due to faulty induction by the underlying notochord or because of the action of teratogenic agents on the neuroepithelial cells in the neural folds. The neural and vertebral defects may be extensive (Fig. 15–10) or may be restricted to a small area (see Fig. 18–15).

Cleft Sternum. Minor sternal clefts (e.g., a notch or foramen in the xiphoid process) are common and of no clinical concern. A *sternal foramen* of varying size and form occurs occasionally at the junction of the third and fourth sternebrae. This insignificant foramen is the result of incomplete fusion of the cartilaginous sternal bars during the embryonic period.

Skull Anomalies. These abnormalities range from major defects that are incompatible with life to those that are minor and insignificant. With large defects, there is often herniation of the meninges and/or brain (see Figs. 18–30 and 18–31).

Acrania (Fig. 15–10). In this condition the calvaria is absent, and extensive defects of the vertebral column are often present. Acrania associated with *meroanencephaly* (partial absence of the brain [often called anencephaly]) occurs about once in 1000 births and is incompatible with

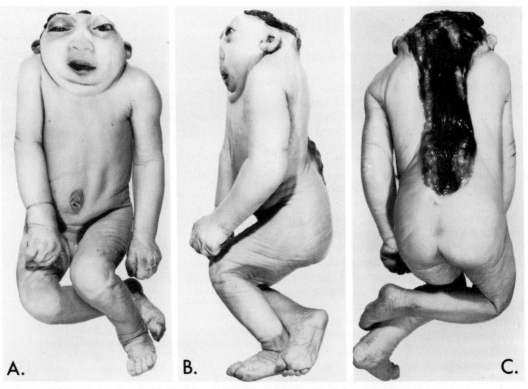

Figure 15–10. Photographs of anterior, lateral, and posterior views of a newborn infant with acrania (absence of the calvaria), meroanencephaly (partial absence of the brain), rachischisis (extensive cleft in the vertebral column), and myeloschisis (severe malformation of the spinal cord). Infants with these severe craniovertebral malformations involving the brain and spinal cord usually die within a few days after birth. For more information about meroanencephaly and spina bifida with myeloschisis, see Chapter 18.

life. This anomaly is the result of failure of the cranial end of the neural tube to close during the fourth week. This defect causes subsequent failure of the calvaria to form (acrania).

Craniosynostosis (Figs. 15–11 and 15–12). Several skull deformities result from premature closure of the skull sutures. Prenatal closure results in the most severe abnormalities. The cause of craniosynostosis is unknown, but genetic factors appear to be important. These abnormalities are much more common in males than in females, and they are often associated with other skeletal anomalies. The type of deformed skull produced depends upon which sutures close prematurely. If the sagittal suture closes early, the skull becomes long, narrow and wedge-shaped (*scaphocephaly* [Fig. 15–11]). This type constitutes about half the cases of craniosynostosis. Another 30 per cent of cases involve premature closure of the coronal suture. This results in a high, towerlike skull (*oxycephaly* or turricephaly [Fig. 15–12*A*]). If the coronal or lambdoid suture closes prematurely on one side only, the skull is twisted and asymmetrical (*plagiocephaly* [Fig. 15–12*B*]).

Microcephaly (see Fig. 18–33). Infants with this condition are born with a normal-sized or slightly small calvaria. The fontanelles close during early infancy, and the sutures close during the first year. This anomaly is not caused by premature closure of sutures. Microcephaly is the result of abnormal development of the central nervous system in which the brain and, consequently, the skull fail to grow. Generally, microcephalics are severely mentally retarded. This CNS anomaly is discussed in Chapter 18.

Anomalies at the Craniovertebral Junction. Congenital abnormalities at the craniovertebral junction are present in about one per cent of newborn infants, but they may not produce symptoms until adult life. The following are examples of these malformations: *basilar invagination* (superior displacement of the bone around the foramen magnum); *assimilation of the atlas* (nonsegmentation at the junction of the atlas and occipital bone); *atlantoaxial dislocation*; Arnold-Chiari malformation (see Chapter 18); and *separate dens* or odontoid process (failure of the centers in the dens to fuse with the centrum of the axis).

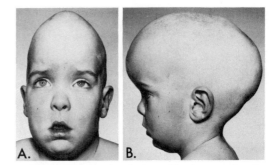

Figure 15–11. Photographs of a boy with a long, wedge-shaped skull (scaphocephaly) resulting from craniosynostosis or premature closure of the sagittal suture. (From Laurence KM, Weeks R: *In* Norman AP [ed]: *Congenital Abnormalities of Infancy.* 2nd ed. 1971. Courtesy of Blackwell Scientific Publications.)

Ossification begins in the long bones by the eighth week of embryonic development and initially occurs in the diaphyses of the bones from *primary centers of ossification* (Fig. 15–3*F* to *J*). By 12 weeks, primary ossification centers have appeared in nearly all bones of the limbs (Fig. 15–14). The clavicles begin to ossify before any other bones in the body. The femora are the next bones to show traces of ossification. The first indication of ossification in the cartilaginous model of a long bone is visible near the center of the future body (shaft); this is the primary center of ossification. Primary centers appear at different times in different bones, but most of them appear between the seventh and twelfth weeks of development. Virtually all of them are present by birth. The part of a bone ossified from a primary center is called the **diaphysis**.

The *secondary ossification centers* of the bones at the knee are the first to appear. The centers for the distal end of the femur and the proximal end of the tibia usually appear during the last month of intrauterine life (34 to 38 weeks after fertilization). Consequently, they are usually present at birth; however,

THE APPENDICULAR SKELETON

The appendicular skeleton consists of the pectoral and pelvic girdles and the limb bones. Mesenchymal bones appear during the fifth week as condensations of mesenchyme appear in the limb buds. During the sixth week the mesenchymal bone models in the limbs undergo chondrification to form hyaline cartilage models (Fig. 15–13*D* and *E*). The clavicle initially develops by intramembranous ossification, but it later develops growth cartilages at both ends. The models of the pectoral girdle (shoulder girdle) and upper limb bones appear slightly before those of the pelvic girdle and lower limb, and the bone models appear in a proximodistal sequence.

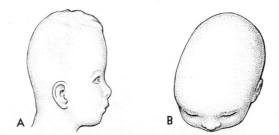

Figure 15–12. Drawings illustrating skull malformations. *A*, Oxycephaly (turricephaly), showing the towerlike skull resulting from premature closure of the coronal suture. *B*, Plagiocephaly, illustrating a type of asymmetrical skull resulting from premature closure of the coronal and lambdoid sutures on the left side.

most secondary centers of ossification appear after birth. The part of a bone ossified from a secondary center is called the **epiphysis**.

The bone formed from the primary center in the diaphysis does not fuse with that formed from the secondary centers in the epiphyses until the bone grows to its adult length. This delay enables lengthening of the bone to continue until the final size is reached. During bone growth, a plate of cartilage known as the *epiphyseal cartilage plate* intervenes between the diaphysis and the epiphysis (Fig. 15–3). The epiphyseal plate is eventually replaced by bone development on each of its two sides, diaphyseal and epiphyseal. When this occurs, growth of the bone ceases.

Bone age is a good index of general maturation. Determination of the number, size, and fusion of epiphyseal centers from radiographs is a commonly used method. A radiologist determines the bone age of a person by assessing the ossification centers using two criteria: *First,* the appearance of calcified material in the diaphysis and/or the epiphysis is specific for each diaphysis and epiphysis and for each bone and sex; *second,* the disappearance of the dark line representing the epiphyseal cartilage plate indicates that the epiphysis has fused with the diaphysis. Fusion of the epiphyseal centers, which occurs at specific times for each epiphysis, happens one to two years earlier in females than in males. Real-time ultrasonography is now increasingly used for the evaluation and measurement of fetal bones as well as for the determination of gestational age (van der Harten, 1990; Filly, 1991b).

Generalized Skeletal Anomalies

Achondroplasia (see Fig. 8–10). This condition is the most common cause of *dwarfism* (shortness of stature). It occurs about once in 10,000 births. The limbs are short because of disturbance of endochondral ossification at the epiphyseal cartilage plates, particularly of long bones, dur-

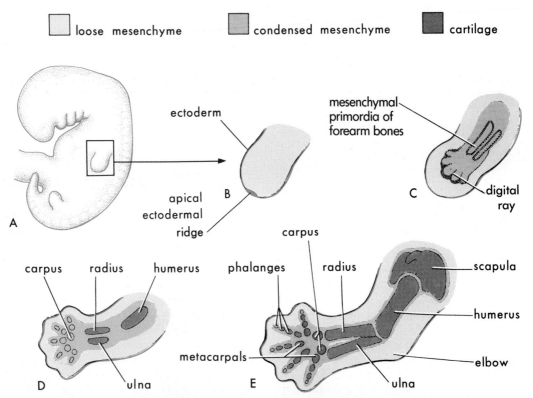

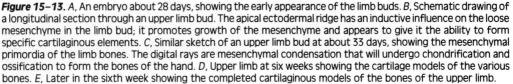

Figure 15–13. *A,* An embryo about 28 days, showing the early appearance of the limb buds. *B,* Schematic drawing of a longitudinal section through an upper limb bud. The apical ectodermal ridge has an inductive influence on the loose mesenchyme in the limb bud; it promotes growth of the mesenchyme and appears to give it the ability to form specific cartilaginous elements. *C,* Similar sketch of an upper limb bud at about 33 days, showing the mesenchymal primordia of the limb bones. The digital rays are mesenchymal condensation that will undergo chondrification and ossification to form the bones of the hand. *D,* Upper limb at six weeks showing the cartilage models of the various bones. *E,* Later in the sixth week showing the completed cartilaginous models of the bones of the upper limb.

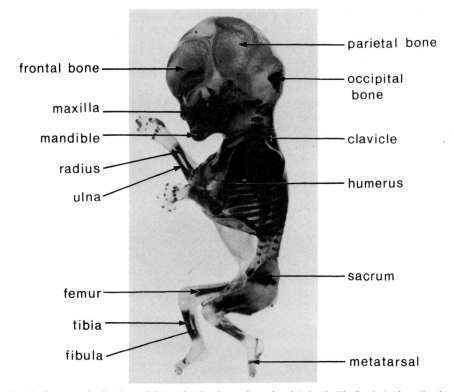

frontal bone

maxilla

mandible

radius

ulna

femur

tibia

fibula

parietal bone

occipital bone

clavicle

humerus

sacrum

metatarsal

Figure 15–14. Photograph of a 12-week fetus that has been cleared and stained with alizarin to show the developing skeleton. Observe the ossification from the primary centers. (Courtesy of Dr. Gary Geddes, Portland, Oregon.)

ing fetal life. The trunk is normal length, but the head may be slightly enlarged with a bulging forehead and "scooped-out" nose. Achondroplasia is an *autosomal dominant disorder*, and about 80 per cent of cases arise from new mutations; the rate increases with paternal age (Strewler, 1985). For details of its inheritance, see Thompson et al. (1991).

Hyperpituitarism. Congenital infantile hyperpituitarism is rare. It causes the infant to grow at an abnormally rapid rate. This may result in *gigantism* (excessive height and body proportions) or *acromegaly* (enlargement of the soft tissues, visceral organs, and bones of the face, hands, and feet). In acromegaly the epiphyseal and diaphyseal centers of the long bones fuse, thereby preventing any elongation of these bones. Both gigantism and acromegaly are the result of an excessive secretion of growth hormone (McCann, 1988).

Hypothyroidism and Cretinism. A severe deficiency of fetal thyroid hormone production results in cretinism, a condition characterized by growth retardation, mental deficiency, skeletal abnormalities, and auditory and neurological disorders. Bone age appears as less than chronological age because epiphyseal development is delayed (Griffin, 1988). Cretinism is very rare except in areas where there is a lack of iodine in the soil and water. Agenesis of the thyroid gland also results in cretinism.

SUMMARY

The skeletal system develops from mesenchyme derived from mesoderm and the neural crest. In most bones, such as the long bones in the limbs, the condensed mesenchyme undergoes chondrification to form cartilage bone models. Ossification centers appear in these models by the end of the embryonic period, and the bones ossify later by *endochondral ossification*. Some bones (e.g., the flat bones of the skull) develop by *intramembranous ossification*. The vertebral column and ribs develop from mesenchymal cells from the sclerotomes of the somites. Each vertebra is formed by fusion of a condensation of the caudal half of one pair of *sclerotomes* with the cranial half of the subjacent pair of sclerotomes.

The developing skull consists of a neurocranium and a viscerocranium, each of which has membranous and cartilaginous components. The neurocranium forms the *calvaria*, a protective case for the brain. The viscerocranium forms the skeleton of the face.

The appendicular skeleton develops from endochondral ossification of the cartilaginous bone models, which form from mesenchyme in the developing limbs.

Joints are classified as: (1) fibrous joints, (2) cartilaginous joints, or (3) synovial joints (Fig. 15–4). They develop from interzonal mesenchyme between the primordia of bones. In a fibrous joint the intervening mesenchyme differentiates into dense fibrous connective tissue. In a cartilaginous joint the mesen-chyme between the bones differentiates into cartilage. In a synovial joint a *synovial cavity* is formed within the intervening mesenchyme by breakdown of the cells. The mesenchyme also gives rise to the synovial membrane and the capsular and other ligaments of the joint.

Although there are numerous types of skeletal anomaly, most of them, except for spina bifida occulta and accessory ribs, are rare.

CLINICALLY ORIENTED QUESTIONS FOR PROBLEM-BASED LEARNING SESSIONS

1. What is the most common congenital anomaly of the vertebral column? Where is the defect usually located? Does this congenital anomaly usually cause symptoms (e.g., back problems)?
2. Occasionally rudimentary ribs are associated with the seventh cervical vertebra and the first lumbar vertebra. Are these accessory ribs of clinical importance? What is the embryological basis of a cervical rib?
3. What vertebral defect can produce scoliosis? Define this condition. What is the embryological basis of the vertebral defect?
4. What is meant by the term *craniosynostosis*? What results from this developmental abnormality? Give a common example.
5. A child presented with characteristics of the Klippel-Feil syndrome. What are the main features of this condition? What vertebral abnormalities are usually present?

The answers to these questions are given on page 465.

References and Suggested Reading

Bagnall KM, Harris PF, Jones PR: A radiographic study of the human fetal spine. *J Anat 123*:777, 1977.

Behrman RE (ed): *Nelson Textbook of Pediatrics.* 14th ed. Philadelphia, WB Saunders, 1992.

Benjamin M, Evans EJ: Fibrocartilage Research Review. *J Anat 171*:1, 1990.

Blechschmidt E, Gasser RF: *Biokinetics and Biodynamics of Human Differentiation.* Springfield, Ill, Charles C Thomas, 1978.

Bruder SP, Caplan AL: Cellular and molecular events during embryonic bone development. *Connect Tissue Res 20*:65, 1989.

Budorick NE, Pretorius DH, Grafe MR, Lou KV: Ossification of the fetal spine. *Radiology 181*:561, 1991.

Caplan AL: Mesenchymal stem cells. *J Orthop Res 9*:641, 1991.

Cohen Jr, MM: Syndrome delineation and its implications for the study of pathogenetic mechanisms. *In* Persaud TVN (ed): *Advances in the Study of Birth Defects.* Vol 5. *Genetic Disorders.* New York, Alan R. Liss, 1982.

Cole DEC, Cohen Jr, MM: Osteogenesis imperfecta. An update. *J Pediatr 119*:73, 1991.

Craig FM, Bayliss MT, Bentley G, Archer CW: A role for hyaluronan in joint development. *J Anat 171*:17, 1990.

Daniels K, Solursh M: Modulation of chondrogenesis by the cytoskeleton and extracellular matrix. *J Cell Sci 100 (Pt. 2)*:249, 1991.

Davis JE, Kalousek DK: Fetal akinesia deformation sequence in previable fetuses. *Am J Med Genet 29*:77, 1988.

Dennison WM: Spina bifida. *In* Mustardé JC (ed): *Plastic Surgery in Infancy and Childhood.* Edinburgh, E & S Livingstone, 1971.

Dhem A, Goret-Nicaise M, Dambrain R, Nyssen-Behets C, Lengele B, Manzanares MC: Skeletal growth and chondroid tissue. *Arch Ital Anat Embriol 94*:237, 1989.

Dziedzic-Goclawska A, Emerich J, Grzesik W, Stachowicz W, Michalik J, Ostrowski K: Differences in the kinetics of the mineralization process in endochondral and intramembranous osteogenesis in human fetal development. *J Bone Miner Res 3*:533, 1988.

Filly RA: The fetus with a CNS malformation: ultrasound evaluation. *In* Harrison MR, Golbus MS, Filly RA (eds): *The Unborn Patient: Prenatal Diagnosis and Treatment.* 2nd ed. Philadelphia, WB Saunders, 1991a.

Filly RA: Sonographic anatomy of the normal fetus. *In* Harrison MR, Golbus MS, Filly RA (eds): *The Unborn Patient. Prenatal Diagnosis and Treatment.* 2nd ed. Philadelphia, WB Saunders, 1991b.

Filly RA, Golbus MS: Ultrasonography of the normal and pathologic fetal skeleton. *Radiol Clin North Am 20*:311, 1982.

Ford EHR: The growth of the foetal skull. *J Anat 90*:63, 1956.

Gasser RF: Evidence that sclerotomal cells do not migrate medially during normal embryonic development of the rat. *Am J Anat 154*:509, 1979.

Gray DJ, Gardner E, O'Rahilly R: The prenatal development of the skeleton and joints of the human hand. *Am J Anat 101*:169, 1957.

Griffin JE: The thyroid. *In* Griffin JE, Ojeda SR (eds): *Textbook of Endrocine Physiology*. New York, Oxford Press, 1988.

Kjaer I: Ossification of the human fetal basicranium. *J Craniofac Genet Dev Biol 10*:29, 1990.

Koenig MP: Endemic goiter and endemic cretinism. *In* Gardner LI (ed): *Endocrine and Genetic Diseases of Childhood and Adolescence*. 2nd ed. Philadelphia, WB Saunders, 1975.

Marin-Padilla M: Cephalic axial skeletal-neural dysraphic disorders: embryology and pathology. *Can J Neurol Sci 18*:153, 1991.

Marks Jr, SC, Popoff SN: Bone cell biology: the regulation of development, structure, and function in the skeleton. *Am J Anat 183*:1, 1988.

McCann SM: The anterior pituitary and hypothalamus. *In* Griffin JE, Ojeda SR (eds): *Textbook of Endocrine Physiology*. New York, Oxford Press, 1988.

McNally E, Sandin B, Wilkins RA: The ossification of the costal element of the seventh cervical vertebra with particular reference to cervical ribs. *J Anat 170*:125, 1990.

Moore KL: *Clinically Oriented Anatomy*. 3rd ed. Baltimore, Williams & Wilkins, 1992.

Noback CR, Robertson GG: Sequences of appearance of ossification centers in the human skeleton during the first five prenatal months. *Am J Anat 89*:1, 1951.

O'Rahilly R, Müller F, Meyer DB: The human vertebral column at the end of the embryonic period proper. 3. The thoracicolumbar region. *J Anat 168*:81, 1990a.

O'Rahilly R, Müller F, Meyer DB: The human vertebral column at the end of the embryonic period proper. 4. The sacrococcygeal region. *J Anat 168*:95, 1990b.

Smith MM, Hall BK: Development and evolutionary origins of vertebrate skeletogenic and odontogenic tissue. *Biol Rev Camb Philos Soc 65*:277, 1990.

Sperber GH: *Craniofacial Embryology*. 4th ed. London, Butterworth, 1989.

Stedman H, Sarkar S: Molecular genetics in basic myology: a rapidly evolving perspective. *Muscle Nerve II*:668, 1988.

Strewler GJ: Osteonecrosis, osteosclerosis and other disorders of bone. *In* Wyngaarden JB, Smith Jr, LH (eds): *Cecil Textbook of Medicine*. 17th ed. Philadelphia, WB Saunders, 1985.

Sundaresan M, Wright M, Price AB: Anatomy and development of the fontanelle. *Arch Dis Child 65*:386, 1990.

Thompson MW, McInnes RR, Willard HF: *Thompson & Thompson Genetics in Medicine*. 5th ed. Philadelphia, WB Saunders, 1991.

Uhthoff HK: *The Embryology of the Human Locomotor System*. New York, Springer-Verlag, 1990.

van der Harten HJ, Brons JT, Schipper NW, Dijkstra PF, Meijer CJ, van Geijin HP: The prenatal development of the normal human skeleton: a combined ultrasonographic and post-mortem radiographic study. *Pediatr Radiol 21*:52, 1990.

Williams PL, Warwick R, Dyson M, Bannister LH: *Gray's Anatomy*. 37th ed. London, Churchill Livingstone, 1989.

16
The Muscular System

The muscular system develops from *intraembryonic mesoderm* except for the muscles of the iris, which develop from ectoderm (p. 427). Muscle tissue develops from embryonic cells called *myoblasts*, which are derived from mesenchyme (embryonic connective tissue). Much of the mesenchyme in the head is derived from the neural crest (see Figs. 4–8 and 5–5), particularly the tissue associated with the branchial or pharyngeal apparatus (Chapter 10); however, the original mesenchyme in the arches gives rise to the musculature of the face and neck (see Fig. 10–6 and Table 10–1).

SKELETAL MUSCLE

The myoblasts that form the skeletal muscles of the trunk are derived from mesoderm in the myotome regions of the somites (see Figs. 15–1 and 16–1). The limb muscles develop from mesenchyme in the limb buds that is derived from somatic mesoderm. The tongue muscles form from head mesenchyme; and, many muscles of the face, jaws, neck, and shoulders, develop from mesenchyme in the branchial or pharyngeal arches (Chapter 10).

The first indication of muscle development is the elongation of the nuclei and cell bodies of mesenchymal cells as they differentiate into *myoblasts*. Soon these primordial muscle cells begin to fuse with one another to form elongated, multinucleated, cylindrical structures called *myotubes*. For a review of recent work on muscle protein genetics and the genetic control and regulation of muscle differentiation, see Stedman and Sarkar (1988), Olson (1990), and Sutherland et al. (1991).

Muscle growth is the result of fusion of myoblasts and myotubes. Myofilaments develop in the cytoplasm of the myotubes during or soon after fusion of the myoblasts. Soon, myofibrils and other organelles characteristic of striated muscle cells develop. Because muscle cells are long and narrow, it is customary to call them muscle fibers. As the myotubes differentiate into muscle fibers, they become invested with external laminae, individually or in groups, which segregates them from the surrounding connective tissue.

Most skeletal muscle develops before birth, and almost all the remaining ones are formed by the end of the first year. Increase in the size of a muscle occurs as the result of an increase in the diameter of the fibers through the formation of more myofilaments. After birth, muscles increase in length and width in order to grow with the skeleton. Their ultimate size depends on the amount of exercise that is performed. Not all embryonic muscle fibers persist; many of them fail to establish themselves as necessary units of the muscle and soon degenerate.

Myotomes. Each typical myotome divides into a small dorsal *epaxial division* and a larger ventral *hypaxial division* (Fig. 16–1B). Each developing spinal nerve also divides and sends a branch to each division, the dorsal primary ramus supplying the epaxial division, and the ventral primary ramus supplying the hypaxial division. Some muscles remain segmentally arranged like the somites (e.g., the intercostal muscles), but most myoblasts migrate away from the myotomes and form nonsegmented muscles.

Derivatives of the Epaxial Divisions of Myotomes (Fig. 16–2). Myoblasts from these parts of the myotomes form the extensor muscles of the neck, the extensor muscles of the vertebral column, and the lumbar extensor musculature. The extensor muscles derived from the sacral and coccygeal myotomes degenerate; their adult derivatives are the dorsal sacrococcygeal ligaments.

Derivatives of the Hypaxial Divisions of Myotomes (Fig. 16–2). Myoblasts from the cervical myotomes form the scalene, prevertebral, geniohyoid, and infrahyoid muscles. The thoracic myotomes form the lateral and ventral flexor muscles of the vertebral column, and the lumbar myotomes form the quadratus lumborum muscle. The sacrococcygeal myotomes form the muscles of the pelvic diaphragm and probably the striated muscles of the anus and sex organs.

Branchial or Pharyngeal Arch Muscles (see Fig. 10–5). The migration of myoblasts from these arches to form the muscles of mastication, facial expression,

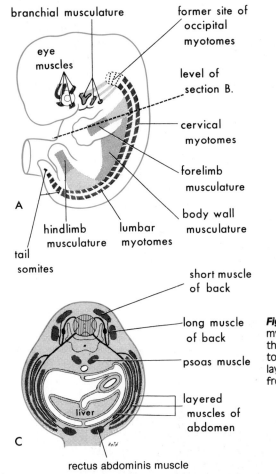

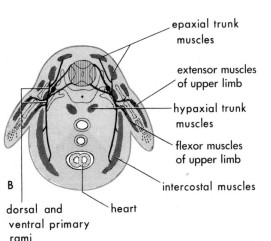

Figure 16–1. *A*, Sketch of an embryo (about 41 days), showing the myotomes and developing muscular system. *B*, Transverse section of the embryo, illustrating the epaxial and hypaxial derivatives of a myotome. *C*, Similar section of a seven-week embryo, showing the muscle layers formed from the myotomes. The limb muscles develop in situ from somatic mesoderm.

pharynx, and larynx is described in Chapter 10 (see Fig. 10–6 and Table 10–1). These muscles are innervated by branchial arch nerves (see Fig. 10–7).

The Ocular Muscles (Figs. 16–1 and 16–2). The origin of the extrinsic eye muscles is unclear, but it is thought that they may be derived from mesenchymal cells near the prochordal plate (Gilbert, 1957). The mesoderm in this area is thought to give rise to the three *preotic myotomes* (Fig. 16–2*A*). Myoblasts differentiate from mesenchymal cells in these myotomes. Groups of myoblasts, each supplied by its own nerve (CN III, CN IV, or CN VI), form the extrinsic muscles of the eye.

The Tongue Muscles (see Fig. 10–6). Initially there are four indistinct *occipital myotomes*; the first pair disappears. Myoblasts from the remaining three myotomes form the tongue muscles, which are innervated by the hypoglossal nerve (CN XII).

The Limb Muscles (see Figs. 15–13 and 16–1). The musculature of the limbs develops in situ from the mesenchyme surrounding the developing bones.

This mesenchyme is derived from the somatic layer of lateral mesoderm. There is no apparent migration of myotomic mesoderm into the human limb buds (Williams et al., 1989)[1].

SMOOTH MUSCLE

Smooth muscle fibers differentiate from the splanchnic mesenchyme surrounding the endoderm of the primitive gut and its derivatives (see Fig. 15–1). The smooth muscle in the walls of many blood and lymphatic vessels arises from somatic mesoderm. The muscles of the iris (sphincter and dilator pupillae) and the myoepithelial cells of mammary and sweat glands are thought to be derived from mesenchymal cells that originate from ectoderm.

---

[1] It is now generally maintained that the somites do not contribute to the limb buds of human embryos (O'Rahilly and Gardner 1975). The somite origin of limb musculature in the avian limb is well established.

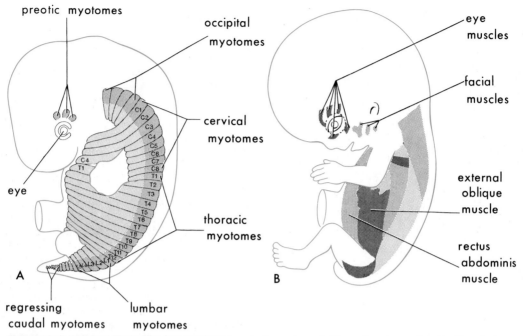

preotic myotomes

occipital
myotomes

eye
muscles

facial
muscles

cervical
myotomes

eye

external
oblique
muscle

thoracic
myotomes

rectus
abdominis
muscle

A

B

regressing
caudal myotomes

lumbar
myotomes

Figure 16–2. Drawings illustrating the developing muscular system. *A,* Six-week embryo, showing the myotome regions of the somites that give rise to most skeletal muscles. *B,* Eight-week embryo, showing the developing superficial trunk musculature. The limb muscles are not illustrated in these drawings (see Fig. 16–1*A* and *B*).

The first sign of differentiation of smooth muscle is the development of elongated nuclei in spindle-shaped cells called myoblasts. During early development, new myoblasts continue to differentiate from mesenchymal cells. During later development, division of existing myoblasts gradually replaces the differentiation of new myoblasts in the production of new smooth muscle tissue. As smooth muscle cells differentiate, filamentous contractile elements develop in their cytoplasm, and the external surface of each cell acquires a surrounding external lamina. As the smooth muscle fibers develop into sheets or bundles, the fibroblasts and/or muscle cells synthesize and lay down collagenous, elastic, and reticular fibers.

CARDIAC MUSCLE

Cardiac muscle develops from splanchnic mesoderm surrounding the developing heart (see Figs. 14–6 and 14–7). Cardiac myoblasts differentiate from the primitive myocardium. Heart muscle is recognizable in the fourth week. Immunohistochemical studies have revealed a spatial distribution of "tissue-specific" antigens (myosin heavy chain isoforms) in the embryonic heart between the fourth and eighth weeks of development (Wessels et al., 1991).

Cardiac muscle fibers arise by differentiation and growth of single cells unlike striated skeletal muscle fibers that develop by fusion of cells. Growth of cardiac muscle fibers is the result of the formation of new myofilaments. The myoblasts adhere to each other as in developing skeletal muscle, but the intervening cell membranes do not disintegrate; these areas of adhesion give rise to the *intercalated discs* (Cormack, 1993).

Late in the embryonic period, special bundles of muscle cells develop with relatively few myofibrils and relatively larger diameters than typical cardiac muscle fibers. These atypical cardiac muscle cells called *Purkinje fibers* form the conducting system of the heart (see Fig. 14–21*D*).

ANOMALIES OF MUSCLES

Absence of one or more muscles is more common than is generally recognized. Usually only a single muscle is absent on one side of the body or only a portion of the muscle fails to develop. Occasionally the same muscle or muscles may be absent on both sides of the body. Any muscle in the body may occasionally be absent; common examples are the sternocostal head of the pectoralis major (Fig. 16–3), the palmaris longus, the trapezius, the serratus anterior, and the quadratus femoris (Moore, 1992).

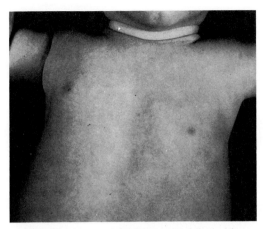

Figure 16–3. Photograph of the thorax of an infant with congenital absence of the left pectoralis major muscle. Note the absence of the anterior axillary fold on the left and the low location of the left nipple. (From Behrman RE: *Nelson Textbook of Pediatrics.* 14th ed. Philadelphia, WB Saunders, 1992).

Absence of the pectoralis major muscle, often its sternal portion, is often associated with syndactyly (fusion of the digits). These anomalies are part of the *Poland syndrome.* Absence of the pectoralis major is occasionally associated with absence of the mammary gland and/or hypoplasia of the nipple (Fig. 16–3).

In rare instances, failure of normal muscle development may be widespread, leading to immobility of multiple joints, a condition known as *arthrogryposis multiplex congenita* (Behrman, 1992). Persons with this disorder have congenital stiffness of one or more joints associated with hypoplasia of the associated muscles.

Some muscular anomalies are of a more serious nature. These include congenital absence of the diaphragm, which is usually associated with severe *pulmonary atelectasis* and pneumonia, and absence of muscle(s) of the anterior abdominal wall, which may be associated with severe gastrointestinal and genitourinary anomalies (see Figs. 13–16 and 13–17). Occasionally individuals with congenital absence of a muscle develop *muscular dystrophy* in later life. The most common association is between congenital absence of the pectoralis major muscle and the Landouzy-Déjérine facioscapulohumeral form of muscular dystrophy (Mastaglia, 1974).

Variations in Muscles

All muscles are subject to a certain amount of variation, but some are affected more often than others. Certain muscles are functionally vestigial (e.g., those of the external ear and scalp). Some muscles present in other primates appear in only some humans (e.g., the sternalis muscle). Variations in the form, position, and attachments of muscles are common and are usually functionally insignificant (Moore, 1992).

The sternocleidomastoid muscle is sometimes injured at birth, resulting in a condition known as *congenital torticollis* (Moore, 1992). There is fixed rotation and tilting of the head due to fibrosis and shortening of the sternocleidomastoid muscle on one side (Fig. 16–4). Some cases of torticollis (wryneck) result from tearing of fibers of the sternocleidomastoid muscle during delivery of the infant. Bleeding into the muscle occurs in a localized area, forming a small swelling called a *hematoma.* Later, a mass develops due to necrosis of muscle fibers and fibrosis (formation of fibrous tissue). Shortening of the muscle usually follows; this causes lateral bending of the head to the affected side and a slight turning away of the head from the side of the short muscle. Although birth trauma is commonly considered as the cause of congenital torticollis, the fact that the condition has been observed in infants delivered by cesarean section suggests that there are other causes in some cases (Behrman, 1992).

SUMMARY

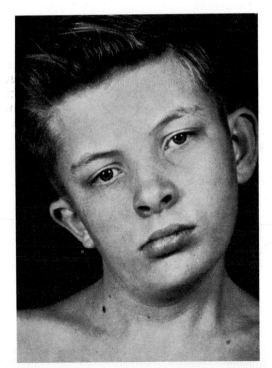

Figure 16–4. Photograph of the head and neck of a 12-year-old boy with congenital torticollis (wryneck). Shortening of the right sternocleidomastoid muscle has caused tilting of the head to the right and turning of the chin to the left. There is also asymmetric development of the face and skull. (From Behrman RE, Vaughan VC, III: *Nelson Textbook of Pediatrics.* 13th ed. Philadelphia, WB Saunders, 1987.)

Most skeletal muscle is derived from the myotome regions of somites. Some head and neck muscles are derived from branchial or pharyngeal arch meso-derm. The limb muscles develop in situ from mesen-chyme derived from somatic mesoderm. Cardiac muscle and most smooth muscle are derived from splanchnic mesoderm. Absence or variation of some muscles is common and is usually of little conse-quence.

CLINICALLY ORIENTED PROBLEMS FOR PROBLEM-BASED LEARNING SESSIONS

1. An infant presented with absence of the left anterior axillary fold. In addition, the left nipple was much lower than usual. Absence of which muscle probably caused these unusual observations? What syndrome would you suspect may be present? For what features would you look? Would the infant be likely to suffer any disability if absence of this muscle was the only anomaly present?

2. A medical student was concerned when she learned that she had only one palmaris longus muscle. Is this a common occurrence? What is its incidence? Does the absence of this muscle cause a disability?

3. The parents of a four-year-old girl observed that she always held her head slightly tilted to the right side and that one of her neck muscles was more prominent than the others. Name the muscle that was likely prominent. Did it pull the child's head to the right side? What is this deformity called? What probably caused the muscle shortening that resulted in this condition?

4. Failure of striated muscle to develop in the median plane of the anterior abdominal wall is associated with the formation of a severe congenital anomaly of the urinary system. What is this anomaly called? What is the probable embryological basis of the failure of muscle to form in these persons?

The answers to these questions are given on page 466.

References

Arey LB: The history of the first somite in human embryos. *Contr Embryol Carneg Instn* 27:235, 1938.

Behrman RE: *Nelson Textbook of Pediatrics.* 14th ed. Philadelphia, WB Saunders, 1992.

Caplan AL: Mesenchymal stem cells. *J Orthop Res* 9:641, 1991.

Cormack DH: *Essential Histology.* Philadelphia, JB Lippincott, 1993.

Deuchar EM: Experimental demonstration of tongue muscle origin in chick embryos. *J Embryol Exp Morphol* 6:527, 1958.

Dubowitz V: *Muscle Disorders in Childhood.* Philadelphia, WB Saunders, 1978.

Gasser RF: The development of the facial muscles in man. *Am J Anat* 120:357, 1967.

Gilbert PW: The origin and development of the human extrinsic ocular muscles. *Contr Embryol Carneg Instn* 36:59, 1957.

Godman JC: On the regeneration and redifferentiation of mammalian striated muscles. *J Morphol* 100:27, 1957.

Kamieniecka Z: The stages of development of human foetal muscles with reference to some muscular diseases. *J Neurol Sci* 7:319, 1968.

Levi AC, Borghi F, Garavoglia M: Development of the anal canal muscles. *Dis Colon Rectum* 34:262, 1991.

Mastaglia FL: The growth and development of skeletal muscles. *In* Davis JA, Dobbing J (eds): *Scientific Foundations of Paediatrics.* Philadelphia, WB Saunders, 1974.

Moore KL: *Clinically Oriented Anatomy.* 3rd ed. Baltimore, Williams & Wilkins., 1992.

Murakami G, Nakamura H: Somites and pattern formation of trunk muscles–a study in quail-chick chimera. *Arch Histol Cytol* 54:249, 1991.

Noden DM: Vertebrate craniofacial development—the relation between ontogenetic process and morphological outcome. *Brain Behav Envol* 38:190, 1991.

Olson EN: MyoD family: a paradigm for development? *Genes Dev* 4:1454, 1990.

O'Rahilly R, Gardner E: The timing and sequence of events in the development of the limbs of the human embryo. *Anat Embryol* 148:1, 1975.

Stedman H, Sarkar S: Molecular genetics in basic myology: A rapidly evolving perspective. *Muscle Nerve* 11:668, 1988.

Sutherland CJ, Elsom VL, Gordon ML, Dunwoodie SL, Hardeman EC: Coordination of skeletal muscle gene expression occurs late in mammalian development. *Dev Biol* 146:167, 1991.

Wessels A, Vermeulen JL, Viragh S, Kalman F, Lamers WH, Moorman AF: Spatial distribution of "tissue-specific" antigens in the developing heart and skeletal muscle. II. An immunohistochemical analysis of myosin heavy chain isoform expression patterns in the embryonic heart. *Anat Rec* 229:355, 1991.

Williams PL, Warwick R, Dyson M, Bannister LH: *Gray's Anatomy.* 37th ed. Edinburgh, Churchill Livingstone, 1989.

17

The Limbs

The general features of limb development are described and illustrated in Chapter 5. Development of the limb bones is described in Chapter 15, and formation of the limb musculature is outlined in Chapter 16. The purpose of this chapter is to consolidate this material.

The **limb buds** first appear as small elevations of the ventrolateral body wall during the fourth week (Fig. 17–1). The upper limb buds are visible by day 26 or 27, and the lower limb buds begin to appear on day 27 or 28. Each limb bud consists of a mass of mesenchyme covered by ectoderm. This mesenchyme is derived from the somatic layer of lateral mesoderm. The limb buds elongate by the proliferation of the mesenchyme within them. The upper limb buds appear disproportionately low on the embryo's trunk because of the early development of the cranial half of the embryo.

The early stages of limb development are alike for the upper and lower limbs (Figs. 17–2 and 17–3) except that development of the upper limb buds precedes that of the lower limb buds by about two days. The upper limb buds develop opposite the caudal cervical segments, and the lower limb buds form opposite the lumbar and cranial sacral segments (Figs. 17–4 and 17–5). At the tip of each limb bud the ectoderm becomes thickened to form an apical ectodermal ridge (see Fig. 15–13*B*). Interaction between this ridge and the mesenchymal cells in the limb bud is essential to limb development.

The *apical ectodermal ridge* (AER) exerts an inductive influence on the limb mesenchyme that promotes growth and development of the limbs. The mesenchyme adjacent to the AER consists of undifferentiated, rapidly proliferating cells; whereas, the mesenchymal cells proximal to it differentiate into muscle and the cartilage models of bones. The limb buds elongate by proliferation of the mesenchyme within them. The distal ends of the flipperlike limb buds soon flatten into paddlelike hand or foot plates (Fig. 17–3). Recent experimental studies have shown that endogenous *retinoic acid* is involved in limb development and pattern formation (see Tabin [1991] for a review of the role of retinoids in limb morphogenesis).

By the end of the sixth week, the mesenchymal tissue in the **hand plates** has condensed to form *digital (finger) rays*. These mesenchymal condensations outline the pattern of the digits (fingers). During the seventh week, similar condensations of mesenchyme form *digital (toe) rays* in the **foot plates**. At the tip of each digital ray is a portion of the apical ectodermal ridge. It induces development of the mesenchyme into the primordia of the bones (phalanges) in the digits. The intervals between the digital rays are occupied by loose mesenchyme. Soon, the intervening regions of mesenchymal tissue break down, forming

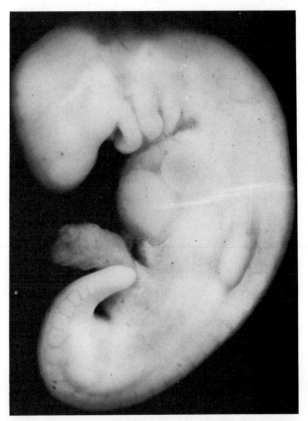

Figure 17–1. Photograph of a human embryo of about 28 days. The upper limb bud appears as an elevation *(arrow)* on the ventrolateral body wall. The lower limb bud is present but is not recognizable (see Fig. 5–8 *E*).

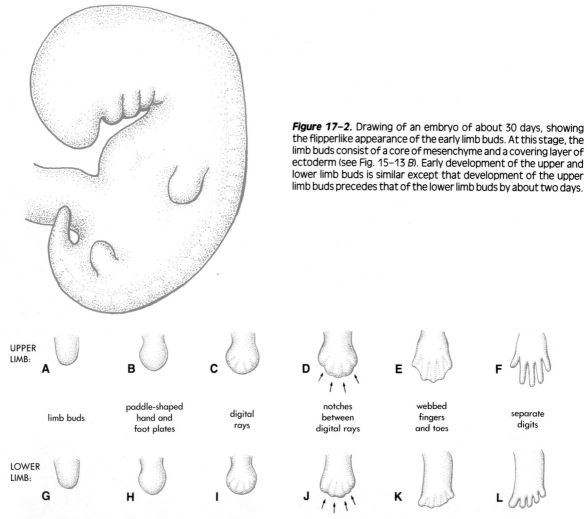

Figure 17–2. Drawing of an embryo of about 30 days, showing the flipperlike appearance of the early limb buds. At this stage, the limb buds consist of a core of mesenchyme and a covering layer of ectoderm (see Fig. 15–13 B). Early development of the upper and lower limb buds is similar except that development of the upper limb buds precedes that of the lower limb buds by about two days.

UPPER LIMB:

A   B   C   D   E   F

limb buds   paddle-shaped hand and foot plates   digital rays   notches between digital rays   webbed fingers and toes   separate digits

LOWER LIMB:

G   H   I   J   K   L

Figure 17–3. Drawings illustrating stages in the development of the hands and feet between the fourth and eighth weeks. The early stages of limb development are alike except that development of the hands precedes that of the feet by a day or so. A, 27 days. B, 32 days. C, 41 days. D, 46 days. E, 50 days. F, 52 days. G, 28 days. H, 36 days. I, 46 days. J, 49 days. K, 52 days. L, 56 days.

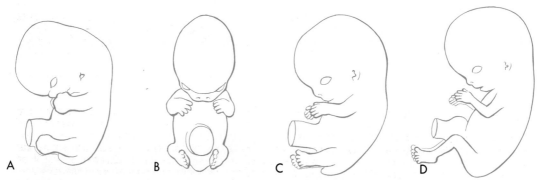

Figure 17–4. Drawings illustrating positional changes of the developing limbs. A, About 48 days, showing the limbs extending ventrally and the hand and foot plates facing each other. B, About 51 days, showing the upper limbs bent at the elbows and the hands curved over the thorax. C, About 54 days, showing the soles of the feet facing medially. D, About 56 days. Note that the elbows now point caudally and the knees cranially.

notches between the digital rays (Fig. 17–3D). As this tissue breakdown progresses, separate digits are produced by the end of the eighth week. If this process is incomplete or is arrested, varying degrees of webbing (*syndactyly*) result (Fig. 17–9).

As the limbs elongate the bones and muscles form. Mesenchymal models of the bones are formed by cell aggregations in the limb during the early part of the fifth week (see Fig. 15–13). *Chondrification centers* appear later in the fifth week. By the end of the sixth week, the entire limb skeleton is cartilaginous (see Fig. 15–13D). *Osteogenesis* of the long bones of the limbs begins in the seventh week from primary ossification centers in the middle of the cartilaginous models of the long bones. Ossification of the carpal (wrist) bones begins during the first year after birth.

As the bones form, myoblasts aggregate and develop a large muscle mass in each limb bud. In general, this muscle mass separates into dorsal (extensor) and ventral (flexor) components. The limb musculature develops in situ from the mesenchyme surrounding the developing bones. The limbs receive no mesenchymal contributions from the myotome regions of the somites. The cervical and lumbosacral myotomes probably contribute to the muscles of the pectoral and pelvic girdles.

Early in the seventh week the limbs extend ventrally. The developing upper and lower limbs then rotate in opposite directions and to different degrees (Fig. 17–4). Originally, the flexor aspect of the limbs is ventral and the extensor aspect dorsal, and the preaxial and postaxial borders are cranial and caudal, respectively (Fig. 17–5A and D).

The upper limbs rotate laterally through 90 degrees on their longitudinal axes; thus, the future elbows point backward or posteriorly, and the extensor muscles come to lie on the lateral and posterior aspects of the limb. *The lower limbs rotate medially* through almost 90 degrees; thus, the future knees face forward or anteriorly, and the extensor muscles lie on the anterior aspect of the lower limb. It should also be clear that the radius and the tibia are homologous bones, as are the ulna and fibula, just as the thumb and great toe are homologous digits.

By the end of the embryonic period, all the cartilage bones of the limbs are present and endochondral ossification of them has begun. Synovial joints appear at the beginning of the fetal period, coinciding with the

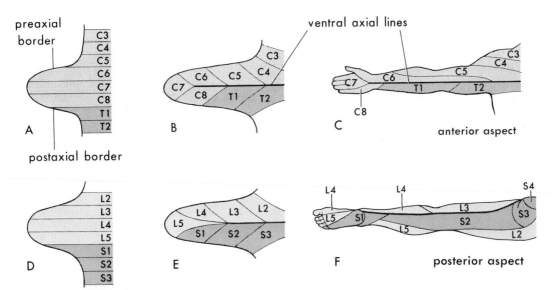

Figure 17–5. Diagrams illustrating development of the dermatomal patterns of the limbs. The axial lines indicate where there is no sensory overlap. *A* and *D,* Ventral aspect of the limb buds early in the fifth week. At this stage the dermatomal patterns show the primitive segmental arrangement. *B* and *E,* Similar views later in the fifth week, showing the modified arrangement of dermatomes. *C* and *F,* The dermatomal patterns in the adult upper and lower limbs. The primitive dermatomal pattern has disappeared, but an orderly sequence of dermatomes can still be recognized. In *F,* note that most of the original ventral surface of the lower limb lies on the back of the adult limb. This is the result of medial rotation of the lower limb that occurs toward the end of the embryonic period. In the upper limb, the ventral axial line extends along the anterior surface of the arm and forearm. In the lower limb, the ventral axial line extends along the medial side of the thigh and knee to the posteromedial aspect of the leg to the heel.

functional differentiation of the limb muscles and their innervation (Kabak and Boizow, 1990).

Dermatomes and Cutaneous Innervation of the Limbs

Because of its relationship to the growth and rotation of the limbs, the cutaneous segmental nerve supply of the limbs is considered in this chapter (Fig. 17–5) rather than in the chapter dealing with the nervous system or the integumentary system. See Lamb (1988) for details of the embryology of the peripheral nerves in relation to the innervation of the muscle fibers in the limbs.

A **dermatome** is defined as the area of skin supplied by a single spinal nerve and its spinal ganglion. During the fifth week, the peripheral nerves grow from the limb plexuses (brachial and lumbosacral) into the mesenchyme of the limb buds. The spinal nerves are distributed in segmental bands, supplying both dorsal and ventral surfaces of the limb buds. As the limbs elongate, the cutaneous distribution of the spinal nerves migrates along the limbs and no longer reaches the surface in the distal part of the limbs. Although the original dermatomal pattern changes during growth of the limbs, an orderly sequence of distribution can still be recognized in the adult (Fig. 17–5C and F). In the upper limb, observe that the areas supplied by C5 and C6 adjoin the areas supplied by T2, T1, and C8, but the overlap between them is minimal at the *ventral axial line* (Fig. 17–5C).

A **cutaneous nerve area** is the area of skin supplied by a peripheral nerve. Both cutaneous nerve areas and dermatomes show considerable overlapping. The dermatomal patterns indicate that, if the dorsal root of that segment is cut, there may be a slight deficit in the area indicated. Because there is overlapping of dermatomes, however, a particular area is not exclusively innervated by a single segmental nerve. The limb dermatomes may be traced progressively down the lateral aspect of the upper limb and back up its medial aspect.

A comparable distribution of dermatomes occurs in the lower limbs, which may be traced down the ventral aspect and then up the dorsal aspect of the lower limb. When the limbs descend, they carry their nerves with them; this explains the oblique course of the nerves of the brachial and lumbosacral plexuses.

LIMB ANOMALIES

Minor limb defects are relatively common, but they can usually be corrected surgically. Although minor anomalies are usually of no serious medical consequence, they may serve as indicators of more serious abnormalities; i.e., they may be part of a specific pattern of malformation (Jones, 1988).

The most *critical period of limb development* is from 24 to 36 days after fertilization (see Fig. 8–13). This estimate is based on clinical studies of infants exposed to thalidomide, a potent human teratogen (Newman, 1986). Exposure to a teratogen before day 33 causes severe anomalies (e.g., absence of the hands). Exposure to a teratogen from days 34 to 36 causes absence or hypoplasia of the thumbs. Consequently, a teratogen that could cause absence of the limbs or parts of them would have to act before the end of this period (Lenz, 1971).

Many severe limb defects occurred from 1957 to 1962 as a result of maternal ingestion of *thalidomide* (Fig. 17–6). This drug, widely used as a sedative and antinauseant, was withdrawn from the market in December 1961. Since that time, similar limb anomalies have rarely been observed. Overall, major limb anomalies are now found about twice in 1000 newborns (Connor and Ferguson-Smith, 1988). Most of these defects are caused by genetic factors. Several unrelated congenital anomalies of the lower limb were found to be associated with a similar aberrant arterial pattern, which might be of some importance in the pathogenesis of these defects (Levinsohn et al., 1991).

The terminology used to describe limb deficiencies in this text follows the international nomenclature in which only two basic descriptive terms are used: (1) *amelia*, complete absence of a limb or limbs (Fig. 17–6A), and (2) *meromelia* (Gr. *meros*, part, and *melos*, extremity), partial absence of a limb or limbs (Fig. 17–6B and C). Descriptive terms such as hemimelia, peromelia, ectromelia, and phocomelia are not used in current nomenclature because of their imprecision.

Cleft Hand and Cleft Foot (Lobster-Claw Deformities; Fig. 17–7E and F). In these rare anomalies there is absence of one or more central digits resulting from failure of development of one or more digital rays (see Fig. 15–13C). The hand or foot is thus divided into two parts that oppose each other like lobster claws. The remaining digits are partially or completely fused (syndactyly).

Congenital Absence of the Radius. The radius is partially or completely absent. The hand deviates radially (laterally), and the ulna bows with the concavity on the lateral side of the forearm. This anomaly is the result of failure of the mesenchymal primordium of the radius to form during the fifth week of development (see Fig. 15–13C). Absence of the radius is usually caused by genetic factors.

Brachydactyly (Fig. 17–8A). Shortness of the digits (fingers or toes) is uncommon and is the result of reduction in the length of the phalanges. It is usually inherited as a dominant trait and is often associated with shortness of stature.

Polydactyly (Fig. 17–8C and D). Supernumerary digits are common. Often the extra digit is incompletely formed and lacks proper muscular development; it is thus useless. If the hand is affected, the extra digit is most commonly medial or lateral rather than central. In the foot the extra toe is usually on the lateral side. Polydactyly is inherited as a dominant trait.

Syndactyly (Fig. 17–9). Syndactyly occurs in 1 to 2200 births (Behrman, 1992). Cutaneous syndactyly (simple webbing of the digits) is the most common limb anomaly. It is more frequent in the foot than in the hand. *Cutaneous syndactyly* is the result of failure of the webs to degenerate between two or more digits. In severe cases there is fusion of the digits (Fig. 17–9B, E, and F). In some cases there is also fusion of the bones (synostosis). *Osseous syndactyly* occurs when the notches between the digital rays fail to develop during the seventh week (Fig. 17–3D and J). As a result, separation of the digits does not occur during the eighth week (Fig. 17–3F and L). Syndactyly is most frequently observed between the third and fourth fingers and between the second and third toes. It is inherited as a simple dominant or simple recessive trait.

Congenital Clubfoot (Fig. 17–9C). Any deformity of the foot involving the talus (ankle bone) is called clubfoot or talipes (L. *talus*, heel, ankle + *pes*, foot). Clubfoot is a common deformity, occurring about once in 1000 births. It is characterized by an abnormal position of the foot that prevents normal weight bearing. As the child develops, he or she tends to walk on the ankle rather than on the sole of the foot; hence, the name talipes. *Talipes equinovarus* (Fig. 17–9C), the most common type of clubfoot, occurs about twice as frequently in males. The sole of the foot is turned medially and the foot is inverted.

There is much uncertainty about the cause of clubfoot. Although it is commonly stated that this condition is the result of abnormal positioning or restricted movement of the fetus's lower limbs in utero, the evidence for this is

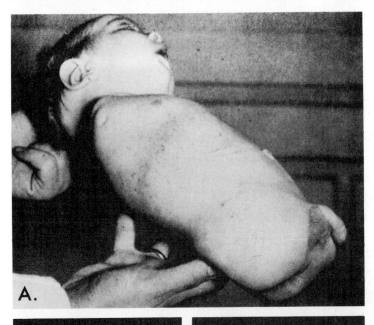

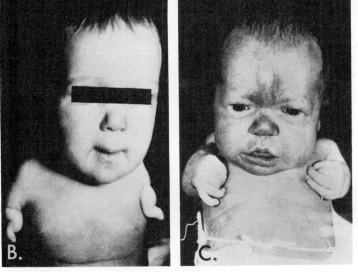

Figure 17–6. Limb malformations caused by thalidomide. *A*, Quadruple amelia. The upper and lower limbs are absent. *B*, Meromelia of the upper limbs. The upper limbs are represented by rudimentary stumps. *C*, Meromelia with the rudimentary upper limbs attached directly to the trunk. (From Lenz W, Knapp K: *Ger Med Mon 7*:253, 1962). See also Figure 8–19.

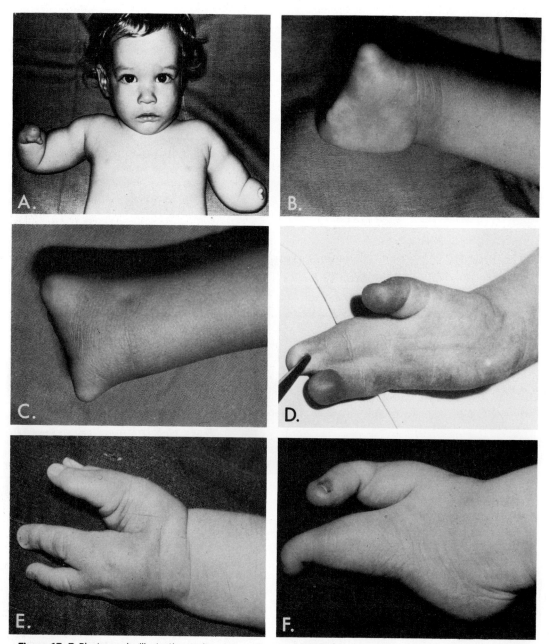

Figure 17–7. Photographs illustrating various types of meromelia. Meromelia denotes partial absence of a limb. It may be terminal (e.g., absence of the hand as in C). A, Absence of the hands and most of the forearms. B, Absence of the phalanges. C, Absence of the hand. D, Absence of the fourth and fifth phalanges and metacarpals. There is also syndactyly. E, Absence of the third phalanx resulting in a cleft hand (lobster claw). F, Absence of the second and third toes resulting in a cleft foot. (D is from Swenson O: *Pediatric Surgery*. 1958. Courtesy of Appleton-Century-Crofts).

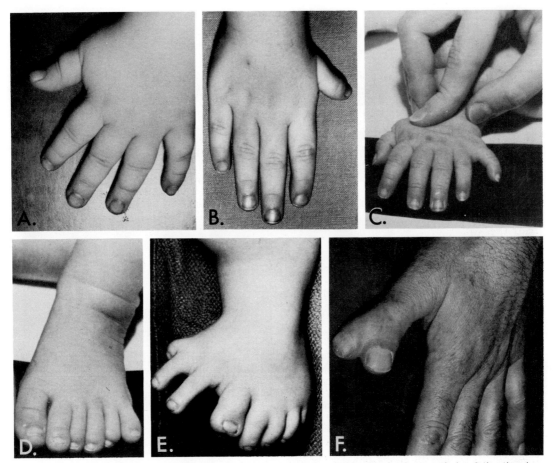

Figure 17–8. Photographs of various types of limb anomaly. *A,* Brachydactyly. *B,* Hypoplasia of the thumb. *C,* Polydactyly, showing a supernumerary finger. *D,* Polydactyly, showing a supernumerary toe. *E,* Partial duplication of the foot. *F,* Partial duplication of the thumb. (*C* and *D* are from Swenson O: *Pediatric Surgery.* 1958. Courtesy of Appleton-Century-Crofts).

inconclusive. Hereditary factors are involved in some cases, and it appears that environmental factors are involved in most cases. Clubfoot appears to follow a multifactorial pattern of inheritance (p. 168); hence, any intrauterine position that results in abnormal positioning of the feet may cause clubfeet if the fetus is genetically predispositioned to this deformity.

Congenital Dislocation of the Hip. This deformity occurs in about one of every 1500 newborn infants and is more common in females than in males. The capsule of the hip joint is very relaxed at birth, and there is underdevelopment of the acetabulum of the hip bone and the head of the femur. The actual dislocation almost always occurs after birth. Two causative factors are commonly suggested:

1. *Abnormal development of the acetabulum.* About 15 per cent of infants with congenital dislocation of the hip are breech deliveries, suggesting that breech posture during the terminal months may result in abnormal development of the acetabulum and the head of the femur.

2. *Generalized joint laxity* appears to be associated with congenital dislocation of the hip. Joint laxity is often a dominantly inherited condition. Congenital dislocation of the hip follows a multifactorial pattern of inheritance (Thompson et al., 1991).

Causes of Limb Anomalies

Abnormalities of the limbs originate at different stages of development. Suppression of limb development during the early part of the fourth week results in absence of the limbs, which is known as *amelia* (Fig. 17–6*A*). Arrest or disturbance of differentiation or growth of the limbs during the fifth week results in various types of *meromelia* (Figs. 17–6*B* and *C* and 17–7). Meromelia denotes the partial absence of a limb, which may be terminal, e.g., absence of the hand (Fig. 17–7*C*).

Like other anomalies, some limb defects are caused by genetic factors, e.g., chromosomal abnormalities as in trisomy 18 (see Fig. 8–4), or mutant genes as in brachydactyly

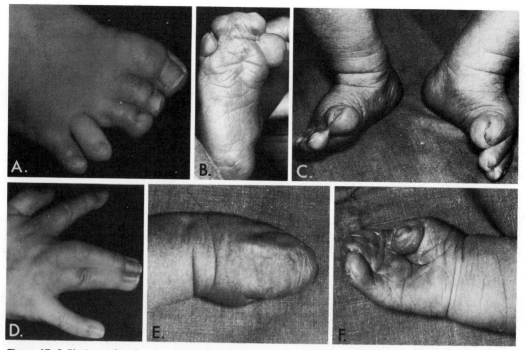

Figure 17–9. Photographs of various types of limb anomaly. *A,* Cutaneous syndactyly, showing skin webs between the first and second and the second and third toes. *B,* Severe cutaneous syndactyly involving fusion of all the toes except the fifth. *C,* Cutaneous syndactyly associated with clubfoot (talipes equinovarus). *D,* Cutaneous syndactyly involving webbing of the third and fourth fingers. *E* and *F,* Dorsal and palmar views of a child's right hand, showing osseous syndactyly (fusion) of the second to fifth fingers. (*A* and *D* are from Swenson O: *Pediatric Surgery.* 1958. Courtesy of Appleton-Century-Crofts).

(Fig. 17–8*A*) or osteogenesis imperfecta (Cole and Cohen Jr., 1991); by environmental factors, e.g., thalidomide (Fig. 17–6); or by a combination of genetic and environmental factors (*multifactorial inheritance*), e.g., congenital dislocation of the hip (Thompson et al., 1991). Vascular disruption may also lead to limb reduction defects (Van Allen, 1992).

Experimental studies support the suggestion that mechanical influences during intrauterine development may cause some limb deformities (Kennedy and Persaud, 1977, 1979). A reduced quantity of amniotic fluid (oligohydramnios) is commonly associated with limb deformities (Dunn, 1976); however, the significance of mechanical influences while in the uterus on congenital postural deformities is still open to question (McKeown, 1976).

SUMMARY

The limbs begin to appear toward the end of the fourth week as slight elevations of the ventrolateral body wall. The upper limb buds develop about two days before the lower limb buds. The tissues of the limb buds are derived from two main sources: somatic mesoderm and ectoderm.

The *apical ectodermal ridge* (AER) exerts an inductive influence on the limb mesenchyme that promotes growth and development of the limbs. The limb buds elongate by proliferation of the mesenchyme within them.

Initially, the developing limbs are directed caudally; later, they project ventrally, and finally, they rotate on their longitudinal axes. The upper and lower limbs rotate in opposite directions and to different degrees.

The majority of limb anomalies appear to be caused by genetic factors; however, many limb defects probably result from an interaction of genetic and environmental factors (multifactorial inheritance). Relatively few congenital anomalies of the limbs can be attributed to specific environmental teratogens except those resulting from thalidomide.

CLINICALLY ORIENTED QUESTIONS FOR PROBLEM-BASED LEARNING SESSIONS

1. Do more female infants have congenital dislocation of the hip than male infants? Are the hip joints of these infants usually dislocated at birth? What are the probable causes of congenital dislocation of the hip?
2. Are limb anomalies similar to those caused by the drug thalidomide common? What was the characteristic *syndrome* produced by thalidomide? Name the limb defects commonly associated with this syndrome.
3. What is the most common type of clubfoot (talipes)? How common is it? Describe the feet of infants born with this anomaly.
4. Is syndactyly common? Does it occur more often in the hands than in the feet? What is the embryological basis of syndactyly?

The answers to these questions are given on page 466.

References and Suggested Reading

Behrman RE: *Nelson Textbook of Pediatrics.* 14th ed. Philadelphia, WB Saunders, 1992.

Bernhardt DB: Prenatal and postnatal growth and development of the foot and ankle. *Phys Ther 68*:1831, 1988.

Blechschmidt E: The early stages of human limb development. *In* Swinyard CA (ed): *Limb Development and Deformity: Problems of Evaluation and Rehabilitation.* Springfield, Ill, Charles C Thomas, 1969.

Cole DEC, Cohen Jr., MM: Osteogenesis imperfecta: an update. *J Pediatr 119*:73, 1991.

Connor JM, Ferguson-Smith MA: *Essential Medical Genetics.* 2nd ed. Oxford, Blackwell Scientific Publications, 1988.

Dunn PM: Congenital postural deformities. *Br Med Bull 32*:65, 1976.

Filly RA: Sonographic anatomy of the normal fetus. *In* Harrison MR, Golbus MS, Filly RA (eds): *The Unborn Patient: Prenatal Diagnosis and Treatment.* 2nd ed. Philadelphia, WB Saunders, 1991.

Frantz CH, O'Rahilly R: Congenital skeletal limb deficiencies. *J Bone Joint Surg 43A*:1202, 1961.

German RZ, Meyers LL: The role of time and size in ontogenetic allometry: II. An empirical of human growth. *Growth Dev Aging 53*:107, 1989.

Hartwig NG, Vermeij-Keers C, DeVries HE, Kagie M, Kragt H: Limb body wall malformation complex: an embryologic etiology? *Hum Pathol 20*:1071, 1989.

Jones KL: *Smith's Recognizable Patterns of Human Malformation.* 4th ed. Philadelphia, WB Saunders, 1988.

Kabak S, Boizow L: Organogenese des Extremitätenskeletts und der Extremitätengelenke beim Menschenembryo. *Anat Anz 170*:349, 1990.

Keegan JJ, Garrett FD: The segmental distribution of the cutaneous nerves in the limbs of man. *Anat Rec 102*:409, 1948.

Kennedy LA, Persaud TVN: Experimental amniocentesis and teratogenesis: clinical implications. *In* Persaud TVN (ed): *Advances in the Study of Birth Defects.* Vol 1. *Teratogenic Mechanisms.* New York, Alan R. Liss, 1979.

Kennedy LA, Persaud TVN: Pathogenesis of developmental defects induced in the rat by amniotic sac puncture. *Acta Anat 97*:23, 1977.

Lamb AH: Aspects of peripheral motor system development. *Aust Paediatr J 24 (Suppl 1)*:37, 1988.

Lamy M, Maroteaux P: The genetic study of limb malformations. *In* Swinyard CA (ed): *Limb Development and Deformity: Problems of Evaluation and Rehabilitation.* Springfield, Ill, Charles C Thomas, 1969.

Lenz W: How can the teratogenic action of a factor be established in man? *South Med J Suppl 64*:41, 1971.

Lenz W, Knapp K: Foetal malformations due to thalidomide. *Ger Med Mon 7*:253, 1962.

Levinsohn EM, Hootnick DR, Packard Jr, DS: Consistent arterial abnormalities associated with a variety of congenital malformations of the lower limb. *Invest Radiol 26*:364, 1991.

Lubinsky MS: Explaining certain limb anomalies and the limb-hematopoiesis community of syndromes using a model of determination. *Teratology 43*:295, 1991.

Mahony BS, Filly RA: High-resolution sonographic assessment of the fetal extremities. *J Ultrasound Med 3*:489, 1984.

Maini PK, Solursh M: Cellular mechanisms of pattern formation in the developing limb. *Int Rev Cytol 129*:91, 1991.

Martin JH: Anatomical substrates for somatic sensation. *In* Kandel ER, Schwartz JH (eds): *Principles of Neural Science.* New York, Elsevier, 1985.

McCarthy D: The developmental anatomy of pes valgo planus. *Clin Podiatr Med Surg 6*:491, 1989.

McKeown T: Human malformations: Introduction. *Br Med Bull 32*:1, 1976.

Moore KL: The vulnerable embryo: Causes of malformation in man. *Manit Med Rev 43*:306, 1963.

Newman CGH: Clinical aspects of thalidomide embryopathy–a continuing preoccupation. *Teratogen Update. Environmentally Induced Birth Risks.* New York, Alan R. Liss, 1986.

O'Rahilly R, Gardner E: The timing and sequence of events in the development of the limbs in the human embryo. *Anat Embryol 148*:1, 1975.

O'Rahilly R, Müller F: *Developmental Stages in Human Embryos.* Washington, Carnegie Institution of Washington, 1987.

Oransky M, Canero G, Maiotti M: Embryonic development of the posterolateral structures of the knee. *Anat Rec 225*:347, 1989.

Saunders JW: Control of growth patterns in limb development. *In* Frantz CH (ed): *Normal and Abnormal Embryological Development.* Washington, National Research Council, 1967.

Seyfer AE, Wind G, Martin RR: Study of upper extremity growth and development using human embryos and computer-reconstructed models. *J Hand Surg 14*:927, 1989.

Swinyard CA (ed): *Limb Development and Deformity: Problems of Evaluation and Rehabilitation.* Springfield, Ill, Charles C Thomas, 1969.

Tabin CJ: Retinoids, homeoboxes, and growth factors: Toward molecular models for limb development. *Cell 66*:199, 1991.

Thompson MW, McInnes RR, Willard HF: *Thompson & Thompson Genetics in Medicine.* 5th ed. Philadelphia, WB Saunders, 1991.

Uhthoff HK: *The Embryology of the Human Locomotor System.* New York, Springer-Verlag, 1990.

Van Allen MI: Structural anomalies resulting from vascular disruption. *Pediatr Clin NA 39*:255, 1992.

Wolpert L: Mechanisms of limb development and malformation. *Br Med Bull 32*:65, 1976.

Zwilling E: Abnormal morphogenesis in limb development. *In* Swinyard CA (ed): *Limb Development and Deformity: Problems of Evaluation and Rehabilitation.* Springfield, Ill, Charles C Thomas, 1969.

The Nervous System

The nervous system develops from a thickened, slipper-shaped area of embryonic ectoderm called the **neural plate** (Fig. 18-1*A*), which appears during the third week (p. 61). The underlying notochordal process and adjacent mesoderm induce the overlying ectoderm to differentiate into the neural plate. Formation of the neural folds, neural tube, and neural crest from the neural plate is illustrated in Figure 18-1. (For details on the mechanisms of neural tube formation, see Schoenwolf and Smith, 1990.) The neural plate and **neural folds** are bathed with amniotic fluid. They are dependent on it in part for their nourishment until the primitive vascular system is established at the end of the fourth week.

The **neural tube** slowly differentiates into the *central nervous system* (CNS) consisting of the brain and spinal cord. The **neural crest** gives rise to most of the *peripheral nervous system* consisting of cranial, spinal, and autonomic ganglia and nerves (Fig. 18-8). In addition, *neural crest cells* differentiate into Schwann cells, pigment cells, odontoblasts, meninges, and skeletal and muscular components of the head.

Formation of the neural tube begins during the early part of the fourth week (22 to 23 days) in the region of the fourth to sixth pairs of somites (see Figs. 5-8*A* and 5-9*B*). This is the primordium of the cervical region of the spinal cord. At this stage the cranial two thirds of the neural plate and neural tube, as far caudal as the fourth pair of somites, represent the future brain, and the caudal one third of the neural tube and neural plate represent the future spinal cord.

Fusion of the neural folds proceeds in cranial and caudal directions until only small areas remain open at both ends. Here the lumen of the neural tube *(neural canal)* communicates freely with the amniotic cavity (Figs. 18-1 and 18-2). The cranial opening called the *rostral (anterior) neuropore* closes on about the twenty-fifth day (see Fig. 5-10), and the *caudal (posterior) neuropore* closes about two days later (Fig. 18-2*D*). Closure of the neuropores coincides with the establishment of a blood vascular circulation for the neural tube (Williams et al., 1989). The walls of the neural tube thicken to form the brain and the spinal cord (Fig. 18-3). The lumen of the neural tube is converted into the *ventricular system* of the brain and the *central canal* of the spinal cord.

THE SPINAL CORD

The neural tube caudal to the fourth pair of somites develops into the spinal cord (Figs. 18-3 and 18-4). The lateral walls of the neural tube thicken, gradually reducing the size of its lumen until only a minute *central canal of the spinal cord* is present at nine weeks (Fig. 18-4*C*).

Initially the wall of the neural tube is composed of a thick, pseudostratified, columnar neuroepithelium (Fig. 18-4*A* and *D*). These neuroepithelial cells constitute the *ventricular zone* (ependymal layer) and give rise to all neurons and macroglial cells (macroglia) in the spinal cord (Fig. 18-5). Macroglial cells are the larger types of neuroglial cell (e.g., astrocytes and oligodendrocytes). Soon, a *marginal zone* composed of the outer parts of the neuroepithelial cells becomes recognizable (Fig. 18-4*E*). This zone gradually becomes the *white matter of the spinal cord* as axons grow into it from nerve cell bodies in the spinal cord, spinal ganglia, and brain.

Some dividing neuroepithelial cells in the ventricular zone differentiate into primitive neurons called **neuroblasts**. These embryonic nerve cells form an *intermediate zone* (mantle layer) between the ventricular and marginal zones (Fig. 18-4*E*). Neuroblasts become neurons as they develop cytoplasmic processes (Fig. 18-5).

The primitive supporting cells of the central nervous system called **glioblasts** (spongioblasts) differentiate from neuroepithelial cells, mainly after neuroblast formation has ceased. The glioblasts migrate from the ventricular zone into the intermediate and marginal zones. Some glioblasts become *astroblasts* and then *astrocytes*; whereas, others become *oligodendroblasts* and eventually *oligodendrocytes*. When the neuroepithelial cells cease producing neuroblasts and glioblasts, they differentiate into *ependymal cells*, which form the *ependyma* (ependymal epithelium) lining the central canal of the spinal cord.

Text continues on page 391.

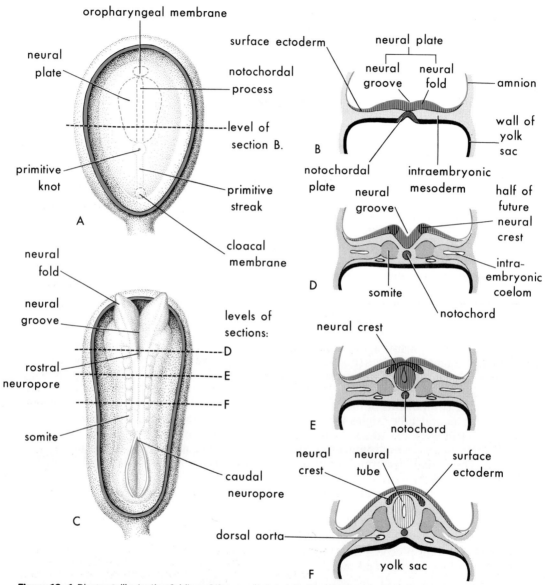

Figure 18–1. Diagrams illustrating folding of the neural plate into the neural tube and formation of the neural crest. *A,* Dorsal view of an embryo of about 18 days, exposed by removing the amnion. *B,* Transverse section of this embryo, showing the neural plate and early development of the neural groove. The developing notochord is also shown (for details of its development, see p. 57). *C,* Dorsal view of an embryo of about 22 days. The neural folds have fused opposite the somites but are widely spread out at both ends of the embryo. The rostral and caudal neuropores are indicated. *D to F,* Transverse sections of this embryo at the levels shown in *C,* illustrating formation of the neural tube and its detachment from the surface ectoderm. Note that some neuroectodermal cells are not included in the neural tube but remain between it and the surface ectoderm as the neural crest.

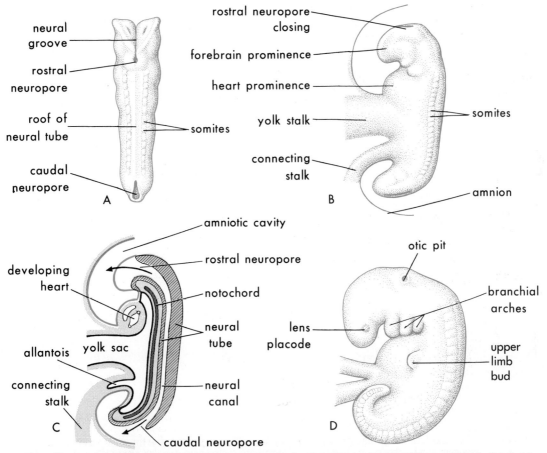

Figure 18-2. *A*, Dorsal view of an embryo of about 23 days, showing advanced fusion of the neural folds. *B*, Lateral view of an embryo of about 24 days, showing the forebrain prominence and closing of the rostral neuropore. *C*, Sagittal section of this embryo, showing the transitory communication of the neural canal with the amniotic cavity *(arrows)*. *D*, Lateral view of an embryo of about 27 days. Note that the neuropores shown in *B* are closed.

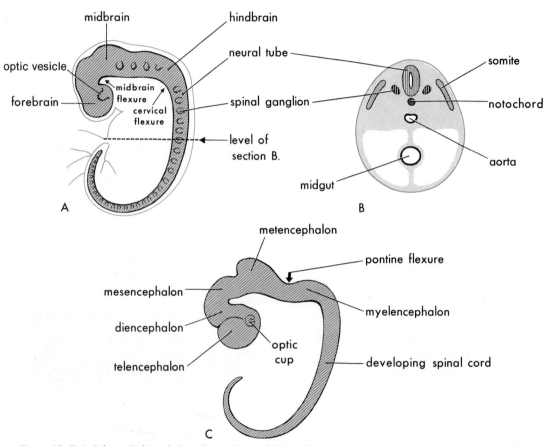

Figure 18–3. *A*, Schematic lateral view of an embryo of about 28 days, showing the three primary brain vesicles: forebrain, midbrain, and hindbrain. The two flexures demarcate the primary divisions of the brain. *B*, Transverse section of this embryo, showing the neural tube that will develop into the spinal cord in this region. The spinal (dorsal root) ganglia derived from the neural crest are also shown. *C*, Schematic lateral view of the central nervous system of a six-week embryo, showing the secondary brain vesicles and pontine flexure. The flexures occur as the brain grows rapidly. They are important factors in determining the final shape of the brain.

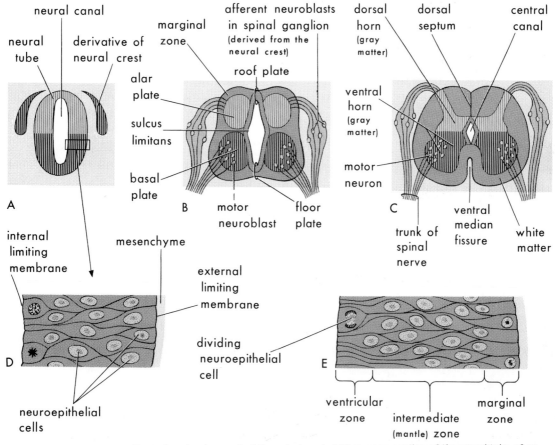

Figure 18–4. Diagrams illustrating development of the spinal cord. *A*, Transverse section of the neural tube of an embryo of about 23 days. *B* and *C*, Similar sections at six and nine weeks, respectively. *D*, Section of the wall of the neural tube shown in *A*. *E*, Section of the wall of the developing spinal cord showing its three zones. In *A* to *C*, note that the neural canal of the neural tube is converted into the central canal of the spinal cord.

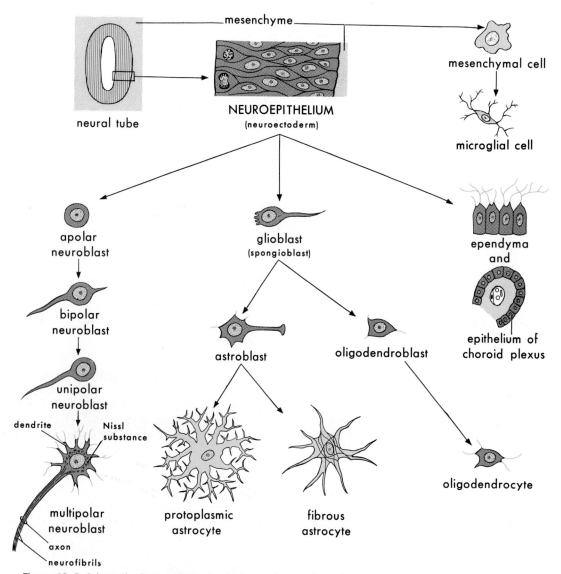

Figure 18–5. Schematic diagram illustrating histogenesis of cells in the central nervous system. After further development the multipolar neuroblast *(lower left)* becomes a nerve cell or neuron. Neuroepithelial cells give rise to all neurons and macroglial cells. Microglial cells are derived from mesenchymal cells that invade the developing nervous system with the developing blood vessels.

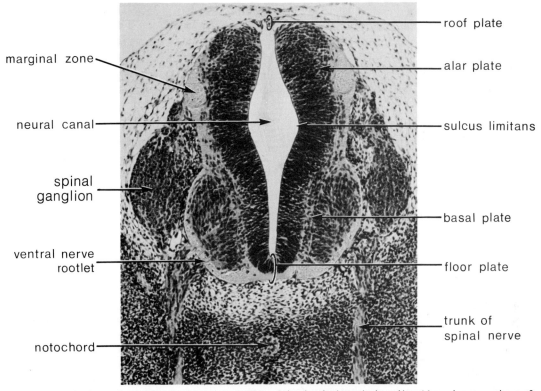

marginal zone

neural canal

spinal
ganglion

ventral nerve
rootlet

notochord

roof plate

alar plate

sulcus limitans

basal plate

floor plate

trunk of
spinal nerve

Figure 18-6. Photomicrograph of a transverse section of the developing spinal cord in a 14-mm human embryo of about 44 days (×75). The roof plate and floor plate contain no neuroblasts and are relatively thin. (Courtesy of Dr. J.W.A. Duckworth, Professor Emeritus of Anatomy and Cell Biology, University of Toronto.)

The *microglial cells* (microglia),[1] which are scattered through the gray and white matter, are small cells that are derived from *mesenchymal cells* (Fig. 18-5); however, there has been much controversy concerning the origin of microglia (Cormack, 1993). These cells invade the central nervous system rather late in the fetal period after it has been penetrated by blood vessels. A current view is that microglia develop from monocytes entering from the circulation during the fetal period (Fitzgerald, 1992).

Proliferation and differentiation of neuroepithelial cells in the developing spinal cord produce thick walls and thin roof and floor plates (Fig. 18-4*B*). Differential thickening of the lateral walls of the spinal cord soon produces a shallow, longitudinal groove on each side called the *sulcus limitans* (Figs. 18-4*B* and 18-5). This groove separates the dorsal part called the *alar plate* (lamina) from the ventral part called the

basal plate (lamina). The alar and basal plates produce longitudinal bulges extending through most of the length of the developing spinal cord. This regional separation is of fundamental importance because the alar and basal plates are later associated with afferent and efferent functions, respectively.

The Alar Plates (Figs. 18-4, 18-6, and 18-7). Cell bodies in the alar plates form the *dorsal gray matter* in columns that extend the length of the spinal cord. In transverse sections of the spinal cord these columns are called *dorsal gray horns*. Neurons in these columns constitute afferent nuclei, and groups of these nuclei form the *dorsal gray columns*. As the alar plates enlarge, the *dorsal septum* forms.

The Basal Plates (Figs. 18-4, 18-6, and 18-7). Cell bodies in the basal plates form the ventral and lateral gray columns. In transverse sections of the spinal cord these columns are commonly called *ventral gray horns* and *lateral gray horns*, respectively. Axons of ventral horn cells grow out of the spinal cord and form bundles called the *ventral roots* of the spinal nerves. As the basal plates enlarge, they bulge ventrally on each side of the median plane. As this occurs, the *ventral median septum* forms, and a deep longitudinal

---

[1] Microglia can transform into actively phagocytic *macrophages* in response to CNS damage. Such cells are believed to be the primary means by which necrotic (dead) tissue is cleared away (Cormack, 1993).

groove known as the *ventral median fissure* develops on the ventral surface of the spinal cord.

The Spinal Ganglia (Figs. 18–6 and 18–7). The unipolar neurons in the spinal ganglia are derived from *neural crest cells* (Figs. 18–1*F*, 18–8, and 18–9). Because these ganglia form swellings on the dorsal roots of spinal nerves, they are often called *dorsal root ganglia*. The axons of cells in the spinal ganglia are at first bipolar, but the two processes soon unite in a T-shaped fashion (Fig. 18–9). Both processes of spinal ganglion cells have the structural characteristics of axons, but the peripheral process is a dendrite in that there is conduction toward the cell body. The peripheral processes of spinal ganglion cells pass in the spinal nerves to sensory endings in somatic or visceral structures (Figs. 18–6 and 18–8). The central processes enter the spinal cord and constitute the *dorsal roots of the spinal nerves* (Figs. 18–7 and 18–8).

The Spinal Meninges. The mesenchyme surrounding the neural tube condenses to form a membrane called the primitive meninx. The external layer of this membrane thickens to form the *dura mater*. The inner layer remains thin and forms the *pia-arachnoid*, composed of pia mater and arachnoid mater; together these layers constitute the *leptomeninges*. Fluid-filled spaces appear within the leptomeninges that soon coalesce to form the *subarachnoid space* (Fig. 18–10). The origin of the pia mater and arachnoid from a single layer is indicated in the adult by the numerous delicate strands of connective tissue (*arachnoid trabeculae*) that pass between them (Moore, 1992). Embryonic *cerebrospinal fluid* (CSF) begins to form during the fifth week.

Positional Changes of the Spinal Cord

The spinal cord in the embryo extends the entire length of the vertebral canal, and the spinal nerves pass through the intervertebral foramina near their levels of origin (Fig. 18–10*A*). Because the vertebral column and dura mater grow more rapidly than the spinal cord, this relationship does not persist. The caudal end of the spinal cord gradually comes to lie at relatively higher levels. At six months it lies at the level of the first sacral vertebra (Fig. 18–10*B*).

In the newborn infant the spinal cord terminates at the level of the second or third lumbar vertebra (Fig. 18–10*C*); and, in the adult, the spinal cord usually terminates at the inferior border of the first lumbar vertebra (Fig. 18–10*D*). This is an average level because the caudal end of the spinal cord may be as superior as the twelfth thoracic vertebra or as inferior as the third lumbar vertebra (Moore, 1992). As a result, the spinal nerve roots, especially those of the lumbar and sacral segments, run obliquely from the spinal cord to the corresponding level of the vertebral column. The dorsal and ventral nerve roots inferior to the end of the cord, represented by the *conus medullaris*, form a sheaf of nerve roots called the **cauda equina** ("horse's tail"; Fig. 18–10*D*). Although the dura mater extends the entire length of the vertebral column in the adult, the other layers of the meninges

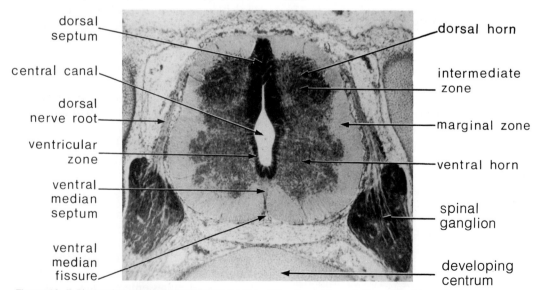

Figure 18–7. Photomicrograph of a transverse section of the developing spinal cord in a 20-mm human embryo of about 50 days (×60). (Courtesy of Professor Jean Hay, Department of Anatomy, University of Manitoba, Winnipeg, Canada.)

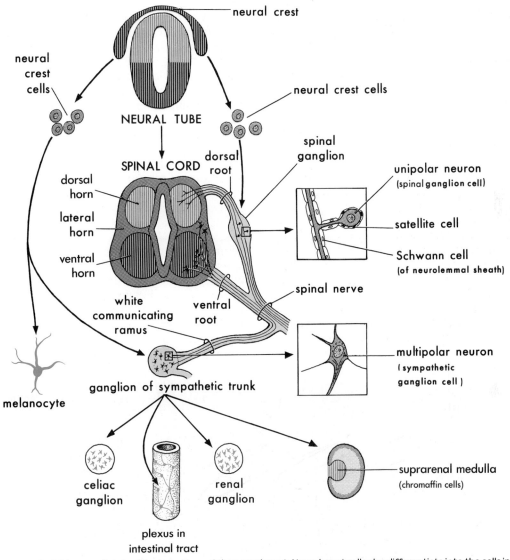

Figure 18–8. Diagram showing the derivatives of the neural crest. Neural crest cells also differentiate into the cells in the afferent ganglia of cranial nerves. The formation of a spinal nerve is also illustrated.

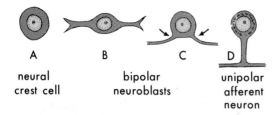

A   B   C   D

neural
crest cell

bipolar
neuroblasts

unipolar
afferent
neuron

Figure 18–9. Diagrams illustrating successive stages in the differentiation of a neural crest cell to form a unipolar afferent neuron of a spinal ganglion.

do not. Distal to the caudal end of the spinal cord, the pia mater forms a long, fibrous thread called the *filum terminale* (Fig. 18–1*D*). This thread extends from the conus medullaris and attaches to the periosteum of the first coccygeal vertebra. The filum terminale also indicates the line of regression of the embryonic spinal cord.

Myelination of Nerves (Fig. 18–11). Myelin sheaths begin to form in the spinal cord during the late fetal period and continue to form during the first postnatal year. In general, fiber tracts become myelinated at about the time they become functional. The *myelin sheaths* surrounding nerve fibers within the

spinal cord are formed by *oligodendrocytes*. The plasma membranes of the oligodendrocytes wrap around the axon, forming a number of layers (Fig. 18–11*F* to *G*).

The myelin sheaths around the axons of peripheral nerve fibers are formed by the plasma membranes of *Schwann cells* (Fig. 18–11*E*). These neuroglial cells are derived from *neural crest cells* that migrate peripherally and wrap themselves around the axons of somatic motor neurons (Fig. 18–8) and preganglionic autonomic motor neurons as they pass out of the central nervous system. These cells also wrap themselves around both the central and peripheral processes of the somatic and visceral sensory neurons as well as around the axons of postganglionic autonomic motor neurons (Fig. 18–11*A* to *F*). For more details of this process, see Cormack (1993) and Barr and Kiernan (1988). Beginning at about 20 weeks, the nerve fibers have a whitish appearance due to the deposition of myelin.

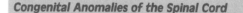

Congenital Anomalies of the Spinal Cord

Most congenital anomalies of the spinal cord are the result of defective closure of the neural tube during the fourth

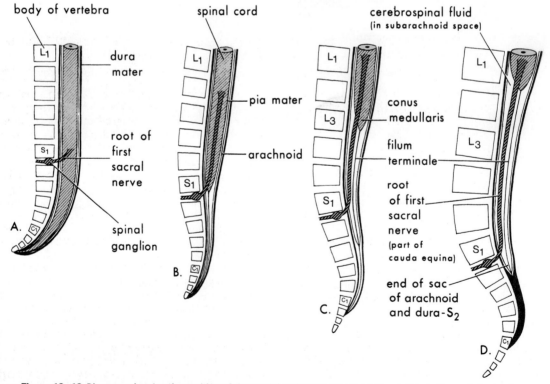

Figure 18–10. Diagrams showing the position of the caudal end of the spinal cord in relation to the vertebral column and meninges at various stages of development. The increasing inclination of the root of the first sacral nerve is also illustrated. *A*, Eight weeks. *B*, 24 weeks. *C*, Newborn. *D*, Adult.

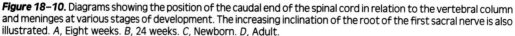

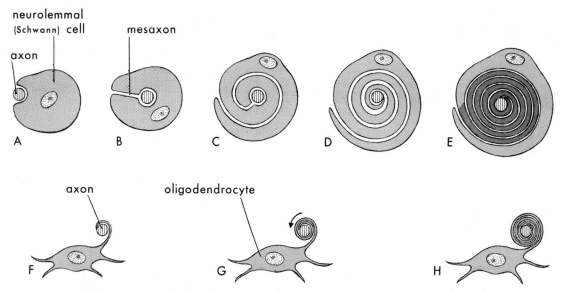

Figure 18–11. Diagrammatic sketches illustrating myelination. *A to E,* Successive stages in the myelination of a peripheral nerve fiber or axon by a neurolemmal or Schwann cell. The axon first indents the cell; the Schwann cell then rotates around the axon as the mesaxon (site of invagination) elongates. The cytoplasm between the layers of cell membrane gradually condenses. Cytoplasm remains on the inside of the sheath between the myelin and axon. *F to H,* Successive stages in the myelination of a nerve fiber in the central nervous system by an oligodendrocyte. A process of the neuroglial cell wraps itself around an axon, and the intervening layers of cytoplasm move to the body of the cell. Myelination in the brain begins in the brain stem and reaches the level of the cerebral hemispheres by birth.

week of development. The resulting **neural tube defects (NTDs)** also involve the tissue overlying the spinal cord: meninges, vertebral arch, muscles, and skin (Figs. 18–12*B* to *D* and 18–17). Anomalies involving the vertebral arches are referred to as **spina bifida**. This term denotes *nonfusion of the embryonic halves of the vertebral arches* that is common to all types of spina bifida. Severe anomalies also involve the spinal cord (Fig. 18–12). Spina bifida ranges from clinically significant types to minor anomalies that are clinically unimportant.

Spina Bifida Occulta (Fig. 18–12*A*). This *defect in the vertebral arch* (neural arch) is the result of failure of the embryonic halves of the arch to grow normally and fuse in the median plane (see Fig. 15–6). Spina bifida occulta occurs in L5 or S1 vertebrae in about ten per cent of otherwise normal people (Moore, 1992). In its most minor form, the only evidence of its presence may be a small dimple with a tuft of hair arising from it (Fig. 18–12*A*). Spina bifida occulta usually produces no clinical symptoms; however, a small per centage of affected infants have functionally significant defects of the underlying spinal cord and spinal roots (Behrman, 1992).

Spinal Dermal Sinus (Fig. 18–13). A posterior skin dimple in the median plane of the sacral region may be associated with a spinal dermal sinus. These dimples indicate the region of closure of the caudal neuropore at the end of the fourth week and therefore represent the last place of separation between the surface ectoderm and the neural

tube. In some cases the dimple is connected with the dura mater by a fibrous cord (Fig. 18–13*B*).

Spina Bifida Cystica (Figs. 18–12*B* to *D*, 18–14, and 18–15). Severe types of spina bifida, involving protrusion of the spinal cord and/or meninges through the defect in the vertebral arch, are often referred to collectively as *spina bifida cystica* because of the cystlike sac that is associated with these anomalies. Spina bifida cystica occurs about once in every 1000 births. When the sac contains meninges and cerebrospinal fluid, the condition is called *spina bifida with meningocele* (Fig. 18–12*B*). The spinal cord and spinal roots are in their normal position, but there may be spinal cord abnormalities. If the spinal cord and/or nerve roots are included in the sac, the malformation is called *spina bifida with meningomyelocele* (Figs. 18–12*C* and 18–14*A*). *Myelo* refers to the spinal cord, which used to be called the spinal medulla (Gr. *myelos,* medulla).

Meningomyeloceles are often associated with a marked *neurological deficit* inferior to the level of the protruding sac. This deficit occurs because nervous tissue is incorporated in the wall of the sac, which impairs the development of nerve fibers. Meningomyeloceles may be covered by skin or a thin, easily ruptured membrane (Fig. 18–14). Spina bifida with meningomyelocele is a more common and much more severe anomaly than spina bifida with meningocele. Meningoceles and meningomyeloceles may occur anywhere along the vertebral column, but they are most common in the lumbar region (Fig. 18–14).

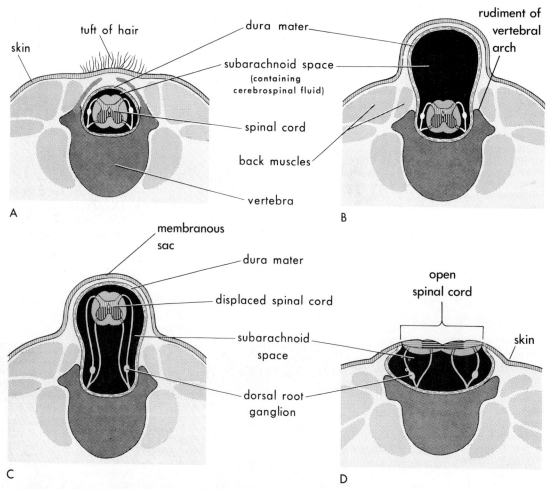

Figure 18–12. Diagrammatic sketches illustrating various types of spina bifida and the commonly associated anomalies of the nervous system. *A,* Spina bifida occulta. *B,* Spina bifida with meningocele. *C,* Spina bifida with meningomyelocele. *D,* Spina bifida with myeloschisis. The types illustrated in *B* to *D* are often referred to collectively as spina bifida cystica because of the cystlike sac that is associated with them (see Fig. 18–14).

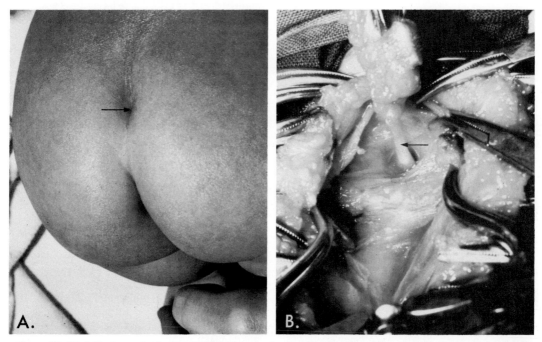

Figure 18-13. *A*, Photograph of a skin dimple in the sacral region. The opening of the spinal dermal sinus is indicated by an arrow. *B*, Photograph taken during removal of this sinus showing a cord *(arrow)* connecting the dimple to the spinal dura mater. (Courtesy of Dr. Dwight Parkinson, Children's Centre, Winnipeg, Canada.)

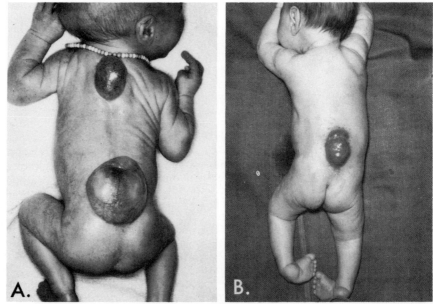

Figure 18-14. Photographs of infants with spina bifida cystica. *A*, Spina bifida with meningomyelocele in the thoracic and lumbar regions. *B*, Spina bifida with myeloschisis in the lumbar region (see also Figs. 18-12*D* and 18-15). Note that the nerve involvement has affected the lower limbs. These anomalies result from incomplete closure of the neural tube during the fourth week of development. As a result, there is a defect in the arches of the associated vertebrae (see Fig. 18-12). (Courtesy of Dr. Dwight Parkinson, Children's Centre, Winnipeg, Canada.)

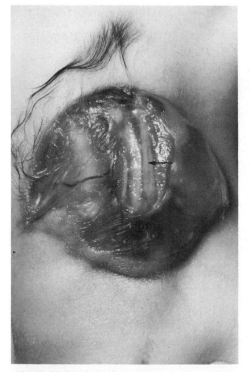

Figure 18-15. Photograph of an infant's back, exhibiting spina bifida with myeloschisis in the lumbar region. The open spinal cord (arrow) is covered by a delicate, semitransparent membrane. This anomaly is the result of a defect in closure of the neural tube during the fourth week (see Fig. 18-12D). Note the tufts of hair on the surrounding skin. (From Laurence KM, Weeks R: Abnormalities of the central nervous system. In Norman AP (ed): Congenital Abnormalities in Infancy. 2nd ed. 1971. Courtesy of Blackwell Scientific Publications.)

Spina bifida cystica shows considerable geographical variation in incidence. In the British Isles, for example, the incidence varies from 4.2 per 1000 newborn infants in South Wales to 1.5 per 1000 in southeastern England (Laurence and Weeks, 1971). Severe cases of spina bifida with meningomyelocele involving several vertebrae are often associated with partial absence of the brain, a severe anomaly known as meroanencephaly or anencephaly (Fig. 18-17).

The most severe type of spina bifida is called *spina bifida with myeloschisis* (also known as spina bifida with myelocele [Figs. 18-12D and 18-15]). In these cases the spinal cord is open because the neural folds failed to fuse during the fourth week (Gr. *schisis*, a cleaving). As a result, the spinal cord in the concerned area is represented by a flattened mass of nervous tissue. Spina bifida with myeloschisis may result from a neural tube defect (NTD) that is caused by a local overgrowth of the neural plate (Fig. 18-16). As a result, the caudal neuropore fails to close at the end of the fourth week.

Spina bifida cystica shows varying degrees of neurological deficit depending on the position and extent of the lesion. There is usually a corresponding dermatome loss of sensation along with complete or partial skeletal muscle paralysis (Fig. 18-14B). The level of the lesion determines the area of anesthesia (area of skin without sensation) and the muscles affected. *Sphincter paralysis* (bladder and/or anal sphincters) is common with lumbosacral meningomyeloceles (Fig. 18-14A). There is almost invariably a *saddle anesthesia* when the sphincters are involved; that is, loss of sensation in the region that impinges on the saddle during riding.

Spina bifida cystica and/or meroanencephaly (anencephaly [Fig. 18-17]) is strongly suspected in utero when there is a high level of alpha-fetoprotein (AFP) in the amniotic fluid (p. 106). In these cases, AFP may also be elevated in the maternal blood serum. *Amniocentesis* (see Fig. 6-14A) is usually performed on pregnant women with high levels of AFP for the determination of the AFP level in the amniotic fluid. An ultrasound scan would also be requested to try to confirm the presence of a NTD that has resulted in spina bifida cystica. The fetal vertebral column can be detected by ultrasound at 10 to 12 weeks' gestation (eight to ten weeks after conception); and, if present, *spina bifida cystica* is sometimes visible as a cystic mass adjacent to the affected area of the vertebral column (Fig. 18-18).

Nutritional and environmental factors undoubtedly play a role in the production of neural tube defects (NTDs). Studies have suggested that vitamins and folic acid supplements taken prior to conception reduce the incidence of NTDs (Wald, 1984; Cockroft, 1991). Certain drugs are known to increase the risk of myelomeningocele (e.g., valproic acid, p. 160). This anticonvulsant causes NTDs in one to two per cent of pregnancies if given during early pregnancy (fourth week of development) when the neural folds are fusing (Holmes, 1992a).

Pregnant animals exposed to hypothermia or vitamin A produce offspring with NTDs (Behrman, 1992). Recent studies have suggested that NTDs might result from specific biochemical abnormalities of the basement membrane, particularly hyaluronate which plays a role in cell division and the shape of the primitive neuroepithelium (Copp and Bernfield, 1988).

THE BRAIN

The neural tube cranial to the fourth pair of somites develops into the brain. Fusion of the neural folds in the cranial region and closure of the rostral neuropore result in the formation of *three primary brain vesicles,* from which the brain develops.

The Brain Vesicles (Figs. 18-3 and 18-19). During the fourth week three primary brain vesicles form: the *forebrain* or prosencephalon, the *midbrain* or mesencephalon, and the *hindbrain* or rhombencephalon. During the fifth week the forebrain partly divides into two vesicles, the *telencephalon* and *diencephalon,* and the hindbrain partly divides into the *metencephalon* and *myelencephalon*. Thus, there are five secondary brain vesicles.

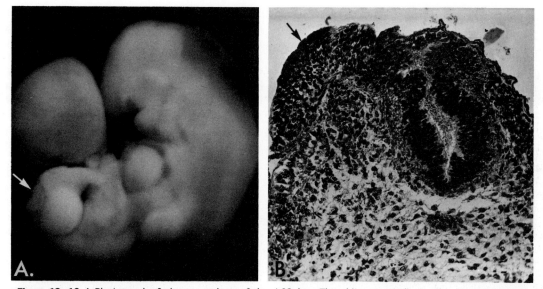

Figure 18–16. *A*, Photograph of a human embryo of about 28 days. The white arrow indicates the site of the neural tube defect (NTD) resulting from failure of closure of the caudal neuropore. Normally the caudal neuropore is closed by day 28. *B*, Photomicrograph of a transverse section through the NTD. The black arrow indicates an abnormal fold of neural tissue extending over the left side of the embryo. It appears that this overgrown neural fold has prevented closure of the neural tube. (From Lemire RJ, Shepard TH, Alvord EJ, Jr: *Anat Rec 152*:9, 1965.)

Figure 18–17. Photograph of an infant with acrania (absence of the calvaria), meroanencephaly, also called anencephaly (absence of part of the brain), rachischisis (failure of fusion of several vertebral arches), and spina bifida with myeloschisis (failure of closure of the neural folds; see Figs. 18–15 and 18–16). These infants are usually stillborn or die shortly after birth.

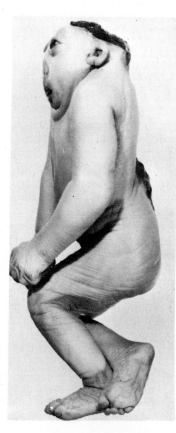

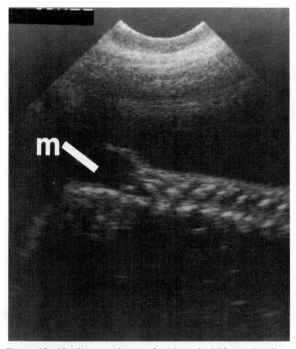

Figure 18–18. Ultrasound scan of a 14-week-old fetus showing a cystlike protrusion representing a meningomyelocele (*m*) in the sacral region of the vertebral column. The well-formed vertebral arches of the vertebrae superior to the neural tube defect are clearly visible. (Courtesy of Dr. Lyndon M. Hill, Magee-Women's Hospital, Pittsburgh, Pennsylvania.)

The Brain Flexures (Figs. 18–3 and 18–20). During the fourth week the embryonic brain grows rapidly and bends ventrally with the head fold (see p. 70 and Fig. 5–2). This produces the *midbrain flexure* in the midbrain region and the *cervical flexure* at the junction of the hindbrain and spinal cord. Later, unequal growth of the brain between these flexures in the hindbrain produces the *pontine flexure* in the opposite direction (Figs. 18–3C and 18–20A). This flexure results in thinning of the roof of the hindbrain (Fig. 18–20D).

Initially, the developing brain has the same basic structure as the developing spinal cord; however, the brain flexures produce considerable variation in the outline of transverse sections at different levels of the brain and in the position of the gray and white matter. The *sulcus limitans* extends cranially to the junction of the midbrain and forebrain, and the alar and basal plates are recognizable only in the midbrain and hindbrain.

The Hindbrain

The *cervical flexure* demarcates the hindbrain from the developing spinal cord (Figs. 18–3A and 18–20A). Later, this junction is arbitrarily defined as the level of the superior rootlet of the first cervical nerve, which is located roughly at the foramen magnum. The *pontine flexure* is located in the future pontine region. This flexure divides the hindbrain into caudal (myelencephalon) and rostral (metencephalon) parts. The myelencephalon becomes the *medulla oblongata* and the metencephalon gives rise to the *pons* and *cerebellum*. The cavity of the hindbrain becomes the fourth ventricle and the central canal in the caudal part of the medulla.

The Myelencephalon (Fig. 18–20). The caudal part of the myelencephalon (closed part of the medulla) resembles the spinal cord both developmentally and structurally. The lumen of the neural tube forms a small central canal. Unlike those of the spinal cord, neuroblasts from the alar plates in the myelencephalon migrate into the marginal zone and form isolated areas of gray matter called the *gracile nuclei* medially and the *cuneate nuclei* laterally. These nuclei are associated with correspondingly named tracts that enter the medulla from the spinal cord. The ventral area of the medulla contains a pair of fiber bundles called *pyramids*, which consist of corticospinal fibers descending from the developing cerebral cortex.

The rostral part of the myelencephalon ("open" part of the medulla) is wide and rather flat especially opposite the pontine flexure (Fig. 18–20C and D). The pontine flexure causes the lateral walls of the medulla to move laterally (outward) like the pages of an open book. It also causes the roof plate to become stretched and greatly thinned. In addition, the cavity of this part of the myelencephalon (part of the future fourth ventricle) becomes somewhat rhomboidal (diamond-shaped). As the walls of the medulla move laterally, the alar plates come to lie lateral to the basal plates. As the positions of the plates change, the motor nuclei generally develop medial to the sensory nuclei (Fig. 18–20C).

Neuroblasts in the basal plates of the medulla, like those in the spinal cord, develop into motor neurons that form nuclei and organize into three cell columns on each side (Fig. 18–20D). From medial to lateral, they are: (1) *general somatic efferent*, represented by neurons of the hypoglossal nerve, (2) *special visceral (branchial) efferent*, represented by neurons innervating muscles derived from the branchial of (pharyngeal) arches (see Chapter 10), and (3) *general visceral efferent*, represented by some neurons of the vagus and glossopharyngeal nerves.

Neuroblasts of the alar plates form neurons that are arranged in four columns on each side. From medial to lateral, they are: (1) *general visceral afferent*, receiving impulses from the viscera; (2) *special visceral afferent*, receiving taste fibers, (3) *general somatic*

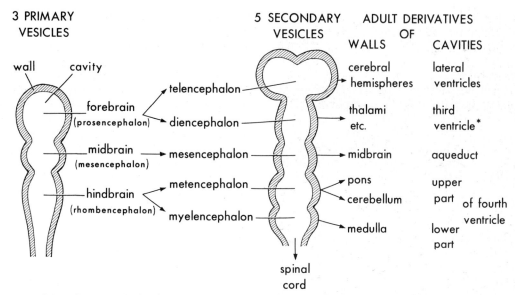

3 PRIMARY VESICLES

5 SECONDARY VESICLES

ADULT DERIVATIVES OF

WALLS

CAVITIES

wall — cavity

forebrain (prosencephalon) → telencephalon → cerebral hemispheres / lateral ventricles

→ diencephalon → thalami etc. / third ventricle*

midbrain (mesencephalon) → mesencephalon → midbrain / aqueduct

hindbrain (rhombencephalon) → metencephalon → pons / cerebellum / upper part of fourth ventricle

→ myelencephalon → medulla / lower part

spinal cord

Figure 18–19. Diagrammatic sketches of the brain vesicles indicating the adult derivatives of their walls and cavities. *The rostral (anterior) part of the third ventricle forms from the cavity of the telencephalon; most of the third ventricle is derived from the cavity of the diencephalon.

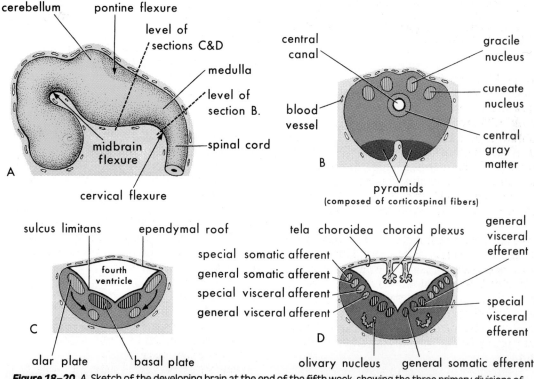

Figure 18–20. A, Sketch of the developing brain at the end of the fifth week, showing the three primary divisions of the brain and the brain flexures. B, Transverse section of the caudal part of the myelencephalon (developing closed part of the medulla). C and D, Similar sections of the rostral part of the myelencephalon (developing "open" part of the medulla), showing the position and successive stages of differentiation of the alar and basal plates. The arrows in C show the pathway taken by neuroblasts from the alar plates to form the olivary nuclei.

afferent, receiving impulses from the surface of the head, and (4) *special somatic afferent*, receiving impulses from the ear. Some neuroblasts from the alar plates migrate ventrally and form the neurons in the olivary nuclei (Fig. 18–20C and D).

The Metencephalon (Fig. 18–21). The walls of the metencephalon form the pons and cerebellum, and its cavity forms the superior part of the fourth ventricle. As in the rostral part of the myelencephalon, the pontine flexure causes divergence of the lateral walls of the pons and spreads the gray matter in the floor of the fourth ventricle. As in the myelencephalon, neuroblasts in each basal plate develop into motor nuclei and organize into three columns on each side.

The **cerebellum** develops from thickenings of dorsal parts of the alar plates. Initially, the cerebellar swellings project into the fourth ventricle (Fig. 18–21B). As the cerebellar swellings enlarge and fuse

in the median plane, they overgrow the rostral half of the fourth ventricle and overlap the pons and medulla (Fig. 18–21D). Some neuroblasts in the intermediate zone of the alar plates migrate to the marginal zone and differentiate into the neurons of the *cerebellar cortex*. Other neuroblasts from these plates give rise to the central nuclei, the largest of which is the *dentate nucleus*. Cells from the alar plates also give rise to the pontine nuclei, the cochlear and vestibular nuclei, and the sensory nuclei of the trigeminal nerve.

Divisions of the Cerebellum (Fig. 18–21C and D). The structure of the cerebellum reflects its phylogenetic development. The *archicerebellum* (flocculonodular lobe), the oldest part phylogenetically, has connections with the vestibular apparatus. The *paleocerebellum* (vermis and anterior lobe) is of more recent development and is associated with sensory data from the limbs. The *neocerebellum* (posterior lobe),

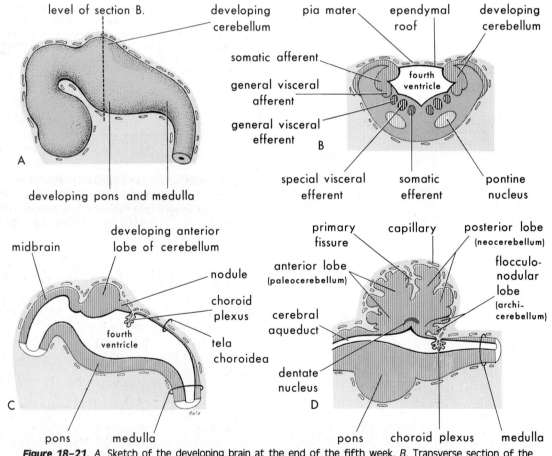

Figure 18–21. *A*, Sketch of the developing brain at the end of the fifth week. *B*, Transverse section of the metencephalon (developing pons and cerebellum), showing the derivatives of the alar and basal plates. *C* and *D*, Sagittal sections of the hindbrain at six and 17 weeks, respectively, showing successive stages in the development of the pons and cerebellum.

the newest part phylogenetically, is concerned with selective control of limb movement.

Nerve fibers connecting the cerebral and cerebellar cortices with the spinal cord pass through the marginal layer of the ventral region of the metencephalon. This region of the *brain stem* is called the *pons* (L. bridge) because of the robust band of nerve fibers that crosses the median plane and forms a bulky ridge on its anterior and lateral aspects.

Choroid Plexuses and Cerebrospinal Fluid (CSF)

The thin ependymal roof of the fourth ventricle is covered externally by *pia mater* derived from the mesenchyme associated with the hindbrain (Figs. 18–20, 18–21, and 18–25). This vascular pia mater, together with the ependymal roof, forms the *tela choroidea*. Because of the active proliferation of the pia mater, the tela choroidea invaginates the fourth ventricle where it differentiates into the *choroid plexus*. Similar choroid plexuses develop in the roof of the third ventricle and in the medial walls of the lateral ventricles.

The choroid plexuses are responsible for the *secretion of ventricular fluid* that becomes CSF when additions are made to it from the surfaces of the brain and spinal cord and from the pia-arachnoid layer of the meninges. The thin roof of the fourth ventricle evaginates in three locations. These outpouchings rupture to form foramina. The median and lateral apertures (foramen of Magendie and foramina of Luschka, respectively) permit the CSF to enter the *subarachnoid space* from the fourth ventricle.

The main site of absorption of CSF into the venous system is through the *arachnoid villi*, which are protrusions of the arachnoid into the dural venous sinuses (Moore, 1992). These villi consist of a thin, cellular layer derived from the epithelium of the arachnoid and the endothelium of the sinus.

The Midbrain

The midbrain (mesencephalon) undergoes less change than any other part of the developing brain except for the most caudal part of the hindbrain. The neural canal narrows and becomes the *cerebral aqueduct* (Fig. 18–21D), a canal that connects the third and fourth ventricles.

Neuroblasts migrate from the alar plates of the midbrain into the *tectum* (roof) and aggregate to form four large groups of neurons, the paired superior and inferior *colliculi*, which are concerned with visual and auditory reflexes, respectively. Neuroblasts from the

basal plates may give rise to groups of neurons in the *tegmentum* (red nuclei, nuclei of the third and fourth cranial nerves, and the reticular nuclei). The *substantia nigra*, a broad layer of gray matter adjacent to the cerebral peduncle, may also differentiate from the basal plate, but some authorities believe it is derived from cells in the alar plate that migrate ventrally.

Fibers growing from the cerebrum form the cerebral peduncles anteriorly. The *cerebral peduncles* become progressively more prominent as more descending fiber groups (corticopontine, corticobulbar, and corticospinal) pass through the developing midbrain on their way to the brain stem and spinal cord (Fig. 18–22E).

The Forebrain

As closure of the rostral neuropore occurs, two lateral outgrowths called *optic vesicles* appear, one on each side of the forebrain (Fig. 18–3A) . The optic vesicles are the primordia of the *retinae* and *optic nerves* (see Chapter 19). A second pair of diverticula soon arise more dorsally and rostrally; these are the *cerebral vesicles* or telencephalic vesicles (Fig. 18–22C). They are the primordia of the **cerebral hemispheres**, and their cavities become the *lateral ventricles*.

The rostral or anterior part of the forebrain, including the primordia of the cerebral hemispheres, is known as the *telencephalon*, and the caudal or posterior part of the forebrain is called the *diencephalon*. The cavities of the telencephalon and diencephalon contribute to the formation of the *third ventricle*, although the cavity of the diencephalon contributes more.

The Diencephalon (Fig. 18–23). Three swellings develop in the lateral walls of the third ventricle which later become the *epithalamus, thalamus*, and *hypothalamus*. The thalamus is separated from the epithalamus by the *epithalamic sulcus* and from the hypothalamus by the *hypothalamic sulcus*. The latter sulcus is not a continuation of the sulcus limitans into the forebrain and does not, like the sulcus limitans, divide sensory and motor areas.

The *thalamus* develops rapidly on each side and bulges into the cavity of the third ventricle, reducing it to a narrow cleft. The thalami meet and fuse in the midline in about 70 per cent of brains, forming a bridge of gray matter across the third ventricle called the *interthalamic adhesion* (massa intermedia).

The *hypothalamus* arises by proliferation of neuroblasts in the intermediate zone of the diencephalic walls ventral to the hypothalamic sulci. Later, a number of nuclei concerned with endocrine activities and homeostasis develop. A pair of nuclei, the *mamillary*

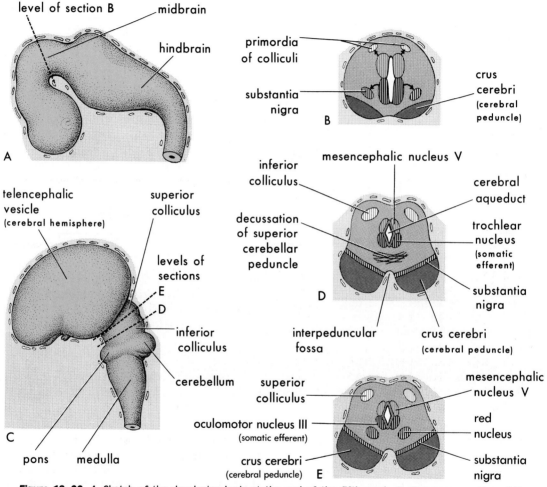

Figure 18-22. *A,* Sketch of the developing brain at the end of the fifth week. *B,* Transverse section of the developing midbrain, showing the early migration of cells from the basal and alar plates. *C,* Sketch of the developing brain at 11 weeks. *D* and *E,* Transverse sections of the developing midbrain at the level of the inferior and superior colliculi, respectively.

bodies, form pea-sized swellings on the ventral surface of the hypothalamus (Fig. 18–23C).

The *epithalamus* develops from the roof and dorsal portion of the lateral wall of the diencephalon. Initially the epithalamic swellings are large, but later they become relatively small.

The *pineal body* (gland) develops as a median diverticulum of the caudal part of the roof of the dien-

cephalon (Fig. 18–23C and D). Proliferation of cells in its walls soon converts it into a solid, cone-shaped gland.

The Pituitary Gland (Figs. 18–24 and 18–25; Table 18–1). The pituitary gland (hypophysis cerebri) is ectodermal in origin. It develops from two different sources: an upgrowth from the *ectodermal roof of the stomodeum* and a downgrowth from the

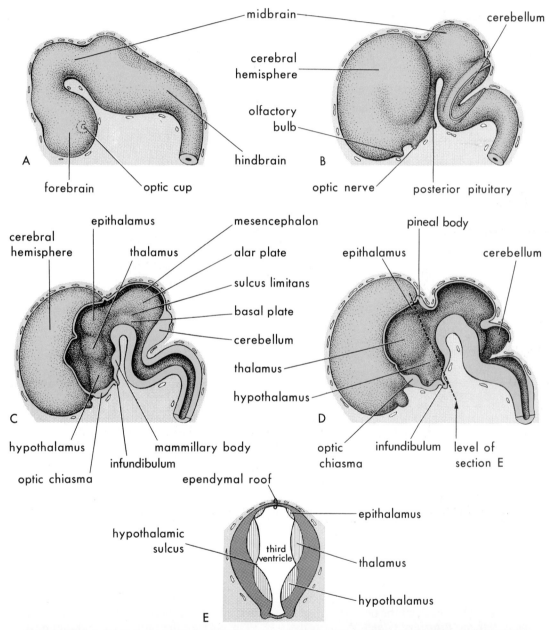

Figure 18–23. *A,* External view of the brain at the end of the fifth week. *B,* Similar view at seven weeks. *C,* Median section of this brain showing the medial surface of the forebrain and midbrain. *D,* Similar section at eight weeks. *E,* Transverse section of the diencephalon, showing the epithalamus dorsally, the thalamus laterally, and the hypothalamus ventrally.

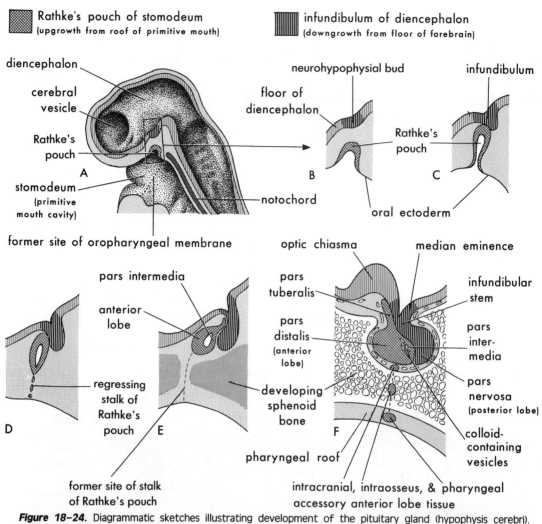

■ Rathke's pouch of stomodeum
(upgrowth from roof of primitive mouth)

▮ infundibulum of diencephalon
(downgrowth from floor of forebrain)

Figure 18–24. Diagrammatic sketches illustrating development of the pituitary gland (hypophysis cerebri). A, Sagittal section of the cranial end of an embryo of about 36 days, showing the hypophysial or Rathke's pouch, an upgrowth from the stomodeum, and the neurohypophysial bud from the forebrain. B to D, Successive stages of the developing pituitary gland. By eight weeks, the Rathke's pouch loses its connection with the oral cavity and is in close contact with the infundibulum, the primordium of the stalk, and the posterior lobe (neurohypophysis) of the pituitary. E and F, Later stages, showing proliferation of the anterior wall of the Rathke's pouch to form the anterior lobe (adenohypophysis) of the pituitary.

neuroectoderm of the diencephalon called *neurohypophysial bud*. This double embryonic origin explains why the gland is composed of two completely different types of tissue. The *adenohypophysis* (glandular portion) or anterior lobe arises from the oral ectoderm, and the *neurohypophysis* (nervous portion) or posterior lobe originates from the neuroectoderm.

Development of the Pituitary Gland. Around the middle of the fourth week, a diverticulum called the *hypophysial or Rathke's pouch* projects dorsally from the roof of the stomodeum and grows toward the

brain (Fig. 18–24A and B). By the fifth week this pouch has elongated and become constricted at its attachment to the oral epithelium, giving it a nipple-like appearance (Fig. 18–24C). By this stage it has come into contact with the *infundibulum* (derived from the neurohypophsial bud), a ventral downgrowth from the diencephalon (Figs. 18–23 to 18–25).

The parts of the pituitary gland that develop from the ectoderm of the stomodeum - pars anterior, pars intermedia, and pars tuberalis - are often referred to as the **adenohypophysis** (Table 18–1). The stalk of

Table 18-1. DERIVATION AND TERMINOLOGY OF THE PITUITARY GLAND (Hypophysis Cerebri)

Oral Ectoderm (From roof of stomodeum) →	Adenohypophysis (glandular portion)	{ Pars distalis { Pars tuberalis { Pars intermedia	Anterior lobe
Neuroectoderm (From floor of diencephalon) →	Neurohypophysis (nervous portion)	{ Pars nervosa { Infundibular stem { Median eminence	Posterior lobe

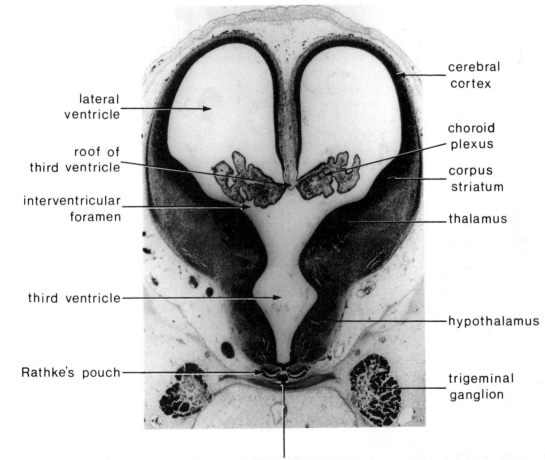

neurohypophysial bud

Figure 18-25. Photomicrograph of a transverse section through the diencephalon and cerebral vesicles of a human embryo (about 50 days) at the level of the interventricular foramina (× 20). This section is through the plane indicated in Figure 18-27A. The choroid fissure is located at the junction of the choroid plexus and the medial wall of the lateral ventricle. (Courtesy of Professor Jean Hay, Department of Anatomy, University of Manitoba, Winnipeg, Canada.)

Rathke's pouch passes between the chondrification centers of the developing presphenoid and basisphenoid bones of the skull (Fig. 18–24*E*). During the sixth week the connection of Rathke's pouch with the oral cavity degenerates and disappears (Fig. 18–24*D* and *E*).

A remnant of the stalk of Rathke's pouch may persist and give rise to a *pharyngeal hypophysis* in the roof of the oropharynx (Fig. 18–24*F*). Very rarely, accessory masses of anterior lobe tissue may develop outside the capsule of the pituitary gland within the sella turcica of the sphenoid bone. A remnant of the site of the stalk of Rathke's pouch called the *basipharyngeal canal* is visible in sections of the newborn sphenoid bone in about one per cent of cases. It can also be identified in a small number of radiographs of the skulls of newborn infants (usually those with skull abnormalities). Occasionally, *craniopharyngiomas* develop in the pharynx or in the basisphenoid from remnants of the stalk of Rathke's pouch, but most often they form in and/or above the sella turcica.

Cells of the anterior wall of Rathke's pouch proliferate actively and give rise to the *pars distalis* of the pituitary gland. Later, a small extension called the *pars tuberalis* grows around the infundibular stem. The extensive proliferation of the anterior wall of Rathke's pouch reduces its lumen to a narrow cleft (Fig. 18–24*E*). This residual cleft is usually not recognizable in the adult gland, but it may be represented by a zone of cysts. Cells in the posterior wall of Rathke's pouch do not proliferate; they give rise to the thin, poorly defined *pars intermedia* (Fig. 18–24*F*).

The part of the pituitary gland that develops from the neuroectoderm of the brain (infundibulum) is often referred to as the **neurohypophysis** (Table 18–1). The infundibulum gives rise to the *median eminence, infundibular stem*, and *pars nervosa* (Fig. 18–24*F*). Initially, the walls of the infundibulum are thin, but the distal end of the infundibulum soon becomes solid as the neuroepithelial cells proliferate. These cells later differentiate into *pituicytes*, which resemble neuroglial cells. Nerve fibers grow into the pars nervosa from the hypothalamic area to which the infundibular stem is attached.

The Telencephalon (Figs. 18–24 to 18–29). The telencephalon consists of a median part and two lateral diverticula, the *cerebral vesicles* (Fig. 18–24*A*). These diverticula are the primordia of the *cerebral hemispheres* (Figs. 18–19 and 18–23). The cavity of the median portion of the telencephalon forms the extreme anterior part of the third ventricle (Fig. 18–25).

At first the cerebral vesicles are in wide communication with the cavity of the third ventricle through the *interventricular foramina* (Fig. 18–25). Along a line known as the *choroid fissure* (Fig. 18–28*A*), part of the medial wall of the developing cerebral hemisphere becomes very thin. Initially, this thin ependymal portion lies in the roof of the hemisphere and is continuous with the ependymal roof of the third ventricle (Fig. 18–26*A*). The *choroid plexus* of the lateral ventricle later forms at this site (Figs. 18–25 and 18–27).

As the **cerebral hemispheres** expand, they successively cover the diencephalon, midbrain, and hindbrain. The cerebral hemispheres eventually meet each other in the midline, flattening their medial surfaces. The mesenchyme trapped in the longitudinal fissure between them gives rise to the *falx cerebri*, a median fold of dura mater (Moore, 1992).

The **corpus striatum** appears during the sixth week as a prominent swelling in the floor of each cerebral hemisphere (Figs. 18–25 and 18–27*B*). The floor of each hemisphere expands more slowly than their thin cortical walls because it contains the rather large corpus striatum; consequently, the cerebral hemispheres become C-shaped (Fig. 18–28).

The growth and curvature of the hemispheres also affect the shape of the lateral ventricles. They roughly become C-shaped cavities filled with CSF. The caudal end of each cerebral hemisphere turns ventrally and then rostrally, forming the temporal lobe; in so doing, it carries the ventricle (forming the temporal horn) and the *choroid fissure* with it (Fig. 18–28). Here, the thin medial wall of the hemisphere is invaginated along the choroid fissure by vascular pia mater to form the *choroid plexus of the temporal (inferior) horn* of the lateral ventricle (Figs. 18–25 and 18–27*B*).

As the cerebral cortex differentiates, fibers passing to and from it pass through the corpus striatum and divide it into the *caudate* and *lentiform nuclei*. This fiber pathway called the **internal capsule** (Fig. 18–27*C*) becomes C-shaped as the hemisphere assumes this form. The caudate nucleus becomes elongated and horseshoe-shaped, conforming to the outline of the lateral ventricle (Fig. 18–28). Its pear-shaped head and elongated body lie in the floor of the frontal (anterior) horn and body of the lateral ventricle; whereas, its tail makes a U-shaped turn to gain the roof of the temporal or inferior horn.

Cerebral Commissures (Fig. 18–27). As the cerebral cortex develops, groups of fibers called commissures connect corresponding areas of the cerebral hemispheres with one another. The most important of these commissures cross in the *lamina terminalis*, the rostral end of the forebrain. This lamina extends from the roof plate of the diencephalon to the optic chiasma. It is the natural pathway from one hemisphere to the other.

The first commissures to form, the *anterior commissure* and the *hippocampal commissure*, are small

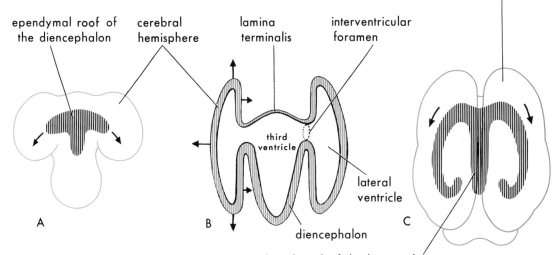

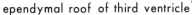

Figure 18-26. *A*, Sketch of the dorsal surface of the forebrain, indicating how the ependymal roof of the diencephalon is carried out to the dorsomedial surface of the cerebral hemispheres. *B*, Diagrammatic section of the forebrain, showing how the developing cerebral hemispheres grow from the lateral walls of the forebrain and expand in all directions until they cover the diencephalon. The arrows indicate some directions in which the hemispheres expand. The rostral wall of the forebrain called the lamina terminalis is very thin. *C*, Sketch of the forebrain as viewed anteriorly, showing how the ependymal roof is finally carried into the temporal lobes as a result of the C-shaped growth pattern of the cerebral hemispheres.

fiber bundles that connect phylogenetically older parts of the brain. The anterior commissure connects the olfactory bulb and related brain areas of one hemisphere with those of the opposite side. The hippocampal commissure connects the hippocampal formations.

The largest cerebral commissure is the *corpus callosum* (Fig. 18–27*A*), connecting neocortical areas. The corpus callosum initially lies in the lamina terminalis, but fibers are added to it as the cortex enlarges; as a result, it gradually extends beyond the lamina terminalis. The rest of the lamina terminalis lies between the corpus callosum and the fornix. It becomes stretched to form the thin *septum pellucidum* (a thin plate of brain tissue [Barr and Kiernan, 1988]). At birth the corpus callosum extends over the roof of the diencephalon. The *optic chiasma*, which develops in the ventral part of the lamina terminalis (Fig. 18–27*A*), consists of fibers from the medial halves of the retinae, which cross to join the optic tract of the opposite side.

Differentiation of the Cerebral Cortex. The walls of the developing cerebral hemispheres initially show the three typical zones of the neural tube (ventricular, intermediate, and marginal); later, a fourth one, the subventricular zone, appears. Cells of the intermediate zone migrate into the marginal zone and give

rise to the cortical layers. The gray matter is thus located peripherally, and axons from its cell bodies pass centrally to form the large volume of white matter known as the *medullary center*.

Initially, the surface of the hemispheres is smooth (Fig. 18–29*A*); but, as growth proceeds, a complex pattern of *sulci* (grooves or furrows) and *gyri* (convolutions or elevations) develops. The sulci and gyri permit a considerable increase in the surface area of the cerebral cortex without requiring an extensive increase in cranial size.

As each cerebral hemisphere grows, the cortex covering the external surface of the corpus striatum grows relatively slowly and is soon overgrown (Fig. 18–29*C*). This buried cortex, hidden from view in the depths of the lateral sulcus (fissure) of the cerebral hemisphere, is known as the *insula* (L. island).

Congenital Anomalies of the Brain

Due to the complexity of its embryological history, abnormal development of the brain is common (about three per 1000 births). Most major congenital anomalies of the brain (e.g., meroanencephaly [anencephaly] and meningoencephalocele) result from defective closure of the rostral neuropore during the fourth week (Figs. 18–17 and 18–30*C*) and involve the overlying tissues (meninges and calvaria). The factors causing the **neural tube defects**

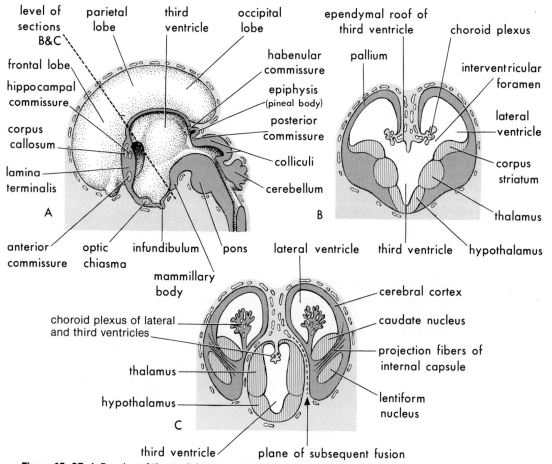

level of
sections
B&C

parietal
lobe

third
ventricle

occipital
lobe

ependymal roof of
third ventricle

choroid plexus

frontal lobe

hippocampal
commissure

corpus
callosum

lamina
terminalis

A

habenular
commissure

epiphysis
(pineal body)

posterior
commissure

colliculi

cerebellum

pallium

interventricular
foramen

lateral
ventricle

corpus
striatum

thalamus

B

anterior
commissure

optic
chiasma

infundibulum

pons

mammillary
body

third ventricle

hypothalamus

lateral ventricle

cerebral cortex

choroid plexus of lateral
and third ventricles

thalamus

hypothalamus

C

third ventricle

plane of subsequent fusion

caudate nucleus

projection fibers of
internal capsule

lentiform
nucleus

Figure 18–27. *A,* Drawing of the medial surface of the forebrain of a ten-week embryo, showing the diencephalic derivatives, the main commissures, and the expanding cerebral hemispheres. *B,* Transverse section of the forebrain at the level of the interventricular foramen, showing the corpus striatum and choroid plexuses of the lateral ventricles. *C,* Similar section at about 11 weeks, showing division of the corpus striatum into caudate and lentiform nuclei by the internal capsule. The developing relationship of the cerebral hemispheres to the diencephalon is also illustrated.

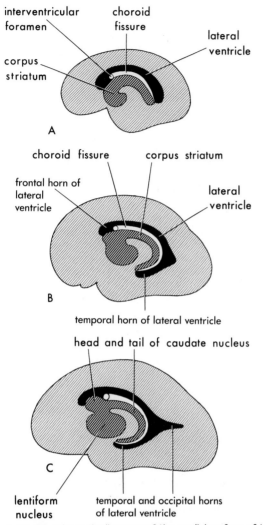

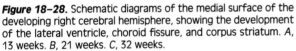

Figure 18–28. Schematic diagrams of the medial surface of the developing right cerebral hemisphere, showing the development of the lateral ventricle, choroid fissure, and corpus striatum. *A*, 13 weeks. *B*, 21 weeks. *C*, 32 weeks.

birth. Cerebral palsy is one of the most crippling conditions of childhood (Behrman, 1992).

Defects in the formation of the cranium (*cranium bifidum*) are often associated with congenital anomalies of the

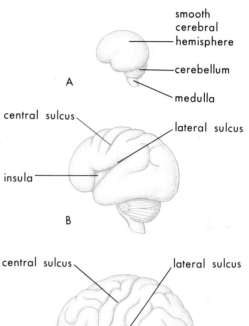

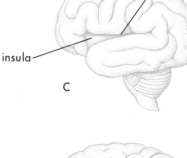

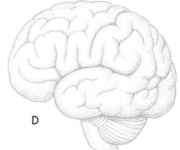

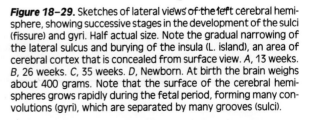

Figure 18–29. Sketches of lateral views of the left cerebral hemisphere, showing successive stages in the development of the sulci (fissure) and gyri. Half actual size. Note the gradual narrowing of the lateral sulcus and burying of the insula (L. island), an area of cerebral cortex that is concealed from surface view. *A*, 13 weeks. *B*, 26 weeks. *C*, 35 weeks. *D*, Newborn. At birth the brain weighs about 400 grams. Note that the surface of the cerebral hemispheres grows rapidly during the fetal period, forming many convolutions (gyri), which are separated by many grooves (sulci).

(NTDs) are genetic and/or environmental in nature. Congenital abnormalities of the brain may be caused by alterations in the morphogenesis or the histogenesis of the nervous tissue or they can result from developmental failures occurring in associated structures (notochord, somites, mesenchyme, and skull).

Abnormal histogenesis of the cerebral cortex can result in various types of congenital mental retardation. Severe **mental retardation** may result from exposure of the embryo/fetus during the 8- to 16-week period of development to certain viruses and high levels of radiation (see Fig. 8–13 and Table 8–5). Prenatal factors may be involved in the development of *cerebral palsy*, but this central motor deficit is most often due to a normal fetus's brain being damaged at brain and/or meninges. Such defects of the cranium are usually in the median plane and usually in the calvaria. The defect is often in the squamous part of the occipital bone and may include the posterior part of the foramen magnum. When the defect in the cranium is small, usually only the meninges herniate, and this condition is called a *cranial meningocele* or cranium bifidum with meningocele (Fig. 18–30*B*).

Some cases of meningomyelocele are associated with *craniolacunia* (defective development of the calvaria). This results in depressed, nonossified areas on the inner surfaces of the flat bones of the calvaria.

When the cranial defect is large, the meninges and part of the brain (Gr. *enkephalos*) herniate, forming a *meningoencephalocele* (Fig. 18–30*C*). If the protruding part of the brain contains part of the ventricular system, the defect is called a *meningohydroencephalocele* (Figs. 18–30*D* and 18–31). The part of the brain that is in the meningeal sac depends on the location of the cranial defect. Cranium bifidum associated with herniation of the brain and/or its meninges occurs about once in every 2000 births.

Exencephaly and Meroanencephaly (Fig. 18–17). These severe anomalies of the brain are the result of failure of the rostral neuropore to close during the fourth week of development (about 25 days after fertilization). As a result, the forebrain primordium is abnormal, and development of the calvaria is defective. Most of the embryo's brain is exposed or extruding from the skull, a condition known as *exencephaly*.

Due to the abnormal structure and vascularization of the embryonic exencephalic brain, the nervous tissue undergoes degeneration. The remains of the brain appear as a spongy, vascular mass mostly consisting of hindbrain structures. Although this neural tube defect (NTD) is often called *anencephaly* (Gr. *an*, without, + *enkephalos*, brain), a rudimentary brain stem (medulla, pons, and midbrain) is present. For this reason, *meroanencephaly* (Gr. *meros*, part) is a better name for this anomaly.

Meroanencephaly (anencephaly) is a common *lethal anomaly*, occurring about once in every 1000 births. It is two to four times more common in females than in males. It is always associated with acrania (absence of the calvaria) and may be associated with *rachischisis* (Fig. 18–17) when defective neural tube closure is extensive. Meroanencephaly accounts for about half of the severe NTDs in Great Britain, and it is the most common serious anomaly seen in stillborn fetuses.

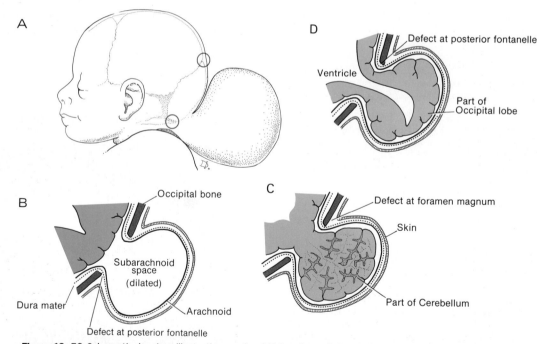

Figure 18–30. Schematic drawings illustrating cranium bifidum (bony defect in the cranium) and the various types of herniation of the brain and/or meninges. *A*, Sketch of the head of a newborn infant with a large protrusion from the occipital region of the skull, similar to that shown in Figure 18–31. The upper red circle indicates a cranial defect at the posterior fontanelle, and the lower red circle indicates a cranial defect near the foramen magnum. *B*, Meningocele consisting of a protrusion of the cranial meninges that is filled with cerebrospinal fluid. *C*, Meningoencephalocele consisting of a protrusion of part of the cerebellum that is covered by meninges and skin. *D*, Meningohydroencephalocele consisting of a protrusion of part of the occipital lobe that contains part of the posterior horn of a lateral ventricle.

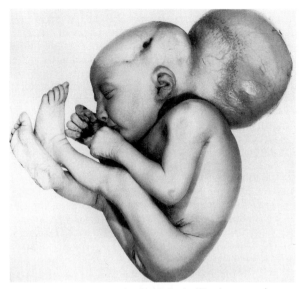

Figure 18–31. Photograph of an infant with a large meningoencephalocele in the occipital area. (Courtesy of Dr. Dwight Parkinson, Children's Centre, Winnipeg, Canada.)

Sustained extrauterine life is impossible in infants born with meroanencephaly. Infants with this severe NTD survive for a few hours after birth at most. Meroanencephaly is suspected in utero when there is an elevated level of alpha-fetoprotein in the amniotic fluid (p. 106). Meroanencephaly can be easily diagnosed by ultrasonography (Fig. 18–32), fetoscopy, and radiography because extensive parts of the brain and calvaria are absent. A therapeutic abortion is usually performed if the mother requests it, when continuation of the pregnancy will result in the birth of a child with severe anomalies, such as meroanencephaly, that are incompatible with life after birth.

Exencephaly and meroanencephaly can be induced experimentally in rats by using various teratogenic agents. Studies of exencephalic human abortuses suggest that the process is similar in humans (see Fig. 8–17). Genetic factors are certainly involved because of the well-established familial incidence of these defects. Meroanencephaly usually has a *multifactorial inheritance* (Thompson et al., 1991). An excess of amniotic fluid (*polyhydramnios*) is often associated with meroanencephaly, possibly because the fetus lacks the neural control for swallowing amniotic fluid; thus, the fluid does not pass into the intestines for absorption and subsequent transfer to the placenta for disposal.

Microcephaly (Fig. 18–33). In this uncommon condition the calvaria and brain are small but the face is of normal size. These infants are *grossly mentally retarded* because the brain is underdeveloped, a condition known as *microencephaly*. Microcephaly (Gr. *mikros*, small, + *kephale*, head) is the result of *microencephaly* (Gr. *mikros*, small, + *enkephalos*, brain) because growth of the *calvaria* is largely due to pressure from the growing brain.

The cause of microcephaly is often uncertain. Some cases appear to be genetic in origin (e.g., trisomy of the autosomes

[p. 146]), and others seem to be associated with environmental factors (Behrman, 1992). Exposure to large amounts of ionizing radiation (p. 167), infectious agents (e.g., cytomegalovirus, rubella, and *toxoplasma gondii* [Greenough et al., 1992]) and drugs (maternal alcohol abuse) during the fetal period are contributing factors in some cases (see Table 8–5).

Microcephaly can be detected in utero by ultrasound. Successive ultrasound scans carried out over the period of gestation are helpful in assessing the rate of growth of the fetal cranium. A small head may result from *premature synostosis* (osseous union) of all the cranial sutures (see Chapter 15), but the calvaria will be thin with exaggerated convolutional markings.

Agenesis of the Corpus Callosum. In this condition there is a complete or partial absence of the corpus callosum, the main neocortical commissure of the cerebral hemispheres. The condition may be asymptomatic, but seizures and mental deficiency are common. In two sisters with agenesis of the corpus callosum, the only symptoms were seizures, which were recurrent in one but only occasional and minor in the other. Their IQs were average. The cause of this anomaly is unknown; there is no evidence that it is inherited. For more information, see Lemire et al., 1975.

Hydrocephalus (Figs. 18–34 and 18–35). Significant enlargement of the head usually occurs due to an imbalance between the production and absorption of cerebrospinal fluid (CSF); as a result, there is **an excess of CSF** in the ventricular system of the brain. Hydrocephalus results from impaired circulation and absorption of CSF or, in very rare

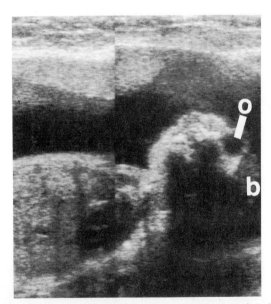

Figure 18–32. Ultrasound scan of a fetus (about 14 weeks) with meroanencephaly (anencephaly); *o* indicates the orbit and *b* represents the remnant of the brain. (Courtesy of Dr. Lyndon M. Hill, Magee-Women's Hospital, Pittsburgh, Pennsylvania.)

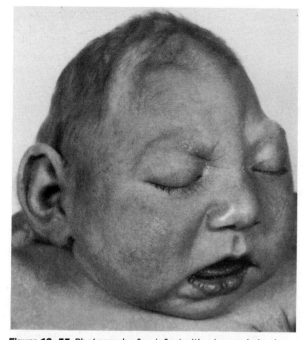

Figure 18–33. Photograph of an infant with microcephaly, showing the typical, normal-sized face and small calvaria covered with loose, wrinkled skin. (From Laurence KM, Weeks R: Abnormalities of the central nervous system. *In* Norman AP (ed): *Congenital Abnormalities in Infancy.* 2nd ed. 1971. Courtesy of Blackwell Scientific Publications.)

tricular system is enlarged. All ventricles are enlarged if the apertures of the fourth ventricle or the subarachnoid space and/or cisterns are blocked; whereas, the lateral and third ventricles are dilated when only the cerebral aqueduct is obstructed (Fig. 18–35). Although rare, obstruction of one interventricular foramen will produce dilation of one ventricle. Hydrocephalus resulting from obliteration of the subarachnoid cisterns or malfunction of the arachnoid villi is called *nonobstructive or communicating hydrocephalus.*

Hydrocephalus almost always is the result of interference with the circulation and absorption of CSF. It is rarely caused by CSF overproduction. Although hydrocephalus may be associated with spina bifida cystica (p. 395), enlargement of the head may not be obvious at birth. Hydrocephalus often produces thinning of the bones of the calvaria, prominence of the forehead, atrophy of the cerebral cortex and white matter, and compression of the basal ganglia and diencephalon.

Hydranencephaly (Fig. 18–36). This extremely rare anomaly may be confused with hydrocephalus. *The cerebral hemispheres are absent* or represented by membranous sacs with remnants of the cerebral cortex dispersed over the meninges (Behrman, 1992). The brain stem (midbrain, pons, and medulla) is relatively intact. These infants gener-

cases, from increased production of CSF by a choroid plexus adenoma (Behrman, 1992).[2]

Impaired circulation of CSF is often the result of *congenital aqueductal stenosis* in which the cerebral aqueduct is narrow or consists of several minute channels. In a few cases aqueductal stenosis is transmitted by an X-linked recessive trait (Behrman, 1992), but most cases appear to result from a *fetal viral infection* (e.g., cytomegalovirus or *Toxoplasma gondii* [p. 166]) or prematurity associated with intraventricular hemorrhage. Blood in the subarachnoid spaces may cause obliteration of the cisterns or arachnoid villi.

Blockage of CSF circulation results in dilation of the ventricles proximal to the obstruction and in pressure on the cerebral hemispheres. This squeezes the brain between the ventricular fluid and the bones of the calvaria. In infants the internal pressure results in an accelerated rate of expansion of the brain and calvaria because the fibrous sutures of the calvaria are not fused (p. 361).

Hydrocephalus usually refers to *obstructive or noncommunicating hydrocephalus* in which all or part of the ven-

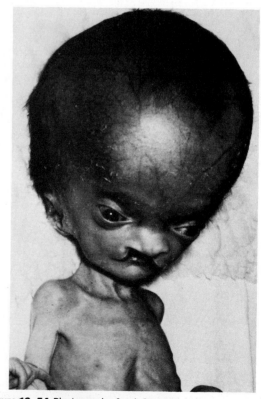

Figure 18–34. Photograph of an infant with hydrocephalus, bilateral cleft lip, and deformed limbs.

---

[2] Persons unfamiliar with the production, circulation, and absorption of CSF would benefit from the clinically oriented account of the ventricular system in the brain described by Moore (1992).

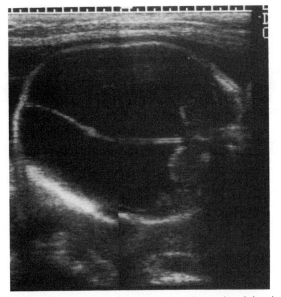

Figure 18–35. Ultrasound scan of a mature fetus's head showing severe hydrocephalus; *v* indicates the enlarged ventricles of the brain containing cerebrospinal fluid. (Courtesy of Dr. Lyndon M. Hill, Magee-Women's Hospital, Pittsburgh, Pennsylvania.)

ally appear normal at birth. The head grows excessively after birth due to the accumulation of CSF. A *ventriculoperitoneal shunt* is usually done to prevent continued enlargement of the calvaria (Behrman, 1992). Mental development fails to occur and there is little or no cognitive development. The cause of this unusual and severe anomaly is uncertain, but there is evidence that it may be the result of early obstruction of blood flow to the areas supplied by the internal carotid arteries (Lemire et al., 1975; Behrman, 1992).

Arnold-Chiari Malformation (Fig. 18–37). This is the most common congenital anomaly involving the lower brain stem and cerebellum. A tonguelike projection formed by elongation of the medulla and inferior displacement of *the vermis of the cerebellum herniates through the foramen magnum* into the vertebral canal (Taeusch and Ballard, 1991). The condition results in a type of communicating hydrocephalus in which there is interference with the absorption of CSF; as a result, the entire ventricular system is distended. The Arnold-Chiari or Chiari malformation occurs about once in every 1000 births and is frequently associated with spina bifida with meningomyelocele, spina bifida with myeloschisis, and hydrocephaly. The cause of the Arnold-Chiari malformation is uncertain; but, in some infants, the posterior cranial fossa is abnormally small. For a discussion of the various hypotheses about the cause of this anomaly, see Lemire et al. (1975).

Mental Retardation

Congenital impairment of intelligence may be the result of various genetically determined conditions (e.g., Down syndrome). It is also well known that mental retardation

may result from the action of a mutant gene or from a chromosomal abnormality (e.g., an extra chromosome 13, 18, or 21). Chromosomal abnormalities and mental deficiency are discussed in Chapter 8. *Maternal alcohol abuse* is thought to be the most common cause of mental retardation (p. 158).

The 8- to 16-week period of human development (Fig. 8–13) is the period of greatest sensitivity for *fetal brain damage resulting from large doses of radiation* (Mole, 1982; Otake and Schull, 1984; Persaud, 1990). By the end of the sixteenth week, most neuronal proliferation and cell migration to form the cerebral cortex are completed. Cell depletion of sufficient degree in the cerebral cortex results in severe mental retardation. Therapeutic abortion is often recommended when exposure exceeds 10,000 mrad (Holmes, 1992b).

Disorders of protein, carbohydrate, or fat metabolism may also cause mental retardation. *Maternal and fetal infections* (e.g., syphilis, rubella virus, toxoplasmosis, and cytomegalovirus) and cretinism are commonly associated with mental retardation (Riley and Vorhees, 1986; Adams, 1989; Persaud, 1990; Greenough et al., 1992).

Retarded mental development throughout the *postnatal growth period* can result from birth injuries, toxins (e.g., lead), cerebral infections (e.g., meningitis), cerebral trauma due to head injuries, and poisoning. For an excellent discussion of mental retardation and its many causes, see Shonkoff (1992).

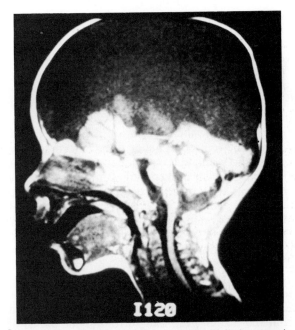

Figure 18–36. MRI of the head of an infant with hydranencephaly, showing the brain stem and spinal cord with remnants of the cerebellum and cerebral cortex. The remainder of the cranium is filled with CSF. (From Behrman RE (ed): *Nelson Textbook of Pediatrics.* 14th ed. Philadelphia, WB Saunders, 1992).

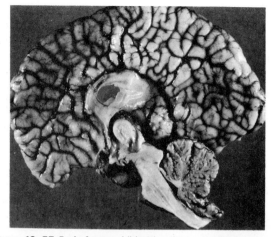

Figure 18–37. Brain from a child with a thoracolumbar meningomyelocele that illustrates the Arnold-Chiari malformation. The anomaly consists of elongation of the medulla with inferior displacement of the inferior part of the vermis of the cerebellum through the foramen magnum into the vertebral canal. (From Taeusch HW, Ballard RA, Avery ME (eds): *Schaffer and Avery's Diseases of the Newborn.* 6th ed. Philadelphia, WB Saunders, 1991.)

THE PERIPHERAL NERVOUS SYSTEM

The peripheral nervous system (PNS) consists of the cranial, spinal, and visceral nerves and the cranial, spinal, and autonomic ganglia. It develops from various sources. All sensory cells (somatic and visceral) of the PNS are derived from *neural crest cells*. The cell bodies of these sensory cells are located outside the central nervous system. With the exception of the cells in the spiral ganglion of the cochlea and in the vestibular ganglion of CN VIII (vestibulocochlear nerve), all the peripheral sensory cells are at first bipolar, but the two processes soon unite to form a single process and a unipolar type of neuron (Fig. 18–9*D*). This process has peripheral and central branches or processes. The peripheral process terminates in a sensory ending; whereas, the central process enters the spinal cord or brain (Fig. 18–8). The sensory cells in the ganglion of CN VIII remain bipolar.

The cell body of each afferent neuron is closely invested by a capsule of modified Schwann cells called *satellite cells* (Fig. 18–8), which are derived from neural crest cells. This capsule is continuous with the neurolemmal sheath of Schwann cells, also derived from the neural crest, that surrounds the axons of afferent neurons. External to the satellite cells is a layer of connective tissue that is continuous with the endoneurial sheath of the nerve fibers. This connective tissue and the endoneurial sheath are derived from mesenchyme.

Neural crest cells in the brain region migrate to form sensory ganglia only in relation to the trigeminal (CN V), the facial (CN VII), the vestibulocochlear (CN VIII), the glossopharyngeal (CN IX), and the vagus (CN X) nerves. Cells of the neural crest also differentiate into multipolar neurons of the *autonomic ganglia* (Fig. 18–8), including ganglia of the sympathetic trunks, that lie along the sides of the vertebral bodies; collateral, or prevertebral, ganglia in plexuses of the thorax and abdomen (e.g., the cardiac, celiac, and mesenteric plexuses); and parasympathetic, or terminal, ganglia in or near the viscera (e.g., the submucosal or Meissner plexus).

Cells of paraganglia called *chromaffin cells* are also derived from the neural crest. The term *paraganglia* includes several widely scattered groups of cells that are similar in many ways to medullary cells of the suprarenal (adrenal) glands. The cell groups largely lie retroperitoneally, often in association with sympathetic ganglia. The carotid and aortic bodies also have small islands of chromaffin cells associated with them. These widely scattered groups of chromaffin cells constitute the *chromaffin system*. Neural crest cells also give rise to melanoblasts (the precursors of the *melanocytes*) and to cells of the medulla of the suprarenal gland (see Fig. 13–19).

The Spinal Nerves

Motor nerve fibers in the spinal cord begin to appear at the end of the fourth week (Figs. 18–4, 18–6, and 18–8). The nerve fibers arise from cells in the *basal plates* of the developing spinal cord and emerge as a continuous series of rootlets along its ventrolateral surface. The fibers destined for a particular developing muscle group become arranged in a bundle, forming a *ventral nerve root*. The myelin sheaths of nerve fibers inside the spinal cord are formed by *oligodendroglia cells*; whereas, outside the spinal cord, the myelin sheaths are formed by *Schwann cells* (Figs. 18–8 and 18–11).

The *dorsal nerve root* is formed by axons of neural crest cells that migrate to the dorsolateral aspect of the spinal cord where they differentiate into the cells of the *spinal ganglion* (Figs. 18–4 and 18–7 to 18–9). The central processes of neurons in the spinal ganglion form a single bundle that grows into the spinal cord opposite the apex of the dorsal horn of gray matter (Fig. 18–4*B* and *C*). The distal processes of spinal ganglion cells grow toward the ventral nerve root and eventually join with it to form a *spinal nerve* (Figs. 18–4, 18–6, and 18–8).

Immediately after being formed, a **mixed spinal nerve** divides into dorsal and ventral primary rami (L. branches). The *dorsal primary ramus*, the smaller division, innervates the dorsal axial musculature (see

Fig. 16–1), vertebrae, posterior intervertebral joints, and part of the skin of the back. The *ventral primary ramus*, the major division of each spinal nerve, contributes to the innervation of the limbs and ventrolateral parts of the body wall. The *major nerve plexuses* (cervical, brachial, and lumbosacral) are formed by ventral primary rami.

As the limb buds develop, the nerves from the spinal cord segments opposite to them elongate and grow into its mesenchyme (see Fig. 17–4) and are distributed to its muscles, which differentiate from the mesenchyme. The skin of the developing limbs is also supplied in a segmental manner. Early in development, successive ventral primary rami are joined by connecting loops of nerve fibers, especially those supplying the limbs (e.g., the *brachial plexus* [Moore, 1992]). The dorsal division of the trunks of these plexuses supply the extensor muscles and the extensor surface of the limbs, and the ventral divisions of the trunks supply the flexor muscles and the flexor surface. The dermatomes and cutaneous innervation of the limbs are described in Chapter 17.

The Cranial Nerves[3]

Twelve pairs of cranial nerves form during the fifth and sixth weeks of development (Fig. 18–38). They are classified into three groups according to their embryological origins.

The Somatic Efferent Cranial Nerves (Fig. 18–38). The trochlear (CN IV), abducent (CN VI), hypoglossal (CN XII), and the greater part of the oculomotor (CN III) nerves are homologous with the ventral roots of spinal nerves. The cells of origin of these nerves are located in the *somatic efferent column* (derived from the basal plates) of the brain stem (Fig. 18–21). Their axons are distributed to the muscles derived from the head myotomes (preotic and occipital; see Fig. 16–2).

The hypoglossal nerve (CN XII) resembles a spinal nerve more than do the other somatic efferent cranial nerves (CN III, CN IV, and CN VI). CN XII develops by the fusion of the ventral root fibers of three or four occipital nerves (Fig. 18–38A). Sensory roots corresponding to the dorsal roots of spinal nerves are absent. The somatic motor fibers originate from the *hypoglossal nucleus* consisting of motor cells resembling those of the ventral horn of the spinal cord. These fibers leave the ventrolateral wall of the medulla in several groups, the *hypoglossal nerve roots*, which converge to form the common trunk of CN XII (Fig. 18–38B). They grow rostrally and eventually innervate the muscles of the tongue which are thought to be

derived from the occipital myotomes (see Fig. 16–2). With development of the neck, the hypoglossal nerve comes to lie at a progressively higher level (Fig. 18–38B).

The abducent nerve (CN VI) arises from nerve cells in the basal plates of the metencephalon (Fig. 18–21). It passes from its ventral surface to the posterior of the three preotic myotomes (see Fig. 16–2A) from which the lateral rectus muscle of the eye is thought to originate.

The trochlear nerve (CN IV) arises from nerve cells in the somatic efferent column in the posterior part of the midbrain (Fig. 18–22). Although a motor nerve, it emerges from the brain stem dorsally and then passes ventrally to supply the superior oblique muscle of the eye.

The oculomotor nerve (CN III) supplies most of the muscles of the eye (i.e., the superior, inferior, and medial recti and the *inferior oblique* muscles) which are thought to be derived from the first preotic myotomes (see Fig. 16–2).

The Nerves of the Branchial or Pharyngeal Arches (see Figs. 10–7A and 18–38A). Cranial nerves V, VII, IX, and X supply the embryonic arches; thus, the structures that develop from them are innervated by these cranial nerves (see Table 10–1).

The trigeminal nerve (CN V) is the nerve of the first arch (see Figs. 10–7A and 18–37A), but it has an ophthalmic division that is not a branchial component. *CN V is chiefly sensory* and is the principal sensory nerve for the head. Its large ganglion lies beside the rostral end of the pons, and its cells are derived from the most anterior part of the neural crest. The central processes of cells in this ganglion form the large sensory root of CN V, which enters the lateral portion of the pons. The peripheral processes of cells in this ganglion separate into three large divisions (the ophthalmic, maxillary, and mandibular nerves). Their sensory fibers supply the skin of the face (see Figs. 10–7B and 18–38B) as well as the lining of the mouth and the nose. The *motor fibers of CN V* arise from cells in the most anterior part of the *special visceral efferent column* in the metencephalon (Fig. 18–21). The motor nucleus of CN V lies at the midlevel of the pons. The fibers leave the pons at the site of the entering sensory fibers and pass to the muscles of mastication and to other muscles that develop in the mandibular prominence of the first arch (see Fig. 10–5 and Table 10–1). The *mesencephalic nucleus of CN V* (Fig. 18–22D) differentiates from cells in the midbrain that extend rostrally from the metencephalon.

The facial nerve (CN VII) is the nerve of the second arch. It consists mostly of motor fibers that arise principally from a nuclear group in the *special visceral efferent column* in the caudal part of the pons (Fig. 18–21). These fibers are distributed to the *muscles of*

---

[3] For a summary of the adult cranial nerves, see Moore (1992).

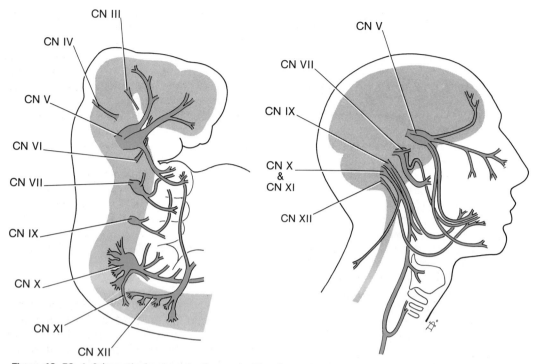

Figure 18–38. *A,* Schematic drawing of a five-week-old embryo, showing the distribution of most of the cranial nerves, especially those supplying the branchial or pharyngeal arches. *B,* Schematic drawing of an adult, showing the general distribution of most of the cranial nerves.

facial expression and to other muscles that develop in the mesenchyme of the second arch (see Fig. 10–5 and Table 10–1). The small general visceral efferent component of CN VII terminates in the peripheral autonomic ganglia of the head. The sensory fibers of CN VII arise from the cells of the *geniculate ganglion.* The central processes of these cells enter the pons, and the peripheral processes pass to the greater superficial petrosal nerve and, via the chorda tympani nerve, to the taste buds in the anterior two thirds of the tongue (see Fig. 10–21).

The glossopharyngeal nerve (CN IX) is the nerve of the third arch. Its motor fibers arise from the special and, to a lesser extent, the general visceral efferent columns of the anterior part of the myelencephalon (Fig. 18–20). CN IX forms from several rootlets that arise from the medulla just caudal to the developing internal ear (otic vesicle; see Fig. 19–13). All fibers from the special visceral efferent column are distributed to the stylopharyngeus muscle, which is derived from mesenchyme in the third arch (see Fig. 10–6 and Table 10–1). The general efferent fibers are distributed to the otic ganglion from which postganglionic fibers pass to the parotid and posterior lingual glands. The *sensory fibers of CN IX* are distributed as

general sensory and special visceral afferent fibers (taste fibers) to the posterior part of the tongue (see Fig. 10–21).

The vagus nerve (CN X) is formed by fusion of the nerves of the fourth and sixth arches (see Table 10–1). It has large visceral efferent and visceral afferent components that are distributed to the heart, the foregut and its derivatives, and to a large part of the midgut (see Chapter 12).

The nerve of the fourth arch becomes the *superior laryngeal nerve* which supplies the cricothyroid muscle and the constrictors of the pharynx. The nerve of the sixth arch becomes the *recurrent laryngeal nerve* which supplies various laryngeal muscles (see Table 10–1).

The accessory nerve (CN XI) has two separate origins (Fig. 18–38). The cranial root is a posterior extension of CN X and the spinal root arises from the cranial five or six cervical segments of the spinal cord. The fibers of the cranial root emerge from the lateral surface of the medulla where they join the vagus nerve and supply the muscles of the soft palate and the intrinsic muscles of the larynx. The fibers of the spinal root supply the sternocleidomastoid and trapezius muscles (Moore, 1992).

The Special Sensory Nerves. The *olfactory nerve (CN I)* arises from the olfactory bulb (see Fig. 10–30). The olfactory cells are bipolar neurons that differentiate from cells in the epithelial lining of the primitive nasal sac (see Fig. 10–26). The axons of the olfactory cells are collected into 18 to 20 bundles around which the *cribriform plate* of the ethmoid bone develops. These unmyelinated nerve fibers end in the olfactory bulb (Moore, 1992).

The optic nerve (CN II) is formed by more than one million nerve fibers that grow into the brain from neuroblasts in the primitive retina (see Fig. 19–2). Because the optic nerve develops from the evaginated wall of the forebrain, it actually represents a fiber tract of the brain. Development of the optic nerve is described in Chapter 19 (p. 426).

The vestibulocochlear nerve (CN VIII) consists of two kinds of sensory fiber in two bundles; these fibers form the vestibular and cochlear nerves. The *vestibular nerve* originates in the semicircular ducts (see Fig. 19–15), and the *cochlear nerve* proceeds from the cochlear duct in which the *spiral organ* (of Corti) develops. The bipolar neurons of the vestibular nerve have their cell bodies in the vestibular ganglion. The central processes of these cells terminate in the *vestibular nuclei* in the floor of the fourth ventricle. The bipolar neurons of the *cochlear nerve* have their cell bodies in the spiral ganglion (see Fig. 19–15*I*). The central processes of these cells end in the ventral and dorsal *cochlear nuclei* in the medulla.

THE AUTONOMIC NERVOUS SYSTEM

Functionally, the autonomic system can be divided into sympathetic (thoracolumbar) and parasympathetic (craniosacral) parts.

The Sympathetic Nervous System

During the fifth week, *neural crest cells* in the thoracic region migrate along each side of the spinal cord where they form paired masses (ganglia) dorsolateral to the aorta (see Figs. 13–20 and 18–8). All these segmentally arranged *sympathetic ganglia* are connected in a bilateral chain by longitudinal nerve fibers. These ganglionated cords called *sympathetic trunks* are located on each side of the vertebral bodies. Some neural crest cells migrate ventral to the aorta and form neurons in the *preaortic ganglia*, such as the celiac and mesenteric ganglia (Fig. 18–8). Other neural crest cells migrate to the area of the heart, lungs, and gastrointestinal tract where they form ter-

minal ganglia in sympathetic organ plexuses located near or within these organs.

After the sympathetic trunks have formed, axons of sympathetic neurons located in the *intermediolateral cell column* (lateral horn) of the thoracolumbar segments of the spinal cord pass via the ventral root of a spinal nerve and a *white ramus communicans* (connecting branch) to a paravertebral ganglion (Fig. 18–8). Here they may synapse with the neurons or ascend or descend in the sympathetic trunk to synapse at other levels. Other preganglionic fibers pass through the paravertebral ganglia without synapsing, forming splanchnic nerves to the viscera. The postganglionic fibers course through a *gray ramus communicans*, passing from a sympathetic ganglion into a spinal nerve; hence, the sympathetic trunks are composed of ascending and descending fibers.

The Parasympathetic Nervous System

The preganglionic parasympathetic fibers arise from neurons in nuclei of the brain stem and in the sacral region of the spinal cord. The fibers from the brain stem leave via the oculomotor (CN III), facial (CN VII), glossopharyngeal (CN IX), and vagus (CN X) nerves. The postganglionic neurons are located in peripheral ganglia or in plexuses near or within the structure being innervated (e.g., the pupil of the eye and the salivary glands).

Congenital Aganglionic Megacolon (Hirschsprung Disease). This condition of extreme dilation and hypertrophy of the colon (described on p. 260) results from failure of neural crest cells to migrate into the wall of the colon and to differentiate into parasympathetic ganglion cells.

SUMMARY

The central nervous system (CNS) develops from a dorsal thickening of ectoderm known as the *neural plate*. This plate appears around the middle of the third week and soon infolds to form a neural groove that has neural folds on each side. When the neural folds fuse to form the *neural tube* beginning during the middle of the fourth week, some neuroectodermal cells are not included in it but remain between the neural tube and the surface ectoderm as the *neural crest*. Development of the neural plate and neural tube is induced by the notochordal process and the associated mesoderm.

The cranial end of the neural tube forms the brain, consisting of the forebrain, midbrain, and hindbrain.

The forebrain gives rise to the cerebral hemispheres and diencephalon. The midbrain becomes the adult midbrain, and the hindbrain gives rise to the pons, cerebellum, and medulla oblongata. The remainder of the neural tube becomes the spinal cord.

The lumen of the neural tube becomes the ventricles of the brain and the central canal of the spinal cord. The walls of the neural tube thicken by proliferation of its neuroepithelial cells. These cells give rise to all nerve and macroglial cells in the central nervous system. The microglia differentiate from mesenchymal cells that enter the central nervous system with the blood vessels.

The *pituitary gland* (hypophysis cerebri) develops from two completely different parts: (1) an ectodermal upgrowth from the stomodeum known as *Rathke's pouch*, and (2) a neuroectodermal downgrowth from the diencephalon called the *neurohypophysial bud*. The *adenohypophysis* arises from the oral ectoderm and the *neurohypophysis* develops from the neuroectoderm (see Table 18–1).

Cells in the cranial, spinal, and autonomic ganglia are derived from the neural crest. Schwann cells, which myelinate the axons external to the spinal cord, also arise from the neural crest. Similarly, most of the autonomic nervous system and all chromaffin tissue, including the suprarenal medulla, develop from neural crest cells.

There are three types of congenital anomaly of the nervous system: (1) structural abnormalities resulting from abnormal organogenesis (e.g., neural tube defects (NTDs) resulting from abnormal development of the neural tube), (2) disturbances in the organization of the cells of the nervous system (e.g., due to the effects of high doses of radiation and severe malnutrition) that result in mental retardation, and (3) errors of metabolism, which are often inherited and can lead to severe mental retardation due to an accumulation of toxic substances (e.g., phenylketonuria) or to a deficiency of essential substances (e.g., congenital hypothyroidism).

Congenital anomalies of the central nervous system are common (about three per 1000 births). Defects in the closure of the neural tube (NTDs) account for most anomalies (e.g., spinal bifida cystica). The anomalies may be limited to the nervous system or they may include the overlying tissues (bone, muscle, and connective tissue).

Some anomalies of the central nervous system (CNS) are caused by genetic abnormalities (e.g., numerical chromosomal abnormalities such as trisomy 21); others result from environmental factors, such as infectious agents, drugs, and metabolic disease. Most CNS defects are probably caused by a combination of genetic and environmental factors. Gross congenital anomalies (e.g., meroanencephaly) are incompatible with life. Other severe defects (e.g., spina bifida with meningomyelocele) often cause functional disability (e.g., muscle paralysis in the lower limbs).

Severe abnormalities of the CNS may result from congenital anomalies of the ventricular system of the brain. There are two main types of hydrocephalus: *obstructive or noncommunicating hydrocephalus* (blockage of cerebrospinal fluid flow in the ventricular system) and *nonobstructive or communicating hydrocephalus* (blockage of cerebrospinal fluid in the subarachnoid space). In most cases congenital hydrocephalus is associated with spina bifida with meningomyelocele.

Mental retardation may result from chromosomal abnormalities arising during gametogenesis, from metabolic disorders, maternal alcohol abuse, or from infections occurring during prenatal life. Various postnatal conditions (e.g., cerebral infection) may also cause abnormal mental development.

CLINICALLY ORIENTED QUESTIONS FOR PROBLEM-BASED LEARNING SESSIONS

1. A pregnant woman developed polyhydramnios over the course of a few days (acute polyhydramnios). Using ultrasonography, a radiologist reported that the fetus had acrania and meroanencephaly. How soon can meroanencephaly (anencephaly) be detected by ultrasound scanning? Why is polyhydramnios associated with meroanencephaly? What other techniques could be used to confirm the diagnosis of meroanencephaly?

2. A male infant was born with a large lumbar meningomyelocele that was covered with a thin membrane. Within a few days the sac ulcerated and began to leak. A marked neurological deficit was detected inferior to the level of the sac. What is the embryological basis of this anomaly? What is the basis of the neurological deficit? What structures would likely be affected?

3. A CT scan of an infant with an enlarged head showed dilation of the lateral and third ventricles. What is this condition called? Where would the block most likely be to produce this abnormal dilation of the ventricles? Is this condition usually recognizable before birth? How do you think this condition might be treated surgically?

4. Is an enlarged head in an infant synonymous with hydrocephalus? What condition is usually associated with an abnormally small head? Is growth of the skull dependent on growth of the brain? What environmental factors are known to cause microencephaly?

5. A radiologist reporting on a pneumoencephalogram stated that the patient's ventricles were dilated posteriorly and that the lateral ventricles were also widely separated by a dilated third ventricle. Agenesis of the corpus callosum was diagnosed. What is the common symptom associated with agenesis of the corpus callosum? Are some patients asymptomatic? What is the basis of the dilated third ventricle?

The answers to these questions are given on page 466.

References and Suggested Reading

Adams J: Prenatal exposure to teratogenic agents and neurodevelopmental outcome. *Research in Infant Assessment (BD:OAS 25:63)*, 1989.

Alvarez IS, Schoenwolf GC: Expansion of surface epithelium provides the major extrinsic force for bending of the neural tube. *J Exp Zool 261*:340, 1992.

Angevine JB Jr, Bodian D, Coulombre AJ, et al.: Embryonic vertebrate central nervous system: revised terminology. *Anat Rec 166*:257, 1970.

Barr ML, Kiernan JA: *The Human Nervous System: An Anatomical Viewpoint.* 5th ed. Philadelphia, JB Lippincott, 1988.

Behrman RE: *Nelson Textbook of Pediatrics.* 14th ed. Philadelphia, WB Saunders, 1992.

Beks JWF: Defects of the lumbar spinal axis. *In* Huffstadt AJC (ed): *Congenital Malformations.* Amsterdam, Excerpta Medica, 1980.

Bell JE: The pathology of central nervous system defects in human fetuses of different gestational ages. *In* Persaud TVN (ed): *Advances in the Study of Birth Defects Vol 7. Central Nervous System and Craniofacial Malformations.* New York, Alan R Liss, 1982.

Bruni JE, Del Bigio MR, Cardoso ER, Persaud TVN: Hereditary hydrocephalus in laboratory animals and humans. *Exp Pathol 35*:239, 1988.

Carpenter MB: *Core Text of Neuroanatomy.* 4th ed. Baltimore, Williams & Wilkins, 1991.

Chuong CM: Adhesion molecules (N-CAM and tenascin) in embryonic development and tissue regeneration. *J Craniofac Genet Dev Biol 10*:147, 1990.

Cockroft DL: Vitamin deficiency and neural tube defects: human and animal studies. *Hum Reprod 6*:148, 1991.

Conel JL: *Postnatal Development of the Human Cerebral Cortex.* Cambridge, Mass, Harvard University Press, 1959.

Copp AJ, Bernfield M: Accumulation of basement membrane-associated hyaluronate is reduced in the posterior neuropore region of mutant (curly tail) mouse embryo developing spinal neural tube defects. *Devel Biol 130*:583, 1988.

Cormack DH: *Ham's Histology.* 9th ed. Philadelphia, JB Lippincott, 1987.

Cormack DH: *Essential Histology.* Philadelphia, JB Lippincott, 1993.

Crelin ES: Development of the Nervous System. A Logical Approach to Neuroanatomy. *Clin Symp, Vol. 26(2)*, 1974.

DeVellis J, Ciment G, Lauder J (eds): *Neuroembryology. Cellular and Molecular Approaches.* New York, Alan R Liss, 1988.

Elder GA, Major EO: Early appearance of type II astrocytes in developing human fetal brain. *Brain Res 470*:146, 1988.

Evrard P: Les troubles du developpement prenatal du cortex cerebral human. *Bull Mem Acad R Med Belg 143*:356, 1988.

Fitzgerald MJT: *Neuroanatomy Basic and Clinical.* 2nd ed. London, Baillière Tindall, 1992.

Flint G: Embryology of the nervous system. *Br J Neurosurg 3*:131, 1989.

Greenough A, Osborne J, Sutherland S (eds): *Congenital, Perinatal and Neonatal Infections.* Edinburgh, Churchill Livingstone, 1992.

Holmes LB: Teratogens. *In* Behrman RE (ed): *Nelson Textbook of Pediatrics.* 14th ed. Philadelphia, WB Saunders, 1992a.

Holmes LB: Radiation. *In* Behrman RE (ed): *Nelson Textbook of Pediatrics.* 14th ed. Philadelphia, WB Saunders, 1992b.

Jacobson M: *Developmental Neurobiology.* 3rd ed. New York, Plenum Publishing, 1992.

Langman J, Guerrant RL, Freeman BG: Behavior of neuroepithelial cells during closure of the neural tube. *J Comp Neurol 127*:399, 1966.

Laurence KM, Carter CO, David PA: The major central nervous system malformations in South Wales. I. Incidence, local variations and geographical factors. *Br J Prev Soc Med 22*:146, 1968.

Laurence KM, Carter CO, David PA: The major central nervous system malformations in South Wales. II. Pregnancy factors, seasonal variations and social class effects. *Br J Prev Soc Med 22*:212, 1968.

Laurence KM, Weeks R: Abnormalities of the central nervous system. *In* Norman AP (ed): *Congenital Abnormalities in Infancy.* 2nd ed. Oxford, Blackwell Scientific Publications, 1971.

Lemire RJ: Variations in development of the caudal neural tube in human embryos (Horizons XIV–XXI). *Teratology 2*:361, 1969.

Lemire RJ, Loeser JD, Leech RW, Alvord EC, Jr: *Normal and Abnormal Development of the Human Nervous System.* Hagerstown, Harper & Row, 1975.

Lemire RJ, Shepard TH, Alvord EC, Jr: Caudal myeloschisis (lumbo-sacral spina bifida cystica) in a five millimeter (Horizon XIV) human embryo. *Anat Rec 152*:9, 1965.

Loggie JMH: Growth and development of the autonomic nervous system. *In* Davis JA, Dobbing J (eds): *Scientific Foundations of Paediatrics*. Philadelphia, WB Saunders, 1974.

Maden M, Ong DE, Chytil F: Retinoid-binding protein distribution in the developing mammalian nervous system. *Development 109*:75, 1990.

Mann RA, Persaud TVN: Histogenesis of experimental open neural defects in the chick embryo. *Anat Anz 146*:171, 1979.

Martinez-Martinez PFA: *Neuroanatomy. Development and Structure of the Central Nervous System*. Philadelphia, WB Saunders, 1982.

Milhorat TH: *Hydrocephalus and the Cerebrospinal Fluid*. Baltimore, Williams & Wilkins, 1972.

Mole RH: Consequences of pre-natal radiation exposure for postnatal development. *Int J Radiat Biol 42*:1, 1982.

Moore KL: *Clinically Oriented Anatomy*. 3rd ed. Baltimore, Williams & Wilkins, 1992.

Müller F, O'Rahilly R: Development of anencephaly and its variants. *Am J Anat 190*:193, 1991.

Müller F, O'Rahilly R: The development of the human brain from a closed neural tube at stage 13. *Anat Embryol (Berl) 177*:55, 1988.

Müller F, O'Rahilly R: The development of the human brain, including the longitudinal zoning in the diencephalon at stage 15. *Anat Embryol (Berl) 177*:55, 1988.

O'Rahilly R, Gardner E: The timing and sequence of events in the development of the human nervous system during the embryonic period proper. *Z Anat Entwicklungsgesch 134*:1, 1971.

O'Rahilly R, Müller F: *Developmental Stages in Human Embryos*. Washington, Carnegie Institution of Washington, 1987.

Otake M, Schull WJ: *In utero* exposure to A-bomb radiation and mental retardation: a reassessment. *Brit J Radiol 52*:409, 1984.

Padget DH.: Neuroschisis and human embryonic maldevelopment. New evidence on anencephaly, spina bifida and diverse mammalian defects. *J Neuropathol Exp Neurol 29*:192, 1970.

Page EW, Villee CA, Villee DB: *Human Reproduction. Essentials of Reproductive and Perinatal Medicine*. 3rd ed. Philadelphia, WB Saunders, 1981.

Parkinson D: The meningomyeloceles and allied malformations. *Manit Med Rev 43*:76, 1963.

Persaud TVN: Abnormal development of the central nervous system. *Anat Anz 150*:44, 1981.

Persaud TVN: *Environmental Causes of Human Birth Defects*. Springfield, Charles C Thomas, 1990.

Peters PW, Dormans JA, Geelan JA: Light microscopic and ultrastructural observations in advanced stages of induced exencephaly and spina bifida. *Teratology 19*:183, 1979.

Prechtl HF: Developmental neurology of the fetus. *Baillieres Clin Obstet Gynaecol 2*:21, 1988.

Riley EP, Vorhees CV (eds): *Handbook of Behavioral Teratology*. New York, Plenum Press, 1986.

Rodier PM: Developmental Toxicology. *Toxicol Pathol 18*:89, 1990.

Rutishauser U, Jessell TM: Cell adhesion molecules in vertebrate neural development. *Physiol Rev 68*:819, 1988.

Sanes JR: Extracellular matrix molecules that influence neural development. *Annu Rev Neurosci 12*:491, 1989.

Sasaki A, Hirato J, Nakazato Y, Ishida Y: Immunohistochemical study of the early human fetal brain. *Acta Neuropathol Berl 76*:128, 1988.

Schnurch H, Risau W: Differentiating and mature neurons express the acidic fibroblast growth factor gene during chick neural development. *Development 111*:1143, 1991.

Schoenwolf GG, Smith JL: Mechanisms of neurulation: traditional viewpoint and recent advances. *Development 109*:243, 1990.

Shager NT, Kelly AB, Wagner JA: Congenital absence of the corpus callosum. *N Engl J Med 256*:1171, 1957.

Shonkoff JP: Mental retardation. *In* Behrman RE (ed): *Nelson Textbook of Pediatrics*. 14th ed. Philadelphia, WB Saunders, 1992.

Smith AS, Blaser SI, Ross JS, Weinstein MA: Magnetic resonance imaging of disturbances in neuronal migration: illustration of an embryonic process. *Radiographics 9*:509, 1989.

Smith DW, Gong BT: Scalp-hair patterning as a clue to early fetal brain development. *J Pediatr 83*:375, 1973.

Taeusch HW, Ballard R, Avery ME (eds): *Schaffer and Avery's Diseases of the Newborn*. 6th ed. Philadelphia, WB Saunders, 1991.

Thompson MW, McInnes RR, Willard HF: *Thompson & Thompson Genetics in Medicine*. 5th ed. Philadelphia, WB Saunders, 1991.

Wald NJ: Neural tube defects and vitamins: The need for a randomized clinical trial. *Br J Obstet Gynecol 91*:516, 1984.

Wald NJ, Cuckle HS: AFP screening in early pregnancy. *In* Spencer JAD (ed): *Fetal Monitoring*. Oxford, Oxford University Press, 1991.

Williams PL, Warwick R, Dyson M, Bannister LH: *Gray's Anatomy*. 37th ed. Edinburgh, Churchill Livingstone, 1989.

19

The Eye and Ear

THE EYE

The visual organs or eyes develop from three sources: (1) neuroectoderm of the forebrain, (2) surface ectoderm of the head, and (3) mesoderm between these layers. The ectodermal outgrowth from the brain becomes the retina, iris, and optic nerve. The surface ectoderm forms the lens, and the surrounding mesoderm gives rise to the vascular and fibrous coats of the eye.

Eye formation is first evident at the beginning of the fourth week of development. Grooves called *optic sulci* appear in the neural folds at the cranial end of the embryo (Fig. 19–1*A* and *B*). As the neural folds fuse to form the forebrain vesicle, the optic sulci evaginate to form hollow diverticula called *optic vesicles*. These vesicles project from the sides of the forebrain into the adjacent mesenchyme (see Figs. 18–3*A* and 19–1*C*). The cavities of the optic vesicles are continuous with the lumen of the forebrain vesicle. The formation of optic vesicles is induced by the mesenchyme adjacent to the developing brain, probably through a chemical mediator. As the bulblike optic vesicles grow laterally, their distal ends expand, and their connections with the forebrain constrict to form hollow *optic stalks* (Fig. 19–1*D*). The optic vesicles soon come in contact with the surface of the ectoderm, and their lateral surfaces become flattened. Concurrently, the surface ectoderm adjacent to the vesicles thickens to form *lens placodes*, which are the primordia of the lenses (Fig. 19–1*C*). The formation of lens placodes is induced by a signal produced by the optic vesicles (see Chapter 5, p. 73).

The central region of each lens placode soon invaginates and sinks deep to the surface, forming a *lens pit* (Fig. 19–1*D*). The edges of the pit gradually approach each other and fuse to form a spherical *lens vesicle* (Fig. 19–1*F*), which is soon pinched off from the surface ectoderm (Fig. 19–1*H*). The lens vesicle develops into the lens of the eye.

As the lens vesicles are developing, the optic vesicles invaginate and become double-walled structures called *optic cups* (see Figs. 18–3*C* and 19–1*H*). The opening of each optic cup is large at first, but the rim of the optic cup infolds and converges around the lens

(Figs. 19–3 and 19–4). By this stage, the lens vesicles have lost their connection with the surface ectoderm and have entered the cavities of the optic cups (Figs. 19–1*H* and 19–4).

Linear grooves called *optic (choroid) fissures* develop on the ventral surface of the optic cups and along the optic stalks (Fig. 19–1*E* to *H*). The optic fissures contain vascular mesenchyme from which the hyaloid blood vessels will develop (Figs. 19–1*F* to *H*, 19–2, and 19–5). The *hyaloid artery*, a branch of the *ophthalmic artery*, supplies the inner layer of the optic cup, the lens vesicle, and the mesenchyme in the optic cup (Fig. 19–1*H*). The *hyaloid vein* returns blood from these structures.

As the edges of the optic fissure approach each other and fuse, the hyaloid vessels are enclosed within the optic nerve (Fig. 19–2*E* and *F*). The distal portions of the hyaloid vessels eventually degenerate (Fig. 19–5*D*), but their proximal portions persist as the *central artery and vein of the retina*.

The Retina

The retina develops from the walls of the optic cup, an outgrowth of the forebrain (Figs. 19–3 to 19–5). The outer, thinner layer of the optic cup becomes the *retinal pigment epithelium*, and the inner, thicker layer differentiates into the complex *neural retina*.

During the embryonic and early fetal periods, the two retinal layers are separated by an *intraretinal space* (Figs. 19–3 to 19–5); it represents the original cavity of the optic cup. This space gradually disappears as the two layers of the retina fuse but this fusion is never firm; hence, when an adult eyeball is dissected, the neural retina is often separated from the retinal pigment epithelium.

The retinal pigment epithelium becomes firmly fixed to the choroid, but its attachment to the neural retina is not so firm; hence, a *detached retina* may follow a blow to the eye, as may occur during boxing matches. Knowledge about eye development makes it clear that, in this clinical condition, it is not a detachment of the entire retina because the retinal pigment epithelium remains firmly attached to the underlying choroid. The detachment is at the site of adherence of

423

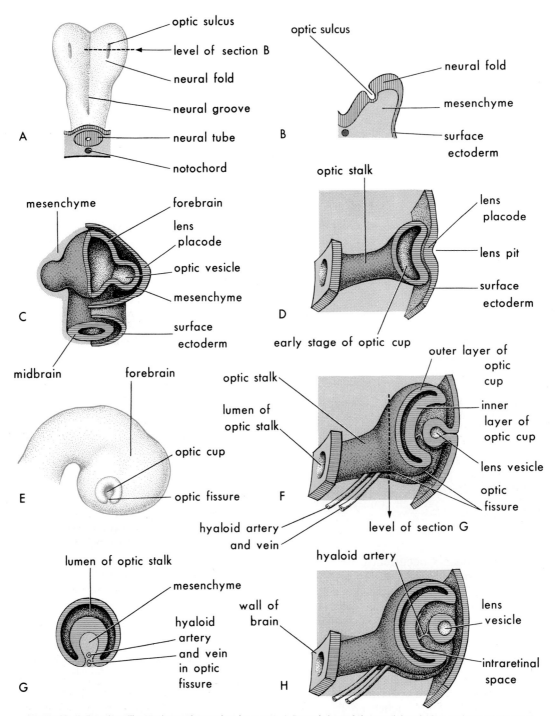

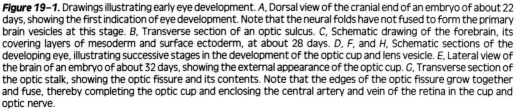

Figure 19–1. Drawings illustrating early eye development. *A,* Dorsal view of the cranial end of an embryo of about 22 days, showing the first indication of eye development. Note that the neural folds have not fused to form the primary brain vesicles at this stage. *B,* Transverse section of an optic sulcus. *C,* Schematic drawing of the forebrain, its covering layers of mesoderm and surface ectoderm, at about 28 days. *D, F,* and *H,* Schematic sections of the developing eye, illustrating successive stages in the development of the optic cup and lens vesicle. *E,* Lateral view of the brain of an embryo of about 32 days, showing the external appearance of the optic cup. *G,* Transverse section of the optic stalk, showing the optic fissure and its contents. Note that the edges of the optic fissure grow together and fuse, thereby completing the optic cup and enclosing the central artery and vein of the retina in the cup and optic nerve.

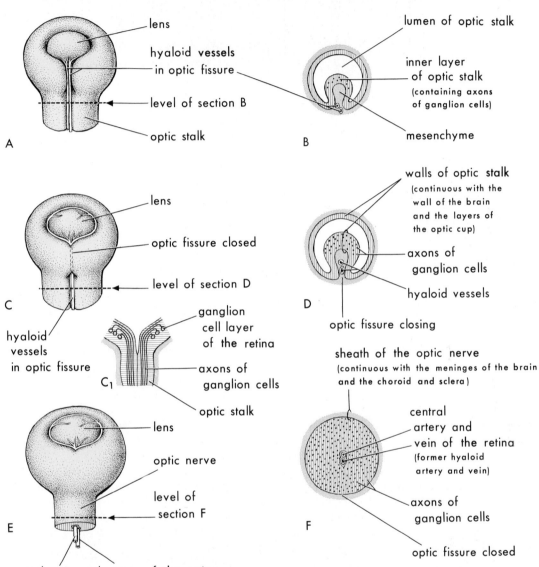

Figure 19–2. Diagrams illustrating closure of the optic fissure and formation of the optic nerve. *A, C,* and *E,* Views of the inferior surface of the optic cup and stalk, showing progressive stages in the closure of the optic fissure. C_1, Schematic sketch of a longitudinal section of a portion of the optic cup and optic stalk, showing axons of ganglion cells of the retina growing through the optic stalk to the brain. *B, D,* and *F,* Transverse sections of the optic stalk, showing successive stages in the closure of the optic fissure and in formation of the optic nerve. The optic fissure normally closes during the sixth week. Defects in closure of the fissure result in colobomata of the iris/retina (Fig. 19–8). Note that the lumen of the optic stalk is gradually obliterated as axons of ganglion cells accumulate in the inner layer of the optic stalk as the optic nerve forms.

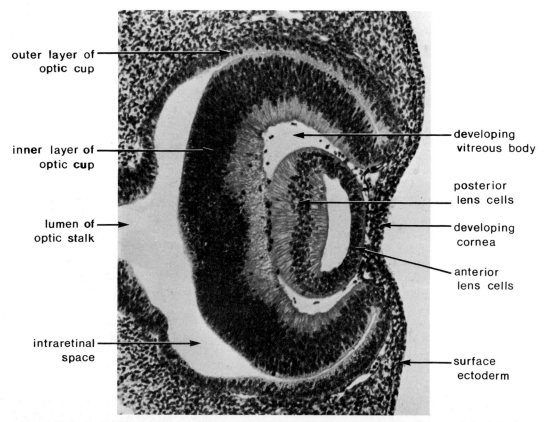

outer layer of
optic cup

inner layer of
optic cup

lumen of
optic stalk

intraretinal
space

developing
vitreous body

posterior
lens cells

developing
cornea

anterior
lens cells

surface
ectoderm

Figure 19–3. Photomicrograph of a sagittal section of the developing eye of a human embryo of about 41 days (×200). The intraretinal space in the optic cup represents the cavity of the original optic vesicle. (Courtesy of Dr. J. W. A. Duckworth, Professor Emeritus of Anatomy and Cell Biology, University of Toronto.)

the outer and inner layers of the optic cup. Although separated from the retinal pigment epithelium, the neural retina retains its blood supply (central artery of the retina) derived from the embryonic hyaloid artery. For details of the development of the blood vessels in the retina, see Penfold et al. (1990).

Because the optic cup is an outgrowth of the forebrain, the layers of the optic cup are continuous with the wall of the brain. Under the influence of the developing lens, the inner layer of the optic cup proliferates and forms a thick neuroepithelium. Subsequently, the cells of this layer differentiate into the light-sensitive region of the eye containing photoreceptors (*rods* and *cones*) and the cell bodies of neurons (e.g., bipolar and ganglion cells).

Because the optic vesicle invaginates as it forms the optic cup, the neural retina is "inverted"; i.e., the light-sensitive parts of the photoreceptor cells are adjacent to the retinal pigment epithelium. As a result, light must pass through most of the retina before reaching the receptors. Because the retina is thin and

transparent, however, it does not produce a barrier to light.

The axons of ganglion cells in the superficial layer of the neural retina grow proximally in the wall of the optic stalk to the brain. As a result, the cavity of the optic stalk is gradually obliterated, and the many axons of ganglion cells form the **optic nerve** (Fig. 19–2B, D, and F).

Myelination of the optic nerve fibers is incomplete at birth. After the eyes have been exposed to light for about ten weeks, myelination is complete, but the process normally stops short of the optic disc (Kwitko, 1979). The normal newborn infant can see, but not too well; it is able to fixate points of contrast. Visual acuity has been estimated to be in the range of 20/600.

The Ciliary Body

The pigmented portion of the epithelium of the ciliary body is derived from the outer layer of the optic cup and is continuous with the retinal pigment epi-

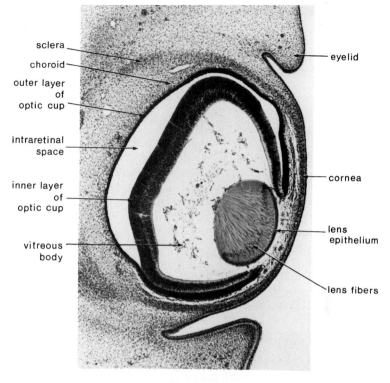

sclera
choroid
outer layer of optic cup
intraretinal space
inner layer of optic cup
vitreous body

eyelid
cornea
lens epithelium
lens fibers

Figure 19–4. Photomicrograph of a sagittal section of the developing eye of a human embryo of about 50 days (×75). The intraretinal space gradually disappears as the inner and outer layers of the optic cup fuse to form the retina (Fig. 19–5). (Courtesy of Professor Jean Hay, Department of Anatomy, University of Manitoba, Winnipeg, Canada.)

thelium (Figs. 19–5 and 19–6). The nonpigmented portion of the ciliary epithelium represents the anterior prolongation of the neural retina in which no neural elements differentiate. The *ciliary muscle* (the smooth muscle responsible for focusing the lens) and the connective tissue in the ciliary body develop from mesenchyme or early fibroblasts located at the edge of the optic cup in the region between the anterior scleral condensation and the ciliary pigment epithelium (Sellheyer and Spitznas, 1988, 1989).

The Iris

The iris develops from the anterior part or rim of the optic cup, which grows inward and partially covers the lens (Figs. 19–5 and 19–6). In this area the two layers of the optic cup have remained thin. The epithelium of the iris represents both layers of the optic cup. It is continuous with the double-layered epithelium of the ciliary body and with the retinal pigment epithelium and the neural retina.

The iris is bluish in most infants. It acquires its definitive color as pigmentation occurs during the first few months. It is the concentration and distribution of pigment-containing cells called *chromatophores* in the spongy, vascular, loose connective tissue of the iris that determine eye color. If the melanin pigment is confined to the *pigmented epithelium* on the posterior surface of the iris, the eye appears blue. If melanin is also distributed throughout the stroma of the iris, the eye appears brown.

The dilator and sphincter pupillae muscles of the iris are derived from the ectoderm of the optic cup. These smooth muscles are the result of a transformation of epithelial cells into smooth muscle fibers. The vascular connective tissue of the iris is derived from mesenchyme located anterior to the rim of the optic cup.

The Lens

The lens develops from the *lens vesicle*, a derivative of the surface ectoderm (Figs. 19–1 and 19–3 to 19–5). The anterior wall of this vesicle, composed of cuboidal epithelium, does not change appreciably as it becomes the *anterior lens epithelium*. The nuclei of the tall columnar cells forming the posterior wall of the lens vesicle undergo dissolution. These cells lengthen considerably to form highly transparent epithelial cells called *primary lens fibers*. As these fibers grow they gradually obliterate the cavity of the lens vesicle (Fig. 19–5A to C).

The rim of the lens is known as the *equatorial zone* or region (Fig. 19–5C) because it is located midway between the anterior and posterior poles of the lens. The cells in the equatorial zone are cuboidal. As these cells elongate, they lose their nuclei and become *secondary lens fibers*. They are added to the external sides of the primary lens fibers that developed from the posterior wall of the lens vesicle. Although secondary lens fibers continue to form during adulthood and the lens continues to increase in diameter, the primary lens fibers (formed during the embryonic period) must last a lifetime.

The developing lens is supplied by the *hyaloid artery* (Figs. 19–1 and 19–5); however, it becomes avascular in the fetal period. Thereafter it depends on diffusion from the aqueous humor in the anterior chamber bathing its anterior surface (Fig. 19–5) and from the vitreous humor around the rest of it.

The developing lens is invested by a vascular mesenchymal layer, the *tunica vasculosa lentis*. The anterior portion of this capsule is called the *pupillary membrane* (Fig. 19–5*B* and *C*). The portion of the hyaloid artery that supplies the tunica vasculosa lentis disappears during the late fetal period. As a result, the tunica vasculosa lentis and the pupillary membrane degenerate (Fig. 19–5*D*), but the *lens capsule* produced by the anterior lens epithelium and the lens fibers persists. The lens capsule represents a greatly thickened basement membrane, which has a lamellar structure because of its development. The former site of the hyaloid artery is indicated by the *hyaloid canal* in the vitreous body (Fig. 19–5*D*). It is usually inconspicuous in the living eye.

The **vitreous body** forms within the cavity of the optic cup (Figs. 19–3 to 19–5). It is composed of vitreous humor, an avascular mass of transparent, gelled, intercellular substance. The original vitreous humor is derived from the vascular mesenchyme in the optic cup. This primary *vitreous humor* does not increase, but it becomes surrounded by a gelatinous secondary vitreous humor, the origin of which is uncertain. It is generally believed to arise from the inner layer of the optic cup.

The Aqueous Chambers and the Cornea

The *anterior chamber of the eye* develops from a cleftlike space that forms in the mesenchyme located between the developing lens and the cornea (Figs. 19–3 and 19–5*A* to *C*). The mesenchyme superficial to this space forms the substantia propria of the cornea and the mesothelium of the anterior chamber. After the lens is established, it induces the surface ectoderm to develop into the epithelium of the cornea and the conjunctiva.

The **cornea** is formed from two sources: surface ectoderm and mesoderm (Sevel and Isaacs, 1989). The surface ectoderm forms the anterior surface of the cornea, which is covered by a stratified squamous, nonkeratinizing epithelium. The substantia propria, composed of dense fibrous connective tissue, and its simple squamous epithelium (corneal endothelium) are derived from the mesenchyme located anterior to the anterior chamber.

The *posterior chamber of the eye* develops from a space that forms in the mesenchyme posterior to the developing iris and anterior to the developing lens. When the pupillary membrane disappears and the pupil forms (Fig. 19–5), the anterior and posterior chambers of the eye are able to communicate with each other.

The Choroid and Sclera

The mesenchyme surrounding the optic cup differentiates into an inner vascular layer, the choroid, and an outer fibrous layer, the sclera (Figs. 19–4 and 19–5). The sclera develops from a condensation of the mesenchyme external to the choroid. Toward the rim of the optic cup, the choroid becomes modified to form the cores of the *ciliary processes*, consisting chiefly of capillaries supported by delicate connective tissue. The first choroidal blood vessels appear during the fifteenth week; and, by the twenty-second week, arteries and veins can be distinguished (Sellheyer, 1990). The sclera is continuous with the substantia propria of the cornea (Fig. 19–5*D*).

At the attachment of the optic nerve to the eye, the choroid is continuous with the pia-arachnoid of the brain, which forms the internal sheath around the optic nerve (Moore, 1992). The sclera is continuous with the dura mater of the brain, which forms the external sheath around this nerve. The continuity of these layers is understandable when it is recalled that the eyes develop from outgrowths of the brain. The subarachnoid space around the brain also extends around the optic nerves as far as their attachment to the eyes. This relationship of the sheaths of the optic nerve to the meninges of the brain and the subarachnoid space is clinically important (Moore, 1992). An increase in cerebrospinal fluid pressure causes edema of the optic disc and slows venous return from the retina. This occurs because the retinal vessels lie in the extension of the subarachnoid space that surrounds the optic nerve.

The Eyelids

The eyelids develop from two surface ectodermal folds containing cores of mesenchyme (Fig. 19–5). The eyelids meet and adhere by about the tenth week and remain adherent until the twenty-sixth week (see Chapter 6). While the eyelids are adherent, a closed *conjunctival sac* exists anterior to the cornea; when the eyes open, the *conjunctiva* covers the "white" of

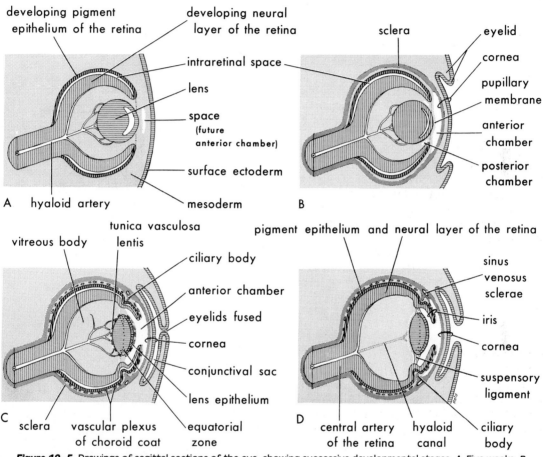

Figure 19–5. Drawings of sagittal sections of the eye, showing successive developmental stages. *A*, Five weeks. *B*, Six weeks. C, 20 weeks. *D*, Newborn. Note that the layers of the optic cup are fused and form the retinal pigment epithelium and neural retina and that they extend anteriorly as the double epithelium of the ciliary body and iris. The retina and optic nerve are formed from the optic cup and optic stalk, which are outgrowths of the brain (Fig. 19–1C). At birth the eye is about three quarters adult size. Most growth occurs during the first year. After puberty, growth of the eye is negligible.

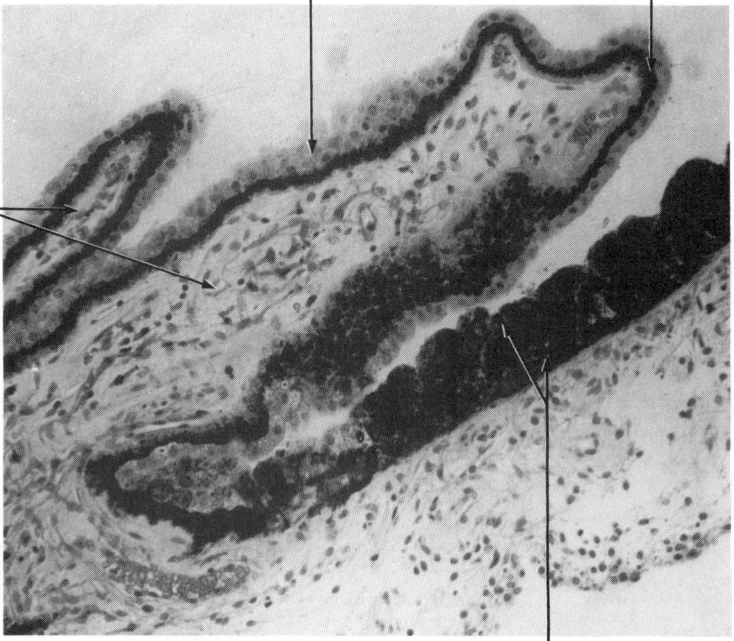

nonpigmented portion of
the ciliary epithelium
(continuous with the
neural layer of the retina)

pigmented portion of
the ciliary epithelium
(continuous with the pigment
epithelium of the retina)

ciliary
processes

Figure 19–6. Photomicrograph of the root of the adult iris (right) and ciliary processes, showing the ciliary and iridial parts of the retina (×215). (From Leeson TS, Leeson CR: *Histology.* 3rd ed. Philadelphia, WB Saunders, 1976.)

double-layered epithelium of the iris
(continuous with the neural and pigmented layers of the retina)

the eye and lines the eyelids. For a detailed account of the development of the eyelids, see Sevel (1988a).

The eyelashes and glands are derived from the surface ectoderm in a manner similar to that described for other parts of the integument (see Chapter 20). The connective tissue and tarsal plates develop from mesenchyme in the developing eyelids. The *orbicularis oculi muscle* is derived from mesenchyme in the second branchial or pharyngeal arch (see Chapter 10). As a result, it is supplied by the seventh cranial nerve (CN VII).

The Lacrimal Glands

At the superolateral angles of the orbits, the lacrimal glands develop from a number of solid buds from the surface ectoderm. These branch and become canalized to form the ducts and alveoli of the glands. The lacrimal glands are small at birth and do not function fully for about six weeks; hence, the newborn infant does not produce tears when it cries.

CONGENITAL ANOMALIES OF THE EYE

Because of the complexity of eye development, many anomalies may occur but most of them are uncommon. The type and severity of the anomaly depend upon the embryonic stage during which development is disrupted. Several environmental teratogens have been reported as causes of congenital eye abnormalities (Stromland et al., 1991). Most common anomalies of the eye are related to *defects in closure of the optic fissure*. This fissure normally closes during the sixth week (Fig. 19–2).

Coloboma of the Eyelid (Fig. 19–7). Defects of the eyelid (*palpebral coloboma*) are uncommon. A coloboma is usually characterized by a small notch in the upper eyelid, but the defect may involve almost the entire lid. Colobomata in the lower eyelid are also uncommon. Palpebral colobomata appear to result from a local developmental disturbance in the growth of the eyelid.

Coloboma of the Iris (Fig. 19–8). In these cases there is a defect in the inferior part of the iris, giving the pupil a keyhole appearance. The notch may be limited to the iris or it may extend deeper and involve the ciliary body and retina.

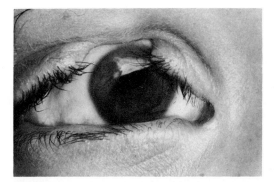

Figure 19–7. Photograph of the eye of a child with a coloboma of the iris and upper eyelid. (From Brown CA: Abnormalities of the eyes and associated structures. In Norman AP [ed]: *Congenital Abnormalities in Infancy.* 2nd ed. 1971. Courtesy of Blackwell Scientific Publications.)

A typical coloboma of the iris is the result of *failure of closure of the optic fissure* during the sixth week. This may be genetically determined or be caused by environmental factors. Simple colobomata of the iris are frequently hereditary and are transmitted as an autosomal dominant characteristic (Behrman, 1992).

Coloboma of the Retina. This defect is characterized by a localized gap in the retina, usually inferior to the optic disc. In most cases the defect is bilateral. A typical coloboma of the retina is the result of *defective closure of the optic fissure.*

Congenital Glaucoma (Fig. 19–9). Abnormal elevation of intraocular pressure in newborn infants is usually the result of abnormal development of the drainage mechanism of the aqueous humor during the fetal period. *Intraocular tension* rises because of an imbalance between production of aqueous humor and its outflow. This imbalance is the result of abnormal development of the *sinus venosus sclerae* (canal of Schlemm) in the iridocorneal angle or angle of the anterior chamber (Fig. 19–5D). Congenital glaucoma is usually caused by recessive mutant genes, but the condition may result from a rubella infection during early pregnancy (see Fig. 8–20B).

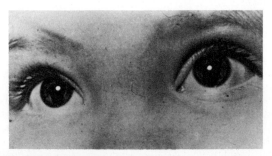

Figure 19–8. Photograph of the eyes of a child showing typical bilateral colobomata of the iris. (From Rahn EK, Scheie HG: The eye. In Rubin A [ed]: *Handbook of Congenital Malformations.* Philadelphia, WB Saunders, 1967.)

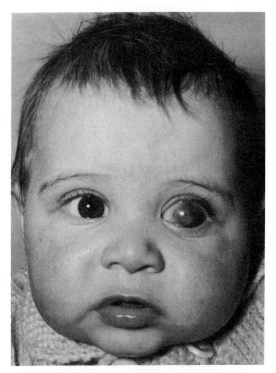

Figure 19–9. Photograph of a child with congenital glaucoma of the left eye. (Courtesy of Dr. C. A. Brown, Consultant Ophthalmologist, Bristol Eye Hospital, England.)

Congenital Cataract (see Fig. 8–20A). In this condition the lens is opaque and frequently appears grayish-white. Blindness results. Many lens opacities are inherited, dominant transmission being more common than recessive or sex-linked transmission (Behrman, 1992). Some congenital cataracts are caused by teratogenic agents, particularly the *rubella virus*, that affect early development of the lenses. They are vulnerable to rubella virus between the fourth and seventh weeks when primary lens fibers are forming (Figs. 19–3 and 19–4). Cataract and other ocular abnormalities caused by the rubella virus could be completely prevented if immunity to rubella were conferred on all women of reproductive age (Warkany, 1981).

Another cause of cataract is an enzymatic deficiency, *congenital galactosemia.* These cataracts are not present at birth, but they appear as early as the second week after birth. Due to enzyme deficiency, large amounts of galactose from milk accumulate in the infant's blood and tissues and cause injury to the lens that results in cataract formation (Crowley, 1974).

Congenital Ptosis of the Eyelid (Fig. 19–10). Drooping of one or both upper eyelids at birth is relatively common. Ptosis may be the result of abnormal development or failure of development of the levator palpebrae superioris muscle (Moore, 1992). Congenital ptosis may also be the result of prenatal injury or abnormal development of the superior division of the oculomotor nerve (CN III), which supplies this muscle. If ptosis is associated with inability to move the

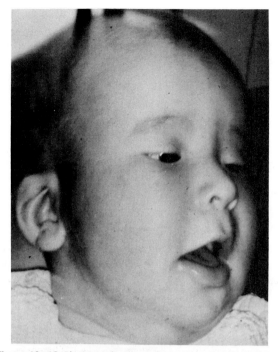

Figure 19–10. Photograph of an infant with congenital bilateral ptosis. Unilateral ptosis is more common. Drooping of the upper eyelid usually results from abnormal development or failure of development of the levator palpebrae superioris, the muscle that elevates the eyelid. In bilateral cases, as here, the infant contracts the frontalis muscle in an attempt to raise the eyelids. (From Taeusch HW, Jr, Ballard RA, Avery ME: *Schaffer and Avery's Diseases of the Newborn.* 6th ed. Philadelphia, WB Saunders, 1991.)

eyeball superiorly, there is also failure of the superior rectus muscle of the eye to develop normally. Congenital ptosis is hereditary, and the isolated defect is usually transmitted as an autosomal dominant trait (Brown, 1971).

Persistent Pupillary Membrane. Remnants of the pupillary membrane, which normally covers the anterior surface of the lens during the early fetal period (Fig. 19–5*B*), may persist as strands of connective tissue over the pupil. This tissue seldom interferes with vision and usually is of no consequence. Very rarely the entire pupillary membrane persists at birth, giving rise to a condition known as *congenital atresia of the pupil.*

Persistence of the Hyaloid Artery. The distal portion of this artery normally degenerates as its proximal part becomes the central artery of the retina. If a small part of the distal portion of the artery persists, it may appear as a freely moving nonfunctional vessel or as a cord projecting from the optic disc into the vitreous body. In some cases a remnant of the hyaloid artery may form a cyst. In unusual cases the entire distal portion of the artery persists and extends from the optic disc through the vitreous body to the lens. In most of these cases, the eye is microphthalmic (very small), but sometimes the eye is otherwise normal.

Congenital Detachment of the Retina. This condition, in which the pigmented and neural layers of the retina are separated, occurs when the inner and outer layers of the optic cup fail to fuse to form the retina and obliterate the intraretinal space (Fig. 19–4). The separation may be partial or complete. This anomaly may occur due to unequal rates of growth of the two layers of the optic cup; as a result, these layers are not in perfect apposition. Sometimes the layers of the optic cup appear to have fused and later separated; such secondary detachments usually occur in association with other anomalies of the eye and head.

Congenital Aphakia. Absence of the lens at birth is extremely rare and is the result of failure of the lens placode to form during the fourth week. This defect is the result of failure of lens induction by the optic vesicle (p. 73).

Congenital Aniridia. This is a congenital anomaly in which there is almost complete absence of the iris. This condition is the result of an arrest of development at the rim of the optic cup during the eighth week. The anomaly may be associated with glaucoma and other eye abnormalities. Aniridia may be familial, the transmission being dominant or sporadic.

Cryptophthalmos. "Hidden eye" occurs due to failure of the eyelids to develop; as a result, skin covers the eye. The eyeball is small and defective, and the cornea and conjunctiva usually do not develop. Fundamentally the defect means absence of the palpebral fissure but usually there is varying absence of eyelashes and eyebrows and eye defects (Jones, 1988). Cryptophthalos is an autosomal recessive condition that is usually part of the *cryptophthalmos syndrome.*

Microphthalmos. The eye may be very small and associated with gross ocular abnormalities or it may be a normal-appearing, miniature eye. The affected side of the face is underdeveloped and the orbit is small. Microphthalmos may be associated with other congenital abnormalities (e.g., facial cleft, p. 222) and be part of a syndrome (e.g., trisomy 13; see Fig. 8–5).

Severe microphthalmos is the result of arrested development of the eye before or shortly after the optic vesicle has formed in the fourth week. In these cases the eye is essentially undeveloped and the lens is not formed. If the interference with development occurs before the optic fissure closes in the sixth week, the eye is larger, but the microphthalmos is associated with gross ocular defects. When eye development is arrested in the eighth week or during the early fetal period, simple microphthalmos occurs (small eye with minor ocular abnormalities).

Some cases of microphthalmos are inherited. The hereditary pattern may be recessive or sex-linked with low penetrance (Smith and Guberina, 1979). Most cases of simple microphthalmia are caused by infectious agents (e.g., rubella virus, *Toxoplasma gondii,* and herpes simplex virus) that cross the placental membrane during the late embryonic and early fetal periods (see Table 8–5 and p. 165).

Anophthalmos (Fig. 19–11). The eyelid forms but no eyeball develops. In some cases eye tissue may be histologically recognizable. Absence of the eye is usually accompanied by other severe craniocerebral anomalies. In *primary anophthalmos,* eye development is arrested early in the fourth week and is the result of failure of the optic vesicle to form. In *secondary anophthalmos,* development of the entire forebrain is suppressed, and absence of the eyes is one of several anomalies.

the result of suppression of median cerebral structures that develop from the cranial part of the neural plate (O'Rahilly and Müller, 1989). Cyclopia is transmitted by recessive inheritance.

THE EAR

The ear consists of three anatomical parts: external, middle, and internal. The external and middle parts are concerned with the transference of sound waves from the exterior to the internal ear, which contains the *vestibulocochlear organ* concerned with equilibration and hearing.

The Internal (Inner) Ear

This is the first of the three anatomical divisions of the ear to develop. Early in the fourth week a thickening of surface ectoderm, the *otic placode*, appears on each side of the myelencephalon, the caudal part of the hindbrain (Figs. 19–13 to 19–15). Each otic placode soon invaginates and sinks deep to the surface ectoderm into the underlying mesenchyme. In so doing, it forms an *otic pit* (Fig. 19–13D). The edges of the otic pit soon come together and fuse to form an *otic vesicle* (otocyst), the primordium of the *membranous labyrinth* (Fig. 19–13G).

The otic vesicle soon loses its connection with the surface ectoderm. A diverticulum grows from this vesicle which elongates to form the *endolymphatic duct and sac* (Figs. 19–14 and 19–15A to E). Two regions of the otic vesicle soon become recognizable: a dorsal *utricular portion*, from which the utricle, semicircular ducts, and endolymphatic duct arise, and a ventral *saccular portion*, which gives rise to the saccule and cochlear duct.

Three flat, disklike diverticula grow from the utricular portion of the developing *membranous labyrinth*. Soon, the central portions of the walls of these diverticula fuse and disappear (Fig. 19–15B to E). The peripheral, unfused portions of the diverticula become the *semicircular ducts*. They are attached to the utricle and are later enclosed in the *semicircular canals* of the bony labyrinth. Localized dilatations, the *ampullae*, develop at one end of each semicircular duct. Sensory nerve endings differentiate in the ampullae (cristae ampullares) and in the utricle and saccule (maculae utriculi and sacculi).

From the ventral saccular portion of the otic vesicle, a tubular diverticulum called the *cochlear duct* grows and coils to form the *membranous cochlea* (Fig. 19–15C to E). The connection of the cochlea with the saccule becomes constricted to form the narrow *ductus reuniens*. The *spiral organ (of Corti)* differentiates from cells in the wall of the cochlear duct (Fig. 19–15F to I). Ganglion cells of the eighth cranial

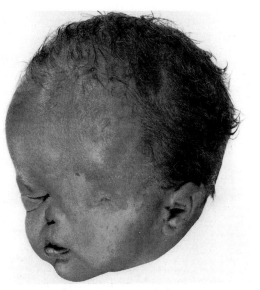

Figure 19–11. Photograph of an infant with anophthalmos and a single nostril.

Cyclopia (Fig. 19–12). In this very rare condition the eyes are partially or completely fused, forming a single, *median eye* enclosed in a single orbit. There is usually a tubular nose (proboscis) superior to the abnormal eye. The abnormality is frequently associated with other severe craniocerebral defects that are incompatible with life. Cyclopia appears to be

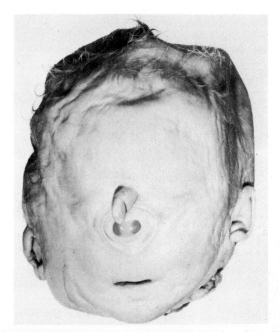

Figure 19–12. Photograph of a newborn infant with cyclopia. The fused eyes are in a single orbit that is surmounted by a proboscis, a tubular structure representing the nose. Because of gross anomalies of the skull, brain, and organs, these severely malformed infants do not survive long after birth.

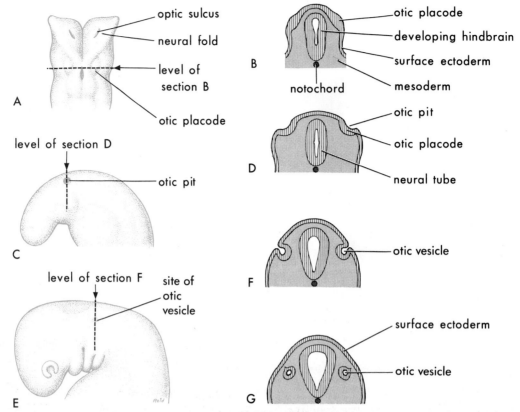

Figure 19–13. Drawings illustrating early development of the internal ear. *A*, Dorsal view of a four-week-old embryo (about 22 days), showing the otic placodes. *B, D, F,* and *G,* Schematic sections, illustrating successive stages in the development of otic vesicles. *C* and *E,* Lateral views of the cranial region of embryos, about 24 and 28 days, respectively.

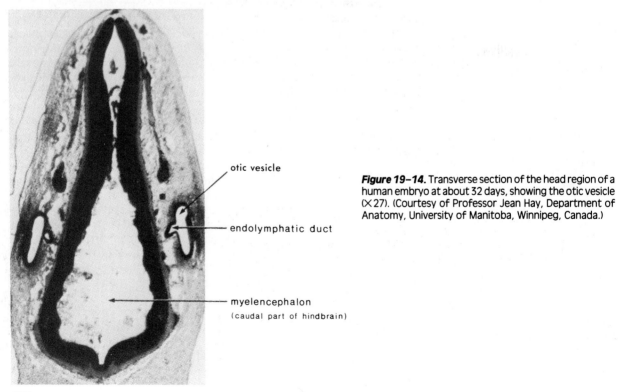

Figure 19–14. Transverse section of the head region of a human embryo at about 32 days, showing the otic vesicle (×27). (Courtesy of Professor Jean Hay, Department of Anatomy, University of Manitoba, Winnipeg, Canada.)

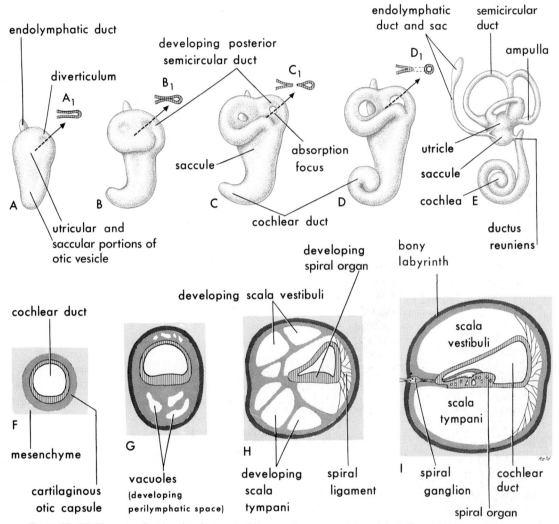

Figure 19–15. Diagrams showing development of the membranous and bony labyrinths of the internal ear. *A to E,* Lateral views showing successive stages in the development of the otic vesicle into the membranous labyrinth from the fifth to eighth weeks. A_1 to D_1, Diagrammatic sketches illustrating the development of a semicircular duct. *F to I,* Sections through the cochlear duct showing successive stages in the development of the spiral organ (of Corti) and the perilymphatic space from the eighth to the twentieth weeks.

nerve migrate along the coils of the cochlea and form the *spiral ganglion* (cochlear ganglion). Nerve processes extend from this ganglion to the *spiral organ* where they terminate on the hair cells. The cells in the spiral ganglion retain their embryonic bipolar condition (see Fig. 18–9*B*); that is, they do not become unipolar like spinal ganglion cells (see Fig. 18–9*D*).

The mesenchyme around the otic vesicle condenses and differentiates into a cartilaginous *otic capsule* (Fig. 19–15*F*). It has recently been suggested from the results of histochemical and *in vitro* studies that transforming growth factor beta (TGF-B1) may play a role in modulating epithelial-mesenchymal interaction in the internal ear and in directing the formation of the otic capsule (Frenz et al., 1991). As the membranous labyrinth enlarges, vacuoles appear in the cartilaginous otic capsule, which soon coalesce to form the *perilymphatic space*. The membranous labyrinth is now suspended in fluid, called *perilymph*, in the perilymphatic space. The perilymphatic space related to the cochlear duct develops two divisions, the *scala tympani* and *scala vestibuli* (Fig. 19–15*H* and *I*). The cartilaginous otic capsule later ossifies to form the *bony labyrinth* of the internal ear. The internal ear reaches its adult size and shape by the middle of the fetal period (20 to 22 weeks).

The Middle Ear

Development of the tubotympanic recess from the first pharyngeal pouch is described in Chapter 10 (p. 193). The distal portion of the tubotympanic recess expands and becomes the *tympanic cavity* (Fig. 19–16). The proximal portion of the tubotympanic

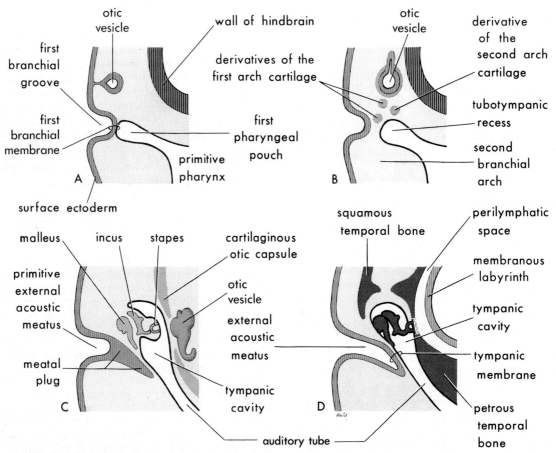

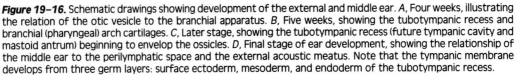

Figure 19–16. Schematic drawings showing development of the external and middle ear. *A*, Four weeks, illustrating the relation of the otic vesicle to the branchial apparatus. *B*, Five weeks, showing the tubotympanic recess and branchial (pharyngeal) arch cartilages. *C*, Later stage, showing the tubotympanic recess (future tympanic cavity and mastoid antrum) beginning to envelop the ossicles. *D*, Final stage of ear development, showing the relationship of the middle ear to the perilymphatic space and the external acoustic meatus. Note that the tympanic membrane develops from three germ layers: surface ectoderm, mesoderm, and endoderm of the tubotympanic recess.

recess becomes restricted to form the *auditory (Eustachian) tube.*

As the tympanic cavity expands it gradually envelops the *auditory ossicles* (malleus, incus, and stapes), their tendons and ligaments, and the chorda tympani nerve. All these structures receive a more or less complete epithelial investment. Even in adults the ossicles are covered with an epithelial layer. From a study of early human embryos and fetuses, it has been suggested that an epithelial-type organizer located at the tip of the tubotympanic recess probably plays a role in the early development of the middle ear and tympanic membrane (Michaels, 1988).

During the late fetal period, expansion of the tympanic cavity gives rise to the *mastoid antrum* located in the petromastoid part of the temporal bone (Moore, 1992). The mastoid antrum is almost adult size at birth; however, no mastoid cells are present in newborn infants. By two years of age the mastoid cells are well-developed and produce conical projections of the temporal bones called *mastoid processes.* The middle ear continues to grow through puberty (Ars, 1989; Behrman, 1992).

The development of the *auditory ossicles* (middle ear bones) is described in Chapter 10 (see Fig. 10–5). The tensor tympani, the muscle attached to the malleus, is derived from mesenchyme in the first branchial (pharyngeal) arch and is innervated by CN V (see Fig. 18–38), the nerve of this arch. The stapedius muscle is derived from the second arch and is therefore supplied by CN VII, the nerve of that arch.

The External Ear

The *external acoustic meatus* develops from the dorsal end of the first branchial (pharyngeal) groove. The ectodermal cells at the bottom of this funnel-shaped tube proliferate and form a solid epithelial plate called the *meatal plug* (Fig. 19–16C). Late in the fetal period, the central cells of this plug degenerate, forming a cavity that becomes the internal part of the external acoustic meatus (external auditory meatus). This meatus is relatively short at birth; and because of this, care must be taken not to injure the tympanic membrane. The external acoustic meatus attains its adult length around the ninth year.

The primordium of the *tympanic membrane* is the first branchial (pharyngeal) membrane, which separates the first branchial (pharyngeal) groove from the first pharyngeal pouch (Fig. 19–16A). As development proceeds, mesenchyme grows between the two parts of the branchial membrane and later differentiates into the collagenic fibers in the tympanic membrane. The external covering (very thin skin) of the tympanic membrane is derived from the surface ecto-

derm; whereas, its internal lining is derived from the endoderm of the tubotympanic recess. The tympanic membrane thus develops from three sources: *ectoderm* of the first branchial (pharyngeal) groove, *endoderm* of the tubotympanic recess from the first pharyngeal pouch, and *mesoderm* of the first and second branchial (pharyngeal) arches.

The *auricle* (pinna) develops from six mesenchymal swellings called *auricular hillocks*, which arise around the margins of the first branchial (pharyngeal) groove (Fig. 19–17A). The mesenchyme in these hillocks is derived from mesoderm in the first and second branchial (pharyngeal) arches. As the auricle grows, the contribution of the first arch becomes relatively reduced (Fig. 19–17B to D). The lobule is the last part of the auricle to develop. The auricles begin to develop in the cranial part of the future neck region (Fig. 19–17A). As the mandible develops, the auricles move to the side of the head and ascend to the level of the eyes (Fig. 19–17B to D). The external ears continue to grow throughout puberty.

The parts of the auricle derived from the first branchial (pharyngeal) arch are supplied by its nerve, the mandibular branch of the trigeminal nerve (CN V), but the parts derived from the second arch are supplied by cutaneous branches of the *cervical plexus*, especially the lesser occipital and greater auricular nerves. The facial nerve (CN VII) of the second arch has few cutaneous branches, but some of its fibers contribute to the sensory innervation of the skin in the mastoid region and probably in small areas on both aspects of the auricle (Moore, 1992).

CONGENITAL ANOMALIES OF THE EAR

Congenital Deafness. Because formation of the internal ear is independent of development of the middle and external ears, congenital impairment of hearing may be the result of maldevelopment of the sound-conducting apparatus of the middle and external ears or of the neurosensory structures of the internal ear.

Most types of congenital deafness are caused by genetic factors. In *deaf-mutism* the ear abnormality is usually perceptive in type. Congenital deafness may be associated with several other head and neck abnormalities as a part of the first arch syndrome (see Fig. 10–14). *Rubella infection* during the critical period of embryonic development of the internal ear, particularly during the seventh and eighth weeks (see Fig. 8–13), can cause maldevelopment of the spiral organ. Congenital deafness may also be associated with maternal goiter, which may result in fetal hypothyroidism.

Congenital fixation of the stapes results in conductive deafness in an otherwise normal ear. Failure of differentiation of the *anular ligament*, which attaches the base of the

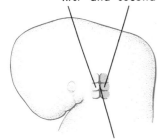

auricular hillocks derived from the
first and second branchial arches

first branchial groove

A

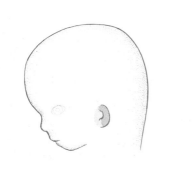

B

C

D

Figure 19-17. Drawings illustrating development of the auricle of the external ear. *A,* Six weeks. Note that three auricular hillocks are located on the first arch and three on the second arch. *B,* Eight weeks. *C,* Ten weeks. *D,* 32 weeks. As the mandible and teeth develop the auricles move from the neck to the side of the head.

stapes to the fenestra vestibuli (Moore, 1992), results in fixation of the stapes to the bony labyrinth. Abnormalities of the malleus and incus are often associated with the *first arch syndrome* (see Fig. 10–14).

Auricular Abnormalities. There is a wide normal variation in the shape of the auricle. Minor deformities of the auricle may be clues to serious congenital anomalies, e.g., renal disorders (Jones, 1988). The auricles are often abnormal in shape and low set in malformed infants (see Figs. 8–4 and 10–14), in infants with chromosomal syndromes (see Table 8–2), and in infants affected by maternal ingestion of certain teratogenic drugs (see Fig. 8–17*C*).

Auricular appendages are common (Fig. 19–18) and result from the development of accessory auricular hillocks. The appendages usually appear anterior to the auricle, more often unilaterally than bilaterally. The appendages (skin tags), often on narrow pedicles, usually consist of skin, but they may be broad-based and contain some cartilage.

Absence of the auricle (anotia) is rare but is commonly associated with the first arch syndrome (p. 199). Anotia is the result of failure of the auricular hillocks to develop.

Microtia (small auricle) results from suppressed development of the auricular hillocks. Atresia of the external acoustic meatus and middle ear abnormalities are commonly associated with microtia.

Preauricular Sinuses (see Figs. 10–10*F* and 19–19). These pitlike, cutaneous depressions or shallow sinuses are commonly located in a triangular area anterior to the auricle. The sinuses are usually narrow tubes or shallow pits that

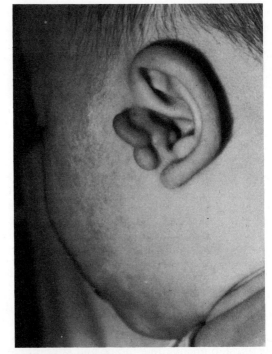

Figure 19-18. Photograph of a child with two auricular appendages, which result from the formation of accessory auricular hillocks. (From Swenson O: *Pediatric Surgery.* 1958. Courtesy of Appleton-Century-Crofts).

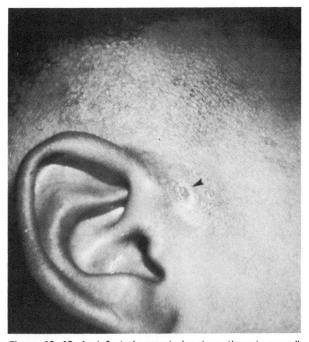

Figure 19–19. An infected preauricular sinus; there is a small patch of chronic granulation tissue at the external orifice of the sinus. (From Raffensperger JG (ed): *Swenson's Pediatric Surgery.* 5th ed. 1990. Courtesy of Appleton & Lange).

Congenital Cholesteatoma. This is a rest[1] of epithelial cells (L. *restare*, to remain) that appears as a white, cystlike structure medial to or within the tympanic membrane. The rest probably consists of cells from the meatal plug that were displaced during its recanalization (Fig. 19–16C). It has been suggested that congenital cholesteatoma may originate from an epidermoid formation which normally involutes by 33 weeks' gestation.

SUMMARY

The eyes and ears begin to develop during the fourth week. These special sense organs are very sensitive to the teratogenic effects of infectious agents (e.g., cytomegalovirus and rubella virus; see Table 8–5). The most serious defects result from disturbances of development during the fourth to sixth weeks, but defects of sight and hearing may result from infection of tissues and organs by certain microorganisms during the fetal period (e.g., rubella virus and *Treponema pallidum*, the microorganism that causes syphilis).

The Eye

The first indication of the eye is the *optic sulcus*, which forms at the beginning of the fourth week. The sulcus soon deepens to form a hollow *optic vesicle* that projects laterally from the forebrain (Fig. 19–1C). The optic vesicle contacts the surface ectoderm and induces development of the *lens placode*, the primordium of the lens. As the lens placode invaginates to form a *lens pit* and a *lens vesicle*, the optic vesicle invaginates to form an *optic cup*. The retina forms from the two layers of the optic cup.

The retina, the optic nerve fibers, the muscles of the iris, and the epithelium of the iris and ciliary body are derived from the *neuroectoderm* of the forebrain. The *surface ectoderm* gives rise to the lens and the epithelium of the lacrimal glands, eyelids, conjunctiva, and cornea. The *mesoderm* gives rise to the eye muscles, except those of the iris, and to all connective and vascular tissues of the cornea, iris, ciliary body, choroid, and sclera. The sphincter and dilator muscles of the iris develop from the ectoderm at the rim of the optic cup.

There are many *ocular anomalies* but most of them are rare. Most anomalies are caused by defective closure of the optic fissure during the sixth week (e.g.,

have pinpoint external openings. Some sinuses may contain a vestigial cartilaginous mass. These defects may be associated with internal anomalies, such as deafness and kidney anomalies. The embryological basis of auricular sinuses is uncertain, but some are related to abnormal development of the auricular hillocks and defective closure of the dorsal part of the first branchial (pharyngeal) groove. Other auricular sinuses appear to represent ectodermal folds that are sequestered during formation of the auricle (Moll, 1991). Preauricular sinuses are familial and frequently bilateral. They are asymptomatic and have only minor cosmetic importance (Raffensperger, 1990); however, they often develop serious infections. *Auricular fistulas* (narrow canals) connecting the exterior with the tympanic cavity or the intratonsillar cleft are extremely rare.

Atresia of the External Acoustic Meatus. Blockage of this canal is the result of failure of the meatal plug to canalize (Fig. 19–16C). Usually, the deep part of the meatus is open, but the superficial part is blocked by bone or fibrous tissue. Most cases are associated with the *first arch syndrome* (see Fig. 10–14). Often, abnormal development of both the first and second branchial (pharyngeal) arches is involved. The auricle is also usually severely affected, and anomalies of the middle and/or internal ear are sometimes present (Parrish and Amedee, 1990). Atresia of the external acoustic meatus can occur bilaterally or unilaterally and usually results from autosomal dominant inheritance.

---

[1] A rest is a group of cells that have become displaced and lies embedded in tissue of another character.

coloboma of the iris). *Congenital cataract* and glaucoma may result from intrauterine infections (e.g., rubella virus), but most congenital cataracts are inherited.

The Ear

The surface ectoderm gives rise to the *otic vesicle* during the fourth week. It develops into the membranous labyrinth of the internal ear. The otic vesicle divides into: (1) a dorsal utricular portion, which gives rise to the utricle, semicircular ducts, and endolymphatic duct, and (2) a ventral saccular portion, which gives rise to the saccule and cochlear duct. The cochlear duct gives rise to the *spiral organ* (of Corti). The *bony labyrinth* develops from the mesenchyme adjacent to the membranous labyrinth.

The epithelium lining the tympanic cavity, mastoid antrum, and auditory tube is derived from the endoderm of the tubotympanic recess that develops from the first pharyngeal pouch. The auditory ossicles (malleus, incus, and stapes) develop from the dorsal ends of the cartilages of the first two branchial (pharyngeal) arches.

The epithelium of the *external acoustic meatus* develops from the ectoderm of the first branchial (pharyngeal) groove. The *tympanic membrane* is derived from three sources: (1) the endoderm of the first pharyngeal pouch, (2) the ectoderm of the first branchial (pharyngeal) groove, and (3) the mesenchyme that grows between these layers.

The auricle develops from six *auricular hillocks*, which result from mesenchymal swellings that develop around the margins of the first branchial (pharyngeal) groove. These hillocks fuse to form the definitive auricle.

Congenital deafness may result from abnormal development of the membranous labyrinth and/or bony labyrinth as well as from abnormalities of the auditory ossicles. Recessive inheritance is the most common cause of congenital deafness, but a rubella virus infection near the end of the embryonic period is a major environmental factor known to cause abnormal development of the spiral organ and defective hearing.

There are many minor, clinically unimportant abnormalities of the auricle, but they alert the clinician to the possible presence of associated major anomalies (e.g., of the heart and kidneys). Low-set, severely malformed ears are often associated with chromosomal abnormalities, particularly trisomy 18 and trisomy 13 (see Chapter 8).

CLINICALLY ORIENTED QUESTIONS FOR PROBLEM-BASED LEARNING SESSIONS

1. An infant was born blind and deaf with congenital heart disease. The mother had had a severe viral infection early in her pregnancy. Considering the congenital anomalies present, name the virus that was probably involved. What is the common congenital cardiovascular lesion found in infants whose mothers have this infection early in pregnancy? Is the history of a rash during the first trimester an essential factor in the development of embryopathy?

2. An infant was born with bilateral ptosis. What is the probable embryological basis of this condition? Are hereditary factors involved? Injury to what nerve could also cause congenital ptosis?

3. An infant has small, multiple calcifications in the brain, microcephaly, and microphthalmia. The mother was known to have a fondness for raw and rare meat. What *protozoon* might be involved? What is the embryological basis of the infant's congenital anomalies? What advice might the doctor give the mother concerning future pregnancies?

4. A mentally retarded female infant had low-set, malformed ears, a prominent occiput, and rocker-bottom feet. A chromosomal abnormality was suspected. What type of chromosomal aberration was probably present? What is the usual cause of this abnormality? How long would the infant likely survive?

5. An infant was born with partial detachment of the retina in one eye. The eye was microphthalmic, and there was persistence of the posterior end of the hyaloid artery. What is the embryological basis of congenital detachment of the retina? What is the usual fate of the hyaloid artery?

The answers to these questions are given on page 467.

References and Suggested Reading

Anson B, Hanson JS, Richany SF: Early embryology of the auditory ossicles and associated structures in relation to certain anomalies observed clinically. *Ann Otol 69*:427, 1960.

Ars B: Organogenesis of the middle ear structures. *J Laryngol Otol 103*:16, 1989.

Aston N: Retinal angiogenesis in the human embryo. *Br Med Bull 26*:103, 1970.

Balfour HH, Jr, Groth KE, Edelman CK: Ra 27/3 rubella vaccine. *Am J Dis Child 134*:350, 1980.

Behrman RE: *Nelson Textbook of Pediatrics.* 14th ed. Philadelphia, WB Saunders, 1992.

Brown CA: Abnormalities of the eyes and associated structures. *In* Norman AP (ed): *Congenital Abnormalities in Infancy.* 2nd ed. Oxford, Blackwell Scientific Publications, 1971.

Cormack DH: *Essential Histology.* Philadelphia, JB Lippincott, 1993.

Crowley LV: *An Introduction to Clinical Embryology.* Chicago, Year Book Medical Publishers, 1974.

Doutreland JJ, Querleu D: Organogenese de l'audition. Developpement de l'oreille. *Rev Fr Gynecol Obstet 83*:23, 1988.

Fraser GR: A study of causes of deafness amongst 2,355 children in special schools. *In* Fisch L (ed): *Research in Deafness in Children.* Oxford, Blackwell Scientific Publications, 1964.

Frenz DA, Van de Water TR, Galinovic-Schwartz V: Transforming growth factor beta: does it direct otic capsule formation. *Ann Otol Rhinol Laryngol 100*:301, 1991.

Hay ED, Meier S: Stimulation of corneal differentiation by interaction between cell surface and extracellular matrix. II. Further studies on the nature and site of transfilter induction. *Dev Biol 52*:141, 1976.

Jain KK, Bhandari GJ, Koronne SP: Histogenesis of the human eyelid. *East Arch Ophthal 3*:8, 1973.

Jones KL: *Smith's Recognizable Patterns of Human Malformation.* 4th ed. Philadelphia, WB Saunders, 1988.

Kendig EL, Jr, Chernick V (eds): *Disorders of the Respiratory Tract in Children.* 4th ed. Philadelphia, WB Saunders, 1987.

Konigsmark BW, Gorlin RJ: *Genetic and Metabolic Deafness.* Philadelphia, WB Saunders, 1976.

Kwitko, ML (ed): *Surgery of the Infant Eye.* New York, Appleton-Century-Crofts, 1979.

Langman J: The first appearance of specific antigens during induction of the lens. *J Embryol Exp Morphol 7*:264, 1959.

Linberg KA, Fisher SK: A burst of differentiation in the outer posterior retina of the eleven-week human fetus: an ultrastructural study. *Vis Neurosci 5*:43, 1990.

Mann IC: *The Development of the Human Eye.* 3rd ed. London, British Medical Association, 1974.

Marles SL, Greenberg CR, Persaud TVN, Shuckett EP, Chudley AE: A new familial syndrome of unilateral upper eyelid coloboma, aberrant anterior hairline pattern and anal anomalies in Manitoba Indians. *Am J Med Genet 42*:793, 1992.

Martyn LJ: Pediatric ophthalmology. *In* Behrman RE (ed): *Textbook of Pediatrics.* 14th ed. Philadelphia, WB Saunders, 1992.

Michaels L: Evolution of the epidermoid formation and its role in the development of the middle ear and tympanic membrane during the first trimester. *J Otolaryngol 17*:22, 1988.

Michaels L, Soucek S: Auditory epithelial migration on the human tympanic membrane. II. The existence of two discrete migratory pathways and their embryologic correlates. *Am J Anat 189*:189, 1990.

Michaels L, Soucek S: Development of the stratified squamous epithelium of the human tympanic membrane and external canal: The origin of auditory epithelial migration. *Am J Anat 184*:334, 1989.

Moll M: Congenital earpits or auricular sinuses. *Acta Path Microbiol Scand 99*:96, 1991.

Moore KL: *Clinically Oriented Anatomy.* 3rd ed. Baltimore, Williams & Wilkins, 1992.

Nordquist D, McLoon SC: Morphological patterns in the developing vertebrate retina. *Anat Embryol 184*:433, 1991.

Norlund JJ: The lives of pigment cells. *Clin Geriatr Med 5*:91, 1989.

Oguni M, Tanaka O, Shinohara H, Yoshioka T, Setogawa T: Ultrastructural study of the retinal pigment epithelium of human embryos, with special reference to the quantitative study on the development of melanin granules. *Acta Anat 140*:335, 1991.

O'Rahilly R: The early development of the eye in staged human embryos. *Contr Embryol Carneg Instn 38*:1, 1966.

O'Rahilly R: The early development of the otic vesicle in staged human embryos. *J Embryol Exp Morphol 11*:741, 1963.

O'Rahilly R: The prenatal development of the human eye. *Exp. Eye Res. 21*:93, 1975.

O'Rahilly R, Müller F: Interpretation of some median anomalies as illustrated by cyclopia and symmelia. *Teratology 40*:409, 1989.

Otto HD, Gerhardt HJ: Kongenitale Epidermoide des Schlafenbeins. *Teil I: Pathogenese HNO 38*:43, 1990.

Parrish KL, Amedee RG: Atresia of the external auditory canal. *J La State Med Soc 142*:9, 1990.

Penfold PL, Provis JM, Madigan MC, van Driel D, Billson FA: Angiogenesis in normal human retinal development: the involvement of astrocytes and macrophages. *Graefes Arch Clin Exp Ophthalmol 228*:255, 1990.

Raffensperger JG (ed): *Swenson's Pediatric Surgery.* 5th ed. Norwalk, Appleton & Lange, 1990.

Repressa JJ, Moro JA, Gato A, Pastor F, Barbosa E: Patterns of epithelial cell death during early development of the human inner ear. *Ann Otol Rhinol Laryngol 99*:482, 1990.

Sellheyer K: Development of the choroid and related structures. *Eye 4(Pt 2)*:255, 1990.

Sellheyer K, Spitznas M: Differentiation of the ciliary muscle in the human embryo and fetus. *Graefes Arch Clin Exp Ophthalmol 226*:281, 1988.

Sellheyer K, Spitznas M: Licht-und elektronenmikroskopische Untersuchungen zur Entwicklung des menschlichen Ziliakorpers. *Fortschr Ophthalmol 86*:392, 1989.

Sellheyer K, Spitznas M: Morphology of the development choroidal vasculature in the human fetus. *Graefes Arch Clin Exp Ophthalmol 226*:461, 1988.

Sevel D: A reappraisal of the development of the eyelids. *Eye 2(Pt 2)*:123, 1988a.

Sevel D: Development of the connective tissue of the extraocular muscles and clinical significance. *Graefes Arch Clin Exp Ophthalmol 226*:246, 1988b.

Sevel D, Isaacs R: A re-evaluation of corneal development. *Trans Am Ophthalmol Soc 86*:178, 1989.

Shah CP, Halperin DS: Congenital deafness. *In* Persaud TVN (ed): *Advances in the Study of Birth Defects. Vol 7. Central Nervous System and Craniofacial Malformations.* New York, Alan R Liss, 1982.

Smith B, Guberina C: Congenital ocular anomalies. *In* Kwitko ML (ed): *Surgery of the Infant Eye.* New York, Appleton-Century-Crofts, 1979.

Stromland K, Miller M, Cook C: Ocular teratology. *Surv Ophthalmol 35*:429, 1991.

Takayama S, Yamamoto M, Hashimoto K, Itoh H: Immunohistochemical study in the developing optic nerves in human embryos and fetuses. *Brain Develop 13*:307, 1991.

Tamura T, Smelser JK: Development of the sphincter and dilator muscles of the iris. *Arch Ophthalmol 89*:332, 1973.

Thould AK, Scowen EF: The syndrome of congenital deafness and goiter. *J Endocrinol 30*:69, 1964.

Tripathi BJ, Tripathi RC, Livingston AM, Borisuth NSC: The role of growth factors in the embryogenesis and differentiation of the eye. *Am J Anat 192*:442, 1991.

Warkany J: Prevention of congenital malformations. *Teratology 23*:175, 1981.

Wilson RS, Char F: Drug-induced ocular malformations. *In* Persaud TVN (ed): *Advances in the Study of Birth Defects. Vol 7. Central Nervous System and Craniofacial Malformations.* New York, Alan R Liss, 1982.

The Integumentary System

This system consists of the skin, sweat glands, nails, hair, sebaceous glands, and arrector pili muscles. It also includes the mammary glands and teeth. The Latin word *integumentum* means "a covering." At the external orifices (e.g., of the digestive tract), the mucous membrane and the integument are continuous.

THE SKIN

The skin is a complex organ system that forms a protective covering on the surface of the embryo. The skin consists of two different layers that are derived from two different germ layers: ectoderm and mesoderm. The superficial layer or epidermis is a specialized epithelial tissue that is derived from the surface ectoderm (Fig. 20–1). The deep, thicker layer or dermis is composed of dense, irregularly arranged, connective tissue that is derived from the mesoderm underlying the ectoderm. See Haake and Lane (1989) and Nanney et al. (1990) for studies of the molecular mechanisms that regulate human fetal skin development.

The Epidermis

During the first and second trimesters, epidermal growth occurs in three stages, which result in an increase in epidermal thickness (Foster et al., 1988). The primordium of the epidermis consists of a single layer of ectodermal cells. These cells proliferate and form a second layer of squamous epithelium called the *periderm*. The cells of this layer continually undergo keratinization and desquamation and are replaced by cells arising from the *basal layer* (Fig. 20–1B). The exfoliated peridermal cells form part of the *vernix caseosa*, a white, greasy substance that covers the fetal skin (Fig. 20–2D). The vernix caseosa also contains sebum from the sebaceous glands (p. 444) which protects the skin of the fetus from constant exposure to amniotic fluid with its urine content during the fetal period. In addition, it facilitates birth of the fetus due to its slippery nature.

The basal layer of the epidermis is later called the *stratum germinativum* because it produces new cells that are displaced into the layers superficial to it. By 11 weeks, cells from the stratum germinativum have formed an intermediate layer (Fig. 20–1C). All layers of the adult epidermis are present at birth (Fig. 20–1D). Replacement of peridermal cells continues until about the twenty-first week; thereafter, the periderm gradually disappears as the stratum corneum forms.

Proliferation of cells in the stratum germinativum also forms *epidermal ridges*, which extend into the developing dermis (Fig. 20–1C). These ridges begin to appear in embryos of about ten weeks and are permanently established by the seventeenth week. The developing afferent nerve fibers apparently play an important role in the spatial and temporal sequence of papillary ridge formation (Moore and Munger, 1989).

The epidermal ridges produce ridges and grooves on the surface of the palms of the hands and the soles of the feet, including the digits. The type of pattern that develops is determined genetically and constitutes the basis for using fingerprints in criminal investigations and medical genetics. Study of the patterns of the epidermal ridges of the skin is called *dermatoglyphics*. Abnormal chromosome complements affect the development of the ridge patterns; e.g., infants with Down syndrome have distinctive patterns on their hands and feet that are of diagnostic value. For details about the use of dermatoglyphics in medical genetics, see Hirschhorn (1992).

During the early fetal period, cells from the *neural crest* differentiate into *melanoblasts* (see Fig. 18–8) and migrate to the dermoepidermal junction where they differentiate into *melanocytes* (Fig. 20–1D). Recent studies have shown that melanocytes appear in the developing skin between 40 to 50 days immediately after the formation and migration of the neural crest cells (Holbrook et al., 1989). In white races, the cell bodies of the melanocytes are usually confined to basal layers of the epidermis, but their dendritic processes extend between the epidermal cells. Only a few melanin-containing cells are normally present in the dermis (Cormack, 1993).

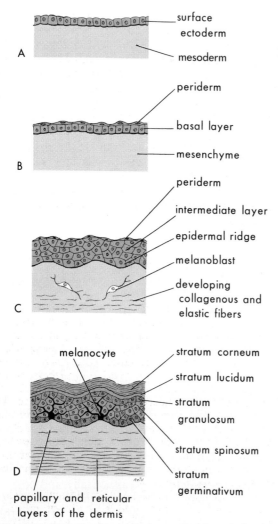

surface
ectoderm

mesoderm

A

periderm

basal layer

mesenchyme

B

periderm

intermediate layer

epidermal ridge

melanoblast

developing
collagenous and
elastic fibers

C

melanocyte

stratum corneum

stratum lucidum

stratum
granulosum

stratum spinosum

stratum
germinativum

D

papillary and reticular
layers of the dermis

Figure 20–1. Drawings illustrating successive stages in the development of thick skin. *A*, Four weeks. *B*, Seven weeks. *C*, 11 weeks. The cells of the periderm continually undergo keratinization and desquamation. The exfoliated peridermal cells form part of the vernix caseosa, a white greasy substance that coats the fetal skin. *D*, Newborn. Note the position of the melanocytes in the basal layer of the epidermis and the way their branching dendritic processes extend between the epidermal cells to supply them with melanin.

The melanocytes begin producing melanin (Gr. *melas*, black) before birth and distribute it to the epidermal cells. Active pigmentary activity can be observed prenatally in the epidermis of dark-skinned races, but there is little evidence of such activity in light-skinned fetuses. Increased amounts of melanin are produced as a response to ultraviolet light. The relative content of melanin in the epidermis accounts for different skin colors.

The Dermis

The dermis is derived from the mesoderm underlying the surface ectoderm. Most of the mesenchyme that differentiates into the connective tissue of the dermis originates from the somatic layer of lateral mesoderm, but some of it is derived from the dermatomes of the somites (see Chapter 15).

By 11 weeks the mesenchymal cells have begun to produce collagenous and elastic connective tissue fibers (Fig. 20–1D). As the epidermal ridges form, the dermis projects into the epidermis and forms *dermal papillae*. Capillary loops develop in some of these papillae and provide nourishment for the epidermis. Sensory nerve endings form in others. The development of the *dermatomal pattern* of innervation of the skin has been described (page 378).

The first blood vessels in the dermis begin as simple, endothelium-lined structures that differentiate from mesenchyme. As the skin grows, new capillaries grow out from the simple vessels. Such small, capillary-like vessels have been observed in the dermis by the end of the fifth week. Some capillaries acquire muscular coats through differentiation of myoblasts from the surrounding mesenchyme and become arterioles and arteries. Other capillaries, through which a return flow of blood is established, acquire muscular coats and become venules and veins. As new blood vessels form, some transitory ones normally disappear. By the end of the first trimester the major vascular organization of the fetal dermis is established (Johnson and Holbrook, 1989).

Glands of the Skin

Two kinds of gland occur in the skin: sebaceous glands and sweat glands.

Sebaceous Glands (Fig. 20–2). Most of these glands develop as buds from the sides of the developing epithelial root sheaths of hair follicles (Fig. 20–2C). The glandular buds grow into the surrounding connective tissue and branch to form the primordia of several alveoli and their associated ducts (Fig. 20–2D). The central cells of the alveoli subsequently break down, forming an oily secretion called *sebum*. The sebum is extruded into the hair follicle and onto the surface of the skin. Here, it mixes with desquamated peridermal cells to form *vernix caseosa*, the greasy, white, cheeselike material that covers and protects the skin. Sebaceous glands independent of hair follicles (e.g., in the glans penis and labia minora) develop in a similar manner from buds that arise from the epidermis.

Sweat Glands (Fig. 20–3). Most sweat glands develop as solid epidermal downgrowths into the underlying mesenchyme (future dermis). As a bud elongates, its end coils, forming the primordium of the secretory portion of the gland. The epithelial attachment of the developing gland to the epidermis forms the primordium of the duct. The central cells of these

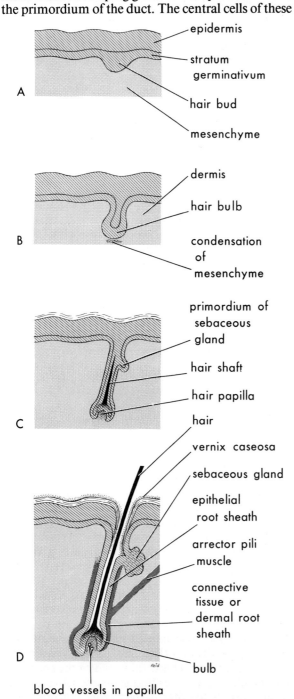

Figure 20–2. Drawings showing successive stages in the development of a hair and its associated sebaceous gland. *A*, 12 weeks. *B*, 14 weeks. *C*, 16 weeks. *D*, 18 weeks. Note that the sebaceous gland develops as an outgrowth from the side of the hair follicle.

primordia degenerate, forming a lumen. The peripheral cells of the secretory portion of the gland differentiate into secretory and *myoepithelial cells.* The myoepithelial cells, derived from ectoderm, are thought to be specialized smooth muscle cells that aid in expelling sweat from the glands.

The distribution of *large sweat glands* in humans is limited. They are mostly confined to the axilla, pubic region, and areolae of the breasts (Fig. 20–7). They develop from the downgrowths of the stratum germinativum of the epidermis that give rise to hair follicles. As a result, the ducts of these glands open, not onto the skin surface as do ordinary sweat glands, but into hair follicles superficial to the openings of the sebaceous glands.

Congenital Anomalies of the Skin

The developmental basis of abnormalities of the skin is not well understood.

Disorders of Keratinization. Ichthyosis (Gr. *ichthys,* fish) is a general term that is applied to a group of disorders resulting from excessive keratinization. They are characterized by dryness and fishskin-like scaling of the skin, which may involve the entire body surface (Fig. 20–4). A *harlequin fetus* results from a rare keratinizing disorder that is inherited as an autosomal recessive trait (Behrman, 1992). The skin is markedly thickened, ridged, and cracked. Affected infants have a grotesque appearance, and most of them die within the first week of life. A *collodion baby* is covered at birth by a thick, taut membrane that resembles collodion. This membrane cracks with the first respiratory efforts and begins to fall off in large sheets, but complete shedding may take several weeks.

Lamellar ichthyosis (Fig. 20–4) is an autosomal recessive disorder. A newborn infant with this condition may first appear to be a "collodion baby," but the scaling persists. Growth of hair may be curtailed and development of sweat glands is often impeded. Affected infants often suffer severely in hot weather due to their inability to sweat.

Congenital Ectodermal Dysplasia. In this rare hereditary disorder there is partial failure of the epidermis and its appendages to develop. In severe cases, there are dental abnormalities and absence of body hair (Moynahan, 1971).

Angiomas of the Skin. These vascular anomalies are developmental defects in which some transitory and/or surplus primitive blood or lymph vessels persist. These anomalies are called *angiomas* even though they may not be true tumors. Those composed of blood vessels may be mainly arterial, mainly venous, or mainly cavernous, but they are often of a mixed type. Angiomas composed of lymphatics are called cystic *lymphangiomas* or cystic hygromas (see page 350).

True angiomas are benign tumors of endothelial cells usually composed of solid or hollow cords; the hollow cords contain blood. Various terms are used to describe angiomatous anomalies ("birthmarks"). *Nevus flammeus* denotes a flat, pink or red, flamelike blotch that often appears on the

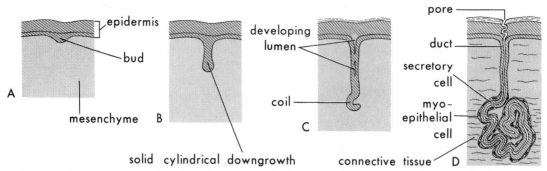

Figure 20–3. Diagrams illustrating successive stages in the development of a sweat gland. The gland develops at about 20 weeks as a solid growth of epidermal cells into the mesenchyme. Its terminal part coils and forms the body of the gland. The central cells degenerate to form the lumen of the gland, and the peripheral cells differentiate into secretory cells and contractile myoepithelial cells.

posterior surface of the neck. A *port-wine stain* or **hemangioma** is a larger and darker angioma than nevus flammeus, and it is nearly always anterior or lateral on the face and/or neck. It is sharply demarcated when it is near the median plane, whereas the common angioma (pinkish-red blotch) may cross the median plane. A port-wine stain in the area of distribution of the trigeminal nerve (see Fig. 10–7*B*) is sometimes associated with a similar type of angioma of the meninges of the brain *(Sturge-Weber syndrome)*. A hemangioma is among the most common neoplasms found in infants and children (Behrman, 1992).

Albinism. In generalized albinism, an autosomal recessive trait, the skin, hair, and retina lack pigment, but the iris usually shows some pigmentation. The condition occurs when the melanocytes fail to produce melanin due to the lack of the enzyme tyrosinase. In localized albinism, or *piebaldism*, an autosomal dominant trait, there is a lack of melanin in patches of skin and/or hair.

Absence of Skin. In rare cases, small areas of skin fail to form, giving the appearance of ulcers. The area usually heals by scarring unless a skin graft is performed. Absence of patches of skin is most common in the scalp.

HAIR

Hairs begin to develop early in the fetal period (ninth to twelfth week), but they do not become easily recognizable externally until about the twentieth week (see Fig. 6–1). Hairs are first recognizable on the eyebrows, upper lip, and chin. A hair follicle begins as a proliferation of the stratum germinativum of the epidermis and extends into the underlying dermis (Fig. 20–2*A*). The deepest part of the embryonic hair follicle or *hair bud* soon becomes club-shaped to form a *hair bulb* (Fig. 20–2*B*). The epithelial cells of the hair bulb constitute the *germinal matrix*, which later gives rise to the hair.

The hair bulb is soon invaginated by a small *mesenchymal hair papilla* (Fig. 20–2*C*). The peripheral cells of the developing hair follicle form the *epithelial root sheath*, and the surrounding mesenchymal cells differentiate into the *dermal root sheath* (Fig. 20–2*D*). As cells in the germinal matrix proliferate, they are pushed toward the surface where they become keratinized to form the *hair shaft* (Fig. 20–2*C*).

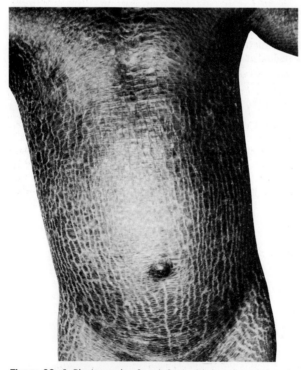

Figure 20–4. Photograph of an infant with lamellar ichthyosis, a congenital disorder of keratinization that is characterized by pronounced scaling involving the entire body. (From Behrman RE [ed]: *Nelson Textbook of Pediatrics.* 14th ed. Philadelphia, WB Saunders, 1992.)

The hair grows through the epidermis on the eyebrows and upper lip by the end of the twelfth week.

The first hairs that appear, called *lanugo* (L. *lana*, fine wool) or lanugo hairs, are fine and colorless. They are replaced during the perinatal period by coarser hairs. This hair persists over most of the body, except in the axillary and pubic regions, where it is replaced at puberty by even coarser terminal hairs. In males similar coarse hairs also appear on the face and often on the chest. *Melanoblasts* migrate into the hair bulb and differentiate into melanocytes. The melanin produced by these cells is transferred to the hair-forming cells in the germinal matrix several weeks before birth. The relative content of melanin accounts for different hair colors.

The *arrector pili muscle*, a small bundle of smooth muscle fibers, differentiates from the surrounding mesenchyme and becomes attached to the dermal root sheath of the hair follicle and the papillary layer of the dermis (Fig. 20–2D). The arrector pili muscles (erectors of the hairs) are poorly developed in the hairs of the axilla and in certain parts of the face. The hairs forming the eyebrows and the cilia forming the eyelashes have no arrector pili muscles.

Abnormalities of Hair

"Gray" hair in infants is associated with *albinism* (p. 446), which results from lack of melanin in the skin. The lack of pigment in the melanocytes of the bulbs of the hairs accounts for the lack of color in the hairs.

Congenital Alopecia (Atrichia Congenita). Absence or loss of hair may occur alone or with other abnormalities of the skin and its derivatives. The hair loss may be caused by failure of hair follicles to develop or it may result from follicles producing poor-quality hairs.

Hypertrichosis. Excessive hairiness results from the development of supernumerary hair follicles or from the persistence of hairs that normally disappear during the perinatal period. It may be localized (e.g., on the shoulders and back) or diffuse. Localized hypertrichosis is often associated with spina bifida occulta (see Fig. 18–12A).

Pili Torti. In this familial disorder the hairs are twisted and bent (L. *tortus*, twisted). Other ectodermal defects (e.g., distorted nails) may be associated with this condition. Pili torti is usually first recognized at two to three years of age.

NAILS

Toenails and fingernails begin to develop at the tips of the digits at about ten weeks (Fig. 20–5). Development of fingernails precedes that of toenails by about four weeks (see Table 6–2). The primordia of the nails first appear as thickened areas or fields of epidermis at the tip of each digit. Later, these fields migrate onto the dorsal surface, carrying their innervation from the ventral surface.

The *nail fields* are surrounded laterally and proximally by folds of epidermis called *nail folds*. Cells from the proximal nail fold grow over the nail field and become keratinized and consolidated to form the *nail plate*, the primordium of the nail.

At first the developing nail is covered by superficial layers of epidermis called the *eponychium*. This later degenerates, exposing the nail except at the base of the nail where it persists as the *cuticle*. The skin under the free margin of the nail is called the *hyponychium*. The fingernails reach the fingertips by about 32 weeks; the toenails reach the toetips by about 36 weeks (see Fig. 6–11). Nails that have not reached the tips of the digits at birth indicate prematurity.

Anomalies of the Nails

Anonychia. Absence of nails may occur but this condition is extremely rare. Anonychia is the result of failure of the nail fields to form or from failure of the proximal nail folds to give rise to nail plates. The abnormality is permanent. It may be associated with congenital absence or extremely poor development of the hair and with

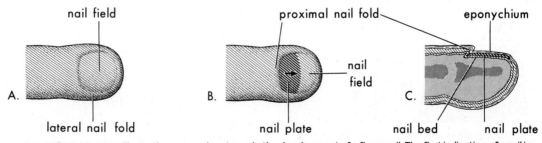

Figure 20–5. Diagrams illustrating successive stages in the development of a fingernail. The first indication of a nail is a thickening of the epidermis, the nail field, at the tip of the digit. The nail field grows proximally to occupy the normal position of the nail (A). As the nail develops it slowly grows toward the tip of the digit (B), which it reaches before birth (i.e., fingers, 32 weeks; toes, 36 weeks).

abnormalities of the teeth. Anonychia may be restricted to one or more nails of the digits of the hands and/or feet.

Deformed Nails. This disorder occurs occasionally and may be a manifestation of a generalized skin disease or systemic disease. There are a number of congenital diseases with nail defects (for details, see Behrman, 1992).

MAMMARY GLANDS

The mammary glands begin to develop during the sixth week as solid growths of the epidermis into the underlying mesenchyme (Fig. 20–6C). These ingrowths occur along the *mammary (milk) ridges*, which are thickened strips of ectoderm that extend from the axillary to the inguinal regions (Fig. 20–6A). The mammary ridges appear during the fourth week but normally persist in humans only in the pectoral area where the breasts are located.

Each primary mammary bud soon gives rise to several secondary buds that develop into *lactiferous ducts* and their branches (Fig. 20–6D and E). Canalization of these buds to form ducts is induced by placental sex hormones entering the fetal circulation. This process continues until late gestation and, by term, 15 to 20 lactiferous ducts are formed. The fibrous connective tissue and fat of the mammary gland develop from the surrounding mesenchyme.

During the late fetal period the epidermis at the site of origin of the mammary gland becomes depressed, forming a shallow *mammary pit* (Fig. 20–6E). The nipples are poorly formed and depressed in newborn infants. Soon after birth the nipples usually rise from the mammary pits due to proliferation of the surrounding connective tissues of the *areola*, the circular area of skin around the nipple. The smooth muscle fibers of the nipple and areola differentiate from surrounding mesenchymal cells.

The rudimentary mammary glands of newborn males and females are identical and are often enlarged. Some secretion, often called "witch's milk," may be produced. These transitory changes are

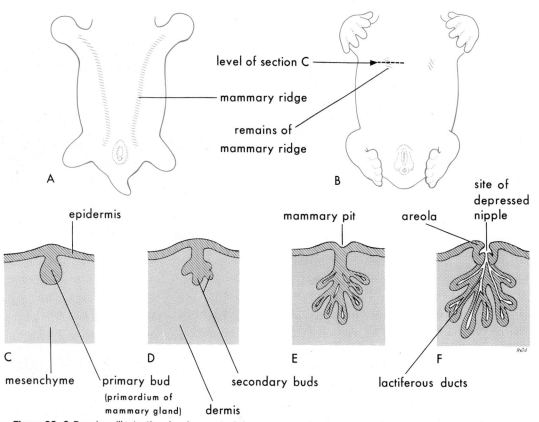

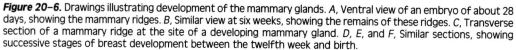

Figure 20–6. Drawings illustrating development of the mammary glands. *A,* Ventral view of an embryo of about 28 days, showing the mammary ridges. *B,* Similar view at six weeks, showing the remains of these ridges. *C,* Transverse section of a mammary ridge at the site of a developing mammary gland. *D, E,* and *F,* Similar sections, showing successive stages of breast development between the twelfth week and birth.

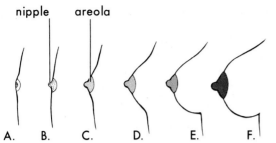

nipple   areola

A.   B.   C.   D.   E.   F.

Figure 20–7. Sketches showing progressive stages in the post-natal development of the female breast. *A*, Newborn. *B*, Child. *C*, Early puberty. *D*, Late puberty. *E*, Young adult. *F*, Pregnant female. Note that the nipple is depressed or inverted at birth, but it normally becomes elevated during childhood to form a true nipple. Failure of this process to occur gives rise to an inverted nipple, which may cause difficulty during breast-feeding later in life. At puberty (12 to 15 years), the breasts enlarge due to development of the mammary glands and to the increased deposition of fat.

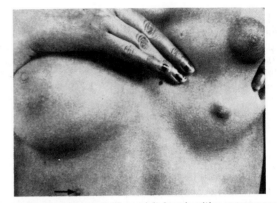

Figure 20–8. Photograph of an adult female with a supernumerary nipple on the right *(arrow)* and a small supernumerary breast inferior to the normal left one. (From Haagensen CD: *Diseases of the Breast.* 3rd ed. Philadelphia, WB Saunders, 1986.)

caused by maternal hormones passing through the placental membrane into the fetal circulation.

Only the main lactiferous ducts are formed at birth, and the mammary glands remain underdeveloped until puberty. In females the glands enlarge rapidly during this period (Fig. 20–7), mainly because of fat and other connective tissue development. Growth of the duct system occurs due to raised levels of circulating estrogens. Progestogens, prolactin, corticoids, and growth hormone also play a role (Beck et al., 1985).

If pregnancy occurs, the mammary glands complete their development due to raised estrogen levels and to the sustained increase in the levels of progesterone. The intralobular ducts undergo rapid development, forming buds that become alveoli. The breasts become hemispherical in shape (Fig. 20–7*D*), largely because of deposition of fat.

The mammary glands in males normally undergo no postnatal development. *Gynecomastia* (Gr. *gynē*, woman, + *mastos*, breast) refers to excessive development of the male mammary glands, e.g., as may occur with Klinefelter syndrome (p. 149).

Anomalies of the Mammary Glands

Absence of the Nipples (Athelia) and Absence of the Breasts (Amastia). These rare congenital anomalies may occur bilaterally or unilaterally. They are the result of failure of development or from complete disappearance of the mammary ridges. These conditions may also be the result of failure of a mammary bud to form. More common is hypoplasia of the breast, often found in association with gonadal agenesis and Turner syndrome (Chapter 8).

Aplasia of the Breast. The breasts of a postpubertal female often differ somewhat in size. Marked differences are regarded as deformities because both glands are exposed to

the same hormones at puberty. In these cases there is often associated rudimentary development of muscles, usually the pectoralis major (see Fig. 16–3).

Supernumerary Breasts and Nipples (Figs. 20–8 and 20–9). An extra breast *(polymastia)* or nipple *(polythelia)* occurs in about one per cent of the female population and is an inheritable condition (Haagensen, 1986). Supernumerary nipples are also relatively common in males. They are often mistaken for moles (nevi). An extra breast or nipple usually develops just inferior to the normal breast.

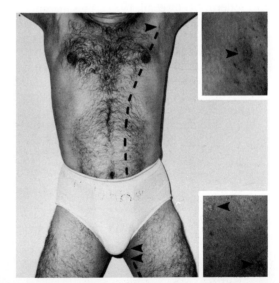

Figure 20–9. Photograph of an adult male with bilateral nipples in the axillary and thigh regions. The inset photographs are enlargements of the nipples on the left *(arrows)*. The broken line indicates the original position of the left mammary ridge along which the extra nipples have developed. (Courtesy of Dr. Kunwar Bhatnagar, Professor of Anatomy, School of Medicine, University of Louisville, Louisville, Kentucky.)

Less commonly, extra mammary glands or nipples appear in the axillary or abdominal regions. In these positions the nipples or breasts develop from extra mammary buds that develop along the mammary ridges. They usually become obvious in women when pregnancy occurs. About one third of affected persons have two extra nipples or breasts. Supernumerary mammary tissue very rarely occurs in a location other than along the course of the mammary ridges. It probably develops from tissue that was displaced from the mammary ridge(s).

Inverted Nipples. Sometimes the nipples fail to elevate above the skin surface, i.e., they remain in their newborn location (Figs. 20–6F and 20–7A). Inverted nipples may make breast-feeding of an infant difficult, but a special exercise can be used to prepare the nipple for feeding an infant.

THE TEETH

Two sets of natural teeth normally develop: the primary dentition or *deciduous teeth* and the secondary dentition or *permanent teeth*. As the mandible and maxilla grow to accommodate the developing teeth, the shape of the face changes. The teeth develop from ectoderm and mesoderm. The enamel is derived from ectoderm of the oral cavity; all other tissues differentiate from the surrounding mesenchyme, a derivative of mesoderm.

Tooth development appears to be initiated by the inductive influence of the mesenchyme on the overlying ectoderm (Kelly et al., 1984). This mesenchyme is of neural crest origin. Tooth development is a continuous process, but it is usually divided into stages for descriptive purposes (bud, cap, and bell stages) on the basis of the appearance of the developing tooth. Not all teeth begin to develop at the same time. The first tooth buds appear in the anterior mandibular region; later tooth development occurs in the anterior maxillary region and then progresses posteriorly in both

Table 20–1. THE ORDER AND USUAL TIME OF ERUPTION OF TEETH AND THE TIME OF SHEDDING OF DECIDUOUS TEETH

Tooth	Eruption Time	Shedding Time
Deciduous		
Medial incisor	6–8 mos	6–7 yr
Lateral incisor	8–10 mos	7–8 yr
Canine	16–20 mos	10–12 yr
First molar	12–16 mos	9–11 yr
Second molar	20–24 mos	10–12 yr
Permanent		
Medial incisor	7–8 yr	*
Lateral incisor	8–9 yr	
Canine	10–12 yr	
First premolar	10–11 yr	
Second premolar	11–12 yr	
First molar	6–7 yr	
Second molar	12 yr	
Third molar	13–25 yr	

(Adapted from Moore, K. L.: *Clinically Oriented Anatomy.* 3rd ed. Baltimore, The Williams & Wilkins Company, 1992.)

* The permanent teeth are not shed. If they are not properly cared for, or disease of the gingiva occurs, they may have to be extracted.

jaws. Tooth development continues for years after birth (Table 20–1).

The first indication of tooth development occurs early in the sixth week as a thickening of the oral epithelium, a derivative of the surface ectoderm. These U-shaped bands called **dental laminae** follow the curves of the primitive jaws (Figs. 20–10 to 20–12).

The Bud Stage (Figs. 20–10B and 20–11B). Each dental lamina soon develops ten centers of proliferation from which swellings called *tooth buds* grow into the underlying mesenchyme. These tooth buds develop into the first teeth. They are called deciduous teeth because they are shed during childhood (Table

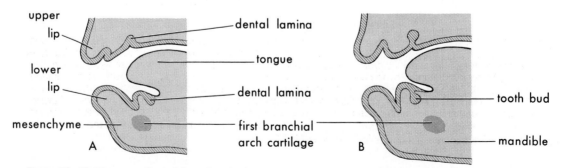

Figure 20–10. Diagrammatic sketches of sagittal sections through the developing jaws illustrating early development of the teeth. *A,* Early in the sixth week, showing the dental lamina. *B,* Later in the sixth week, showing tooth buds arising from the dental laminae.

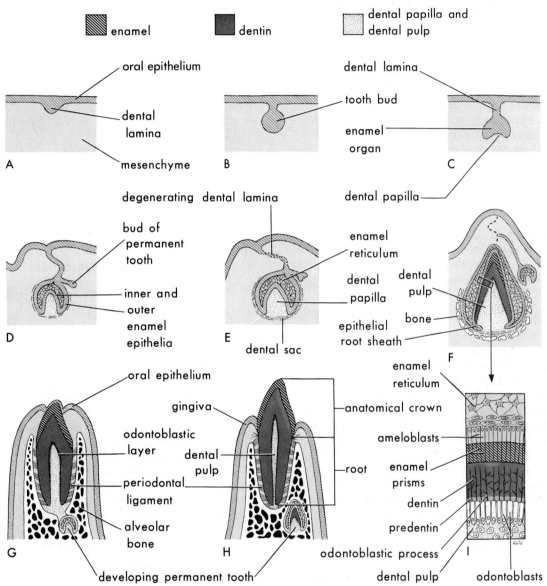

Figure 20–11. Schematic drawings of sagittal sections, showing successive stages in the development and eruption of an incisor tooth. *A*, Six weeks, showing the dental lamina. *B*, Seven weeks, showing the tooth bud developing from the dental lamina. *C*, Eight weeks, showing the cap stage of tooth development. *D*, Ten weeks, showing the early bell stage of the deciduous tooth and the bud stage of the developing permanent tooth. *E*, Fourteen weeks, showing the advanced bell stage of the enamel organ. Note that the connection (dental lamina) of the tooth to the oral epithelium is degenerating. *F*, 28 weeks, showing the enamel and dentin layers. *G*, Six months postnatal, showing early tooth eruption. *H*, 18 months postnatal, showing a fully erupted deciduous incisor tooth. The permanent incisor tooth now has a well-developed crown. *I*, Section through a developing tooth, showing the ameloblasts (enamel producers) and the odontoblasts (dentin producers).

20–1). There are ten tooth buds in each jaw, one for each deciduous tooth.

The tooth buds for permanent teeth that have deciduous predecessors begin to appear at about ten fetal weeks from deep continuations of the dental lamina. They develop lingual to (i.e., toward the tongue) the deciduous tooth buds (Fig. 20–11*D*). The permanent molars that have no deciduous predecessors develop as buds from posterior extensions of the dental laminae. The tooth buds for the permanent teeth appear at different times, mostly during the fetal period. The buds for the second and third permanent molars develop after birth.

The Cap Stage (Figs. 20–11*C* and 20–12*A*). As each tooth bud grows, it becomes cap-shaped due to invagination by mesenchyme. Its ectodermal part becomes known as the *enamel organ* (dental organ) because it produces enamel. The internal part of each cap-shaped tooth bud, which was invaginated by mesenchyme, is called the *dental papilla*. It is the primordium of the *dental pulp*.

The outer cell layer of the enamel organ is called the *outer enamel epithelium*, and the inner cell layer lin-

ing the "cap" is called the *inner enamel epithelium* (Fig. 20–11*D*). The central core of loosely arranged cells between the layers of enamel epithelium is called the *enamel (stellate) reticulum*. As the enamel organ and dental papilla form, the mesenchyme surrounding the developing tooth condenses to form a capsule-like structure called the *dental sac* (Fig. 20–11*E*). It is the primordium of the cementum and periodontal ligament.

The Bell Stage (Figs. 20–11*D* and *E*, 20–12*B*, and 20–13). As the enamel organ differentiates, the developing tooth assumes the shape of a bell. The mesenchymal cells in the dental papilla adjacent to the inner enamel epithelium differentiate into *odontoblasts*, which produce predentin and deposit it adjacent to the inner enamel epithelium. Later, the *predentin* calcifies and becomes **dentin**. As the dentin thickens, the odontoblasts regress toward the center of the dental papilla, but their cytoplasmic processes called *odontoblastic (Tomes') processes* remain embedded in the dentin (Fig. 20–11*F* and *I*).

Cells of the inner enamel epithelium differentiate into *ameloblasts*. They produce **enamel** in the form of

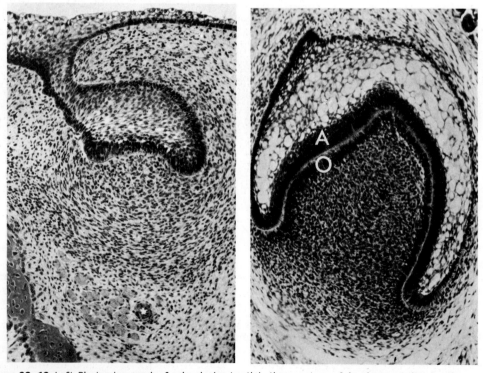

Figure 20–12. *Left*: Photomicrograph of a developing tooth in the cap stage of development showing the enamel organ attached to the oral mucosa by the dental lamina (✕100). Compare with Figure 20–11*C*. *Right*: Photomicrograph of a developing tooth in the late bell stage with ameloblasts (inner enamel epithelium [*A*]) differentiated and in contact with odontoblasts (*O*). Compare with Figure 20–11*E*. (From Leeson CR, Leeson TS: *Histology.* 5th ed. Philadelphia, WB Saunders, 1985.)

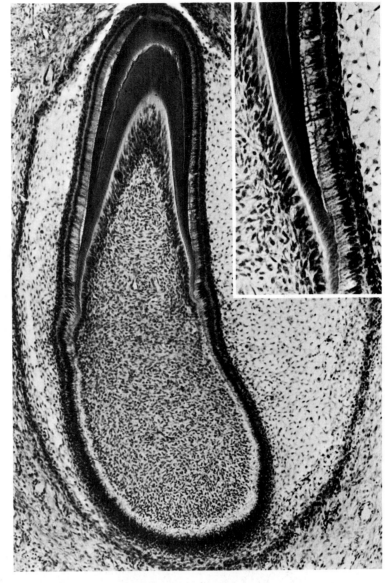

Figure 20–13. Photomicrograph of a developing tooth at the stage during which crown formation is well advanced. (Compare with Figure 20–11F.) Enamel and dentin are present with a thin layer of predentin in relation to the odontoblasts (×75). Upper right insert: A higher magnification of part of the tooth, showing, from left to right, pulp, odontoblasts, predentin, dentin, enamel (black), ameloblasts, stratum intermedium, and enamel reticulum (×175). (From Leeson CR, Leeson TS, Paparo AA: *Text/Atlas of Histology*. Philadelphia, WB Saunders, 1988.)

prisms (rods) over the dentin. As the enamel increases, the ameloblasts regress toward the outer enamel epithelium. Enamel and dentin formation begins at the tip (cusp) of the tooth and progresses toward the future root.

The *root of the tooth* begins to develop after dentin and enamel formation is well advanced. The inner and outer enamel epithelia come together in the neck region of the tooth; here, they form a fold called the *epithelial root sheath*. This sheath grows into the mesenchyme and initiates root formation. The odontoblasts adjacent to the epithelial root sheath form dentin that is continuous with that of the crown. As the

dentin increases, it reduces the pulp cavity to a narrow *root canal* through which the vessels and nerves pass. The inner cells of the dental sac differentiate into *cementoblasts*, which produce **cementum**. This substance is deposited over the dentin of the root and meets the enamel at the neck of the tooth *(the cementoenamel junction)*.

As the teeth develop and the jaws ossify, the outer cells of the dental sac also become active in bone formation. Each tooth soon becomes surrounded by bone except over its crown. The tooth is held in its *alveolus* (bony socket) by the strong *periodontal ligament*, a derivative of the dental sac (Fig. 20–11*G*).

Some parts of its fibers are embedded in the cementum; other parts are embedded in the bony wall of the alveolus.

Tooth Eruption (Figs. 20–11*G* and 20–14; Table 20–1). As the teeth develop they begin a continuous movement externally. The mandibular teeth usually erupt before the maxillary teeth, and girls' teeth usually erupt sooner than boys' teeth. The child's dentition contains 20 deciduous teeth. The complete adult dentition consists of 32 teeth. As the root of the tooth grows, the crown gradually erupts through the oral epithelium (Fig. 20–11*G* and *H*).

The part of the oral mucosa around the erupted crown becomes the *gingiva* (gum). Eruption of the deciduous teeth usually occurs between the sixth and twenty-fourth months after birth (Table 20–1). The mandibular medial or central incisors usually erupt six to eight months after birth, but this process may not begin until twelve or thirteen months in some normal children. Despite this, all 20 deciduous teeth are usually present by the end of the second year in healthy children. Delayed eruption of all teeth may indicate a systemic or nutritional disturbance, such as hypopituitarism or hypothyroidism (Behrman, 1992).

The permanent teeth develop in a manner similar to that just described for deciduous teeth. As a permanent tooth grows, the root of the corresponding deciduous tooth is gradually resorbed by osteoclasts. Consequently, when the deciduous tooth is shed, it consists of only the crown and the uppermost portion of the root. The permanent teeth usually begin to erupt during the sixth year and continue to appear until early adulthood (Table 20–1).

The development of the face is affected by the development of the paranasal sinuses (see Chapter 10) and by the growth of the maxilla and mandible to accommodate the teeth. It is the lengthening of the *alveolar processes* (the bony sockets which support the teeth) that results in the increase in the depth of the face during childhood.

Abnormalities of Teeth

Natal Teeth. These are teeth that are erupted at birth. They are observed in about one in 2000 newborn infants (Behrman, 1992). There are usually two in the position of the mandibular incisors. This suggests that early eruption of the other teeth may occur. Obviously, natal teeth may produce maternal discomfort due to biting of the nipple during breast-feeding. In addition, the infant's tongue may be lacerated or the teeth may detach and be aspirated; for these reasons, natal teeth are sometimes extracted.

Enamel Hypoplasia (Fig. 20–15). Defective enamel formation causes pits and/or fissures in the enamel. These defects are the result of temporary disturbances in enamel formation. Various factors may injure the ameloblasts (e.g., nutritional deficiency, tetracycline therapy, and infectious diseases, such as measles).

Rickets during the critical period of permanent tooth development is the most common known cause of enamel hypoplasia. Rickets is caused by a deficiency of vitamin D, especially during infancy and childhood, and is characterized by a disturbance of ossification.

Abnormalities of Shape (Fig. 20–15*A* to *G*). Abnormally shaped teeth are relatively common. Occasionally, spherical masses of enamel called *enamel pearls* are attached to the tooth. They are formed by aberrant groups of ameloblasts. The maxillary lateral incisor teeth may assume a slender, tapering shape (peg-shaped lateral incisors). *Congenital syphilis* affects the differentiation of the permanent teeth resulting in screwdriver-shaped incisors with central notches in their incisive edges.

Numerical Abnormalities (Fig. 20–15*H* and *I*). One or more supernumerary teeth may develop or the normal number of teeth may fail to form. *Supernumerary teeth* usually appear in the area of the maxillary incisors where they disrupt the position and eruption of normal teeth. The extra teeth commonly erupt posterior to the normal ones. In partial *anodontia*, one or more teeth are absent. Congenital absence of one or more teeth is often a familial trait. In total anodontia, no teeth develop; this very rare condition is usually associated with *congenital ectodermal dysplasia* (Behrman, 1992).

Abnormal Size of the Teeth. Disturbances during the differentiation of teeth may result in gross alterations of dental morphology, e.g., macrodontia (large teeth) and microdontia (small teeth).

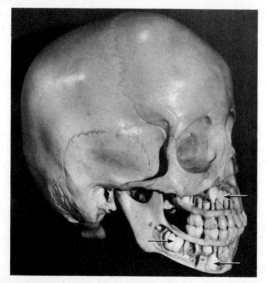

Figure 20–14. Photograph of a child's skull in the fourth year. The bone has been removed to show the relations of the developing permanent teeth *(arrows)* to the erupted deciduous teeth.

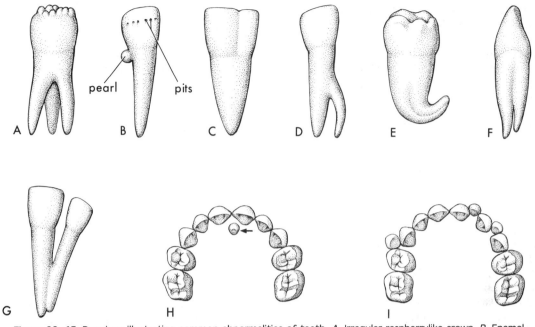

Figure 20–15. Drawings illustrating common abnormalities of teeth. *A*, Irregular raspberrylike crown. *B*, Enamel pearl and pits. *C*, Incisor tooth with a double crown. *D*, Abnormal division of root. *E*, Distorted root. *F*, Branched root. *G*, Fused roots. *H*, Hyperdontia with a supernumerary incisor tooth in the anterior region of the palate *(arrow)*. *I*, Hyperdontia with 13 deciduous teeth in the maxilla (upper jaw) instead of the normal ten.

Fused Teeth (Fig. 20–15*C* and *G*). Occasionally a tooth bud divides or two buds partially fuse to form fused teeth. This condition is commonly observed in the mandibular incisors of the primary dentition. "Twinning" of teeth is the result of division of the tooth bud. In some cases the perma-

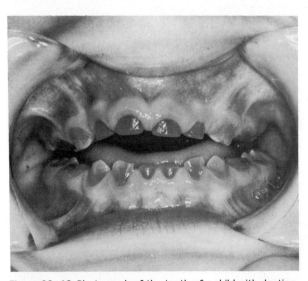

Figure 20–16. Photograph of the teeth of a child with dentinogenesis imperfecta. (From Thompson MW: *Genetics in Medicine.* 4th ed. Philadelphia, WB Saunders, 1986.)

nent tooth does not form; this suggests that the deciduous and permanent tooth primordia fused to form the primary tooth.

Dentigerous Cyst (Tooth-Bearing Cyst). In rare cases a cyst develops in the mandible, maxilla, or maxillary sinus that contains an unerupted tooth. The cyst develops due to cystic degeneration of the enamel reticulum of the enamel organ of an unerupted tooth. Most of these cysts are deeply situated in the jaw and are associated with misplaced or malformed secondary teeth that have failed to erupt.

Amelogenesis Imperfecta. The enamel is soft and friable because of hypocalcification and the teeth are yellow to brown in color. This autosomal dominant trait affects about one in every 20,000 children. For details of this condition, see Behrman (1992).

Dentinogenesis Imperfecta (Fig. 20–16). This condition is relatively common in white children. The teeth are brown to gray-blue with an opalescent sheen. The enamel tends to wear down rapidly, exposing the dentin. This anomaly is inherited as an autosomal dominant trait (Thompson et al., 1991).

Discolored Teeth. Foreign substances incorporated into the developing enamel will cause discoloration of the teeth. The hemolysis (liberation of hemoglobin) associated with erythroblastosis fetalis or HDN (p. 121) may produce blue to black discoloration of the primary teeth. *All tetracyclines are extensively incorporated into the enamel of teeth.* These drugs may produce brownish-yellow discoloration (mottling) and hypoplasia of the enamel because they interfere with the metabolic processes of the ameloblasts. The primary teeth are affected if the tetracyclines are given from 18 weeks (prenatal) to ten months (postnatal), and the permanent teeth are affected from 18 weeks (prenatal) to 12 years. **Tetracyclines** should not be administered to pregnant women or to children if they can be avoided because these drugs adversely affect tooth development (Shepard, 1992).

SUMMARY

The skin and its appendages develop from ectoderm and mesoderm. The epidermis is derived from ectoderm. The melanocytes are derived from *neural crest cells* that migrate into the epidermis. The dermis develops from mesenchyme that differentiates from mesoderm. Cast-off cells from the epidermis mix with secretions of the sebaceous glands to form a whitish, greasy coating for the skin known as *vernix caseosa*. It protects the epidermis, probably making it more waterproof, and facilitates birth due to its slipperiness.

Hairs develop from downgrowths of the epidermis into the dermis. By about 20 weeks the fetus is completely covered with fine, downy hairs called *lanugo*. These hairs are shed by birth or shortly thereafter and are replaced by coarser hairs. Most sebaceous glands develop as outgrowths from the side of hair follicles. Some sebaceous glands develop as downgrowths of the epidermis into the dermis. Sweat glands also develop from epidermal downgrowths into the dermis. Mammary glands develop in a similar manner.

Congenital anomalies of the skin are mainly *disorders of keratinization* (ichthyosis) and pigmentation (albinism). Abnormal blood vessel development results in various types of *angioma*. Nails may be absent or malformed. Hair may be absent or excessive. Absence of mammary glands is rare, but supernumerary breasts (polymastia) or nipples (polythelia) are relatively common.

Teeth also develop from ectoderm and mesoderm. The enamel is produced by *ameloblasts*, which are derived from the oral ectoderm; all other dental tissues develop from mesoderm. The common congenital anomalies of teeth are defective formation of enamel and dentin, abnormalities in shape, and variations in number and position. All tetracyclines are extensively incorporated into the enamel of developing teeth and produce brownish-yellow discoloration and hypoplasia of the enamel. Consequently, they are not used during pregnancy and in children under 12 years of age.

CLINICALLY ORIENTED QUESTIONS FOR PROBLEM-BASED LEARNING SESSIONS

1. A newborn infant had two erupted mandibular incisor teeth. What are these teeth called? How common is this? Are they supernumerary teeth? What problems and/or danger might be associated with the presence of teeth at birth?
2. The primary dentition of an infant had a brownish-yellow color and some hypoplasia of the enamel. The mother recalled that she had been given antibiotics during the second trimester of her pregnancy. What is the probable cause of the infant's tooth discoloration? Dysfunction of what cells would cause the hypoplasia of enamel? Would the secondary dentition be discolored?
3. An infant was born with a small, irregularly shaped, light red blotch on the posterior surface of the neck; it was level with the surrounding skin and blanched when light pressure was applied. Name this anomaly. What do these observations probably indicate? Is this condition common? Are there other names for this anomaly?
4. A newborn infant had a midline tuft of hair in the lumbosacral region of the back. What does this probably indicate? Is this condition common? Is it clinically important?
5. A newborn infant had a collodion type of covering that fissured and exfoliated shortly after birth. Later, lamellar ichthyosis developed. Briefly describe this condition. Is it common? How is it inherited?

The answers to these questions are given on page 468.

References and Suggested Reading

Avery JK: *Essentials of Oral Histology and Embryology.* St. Louis, Mosby-Year Book, 1992.

Beck F, Moffat DB, Davies DP: *Human Embryology.* 2nd ed. Oxford, Blackwell Scientific Publications, 1985.

Behrman RE (ed): *Nelson Textbook of Pediatrics.* 14th ed. Philadelphia, WB Saunders, 1992.

Beller F: Development and anatomy of the breast. *In* Mitchell Jr, GW, Bassett LW (eds): *The Female Breast and Its Disorders.* Baltimore, Williams & Wilkins, 1990.

Bland KI, Copeland III, EM (eds): *The Breast.* Philadelphia, WB Saunders, 1991.

Booth DH, Persaud TVN: Congenital absence of the breast. *Anat Anz 155:*23, 1984.

Boyd JD: The embryology and comparative anatomy of the melanocyte. *In* Rook A (ed): *Progress in the Biological Sciences in Relation to Dermatology.* London, Cambridge University Press, 1960.

Butler PM, Joysey KA (eds): *Development, Function and Evolution of Teeth.* New York, Academic Press, 1978.

Cormack DH: *Essential Histology.* Philadelphia, JB Lippincott, 1993.

Foster CA, Bertram JF, Holbrook KA: Morphometric and statistical analyses describing the *in utero* growth of human epidermis. *Anat Rec 222:*201, 1988.

Goldenring H, Crelin ES: Mother and daughter with bilateral congenital amastia. *Yale J Biol Med 33:*466, 1961.

Haagensen CD: *Diseases of the Breast.* 3rd ed. Philadelphia, WB Saunders, 1986.

Haake AR, Lane AT: Retention of differentiated characteristics in human fetal keratinocytes *in vitro. In Vitro Cell Dev Biol 25:*592, 1989.

Hale AR: Morphogenesis of volar skin in the human fetus. *Am J Anat 91:*147, 1952.

Hirschhorn K: Dermatoglyphics. *In* Behrman RE (ed): *Nelson Textbook of Pediatrics.* 14th ed. Philadelphia, WB Saunders, 1992.

Holbrook KA, Underwood RA, Vogel AM, Gown AM, Kimball H: The appearance, density and distribution of melanocytes in human embryonic and fetal skin revealed by the anti-melanoma monoclonal antibody. *Anat Embryol 180:*443, 1989.

Horn TD: Developmental defects of the skin. *In* Farmer ER, Hood AF (eds): *Pathology of the Skin.* Norwalk, Appleton & Lange, 1990.

Hunter JAA, Savin JA, Dahl MV: *Clinical Dermatology.* London, Blackwell Scientific Publications, 1990.

Johnson CL, Holbrook KA: Development of human embryonic and fetal dermal vasculature. *J Invest Dermatol 93(Suppl):*105, 1989.

Kelly DE, Wood RL, Enders AC: *Bailey's Textbook of Microscopic Anatomy.* 18th ed. Baltimore, Williams & Wilkins, 1984.

Leeson CR, Leeson TS, Paparo AA: *Text/Atlas of Histology.* Philadelphia, WB Saunders, 1988.

Mackie RM: *Clinical Dermatology.* 3rd ed. Oxford, Oxford University Press, 1991.

Moore KL: *Clinically Oriented Anatomy.* 3rd ed. Baltimore, Williams & Wilkins, 1992.

Moore SJ, Munger BL: The early ontogeny of the afferent nerves and papillary ridges in human digital glabrous skin. *Dev Brain Res 48:*119, 1989.

Moynahan EJ: Abnormalities of the skin. *In* Norman AP (ed): *Congenital Abnormalities in Infancy.* 2nd ed. Oxford, Blackwell Scientific Publications, 1971.

Müller M, Jasmin JR, Monteil RA, Loubiere R: Embryology of the hair follicle. *Early Hum Dev 26:*159, 1991.

Nanney LB, Stoscheck CM, King Jr, LE, Underwood RA, Holbrook KA: Immunolocalization of epidermal growth factor receptors in normal developing human skin. *J Invest Dermatol 94:*742, 1990.

Opitz JM: Pathogenetic analysis of certain developmental and genetic ectodermal defects. *Birth Defects 24:*75, 1988.

Osborne MP: Breast development and anatomy. *In* Harris JR, Hellman S, Henderson IC, Kinne, DW (eds): *Breast Diseases.* 2nd ed. Philadelphia, JB Lippincott, 1991.

Pardo-Castello V: *Diseases of Nails.* Springfield, Ill, Charles C Thomas, Publisher, 1960.

Persaud TVN: *Environmental Causes of Human Birth Defects.* Springfield, Ill. Charles C Thomas, 1990.

Pinkus H: Embryology of hair. *In* Montagne W, Ellis RA (eds): *The Biology of Hair Growth.* New York, Academic Press, 1958.

Rawles ME: Origin of melanophores and their role in the development of color patterns in vertebrates. *Physiol Rev 28:*383, 1948.

Ronchese F: Peculiar nail anomalies. *Arch Dermatol 63:*565, 1951.

Schwarz V: The development of the sweat glands and their function. *In* Davis JA, Dobbing J (eds): *Scientific Foundations of Paediatrics.* Philadelphia, WB Saunders, 1974.

Shafer WG, Hine MG, Levy BM: *A Textbook of Oral Pathology.* 4th ed. Philadelphia, WB Saunders, 1983.

Shepard TH: *Catalog of Teratogenic Drugs.* 6th ed. Baltimore, The Johns Hopkins University Press, 1992.

Smith DW, Gong BT: Scalp-hair patterning: Its origin and significance relative to early brain and upper facial development. *Teratology 9:*17, 1974.

Sperber GH: *Craniofacial Embryology.* 4th ed. London, Butterworth, 1989.

Sperber GH: Genetic mechanisms and anomalies in odontogenesis. *J Can Dent Assoc 33:*433, 1967.

Telford IR, Bridgman CF: *Introduction to Functional Histology.* New York, Harper & Row Publishers, 1990.

Ten Cate AR: Development of the tooth. *In* Ten Cate, AR (ed): *Oral Histology. Structure and Function.* St. Louis, CV Mosby, 1989.

Ten Cate AR, Mills C, Solomon G: The development of the periodontium. A transplantation and autoradiographic study. *Anat Rec 170:*365, 1971.

Termine JD: Development of dental and paradental structures; Enamel. *In* Provenza DV (ed): *Fundamentals of Oral Histology and Embryology.* 2nd ed. Philadelphia, Lea & Febiger, 1988.

Thesleff I: Extracellular matrix and tooth morphogenesis. *In* Pratt RM, Christensen RL (eds): *Current Research Trends in Prenatal Craniofacial Development.* Amsterdam, Elsevier/North Holland, 1980.

Thesleff I: Role of the basement membrane in odontoblast differentiation. *J Biol Buccale 6:*241, 1978.

Thompson MW, McInnes RR, Willard HF: *Thompson & Thompson Genetics in Medicine.* 5th ed. Philadelphia, WB Saunders, 1991.

Trier WC: Complete breast absence. *Plastic Reconstr Surg 36:*430, 1965.

Turner EP: The growth and development of the teeth. *In* Davis JA, Dobbing J (eds): *Scientific Foundations of Paediatrics.* Philadelphia, WB Saunders, 1974.

Wilflingseder P: Skin hemangiomas; aggressive approach. *In* Huffstadt AJC (ed): *Congenital Malformations.* Amsterdam, Excerpta Medica, 1980.

Answers to Clinically Oriented Questions for Problem-Based Learning Sessions

Chapter 1

1. The development of a human being begins with fertilization, a process during which a sperm from a male unites with an oocyte (ovum) from a female. The numbered developmental stages end at eight weeks, but development continues during the fetal period and after birth.

2. At the beginning of its development a human organism is called a zygote. This is an appropriate term because the term *zygōtus* means united and refers to the union of the oocyte (ovum) and sperm. The term *conceptus* refers to all structures that develop from the zygote (e.g., the chorionic sac). The terms, therefore, are not synonymous.

3. The term *conceptus* is used when referring to an embryo and its membranes, i.e., the products of conception. The term *abortus* refers to any product or all products of an abortion, e.g., the embryo (or part of it) and/or its membranes and placenta (or parts of them). An abortus, therefore, is an aborted conceptus.

4. Growth of secondary sexual characteristics occurs, reproductive functions begin, and sexual dimorphism becomes more obvious; consequently, the changes are not the same in males and females. The ages of presumptive puberty are 12 years in girls and 14 years in boys.

5. *Embryology* refers to the study of the normal embryo; but clinically it refers to the study of the embryo and fetus, i.e., the study of prenatal development. *Teratology* refers to the study of the abnormal embryo and/or fetus. Teratology is the branch of embryology concerned with abnormal development and the factors that produce it, e.g., drugs and viruses (Chapter 8). These investigations are applicable to clinical studies because they indicate vulnerable periods of the developing human before birth.

Chapter 2

1. Numerical changes in chromosomes arise chiefly through *nondisjunction,* either during a mitotic division or a meiotic division, usually during meiosis I. Nondisjunction is the failure of two members of a chromosome pair to dissociate during anaphase of cell division; as a result, both chromosomes pass to the same daughter cell and trisomy results. *Trisomy 21* (Down syndrome) is the most common numerical chromosomal disorder resulting in congenital anomalies (see Fig. 8–3). It occurs about once in every 700 births.

2. A morula with an extra set of chromosomes (triploidy) in its cells is usually the result of fertilization of an ovum by two sperms (*dispermy*). A fetus could develop from it and be born, but most trisomic infants die shortly after birth.

3. Blockage of the uterine tubes resulting from infection is one of the major causes of infertility in women. Because this occlusion prevents secondary oocytes from coming into contact with sperms, fertilization cannot occur. Infertility in males is usually the result of inadequate spermatogenesis. Nondescent of the testes is one cause of *aspermatogenesis* (failure of sperm formation to occur), but normally positioned testes may not produce adequate numbers of actively motile sperms.

4. Mosaicism is the result of nondisjunction of a pair of chromosomes during an early cleavage division of the zygote rather than during gametogenesis. As a consequence, the embryo has two cell lines with different chromosome numbers. The persons who develop from these chromosomally abnormal embryos are known as *mosaics.* About one per cent of Down syndrome patients are mosaics. They have relatively mild stigmata of the syndrome and are less retarded than typical patients. *Mosaicism* can be detected before birth by cytogenetic techniques, e.g., amniocentesis and chorionic villus sampling (see Chapter 6).

5. Postcoital birth control pills ("morning after pills") may be available in an emergency (e.g., following sexual abuse) but not for routine use. Ovarian hormones (estrogen) taken in large doses within 72 hours after sexual intercourse will usually prevent implantation of the blastocyst, proba-

bly by causing abnormal development of the endometrium. Understand that they prevent implantation, not fertilization. Consequently, they cannot be called contraceptive pills. Pregnancy occurs but the blastocyst does not implant. The term abortion would not be applied to such an early termination of pregnancy.

Chapter 3

1. Yes, a chest radiograph could be taken because the patient's uterus and ovaries are not in the x-ray beam. The only radiation the ovaries would receive would be a negligible and scattered amount from the irradiated thorax. Furthermore, this small amount of radiation would be highly unlikely to damage the products of conception if the patient happened to be pregnant. Most physicians, however, would defer the radiographic examination if at all possible because, if the woman had an abnormal child, she might sue the doctor, claiming that the x-rays produced the abnormality. A jury may not accept the scientific evidence of the nonteratogenicity of low-dose radiation.

2. Diethylstilbestrol (DES) appears to affect the endometrium by rendering it unsuitable for implantation, a process that is regulated by a delicate balance between estrogen and progesterone. The large doses of estrogen given to the patient upset this balance. Progesterone makes the endometrium grow thick and succulent so that the blastocyst may become embedded and be nourished adequately. DES pills are referred to as "morning after pills" by laypeople. When the media refer to the "abortion pill" they are usually referring to RU486. This drug, developed in France, also interferes with implantation of the blastocyst. It blocks the production of progesterone. Its use has not been authorized in North America (at the time of writing). A pregnancy can be detected at the end of the second week after fertilization using highly sensitive pregnancy tests. Most tests depend on the presence of an early pregnancy factor (EPF) in the maternal serum (p. 32).

3. Over 95 to 97 per cent of ectopic pregnancies are in the uterine tube, and 60 per cent of them are in its ampulla. *Endovaginal sonography* is often used to detect ectopic tubal pregnancies. The doctor would perform a *laparotomy* (incision in the abdomen), removing the uterine tube containing the conceptus.

4. No! Exposure of an embryo during the second week of its development to the slight trauma that might be associated with abdominal surgery would not cause a congenital anomaly of the brain. Furthermore, the anesthetics used during the operation could not induce a gross anomaly of the brain. Teratogens are not known to induce congenital anomalies during the first two weeks of development (see Fig. 8–13).

5. Women over 40 years of age are more likely to have a baby with congenital anomalies, such as occur with Down syndrome (see Table 8–3), but women over 40 can have normal children. Prenatal diagnosis (e.g., using chorionic villus sampling or amniocentesis) is now available in large health centers for women over 35 years of age. This procedure will tell whether the embryo has severe chromosomal abnormalities (e.g., trisomy 13) that would cause its death shortly after birth. In most cases the embryo is normal and the pregnancy continues.

Chapter 4

1. Severe chromosomal abnormalities may have caused the spontaneous abortion. The incidence of chromosomal abnormalities in early abortions is very high. A pronounced increase in polyploidy (cells containing three or more times the haploid number of chromosomes) has been observed in embryos expelled during spontaneous abortions when conception occurred within two months after discontinuing oral contraception. Polyploidy is known to be fatal to the developing embryo. This information suggests that it might be wise to use some other type of contraception for one or two menstrual cycles before attempting pregnancy after discontinuing oral contraceptives. In the present case, the physician probably told the patient that her abortion was a natural screening process; i.e., that it was probably the spontaneous expulsion of an embryo that could not have survived because it likely had severe chromosomal abnormalities.

2. The presence of embryonic and/or chorionic tissue in the endometrial remnants would be an absolute sign of pregnancy, but this tissue would be difficult to find at such an early stage of pregnancy. By five days after the expected menses (i.e., about five weeks after the last menstrual period), the embryo would be in the third week of its development. The blastocyst would be about 2 mm in diameter.

3. The central nervous system (brain and spinal cord) begins to develop during the third week. Anencephaly or meroencephaly, in which most of the brain and calvaria are absent, may be the result of environmental teratogens acting during the third week of development. This severe anomaly of the

brain occurs because of failure of the cranial part of the neural tube to develop normally, which is caused by nonclosure of the rostral neuropore.

4. Sacrococcygeal teratomas arise from remnants of the primitive streak, probably in the region of the primitive knot. Because cells from the primitive streak are pleuripotent, the tumors contain various types of tissue derived from all three germ layers. There is a clear-cut difference in the incidence of these tumors with regard to sex; i.e., they are three to four times more frequent in girls than in boys.

5. Ultrasonography is very important for assessing pregnancy during the third week because the embryo and its membranes can be visualized. It is, therefore, possible to determine if the early embryo is developing normally. A negative pregnancy test in the third week does not rule out an ectopic pregnancy because ectopic pregnancies produce hCG at a slower rate than intrauterine pregnancies. The hormone hCG is the basis of pregnancy tests.

Chapter 5

1. The physician would likely tell the patient that her embryo was undergoing a critical stage of its development and that it would be safest for her baby if she were to stop smoking and avoid taking any unprescribed medication throughout her pregnancy. The physician would also likely tell her that heavy cigarette smoking is known to cause intrauterine growth retardation and underweight babies and that the incidence of prematurity increases with the number of cigarettes smoked. The physician would also recommend that she not consume alcohol during pregnancy because of its known teratogenic effects (see Chapter 8).

2. The embryonic period is the most critical period of development because all the main tissues and organs are forming. It is, therefore, the time during which the embryo is most vulnerable to the injurious effects of environmental agents (e.g., large doses of radiation, drugs, and viruses).

3. One cannot always predict how a drug will affect the human embryo because human and animal embryos may differ in their response to a drug; for example, thalidomide is extremely teratogenic to human embryos but has very little effect on some experimental animals, e.g., rats and mice. Drugs known to be strong teratogens in animals should not be used during human pregnancy, especially during the embryonic period. The germ layers form during the process known as gastrulation. All the tissues and organs of the embryo develop from the three germ layers.

4. Information about the starting date of a pregnancy may be unreliable because it depends upon the patient's remembering an event (last menses) that occurred two or three months earlier. In addition, she may have had some implantation bleeding, or breakthrough bleeding, at the time of her first missed period and may have thought that it was a light menses. Ultrasonography is now reliable for determining embryonic age and the starting date of a pregnancy.

5. No! To cause severe limb defects the teratogens would have to be present during the critical period of limb development (24 to 36 days). Teratogens interfere with differentiation of the tissues, often arresting development of the tissue or organ concerned. See Chapter 8 for more details.

Chapter 6

1. Physicians cannot completely rely on information about the time of the last menstrual period reported by the patient, especially in cases in which determination of gestational age is extremely important (e.g., in high-risk pregnancies in which one might wish to induce labor as soon as possible). One can determine with reasonable accuracy the estimated date of delivery (EDD) using diagnostic ultrasound to estimate the size of the fetal head and/or of the entire fetus. Labor would likely be induced at about 32 weeks using hormones (e.g., prostaglandins).

2. The patient would likely undergo chorionic villus sampling or amniocentesis for study of the fetus's chromosomes. The most common chromosomal disorder detected in fetuses of women over 40 years of age is trisomy 21. If the chromosomes of the patient's fetus were normal but congenital abnormalities of the brain or the limbs were still suspected, fetoscopy or ultrasonography might be performed. These methods allow one to look for morphological abnormalities while scanning the entire fetus. The sex of the fetus could be determined by examining the sex chromosomes or the sex chromatin patterns in the nuclei of cells obtained by amniocentesis. One can often determine fetal sex using ultrasonography. In persons with technical experience, this method can be used to identify the sex (particularly male) with a certainty that approaches 100 per cent after about 30 weeks of gestation.

3. There is a danger when uncontrolled drugs (over-the-counter drugs, e.g., aspirin, cough medicine) are consumed excessively or indiscriminately by pregnant women. Withdrawal seizures have been reported in infants born to mothers who are heavy

drinkers, and the fetal alcohol syndrome is present in some of these infants (see Chapter 8). The physician would likely tell the patient not to take any drugs that he does not prescribe. He might tell her that those drugs that are most detrimental to her fetus are under legal control and that he dispenses them with great care.

4. Many factors (fetal, maternal, and environmental) may reduce the rate of fetal growth. Examples of such factors are intrauterine infections, multiple pregnancies, and chromosomal abnormalities (see Chapters 7 and 8). Cigarette smoking, narcotic addiction, and consumption of large amounts of alcohol are also well-established causes of intrauterine growth retardation. A mother interested in the growth and general well-being of her fetus will consult her doctor frequently, eat a good-quality diet, and will not use narcotics, smoke, or drink alcohol.

5. Amniocentesis is relatively devoid of risk. The chance of inducing an abortion is estimated to be about 0.5 per cent. Chorionic villus sampling can also be used for obtaining cells for chromosome study. PUBS refers to percutaneous umbilical cord blood sampling. The needle is inserted into an umbilical vessel with the guidance of ultrasonography. Chromosome and hormone studies can be performed on this fetal blood.

6. Neural tube defects can be suspected from high levels of AFP. Further studies would be done using ultrasonography. Low levels of AFP may indicate Down syndrome. Chromosome studies would be done to check the chromosome complement.

Chapter 7

1. The common method of estimating the time of delivery, called Nagele's rule, is to count back three months from the first day of the last normal menstrual period (LNMP) and then add one year and seven days. The biparietal diameter of the fetal head could be measured by ultrasonography because this measurement correlates well with fetal age.

2. Polyhydramnios is the accumulation of an excessive amount of amniotic fluid. When it occurs over the course of a few days, there is an associated high risk of severe fetal abnormalities, especially of the central nervous system (meroanencephaly and spina bifida cystica). Fetuses with gross brain defects do not drink the usual amounts of amniotic fluid; hence, the amount of liquid increases. Atresia of the esophagus is almost always accompanied by polyhydramnios because the fetus cannot swal-

low and absorb amniotic fluid. Twinning is also a predisposing cause of polyhydramnios.

3. There is a well-known tendency for twins to "run in families." It appears unlikely that there is a genetic factor in monozygotic twinning, but a disposition to dizygotic twinning is genetically determined. The frequency of dizygotic twinning rises sharply with maternal age up to 35 years and then declines, but the frequency of monozygotic twinning is affected very little by the age of the mother. Determination of twin zygosity can usually be made on the basis of the type of placenta and fetal membranes expelled after birth. One can later determine zygosity by looking for genetically determined similarities and differences in a twin pair. A single difference in a genetic marker proves twins to be dizygotic.

4. A single umbilical artery occurs in about one of every 200 umbilical cords. This abnormality is accompanied by a 15 to 20 per cent incidence of cardiovascular abnormalities.

5. Two zygotes were fertilized by X-bearing sperms. The resulting blastocysts implanted close together and their placentas fused. If two chorionic sacs had been observed during ultrasonography, this type of pregnancy would have been suspected.

6. Amniotic bands form when the amnion tears during pregnancy. The bands surround parts of the embryo's body and produce anomalies, e.g., absence of a hand or deep grooves in a limb.

Chapter 8

1. About seven per cent of congenital anomalies are caused by environmental factors, such as drugs and chemicals. It is difficult for clinicians to assign specific defects to specific drugs because: (1) the drug may be administered as therapy for an illness that itself may cause the anomaly, (2) the fetal anomaly may cause maternal symptoms that are treated with a drug, (3) the drug may prevent the spontaneous abortion of an already malformed fetus, and (4) the drug may be used with another drug that causes the anomaly. Women should know that several drugs cause severe anomalies if taken during pregnancy and that these drugs should be avoided.

2. Women over the age of 35 years are more likely to have a child with Down syndrome or some other chromosomal disorder than are younger women (25 to 30 years); nevertheless, most women over the age of 35 have normal children. The doctor caring for a pregnant, 40-year-old woman would certainly recommend chorionic villus sampling or

amniocentesis to determine whether the infant had some severe chromosomal disorder (e.g., trisomy 13).

3. Penicillin has been widely used during pregnancy for over 25 years without any implication of teratogenicity. Small doses of aspirin and other salicylates are ingested by most pregnant women; and, when they are consumed as directed, the teratogenic risk associated with maternal ingestion of these substances is very low. Chronic consumption of large doses of aspirin during early pregnancy may be harmful. Alcohol and other social drugs should be avoided.

4. The physician would likely tell the mother that there was no danger that her child would develop cataracts as the result of German measles. She would undoubtedly explain that cataracts often develop in embryos whose mothers contract the disease early in pregnancy and occur because of the damaging effect the rubella virus has on the developing lens. The physician might say that it is not necessarily bad for a girl to contract German measles before her childbearing years because this attack would probably confer permanent immunity to the disease. She would, however, likely urge the mother to tell the girl to avoid exposure to German measles should she later become pregnant because of the common permanent defects caused by spread of the infection to the fetus.

5. Cats may be infected with a parasite called *Toxoplasma gondii*. Oocysts of these parasites appear in the feces of cats and can be ingested if one is careless in handling the cat's litter. If the woman is pregnant, the parasite can cause severe anomalies of the central nervous system (e.g., mental retardation and blindness).

Chapter 9

1. A diagnosis of congenital diaphragmatic hernia (CDH) is most likely. The congenital defect in the diaphragm that produces this hernia is the result of failure of the left pericardioperitoneal canal to close completely during the sixth week of development; consequently, herniation of abdominal organs into the thorax occurs. This compresses the lungs, especially the left one, and results in respiratory distress. The diagnosis can usually be established by a radiographic examination of the chest. The anomaly can be detected prenatally using ultrasonography. Characteristically, there are air- and/or fluid-filled loops of intestine in the left hemithorax of a newborn infant afflicted with this condition.

2. In the rare congenital anomaly known as retrosternal hernia, the intestine may herniate into the pericardial sac or, conversely, the heart may be displaced into the superior part of the peritoneal cavity. A hernia through the sternocostal hiatus causes this condition.

3. Posterolateral defect of the diaphragm (CDH), which is usually on the left, occurs about once in every 2000 births. A newborn infant, in whom a diagnosis of this defect is suspected, would immediately be positioned with the head and thorax higher than the abdomen and feet to facilitate the inferior displacement of the abdominal organs that would likely be in the thorax. Newborns with CDH usually die of severe respiratory distress due to poor development of the lungs.

4. Epigastric hernias occur in the median plane of the epigastric region. They are uncommon and resemble umbilical hernias. The defect through which herniation occurs is the result of failure of the lateral body folds to fuse in this region during the fourth week.

Chapter 10

1. The mucoid material was probably discharged from an external branchial (pharyngeal) sinus, a remnant of the second branchial (pharyngeal) groove and/or cervical sinus. Normally, this groove and sinus disappear as the neck of the embryo forms. As evident in this case, the branchial sinus extends superiorly into the subcutaneous tissue.

2. The position of the inferior parathyroid glands is variable. They develop in close association with the thymus gland and are carried caudally with it during its descent through the neck. If the thymus fails to descend to its usual position in the superior mediastinum, one or both inferior parathyroid glands may be located near the bifurcation of the common carotid artery. If an inferior parathyroid gland does not separate from the thymus and adhere to the thyroid gland, it may be carried into the superior mediastinum with the thymus.

3. The patient very likely has a thyroglossal duct cyst that arose from a small remnant of the embryonic thyroglossal duct. When complete degeneration of this duct does not occur, a cyst may form from it anywhere along the median plane of the neck between the foramen cecum of the tongue and the jugular notch. A thyroglossal cyst may be confused with an ectopic thyroid gland; i.e., one that has not descended to its normal position in the neck.

4. The unilateral cleft of the lip resulted from failure of the maxillary prominence on the affected side to

fuse with the merged medial nasal prominences. Clefting of the maxilla anterior to the incisive foramen resulted from failure of the lateral palatine process to fuse with the primary palate. About 60 to 80 per cent of persons who have a cleft lip, with or without cleft palate, are males. When both parents are normal and have had one child with a cleft lip, the chance that the next infant will have the same anomaly is about four per cent.

5. There is substantial evidence that anticonvulsant drugs (e.g., phenytoin, or diphenylhydantoin), when given to epileptic women during pregnancy, increase by two- or threefold the incidence of cleft lip and cleft palate when compared with the general population. Cleft lip with cleft palate is caused by many factors, some genetic and others environmental; i.e., this condition has a multifactorial etiology. In most cases the environmental factor involved is not identifiable.

Chapter 11

1. Inability to pass a catheter through the esophagus into the stomach indicates esophageal atresia. Because this severe anomaly is commonly associated with tracheoesophageal fistula and respiratory distress, the pediatrician would probably suspect a tracheoesophageal fistula. A radiographic examination would demonstrate the esophageal atresia. The presence of this anomaly would be confirmed by imaging the nasogastric tube arrested in the proximal esophageal pouch. If necessary a small amount (1 to 3 ml) of air would be injected to highlight the image. If certain types of tracheoesophageal fistula were present, there would also be air in the stomach that passed there from a connection between the esophagus and the trachea. A combined radiologic, endoscopic, and surgical approach would usually be used to detect a tracheoesophageal fistula.

2. An infant in respiratory distress tries to overcome the ventilatory problem by increasing the rate and depth of respiration. Intercostal, subcostal, or sternal retractions and nasal flaring are prominent signs of respiratory distress. Hyaline membrane disease is a leading cause of the respiratory distress syndrome and death in liveborn, premature infants. A deficiency of pulmonary surfactant is associated with RDS.

3. The most common type of tracheoesophageal fistula connects the trachea with the inferior part of the esophagus. This anomaly is associated with atresia of the esophagus superior to the fistula. Tracheoesophageal fistula is the result of incom-

plete division of the foregut by the tracheoesophageal septum into the esophagus and trachea.

4. In most types of tracheoesophageal fistula, air passes from the trachea through the fistula into the esophagus and stomach. Pneumonitis (pneumonia) resulting from aspiration of oral and nasal secretions into the lungs is a serious complication of this anomaly. Giving the baby water or food by mouth is obviously contraindicated in such cases.

Chapter 12

1. Complete absence of a lumen (duodenal atresia) usually involves the second (descending) and third (horizontal) parts of the duodenum. The obstruction is usually the result of incomplete vacuolization of the lumen of the duodenum during the eighth week. The obstruction causes distention of the stomach and proximal duodenum because the fetus swallows amniotic fluid, and the newborn infant swallows air, mucous, and milk. Duodenal atresia is common in infants with Down syndrome, as are other severe congenital anomalies, e.g., anular pancreas, cardiovascular abnormalities, malrotation of the bowel (midgut loop), and anorectal anomalies. Polyhydramnios occurs because the duodenal atresia prevents normal absorption of amniotic fluid from the fetal intestine distal to the obstruction. The fetus swallows amniotic fluid before birth; but, due to blockage of the duodenum, this fluid cannot pass along the bowel and be absorbed into the fetal circulation and transferred across the placental membrane into the mother's circulation from which it enters her urine.

2. The yolk stalk normally undergoes complete involution by the tenth week of development, at which time the intestines return to the abdomen. In two to four per cent of people, a remnant of this stalk persists as a diverticulum of the ileum known as a Meckel diverticulum, but only a small number of these ever become symptomatic. In the present case, the entire yolk stalk persisted so that the diverticulum was connected to the anterior abdominal wall and the umbilicus by a sinus tract. This anomaly is rare, and its external opening may be confused with a granuloma (inflammatory lesion) of the stump of the umbilical cord.

3. The fistula was likely connected to the blind end of the rectum. The condition, known as imperforate anus with rectovaginal fistula, is the result of failure of the urorectal septum to form a complete separation between the anterior and posterior portions of the urogenital sinus. Because the inferior one third of the vagina forms from the anterior

part of the urogenital sinus, it joins the rectum, which forms from the posterior part of the urogenital sinus.

4. This anomaly is called omphalocele (exomphalos). A small omphalocele, like the one described here, is sometimes called an umbilical cord hernia, but it should not be confused with an umbilical hernia, which occurs after birth and is covered by skin. The thin membrane covering the mass in the present case would be composed of peritoneum and amnion. The mass or hernia would be composed of small intestinal loops. Omphalocele occurs when the intestinal loops fail to return to the abdominal cavity from the umbilical cord during the tenth week of fetal life. In the present case, because the hernia is relatively small, the intestine may have entered the abdominal cavity and then herniated later when the rectus muscles did not approach each other and close the circular defect in the anterior abdominal wall.

5. The ileum was probably obstructed. This condition is called ileal atresia. Congenital atresia of the small bowel involves the ileum most frequently; the next most frequently affected region is the duodenum. The jejunum is involved least often. Some meconium ("fetal feces") is formed from the exfoliated fetal epithelium and mucous in the intestinal lumen and is distal to the obstructed area (atretic segment). At operation the atretic ileum would probably appear as a narrow segment connecting the proximal and distal segments of small bowel. Atresia of the ileum could be the result of failure of recanalization of the lumen; but, more likely, the atresia occurred because of a prenatal interruption of the blood supply to the ileum. Sometimes a loop of small bowel becomes twisted, interrupting its blood supply and causing death of the affected segment. The damaged section of bowel usually becomes a fibrous cord that connects the proximal and distal segments of bowel.

Chapter 13

1. Double renal pelves and ureters are the result of the formation of two metanephric diverticula, or ureteric buds, on one side of the embryo. Subsequently, the primordia of these structures fuse. Both ureters usually open into the urinary bladder. Occasionally, the extra ureter opens into the urogenital tract inferior to the bladder. This occurs when the extra ureter is not incorporated into the base of the bladder with the other ureter; instead, the extra ureter is carried caudally with the mesonephric duct and opens with it into the caudal part of the urogenital sinus. Because this part of the urogenital sinus gives rise to the urethra and the epithelium of the vagina, the ectopic (abnormally placed) ureteric orifice may be located in either of these structures, which accounts for the continual dribbling of urine into the vagina. An ectopic ureteral orifice that opens inferior to the bladder results in urinary incontinence because there is no urinary bladder or urethral sphincter between it and the exterior. Normally, the oblique passage of the ureter through the wall of the bladder allows the contraction of the bladder musculature to act like a sphincter for the ureter, controlling the flow of urine from it.

2. Supernumerary renal arteries are very common. About 25 per cent of kidneys receive two or more branches directly from the aorta, but more than two is exceptional. Supernumerary arteries enter either through the renal sinus or at the poles of the kidney, usually the inferior pole. Accessory renal arteries, more common on the left side, represent persistent, fetal renal arteries which grow out in sequence from the aorta as the kidneys "ascend" from the pelvis to the abdomen. Usually, the inferior vessels degenerate as new ones develop. Supernumerary arteries are about twice as common as supernumerary veins. They usually arise at the level of the kidney. The presence of a supernumerary artery is of clinical importance in other circumstances because it may cross the ureteropelvic junction and hinder the outflow of urine, leading to some dilation of the calices and pelvis on the same side (hydronephrosis). Hydronephrotic kidneys frequently become infected (pyelonephritis); infection may lead to destruction of the kidneys.

3. Rudimentary horn pregnancies are very rare, but they are clinically important because it is difficult to distinguish between this type of pregnancy and a tubal pregnancy. In the present case, the uterine anomaly was the result of retarded growth of the right paramesonephric duct and incomplete fusion of this duct with its partner during development of the uterus. Most anomalies resulting from incomplete fusion of the paramesonephric ducts do not cause clinical problems, but a rudimentary horn that does not communicate with the main part of the uterus may cause pain during the menstrual period because of distention of the horn by blood. Because most rudimentary uterine horns are thicker than uterine tubes, a rudimentary horn pregnancy is likely to rupture much later than a tubal pregnancy.

4. Glandular hypospadias is the term applied to a penile anomaly in which the urethral orifice is on the ventral surface near the glans penis. The ventral curving of the penis is called chordee. Glandu-

lar hypospadias is the result of failure of the uro-genital folds on the ventral surface of the developing penis to fuse completely and establish communication with the terminal part of the spongy urethra within the glans penis. Hypospa-dias may be associated with an inadequate pro-duction of androgens by the fetal testes, or there may be resistance to the hormones at the cellular level in the urogenital folds. Hypospadias is thought to have a multifactorial etiology because close relatives of patients with hypospadias are more likely to have the anomaly than persons in the general population. Hypospadias, a common anomaly of the urogenital tract, occurs in about one of every 300 male infants.

5. The embryological basis of indirect inguinal her-nia is persistence of the processus vaginalis, a fetal outpouching of peritoneum. This fingerlike pouch evaginates the anterior abdominal wall and forms the inguinal canal. A persistent processus vaginalis predisposes to indirect inguinal hernia by creating a weakness in the anterior abdominal wall and a hernial sac into which abdominal contents may herniate if the intra-abdominal pressure becomes very high (as occurs during straining). The hernial sac would be covered by internal spermatic fascia, cremaster muscle, and cremasteric fascia.

Chapter 14

1. Ventricular septal defect (VSD) is the most com-mon cardiac defect. It occurs in about 25 per cent of children with congenital heart disease. Most pa-tients with a large VSD have a massive left-to-right shunt of blood.

2. Patent ductus arteriosus (PDA) is the most com-mon cardiovascular anomaly associated with ma-ternal rubella infection during early pregnancy. When the ductus arteriosus remains patent, aortic blood is shunted into the pulmonary artery. In extreme cases, one half to two thirds of the left ventricular output may be shunted through the patent ductus arteriosus. This extra work for the heart results in cardiac enlargement.

3. The tetrad of cardiac abnormalities present in the tetralogy of Fallot is as follows: pulmonary steno-sis, ventricular septal defect (VSD), overriding aorta, and right ventricular hypertrophy. Angio-cardiography could be used to reveal the malposi-tioned aorta (straddling the ventricular septal de-fect) and the degree of pulmonary stenosis. Cyanosis occurs because of the shunting of unsat-urated blood, but it may not be present at birth. The main aim of therapy is to improve the oxygen-ation of the blood in the infant, usually by surgical

correction of the pulmonary stenosis and closure of the VSD.

4. Cardiac catheterization would probably be used to confirm the diagnosis of transposition of the great arteries (TGA). If this cardiac abnormality were present, a bolus of contrast material injected into the right ventricle would enter the aorta; whereas, contrast material injected into the left ventricle would enter the pulmonary circulation. The infant was able to survive after birth because the ductus arteriosus remains open in these patients, allowing some intermixing of blood between the two circu-lations. In other cases, there is also an ASD or VSD that permits intermixing of blood. Complete transposition of the great arteries is incompatible with life if there are no associated septal defects or a patent ductus arteriosus.

5. This would probably be a secundum type of atrial septal defect (ASD) located in the region of the fossa ovalis because this is the most common type of clinically significant ASD. Large defects, as in the present case, often extend toward the inferior vena cava. The pulmonary artery and its major branches are dilated as the result of the increased blood flow through the lungs and the increased pressure within the pulmonary circulation. In these cases a considerable shunt of oxygenated blood flows from the left atrium to the right atrium. This blood, along with the normal venous return to the right atrium, enters the right ventricle and is pumped to the lungs. Large ASDs may be tolerated for a long time, as in the present case, but progressive dilation of the right ventricle often leads to heart failure.

Chapter 15

1. The common congenital anomaly of the vertebral column is spina bifida occulta. This defect of the vertebral arch of the first sacral and/or the last lumbar vertebra is present in about ten per cent of people. The defect also occurs in cervical and tho-racic vertebrae. The spinal cord and nerves are usually normal, and neurological symptoms are usually absent. Spina bifida occulta does not cause back problems in most people, but it may occa-sionally and is associated with neurological or musculoskeletal disturbances.

2. A rib on the seventh cervical vertebra is of clinical importance because it may compress the subcla-vian artery and/or the brachial plexus, producing symptoms of artery and nerve compression. In most cases, cervical ribs produce no symptoms. They are the result of development of the costal processes of the seventh cervical vertebra into ribs.

3. A hemivertebra can produce an abnormal lateral curvature of the vertebral column (scoliosis). A hemivertebra is composed of one half of a body, a pedicle, and a lamina. This anomaly occurs when the mesenchymal cells from the sclerotomes on one side fail to form the primordium of half of a vertebra. As a result, there are more growth centers on the one side of the vertebral column; this imbalance causes the vertebral column to bend laterally.
4. Craniosynostosis indicates premature closure of one or more of the cranial sutures. This developmental abnormality results in malformations of the skull. Scaphocephaly, or a long narrow skull, results from premature closure of the sagittal suture. This type of craniosynostosis accounts for about 50 per cent of the cases of premature closure of the cranial sutures.
5. The features of Klippel-Feil syndrome are short neck, low hair line, and restricted neck movements. In most cases the number of cervical vertebral bodies is less than normal.

Chapter 16

1. Absence of the sternocostal portion of the left pectoralis major muscle is the cause of the surface abnormalities observed. The costal heads of the pectoralis major and pectoralis minor muscles are usually present. Despite its numerous and important actions, absence of all or part of the pectoralis major muscle usually causes no disability; but the deformity caused by the absence of the anterior axillary fold is striking, as is the inferior location of the nipple. The actions of other muscles associated with the shoulder joint compensate for the absence of this part of the muscle.
2. About 13 per cent of people lack a palmaris longus muscle on one or both sides. Its absence causes no disability.
3. It would be the left sternocleidomastoid muscle that was prominent when tensed. The left one is the unaffected muscle, and it does not pull the child's head to the right side. It is the short, contracted, right sternocleidomastoid that tethers the right mastoid process to the right clavicle and sternum; hence, continued growth of the left side of the neck results in tilting and rotation of the head. This relatively common condition called *congenital torticollis* (wryneck) may occur because of injury to the muscle during birth. Tearing of some muscle fibers probably occurred, resulting in bleeding into the muscle. Over several weeks, necrosis of some fibers occurred, and the blood was replaced by fibrous tissue. This resulted in short-

ening of the muscle and in pulling of the child's head to the side.
4. Absence of striated musculature in the median plane of the anterior abdominal wall of the embryo is associated with exstrophy of the urinary bladder. This severe anomaly is caused by: (1) incomplete midline closure of the inferior part of the anterior abdominal wall, and (2) failure of mesenchymal cells to migrate from the somatic mesoderm between the surface ectoderm and the urogenital sinus during the fourth week of development. The absence of mesenchymal cells in the median plane results in failure of striated muscles to develop.

Chapter 17

1. The number of female infants with dislocation of the hip is approximately eight times that of male infants. The hip joint is not usually dislocated at birth, but the acetabulum is abnormal (i.e., underdeveloped). Dislocation of the hip may not become obvious until the infant attempts to stand up several months after birth. This condition is probably caused by deforming forces acting directly on the hip joint of the fetus.
2. Severe anomalies of the limbs (amelia and meromelia), similar to those produced by thalidomide, are rare and they usually have a genetic basis. The thalidomide syndrome consisted of absence of limbs (amelia), gross defects of the limbs (meromelia) (e.g., hands and feet attached to the trunk by small, irregularly shaped bones), intestinal atresia, and cardiac defects.
3. The most common type of clubfoot is talipes equinovarus, occurring in about one of every 1000 newborn infants. In this deformation, the soles of the feet are turned medially and the feet are sharply plantarflexed. The feet are fixed in the tiptoe position, resembling the foot of a horse (L. *equinus*, horse).
4. Syndactyly (fusion of the digits) is the most common type of limb anomaly. It varies from cutaneous webbing between the digits to synostosis (union of the phalanges, the bones of the digits). Syndactyly is more common in the foot than in the hand. This deformity occurs when separate digital rays fail to form in the fifth week or the webbing between the developing digits fails to break down between the sixth and eighth weeks. As a consequence, separation of the digits does not occur.

Chapter 18

1. Ultrasound scanning of the fetus may detect absence of the calvaria (acrania) as early as 14 weeks.

Fetuses with meroanencephaly (absence of part of the brain) do not drink the usual amounts of amniotic fluid, presumably because of impairment of the neuromuscular mechanism that controls swallowing. Inasmuch as fetal urine is excreted into the amniotic fluid at the usual rate, the amount of amniotic fluid increases. Normally, the fetus swallows amniotic fluid, which is absorbed by its intestines and passed to the placenta for elimination via the mother's blood and kidneys.

Meroanencephaly (partial absence of the brain), often inaccurately called anencephaly (absence of the brain), can be easily and safely detected by a plain radiograph, but radiographs of the fetus are not usually done during the first six months. This severe anomaly could also be detected by ultrasonography (see Fig. 18–32) fetoscopy, or amniocentesis. An elevated level of alpha-fetoprotein in the amniotic fluid indicates an open neural tube defect, such as acrania with meroanencephaly or spina bifida with myeloschisis.

2. A neurological deficit is associated with meningomyelocele because the spinal cord and/or nerve roots are often incorporated into the wall of the protruding sac. This impairs the nerves supplying various structures. Paralysis of the lower limbs often occurs, and there may be incontinence of urine and feces due to paralysis of the sphincters of the anus and urinary bladder.

3. The condition is called internal or obstructive hydrocephalus. The block would most likely be in the cerebral aqueduct of the midbrain. Obstruction at this site (stenosis or atresia) interferes with or prevents passage of ventricular fluid from the lateral and third ventricles to the fourth ventricle. Hydrocephalus is sometimes recognized before birth, but most cases are diagnosed in the first few weeks or months after birth. Hydrocephalus can be recognized using ultrasonography or radiography of the mother's abdomen during the last trimester. Surgical treatment of hydrocephalus usually consists of shunting the excess ventricular fluid via a plastic tube to another part of the body (e.g., into the blood stream or the peritoneal cavity) where it will subsequently be excreted by the infant's kidneys.

4. Hydrocephalus is not synonymous with a large head because a large brain (macroencephalon), a subdural hygroma, or a hematoma can also cause enlargement of the head. Hydrocephalus may or may not enlarge the head. Although it usually does, a condition known as hydrocephalus ex vacuo causes enlargement of the ventricles due to brain destruction, but the head is not enlarged.

Microencephaly (small brain) is usually associated with microcephaly (small calvaria). Because growth of the skull is largely dependent upon growth of the brain, arrest of brain development can cause microcephaly. During the fetal period, environmental exposure to agents such as cytomegalovirus, *Toxoplasma gondii,* herpes simplex virus, and high-level radiation is known to induce microencephaly and microcephaly. Severe mental retardation may occur due to exposure of the embryo/fetus to high levels of radiation during the 8- to 16-week period of development. Measles and mumps occurring after birth can also cause cerebral atrophy and mental retardation.

5. Agenesis of the corpus callosum, partial or complete, is frequently associated with low intelligence in 70 per cent and seizures in 60 per cent of patients. Some patients are asymptomatic and lead normal lives. Agenesis of the corpus callosum may occur as an isolated defect, but it is often associated with other CNS anomalies, such as the holoprosencephalies. As in the present case, a large third ventricle may be associated with agenesis of the corpus callosum. A large third ventricle exists because it is able to rise superior to the roofs of the lateral ventricles when the corpus callosum is absent. The lateral ventricles are usually moderately enlarged.

Chapter 19

1. The mother had certainly contracted German measles during early pregnancy because her infant had the characteristic triad of anomalies resulting from infection of an embryo by the rubella virus. Cataract is common when severe infections occur during the first six weeks of pregnancy because the lens vesicle is forming and separating from the surface ectoderm during this period. Congenital cataract is believed to be the result of invasion of the developing lens by the rubella virus. The most common cardiovascular lesion in infants whose mothers had rubella in early pregnancy is patent ductus arteriosus. Although a history of a rash during the first trimester of pregnancy is helpful for diagnosing the congenital rubella syndrome, embryopathy (embryonic disease) can occur after subclinical maternal rubella infection (i.e., without a rash).

2. Congenital ptosis (drooping of the upper eyelids) is usually caused by abnormal development or failure of development of the levator palpebrae superioris muscle. Congenital ptosis is usually transmitted by autosomal dominant inheritance, but injury to the superior branch of the oculomotor nerve (CN III), which supplies the levator

palpebrae superioris muscle, would also cause drooping of an upper eyelid.

3. The protozoon most likely involved was *Toxoplasma gondii,* an intracellular parasite. The congenital abnormalities are the result of invasion of the fetal blood stream and developing organs by the toxoplasma parasites. These parasites disrupt development of the central nervous system including the eyes, which develop from outgrowths of the brain (optic vesicles). The physician would certainly tell the woman about toxoplasma cysts in meat and advise the woman to cook her meat well, especially if she decided to have more children. She would tell her that toxoplasma oocysts are often found in cat feces and about the importance of carefully washing her hands after handling a cat or its litter box.

4. Very likely the infant had trisomy 18 because the characteristic phenotype is present (see Chapter 8). Low-set, malformed ears associated with severe mental retardation, prominent occiput, congenital heart defect, and failure to thrive are all suggestive of the trisomy 18 syndrome. This numerical chromosomal abnormality results from nondisjunction of the number 18 chromosome pair during gametogenesis. Its incidence is about one in 8000 newborn infants. Probably 95 per cent of trisomy 18 fetuses abort spontaneously. Postnatal survival of these infants is poor with 30 per cent dying within a month of birth; the mean survival time is only two months. Less than ten per cent of these infants survive more than a year.

5. Detachment of the retina is a separation of the two embryonic retinal layers: the neural pigment epithelium derived from the outer layer of the optic cup and the neural retina derived from the inner layer of the optic cup. The intraretinal space, representing the cavity of the optic vesicle, normally disappears as the retina forms. The proximal part of the hyaloid artery normally persists as the central artery of the retina, but the distal part of this vessel normally degenerates.

Chapter 20

1. Natal teeth (L. *natus,* to be born) occur in about one of every 2000 newborn infants. There are usually two teeth in the position of the mandibular medial or central incisors. Natal teeth may be supernumerary ones, but they are often prematurely erupted primary teeth. If it is established radiologically that they are supernumerary teeth, they would probably be removed so that they would not interfere with the subsequent eruption of the normal primary teeth. Natal teeth may cause maternal discomfort due to abrasion or biting of the nipple during nursing. They may also injure the infant's tongue which, because the mandible is relatively small at birth, lies between the alveolar processes of the jaws.

2. The discoloration of the infant's teeth was likely caused by the administration of tetracycline to the mother during her pregnancy. Tetracyclines become incorporated into the developing enamel of the teeth and cause discoloration. Dysfunction of ameloblasts due to tetracycline therapy causes hypoplasia of the enamel (e.g., pitting). It is very likely that the secondary dentition would also be affected because enamel formation begins in the permanent teeth before birth (about 20 weeks in the incisors).

3. This is an angiomatous anomaly of the skin often called a capillary angioma or hemangioma. It is formed by an overgrowth of small blood vessels consisting mostly of capillaries, but there are also some arterioles and venules in it. The blotch is red because oxygen is not taken from the blood passing through it. This type of angioma is quite common, and the mother would be assured that this anomaly is of no significance and requires no treatment. It will fade in a few years. Formerly this type of angioma was called a *nevus flammeus* (flamelike birthmark), but these names are sometimes applied to other types of angiomas; and, to avoid confusion, it is better not to use them. Nevus is not a good term because it is derived from a Latin word meaning a mole or birthmark, which may or may not be an angioma.

4. A tuft of hair in the median plane of the lumbosacral region usually indicates the presence of spina bifida occulta. This is the most common developmental abnormality of the vertebrae and is present in L5 and/or L1 in about ten per cent of otherwise normal people. Spina bifida occulta is usually of no clinical significance, but some infants with this vertebral anomaly also have a developmental defect of the underlying spinal cord and nerve roots.

5. The superficial layers of the epidermis of infants with lamellar ichthyosis, resulting from excessive keratinization, consist of fishlike, grayish-brown scales that are adherent in the center and raised at the edges. Fortunately, the condition is very rare. It is inherited as an autosomal recessive trait.

Appendices

TIMETABLE OF HUMAN PRENATAL DEVELOPMENT
1 to 6 weeks

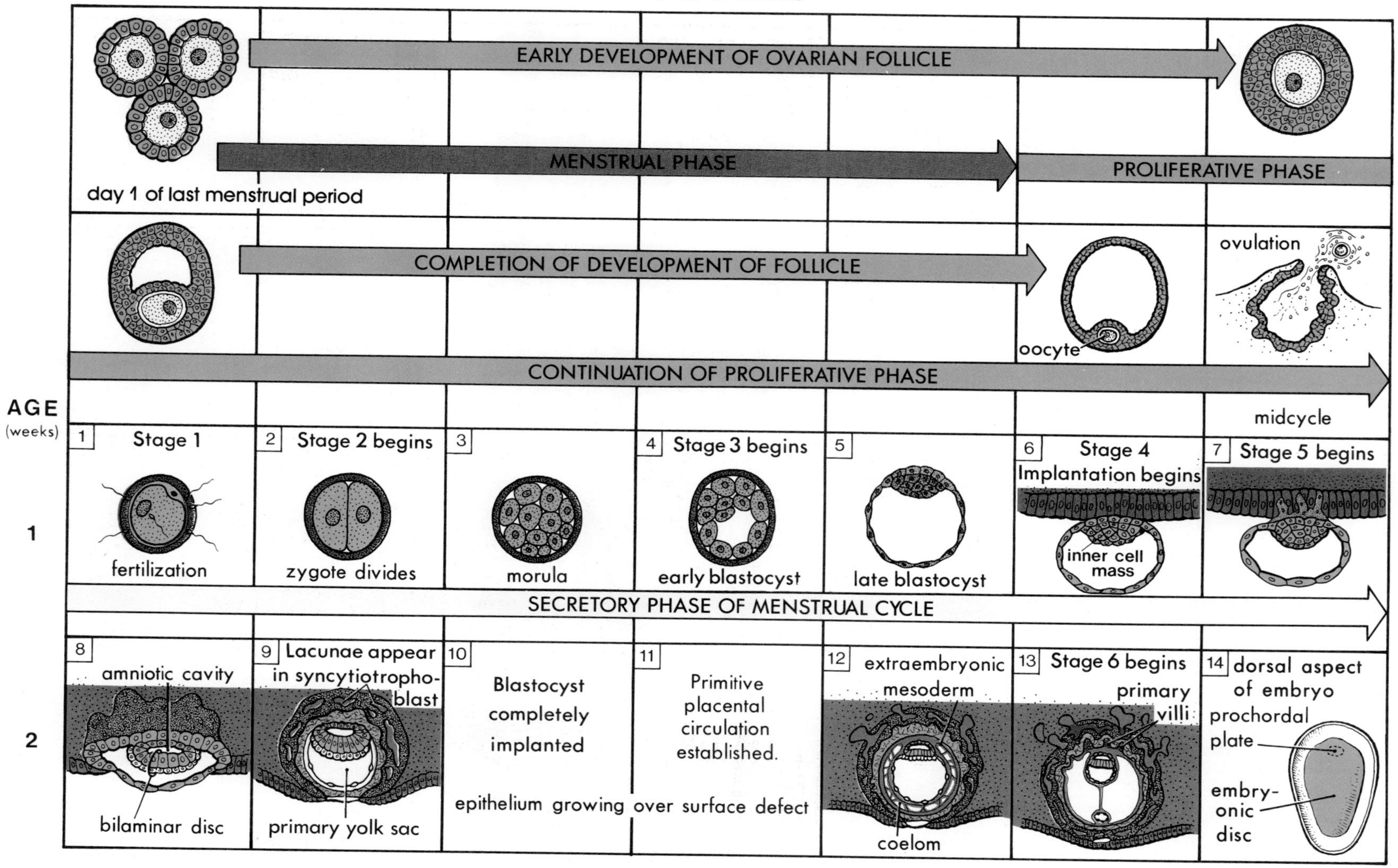

EARLY DEVELOPMENT OF OVARIAN FOLLICLE

MENSTRUAL PHASE

PROLIFERATIVE PHASE

day 1 of last menstrual period

ovulation

midcycle

COMPLETION OF DEVELOPMENT OF FOLLICLE

oocyte

CONTINUATION OF PROLIFERATIVE PHASE

| 1 | Stage 1 | 2 | Stage 2 begins | 3 | 4 | Stage 3 begins | 5 | 6 | Stage 4 Implantation begins | 7 | Stage 5 begins |

fertilization

zygote divides

morula

early blastocyst

late blastocyst

inner cell mass

dorsal aspect of embryo

prochordal plate

embryonic disc

SECRETORY PHASE OF MENSTRUAL CYCLE

| 8 | 9 | Lacunae appear in syncytiotrophoblast | 10 | Blastocyst completely implanted | 11 | Primitive placental circulation established. | 12 | extraembryonic mesoderm | 13 | Stage 6 begins | 14 |

amniotic cavity

bilaminar disc

primary yolk sac

epithelium growing over surface defect

coelom

primary villi

AGE (weeks)

1

2

470

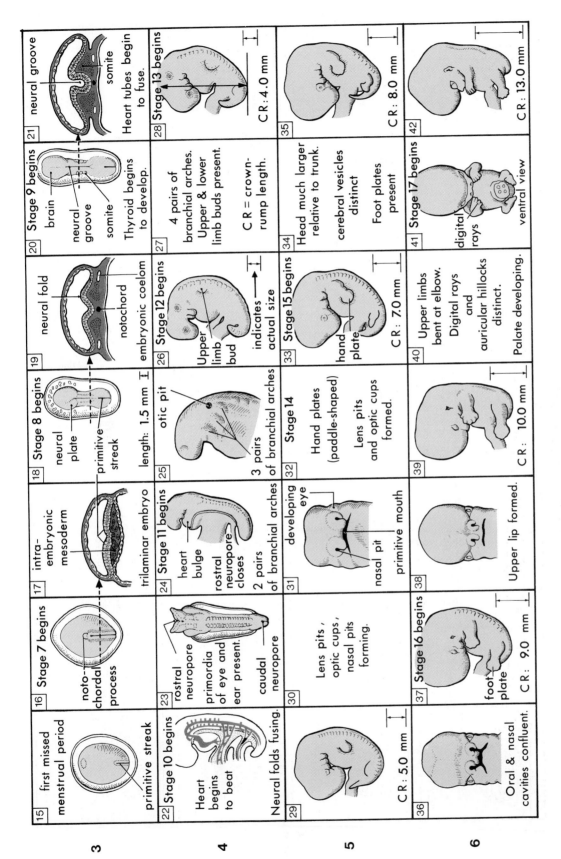

15 first missed menstrual period

primitive streak

16 Stage 7 begins

noto-chordal process

17 intra-embryonic mesoderm

18 Stage 8 begins

neural plate

primitive streak

length: 1.5 mm

19 neural fold

notochord

embryonic coelom

20 Stage 9 begins

brain

neural groove

somite

Thyroid begins to develop.

21 neural groove

somite

Heart tubes begin to fuse.

22 Stage 10 begins

Heart begins to beat

Neural folds fusing.

23 rostral neuropore

primordia of eye and ear present.

caudal neuropore

trilaminar embryo

24 Stage 11 begins

heart bulge

rostral neuropore closes

2 pairs of branchial arches

25 otic pit

3 pairs of branchial arches

26 Stage 12 begins

Upper limb bud

↑ indicates actual size

27 4 pairs of branchial arches.

Upper & lower limb buds present.

C R = crown-rump length.

28 Stage 13 begins

C R : 4.0 mm

29 C R : 5.0 mm

30 Lens pits, optic cups, nasal pits forming.

31 developing eye

nasal pit

primitive mouth

32 Stage 14

Hand plates (paddle-shaped)

Lens pits and optic cups formed.

33 Stage 15 begins

hand plate

C R : 7.0 mm

34 Head much larger relative to trunk.

cerebral vesicles distinct

Foot plates present

35 C R : 8.0 mm

36 Oral & nasal cavities confluent.

37 Stage 16 begins

foot plate

C R : 9.0 mm

38 Upper lip formed.

39 C R : 10.0 mm

40 Upper limbs bent at elbow.

Digital rays and auricular hillocks distinct.

Palate developing.

41 Stage 17 begins

digital rays

ventral view

42 C R : 13.0 mm

3

4

5

6

471

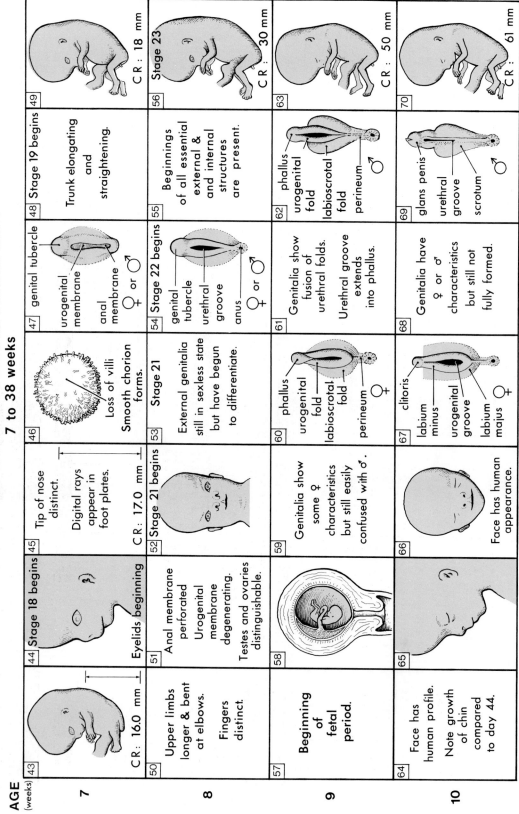

TIMETABLE OF HUMAN PRENATAL DEVELOPMENT
7 to 38 weeks

AGE (weeks)

7

| 43 | 44 Stage 18 begins | 45 | 46 | 47 genital tubercle | 48 Stage 19 begins | 49 |
| CR: 16.0 mm | | Tip of nose distinct. Digital rays appear in foot plates. | Loss of villi Smooth chorion forms. | urogenital membrane anal membrane ♀ or ♂ | Trunk elongating and straightening. | CR: 18 mm |

8

| 50 | 51 Eyelids beginning | 52 Stage 21 begins | 53 Stage 21 | 54 Stage 22 begins | 55 Stage 22 begins | 56 Stage 23 |
| Upper limbs longer & bent at elbows. Fingers distinct. | Anal membrane perforated Urogenital membrane degenerating. Testes and ovaries distinguishable. | CR: 17.0 mm | External genitalia still in sexless state but have begun to differentiate. | genital tubercle urethral groove anus ♀ or ♂ | Beginnings of all essential external & and internal structures are present. | CR: 30 mm |

9

| 57 | 58 | 59 | 60 | 61 | 62 | 63 |
| Beginning of fetal period. | | Genitalia show some ♀ characteristics but still easily confused with ♂. | phallus urogenital fold labioscrotal fold perineum ♀ | Genitalia show fusion of urethral folds. Urethral groove extends into phallus. | phallus urogenital fold labioscrotal fold perineum ♂ | CR: 50 mm |

10

| 64 | 65 | 66 | 67 | 68 | 69 | 70 |
| Face has human profile. Note growth of chin compared to day 44. | | Face has human appearance. | clitoris labium minus urogenital groove labium majus ♀ | Genitalia have ♀ or ♂ characteristics but still not fully formed. | glans penis urethral groove scrotum ♂ | CR: 61 mm |

472

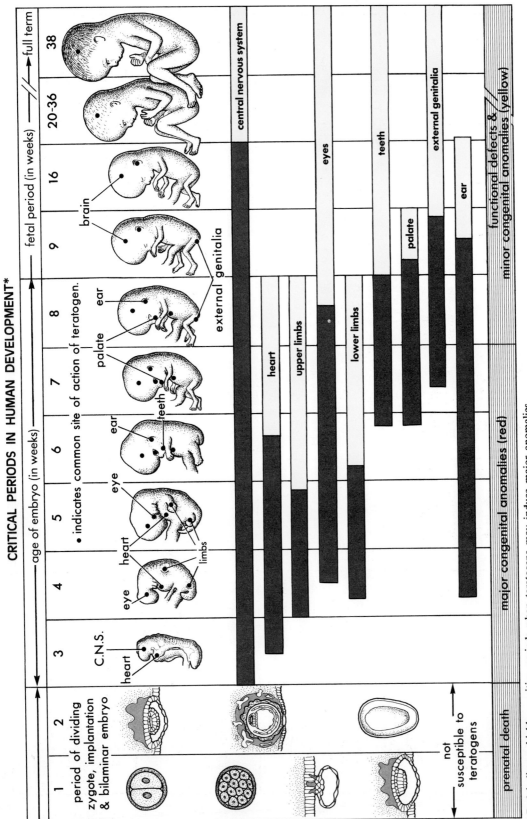

CRITICAL PERIODS IN HUMAN DEVELOPMENT*

* Red indicates highly sensitive periods when teratogens may induce major anomalies.

473

Index

Note: Page numbers in *italics* refer to illustrations; page numbers followed by t refer to tables.